The Palgrave Handbook o
Activity Pro

"With advancing years people find themselves out of breath climbing the stairs or walking uphill, so they take to the lift or the wheels, thereby exacerbating the problem.
I always advocate physical activity whether to be able to keep climbing stairs, regain confidence, or to just feel good. This Handbook provides the latest scientific evidence for why we all need to keep active in later life and the different ways we can support older people to keep active and well."

—Jane Asher, aged 86, is an elite Masters swimmer. She set her first Masters World Record in 1986 in the 55–59 age group and has since set another 186 records across different age groups, strokes, and distances.

"It is evident that we must meet the challenges of old age not only at the level of the individual but also at the level of society. This timely Handbook provides the first interdisciplinary review of physical activity—perhaps our most valuable strategy to enhance wellbeing in late life. With topics ranging from exercise physiology and the well-established clinical benefits to broader issues such as epidemiology, population health, and psychological and social considerations, this volume will be an indispensable reference for researchers, practitioners, and advanced students."

—John W. Rowe, *MD, President, International Association of Gerontology and Geriatrics*

"Given the hugely important topic of physical activity in the context of healthy ageing, this Handbook will be a 'go to' source for some time. It is comprehensive in its coverage and will appeal to students, researchers, and practitioners. In addition to the importance of covering the health outcomes of physical activity among older adults, the Handbook gives appropriately extensive coverage to what physical activity to promote, how to maximize participation, how to implement activities for this population, the social and environmental factors influencing participation, and issues and debates. This is a marvellous resource."

—Professor Stuart Biddle, *University of Southern Queensland*

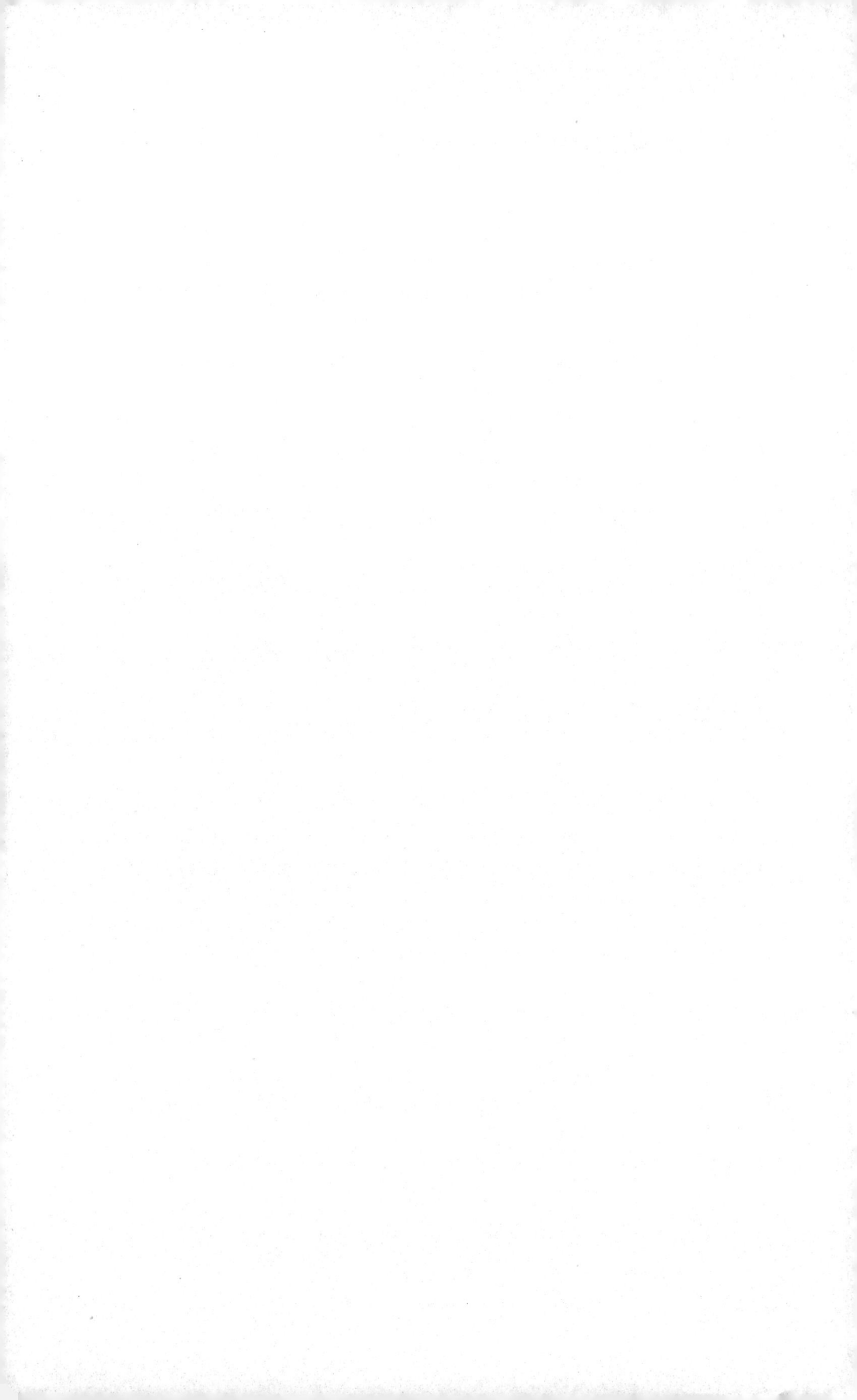

Samuel R. Nyman • Anna Barker
Terry Haines • Khim Horton
Charles Musselwhite
Geeske Peeters • Christina R. Victor
Julia Katharina Wolff
Editors

The Palgrave Handbook of Ageing and Physical Activity Promotion

palgrave
macmillan

Editors
Samuel R. Nyman
Department of Psychology
Bournemouth University
Poole, UK

Terry Haines
Department of Physiotherapy
Monash University
Frankston, VIC, Australia

Charles Musselwhite
Centre for Innovative Ageing
Swansea University
Swansea, UK

Christina R. Victor
College of Health and Life Sciences
Brunel University
Uxbridge, UK

Anna Barker
Epidemiology and Preventive Medicine
Monash University
Melbourne, VIC, Australia

Khim Horton
School of Health Sciences
City, University of London
London, UK

Geeske Peeters
Global Brain Health Institute
Trinity College Dublin
Dublin, Ireland

Julia Katharina Wolff
Institute of Psychogerontology, Friedrich-Alexander-University Erlangen-Nuremberg
Nuremberg, Germany

ISBN 978-3-030-10037-7   ISBN 978-3-319-71291-8   (eBook)
https://doi.org/10.1007/978-3-319-71291-8

© The Editor(s) (if applicable) and The Author(s) 2018, corrected publication 2018
Softcover re-print of the Hardcover 1st edition 2018

This work is subject to copyright. All rights are solely and exclusively licensed by the Publisher, whether the whole or part of the material is concerned, specifically the rights of translation, reprinting, reuse of illustrations, recitation, broadcasting, reproduction on microfilms or in any other physical way, and transmission or information storage and retrieval, electronic adaptation, computer software, or by similar or dissimilar methodology now known or hereafter developed.

The use of general descriptive names, registered names, trademarks, service marks, etc. in this publication does not imply, even in the absence of a specific statement, that such names are exempt from the relevant protective laws and regulations and therefore free for general use.

The publisher, the authors and the editors are safe to assume that the advice and information in this book are believed to be true and accurate at the date of publication. Neither the publisher nor the authors or the editors give a warranty, express or implied, with respect to the material contained herein or for any errors or omissions that may have been made. The publisher remains neutral with regard to jurisdictional claims in published maps and institutional affiliations.

Cover credit: Tom Dunkley/getty images

Printed on acid-free paper

This Palgrave Macmillan imprint is published by the registered company Springer Nature Switzerland AG
The registered company address is: Gewerbestrasse 11, 6330 Cham, Switzerland

Foreword

In my experience, people are more concerned about the problems of ageing than they are enthused about the benefits of advancing years. Common worries are physical and mental decline, losing friends and loved ones, financial limitations, and loss of function and independence. These overshadow the advantages of wisdom, greater freedom in use of time for enjoyable pursuits, opportunity to contribute more to society, emotional equanimity, and ability to put life's inevitable turmoil in perspective. Wouldn't it be great if there was something that could diminish the complications and amplify the joys of ageing? Fortunately, there is one thing that has the ability to grant most people a seemingly impossible long list of wishes. Of course, physical activity is that thing that could make the ageing process less debilitating and more fulfilling.

Unfortunately, people become less active as they grow older, and in some countries the reduction is dramatic. Even worse, industrial and technological forces over the past couple of centuries have produced never-ending innovations to make physical activity unnecessary. Tragically, we have been designing cities, roads, and buildings that make physical activity unpleasant, unsafe, or even impossible. At this historical moment, we are seeing the collision of a global population explosion of older people and a world that is increasingly well designed to discourage physical activity. The result is a global public health train wreck, resulting in needless loss of life and preventable suffering.

The *Palgrave Handbook of Ageing and Physical Activity Promotion* comes at a critical time with the goal of providing evidence-based solutions to some of the world's biggest health and economic problems. Late-life healthcare costs are expected to threaten the viability of not only healthcare systems but national economies as well. Physical activity is a unique solution because of the range of documented benefits that lead to both longer life and better quality of life. However, physical activity also may be unique in the difficulty of intervening effectively. The barriers to physical activity range from biological factors that reduce people's ability to obtain pleasure from movement as they grow older, to cultures that devalue physical activity, to economic forces and environments designed to discourage active living.

This book has many elements of a real solution. It is organised by ecological levels, so the reader will learn about effective approaches at multiple levels. To implement the multi-level interventions that will be needed, multiple disciplines and sectors will need to work together. The interdisciplinary thought leadership of the book editors helps break down disciplinary boundaries that impede integrated solutions. The book has a variety of audiences who will need to understand the problems and solutions so they can design and implement effective interventions: researchers, practitioners, and students from multiple disciplines. Thus, this book can be viewed from distinctly different perspectives, like a 3-D puzzle. The book has a depth of information for each audience, for each discipline, and at each level of intervention.

The reader will learn that research has generated effective interventions at each level. The biggest problem is that very few of the solutions are being implemented widely. This book is a well-designed instrument for putting into practice what we have learned—and doing so across the globe. This book is a big step towards improving physical activity among older adults so they can avoid the decline in quality of life that people fear and enhance physical and mental vigour so people can thrive and enjoy their later years. As you read this book, please consider what contribution you can make, working with interdisciplinary groups, to implement the effective strategies summarized in the following pages.

University of California San Diego James F. Sallis
La Jolla, CA, USA
Institute for Health and Ageing
Australian Catholic University
Melbourne, VIC, Australia

Preface

In this handbook, our aim was, for the first time, to provide a text that brought together the different relevant disciplines required to understand the multi-disciplinary issue of how to promote physical activity among older people. This required a section devoted to each relevant discipline and a co-editor with expertise from that discipline. Therefore, this handbook is organised into sections by an editor who has reviewed every chapter in their section and written an introductory preface. In addition, as the lead editor, Samuel Nyman has reviewed every chapter to provide a second peer-review of the content and to bring consistency across all the chapters and sections for the whole handbook.

This handbook has been a large undertaking, with 83 authors from 15 different countries from 5 continents. We would like to thank the authors of all the chapters for their contributions and for striving to make the nuances of their particular research fields accessible to a wider audience. We also thank the authors who all contributed to the glossary and subject index which has been compiled by the lead editor. In addition, we are grateful to Professor Sallis for his foreward and Jane Asher and Professors Rowe and Biddle for their endorsements. Without the combined effort of such a large and multi-disciplinary team this handbook would not have been possible.

Dr Samuel R. Nyman, and section co-editors: Dr Anna Barker, Professor Terry Haines, Dr Khim Horton, Dr Charles Musselwhite, Dr Geeske Peeters, Professor Christina Victor, and Dr Julia K. Wolff.

Poole, UK	Samuel R. Nyman
Melbourne, VIC, Australia	Anna Barker
Frankston, VIC, Australia	Terry Haines

London, UK   Khim Horton
Swansea, UK   Charles Musselwhite
Dublin, Ireland   Geeske Peeters
Uxbridge, UK   Christina R. Victor
Nuremberg, Germany   Julia Katharina Wolff

Contents

1 **A Multidisciplinary Approach to Promoting Physical Activity Among Older People**   1
Samuel R. Nyman

Section 1   **The Need for Promoting Physical Activity Among Older People**   21

2 **The Problem of Physical Inactivity Worldwide Among Older People**   25
Robert L. Hill and Kristiann C. Heesch

3 **The Benefits of Physical Activity for Older People**   43
Annemarie Koster, Sari Stenholm, and Jennifer A. Schrack

4 **The Benefits of Physical Activity in Later Life for Society**   61
Geeske Peeters, Sheila Tribess, and Jair S. Virtuoso-Junior

Section 2   **Selection of What Physical Activity to Promote Among Older People**   79

5 **Principles of Physical Activity Promotion Among Older People**   83
Melanie K. Farlie, David A. Ganz, and Terry P. Haines

Contents

6 Promotion of Physical Activity for the General Older Population 103
Anne-Marie Hill

7 Promotion of Physical Activity for Older People with Cardiorespiratory Conditions 123
Narelle S. Cox, Jennifer M. Patrick, and Anne E. Holland

8 Promotion of Physical Activity for Older People with Neurological Conditions 145
Monica Rodrigues Perracini, Sandra Maria Sbeghen Ferreira Freitas, Raquel Simoni Pires, Janina Manzieri Prado Rico, and Sandra Regina Alouche

9 Promotion of Physical Activity for Older People with Musculoskeletal Conditions 165
Steven M. McPhail

10 Promotion of Physical Activity for Acutely Unwell Older People 185
Nina Beyer and Charlotte Suetta

Section 3 How to Maximise Participation in Physical Activity Among Older People 207

11 Behaviour Change Theories and Techniques for Promoting Physical Activity Among Older People 211
Karen Morgan and Maw Pin Tan

12 Self-Efficacy and Its Sources as Determinants of Physical Activity among Older People 231
Lisa M. Warner and David P. French

13 Motivational Barriers and Resources for Physical Activity Among Older People 251
Verena Klusmann and Nanna Notthoff

14	**Self-Regulation and Planning Strategies to Initiate and Maintain Physical Activity Among Older People** *Paul Gellert and Andre M. Müller*	271
15	**Making Physical Activity Interventions Acceptable to Older People** *Angela Devereux-Fitzgerald, Laura McGowan, Rachael Powell, and David P. French*	291

Section 4	**Implementation of Physical Activities for Older People**	313
16	**Social Relationships and Promoting Physical Activity Among Older People** *Diane E. Whaley*	317
17	**The Role of the Instructor in Exercise and Physical Activity Programmes for Older People** *Helen Hawley-Hague, Bob Laventure, and Dawn A. Skelton*	337
18	**Promoting Physical Activity Among Older People in Long-Term Care Environments** *Julie Whitney*	359
19	**Promoting Physical Activity Among Older People in Hospital** *Anna Barker and Sze-Ee Soh*	381
20	**Implementing Physical Activity Programmes for Community-Dwelling Older People with Early Signs of Physical Frailty** *Afroditi Stathi, Max Western, Jolanthe de Koning, Oliver Perkin, and Janet Withall*	401

Section 5	**Physical Environmental Factors and Physical Activity Among Older People**	423
21	**Outdoor Mobility and Promoting Physical Activity Among Older People** *Neil Thin, Katherine Brookfield, and Iain Scott*	427

22 Physical Environments That Promote Physical Activity Among Older People 447
Jelle Van Cauwenberg, Andrea Nathan, Benedicte Deforche, Anthony Barnett, David Barnett, and Ester Cerin

23 Indoor Environments and Promoting Physical Activity Among Older People 467
Maureen C. Ashe

24 Restorative Environments and Promoting Physical Activity Among Older People 485
Jenny Roe and Alice Roe

25 Transportation and Promoting Physical Activity Among Older People 507
Charles Musselwhite

Section 6 Sociological Factors and Physical Activity Among Older People 527

26 Physical Activity and the Ageing Body 531
Victoria J. Palmer, Emmanuelle Tulle, and James Bowness

27 Physical Activity Across the Life Course: Socio-Cultural Approaches 551
Adam B. Evans, Anne Nistrup, and Jacquelyn Allen-Collinson

28 The Role of Gender and Social Class in Physical Activity in Later Life 571
Tamar Z. Semerjian

29 Physical Activity Amongst Ethnic Minority Elders: The Experience of Great Britain 589
Christina Victor

30 The Role of Government Policy in Promoting Physical Activity 607
Debra J. Rose and Koren L. Fisher

Section 7	**Current Issues and Debates in Promoting Physical Activity Among Older People**	627
31	**Measurement of Physical Activity Among Older People** *Nicolas Aguilar-Farias and Marijke Hopman-Rock*	631
32	**Reducing Sedentary Behaviour Among Older People** *Gladys Onambele-Pearson, Jodi Ventre, and Jon Adam Brown*	653
33	**The Role of Sport in Promoting Physical Activity Among Older People** *Rachael C. Stone, Rylee A. Dionigi, and Joseph Baker*	673
34	**Physical Activity as a Strategy to Promote Cognitive Health Among Older People** *Teresa Liu-Ambrose*	693
35	**The Potential for Technology to Enhance Physical Activity Among Older People** *Beatrix Vereijken and Jorunn L. Helbostad*	713
	Erratum to: Physical Environments That Promote Physical Activity Among Older People	E1
	Glossary	733
	Index	747

Editors and Contributors

About the Editors

Anna Barker is a physiotherapist (B.Phty, M.Phty (Geriatrics), PhD) with an interest in healthy ageing and care of older people. She has led several research projects in this field with a focus on fall and fracture prevention. She is a National Health and Medical Research Council Career Development fellow and associate professor (Research) at Monash University.

Terry Haines has a background in physiotherapy and health economics (B.Phty Hons, G. Cert. Health Econ, PhD) and has led a diverse programme of research imbedded in health service provision. He has published over 230 full peer-reviewed publications with high-profile papers in *The Lancet*, *BMJ*, *JAMA Internal Medicine*, and *Journal of Clinical Epidemiology*. He has investigated the use of physical activity interventions in oncology, geriatric, orthopaedic, neurological, critical care, and cardiopulmonary populations.

Khim Horton is an experienced registered nurse with specialist interest in social gerontology (BSc (Hons), PhD). With an interest in the sociology of ageing, Dr Horton's initial study on falls among older people focused on the negotiations and gender issues that older people and their family members have in the prevention of falls. The importance of active and healthy ageing has led Dr Horton, with other EU partners, to coordinate Intensive Programmes on Active and Healthy Ageing involving EU students to participate in summer schools in Slovenia and the Netherlands.

Charles Musselwhite's has research interests in ageing; travel and transport; addressing technological, environmental, health, and sustainability contexts of transportation; and built environment studies. Dr Musselwhite is an Executive Committee member of the British Society of Gerontology (BSG), where he is editor of their journal, *Generations Review*. He is associate editor of *Transport & Health* and on the editorial board of *Ageing & Society*.

Samuel R. Nyman has a background in psychological research (BSc, MSc, PhD). His research interests centre on falls prevention and physical activity promotion among older people and people with dementia. He is currently a National Institute for Health Research Career Development fellow and chief investigator for The TACIT Trial: TAi ChI for people with demenTia.

Geeske Peeters has a background in epidemiology, human movement science, and occupational therapy (BA, MSc, PhD). Her research interests are on the prevention of ageing-related problems such as dementia, falls, and frailty. She received a Global Brain Health Institute Fellowship (2016) to develop strategies to optimize physical and cognitive functioning across the adult lifespan.

Christina R. Victor is a social gerontologist with a background in public health. Her research interests focus upon promoting healthy and active ageing. As such she has an established research programme focusing upon the development and evaluation of interventions to promote physical activity among older adults.

Julia Katharina Wolff is a psychologist who combines developmental and health psychology topics in her research. In her scientific career, she developed an intervention to promote physical activity in old age and worked as deputy head of the German Ageing Survey at the German Centre of Gerontology. The main focus of her research is on health and protective factors for health in older adults including personal resources, such as social support, self-perceptions of ageing, as well as health behaviours, such as physical activity.

List of Contributors

Nicolas Aguilar-Farias Departamento de Educación Física, Deportes y Recreación, Universidad de La Frontera, Temuco, Chile

Jacquelyn Allen-Collinson Human Performance Centre, School of Sport & Exercise Science, University of Lincoln, Lincoln, Lincolnshire, UK

Sandra Regina Alouche Universidade Cidade de São Paulo, São Paulo, Brazil

Maureen C. Ashe Center for Hip Health and Mobility, Vancouver, BC, Canada

Joseph Baker School of Kinesiology and Health Science, York University, Toronto, ON, Canada

Anna Barker School of Public Health and Preventive Medicine, Monash University, Melbourne, VIC, Australia

Anthony Barnett Institute for Health and Ageing, Australian Catholic University, Melbourne, VIC, Australia

David Barnett Institute for Health and Ageing, Australian Catholic University, Melbourne, VIC, Australia

Nina Beyer Department Physical & Occupational Therapy, Bispebjerg Hospital, University of Copenhagen, Kongens Lyngby, Denmark

James Bowness Department of Social Sciences, Media and Journalism, Glasgow Caledonian University, Glasgow, UK

Katherine Brookfield Environment Department, University of York, York, UK

Jon Adam Brown Department of Exercise & Sport Science, Manchester Metropolitan University, Crewe, Cheshire, UK

Jelle Van Cauwenberg Department of Public Health, Ghent University, Ghent, Belgium Research Foundation Flanders, Brussels, Belgium

Ester Cerin Institute for Health and Ageing, Australian Catholic University, Melbourne, VIC, Australia

Narelle S. Cox Physiotherapy, La Trobe University, Melbourne, VIC, Australia
Institute for Breathing and Sleep, Heidelberg, VIC, Australia

Benedicte Deforche Department of Public Health, Ghent University, Ghent, Belgium

Angela Devereux-Fitzgerald Manchester Centre for Health Psychology, School of Health Sciences, University of Manchester, Manchester, UK

Rylee A. Dionigi School of Exercise Science, Charles Sturt University, Port Macquarie, NSW, Australia

Adam B. Evans Faculty of Science, Department of Nutrition, Exercise & Sport, University of Copenhagen, København, Denmark

Melanie K. Farlie Allied Health Research Unit, Monash Health, and Faculty of Medicine, Nursing and Health Sciences, Monash University, Cheltenham, VIC, Australia

Koren L. Fisher Center for Successful Aging and Department of Kinesiology, California State University, Fullerton, CA, USA

Sandra Maria Sbeghen Ferreira Freitas Universidade Cidade de São Paulo, São Paulo, Brazil

David P. French Manchester Centre for Health Psychology, School of Health Sciences, University of Manchester, Manchester, UK

David A. Ganz US Department of Veterans Affairs Greater Los Angeles Healthcare System, University of California at Los Angeles, Los Angeles, CA, USA

Paul Gellert Institute of Medical Sociology and Rehabilitation Science, Charité – Universitätsmedizin Berlin, Berlin, Germany

Terry P. Haines Allied Health Research Unit, Monash Health, and Faculty of Medicine, Nursing and Health Sciences, Monash University, Cheltenham, VIC, Australia

Helen Hawley-Hague Division of Nursing, Midwifery and Social Work, School of Health Sciences, Faculty of Biology, Medicine and Health, University of Manchester, Manchester, UK

Kristiann C. Heesch School of Public Health and Social Work and Institute of Health and Biomedical Innovation, Queensland University of Technology, Kelvin Grove, QLD, Australia

List of Contributors

Jorunn L. Helbostad Department of Neuroscience, Norwegian University of Science and Technology, Trondheim, Norway

Anne-Marie Hill School of Physiotherapy and Exercise Science, Curtin University, Bentley, WA, Australia

Robert L. Hill Fairfield, QLD, Australia

Anne E. Holland Physiotherapy, La Trobe University, Melbourne, VIC, Australia
Institute for Breathing and Sleep, Heidelberg, VIC, Australia
Physiotherapy Alfred Health, Melbourne, VIC, Australia

Marijke Hopman-Rock EMGO Institute, VUmc, Amsterdam, MB, The Netherlands

Virtuoso Júnior Department of Sports Science, Institute of Health Sciences, Federal University of Triangulo Mineiro, Uberaba, MG, Brazil

Verena Klusmann Department of Psychology, Psychological Assessment & Health Psychology, University of Konstanz, Konstanz, Germany University of Bremen, Bremen, Germany

Jolanthe de Koning Department for Health, University of Bath, Bath, UK

Annemarie Koster Department of Social Medicine, CAPHRI School for Public Health and Primary Care, Maastricht University, Maastricht, The Netherlands

Bob Laventure Consultant in Physical Activity, Ageing and Health, Amble, Northumberland, UK

Teresa Liu-Ambrose Aging, Mobility and Cognitive Neuroscience Laboratory and Vancouver General Hospital Falls Prevention Clinic, University of British Columbia, Vancouver, BC, Canada

Laura McGowan Manchester Centre for Health Psychology, School of Health Sciences, University of Manchester, Manchester, UK

Steven McPhail Queensland University of Technology and Southern Metropolitan Area Health Service, Queensland Health, Brisbane, QLD, Australia

Karen Morgan Division of Population Health Sciences, Perdana University-Royal College of Surgeons in Ireland School of Medicine, Serdang, Selangor, Malaysia

Andre M. Müller National University of Singapore, Singapore, Singapore

Charles Musselwhite Centre for Innovative Ageing, Swansea University, Swansea, UK

Andrea Nathan Institute for Health and Ageing, Australian Catholic University, Melbourne, VIC, Australia

Anne Nistrup Faculty of Science, Department of Nutrition, Exercise & Sport, University of Copenhagen, København, Denmark

List of Contributors

Nanna Notthoff Institute of Psychology, Humboldt University Berlin, Berlin, Germany

Samuel Nyman Department of Psychology and Ageing and Dementia Research Centre, Bournemouth University, Poole, UK

Gladys Onambele-Pearson Department of Exercise & Sport Science, Manchester Metropolitan University, Crewe, Cheshire, UK

Victoria J. Palmer Institute of Health and Wellbeing, University of Glasgow, Glasgow, UK

Jennifer M. Patrick Cardiac Rehabilitation Unit, Caulfield Hospital, Alfred Health, Melbourne, VIC, Australia

Geeske Peeters Global Brain Health Institute, University of California San Francisco, San Francisco, CA, USA Trinity College Dublin, Dublin 2, Ireland

Oliver Perkin Department for Health, University of Bath, Bath, UK

Monica Rodrigues Perracini Universidade Cidade de São Paulo, São Paulo, Brazil Universidade Estadual de Campinas, Campinas, Brazil

Tan Maw Pin Department of Medicine, Faculty of Medicine, University of Malaya, Kuala Lumpur, Malaysia

Raquel Simoni Pires Universidade Cidade de São Paulo, São Paulo, Brazil

Rachael Powell Manchester Centre for Health Psychology, School of Health Sciences, University of Manchester, Manchester, UK

Janina Manzieri Prado Rico Universidade Cidade de São Paulo, São Paulo, Brazil

Alice Roe Age UK, London, UK

Jenny Roe School of Architecture, University of Virginia, Charlottesville, VA, USA

Debra J. Rose Kinesiology Department, Center for Successful Aging, and Fall Prevention Center of Excellence, California State University, Fullerton, CA, USA

Jennifer A. Schrack Department of Epidemiology & Core Faculty, Center on Aging and Health, Johns Hopkins Bloomberg School of Public Health, Baltimore, MD, USA

Iain Scott Edinburgh College of Art, University of Edinburgh, Edinburgh, UK

Tamar Z. Semerjian Department of Kinesiology, San José State University, San Jose, CA, USA

Dawn A. Skelton School of Health and Life Sciences, Institute for Applied Health Research, Glasgow Caledonian University, Glasgow, UK

Sze-Ee Soh School of Public Health and Preventive Medicine, Monash University, Melbourne, VIC, Australia

List of Contributors

Afroditi Stathi Department for Health, University of Bath, Bath, UK

Sari Stenholm Department of Public Health, University of Turku, Turku, Finland

Rachael C. Stone School of Kinesiology and Health Studies, Queen's University, Kingston, ON, Canada

Charlotte Suetta Department of Clinical Physiology, Nuclear Medine & PET at Rigshospitalet, Faculty of Health and Medical Sciences, University of Copenhagen, Frederiksberg, Denmark

Neil Thin School of Social Political Sciences, University of Edinburgh, Edinburgh, UK Sheila Tribess Department of Sports Science, Institute of Health Sciences, Federal University of Triangulo Mineiro, Uberaba, MG, Brazil

Emmanuelle Tulle Department of Social Sciences, Media and Journalism, Glasgow Caledonian University, Glasgow, UK

Jodi Ventre Department of Exercise & Sport Science, Manchester Metropolitan University, Crewe, Cheshire, UK

Beatrix Vereijken Department of Neuroscience, Norwegian University of Science and Technology, Trondheim, Norway

Christina Victor College of Health and Life Sciences, Department of Clinical Sciences, Healthy Ageing/Brunel Initiative for Ageing Studies (BIAS), Brunel University London, Uxbridge, UK

Lisa M. Warner Department of Health Psychology and Social, Organization and Economic Psychology, Freie Universität Berlin, Berlin, Germany

Max Western Department for Health, University of Bath, Bath, UK

Diane E. Whaley Educational Psychology/Applied Developmental Science Program, University of Virginia, Charlottesville, VA, USA

Julie Whitney Clinical Age Research Unit, King's College Hospital, Cheyne Wing, London, UK

Janet Withall Department for Health, University of Bath, Bath, UK

List of Figures

Fig. 1.1	The main determinants of health (Dahlgren and Whitehead 1991)	9
Fig. 4.1	Theoretical pathway of how physical activity may influence quality of life, health care utilisation and health care costs	62
Fig. 7.1	Components of exercise training in pulmonary rehabilitation (PR) and cardiac rehabilitation (CR). (Sources: The pulmonary rehabilitation toolkit. Alison J et al., The Pulmonary Rehabilitation Toolkit on behalf of The Australian Lung Foundation (2009) www.pulmonaryrehab.com.au; The heart education assessment rehabilitation toolkit. National Heart Foundation of Australia. www.heartonline.org.au)	128
Fig. 7.2	Effect of interventions on increasing daily physical activity relative to quality of evidence	136
Fig. 8.1	Downward spiral of decreased physical activity and sedentary behaviour in older people with neurological conditions	146
Fig. 9.1	Potential cycle of interactions between physical inactivity, body structures, lifestyle-related conditions and chronic diseases, musculoskeletal conditions, ability (and desire) to undertake physical activity	166
Fig. 10.1	Hospital-associated disability. Panel 1 (left) shows the proportion of older medical patients who required personal assistance in daily activities two weeks prior to admission, at admission, and at discharge (Mudge et al. 2010). Panel 2 (right) shows a model for suggested outcomes of 'fast-track treatment' including mobilisation during hospitalisation (A) and 'usual care' (B) for two patients with different functional status at hospital admission	189

List of Figures

Fig. 12.1	Illustration of the social cognitive theory for physical activity in older adults	234
Fig. 12.2	Summary of the modes of induction for the four sources of self-efficacy for physical activity among older adults	243
Fig. 14.1	Feedback loop with physical activity-related examples (Modified after Carver and Scheier 2002, p. 305)	272
Fig. 15.1	Dynamic model of older adults' acceptability of physical activity interventions	295
Fig. 18.1	Recommended activity interventions in LTC with barriers and enablers	368
Fig. 19.1	Barriers to increasing older people's physical activity while in hospital and strategies to address these	386
Fig. 24.1	Urban farmers' markets offer older people a wealth of health opportunities. (Source: The image is © JABA (Jefferson Area Board for Aging))	496
Fig. 32.1	Illustration of the four different types of physical activity patterns in adult humans. 1.0 MET is 1 kcal/kg/hour or 3.5 ml/kg/min of energy cost and is equivalent to sitting quietly	654

List of Tables

Table 5.1	Exercise prescription guidelines for older adults from position statements and recommendation reports	86
Table 8.1	Exercise/PA recommendations for patients with neurological conditions	148
Table 11.1	Experiential and behavioural processes which facilitate movement between stages of change	214
Table 16.1	Summary of major themes and strategies for maximising physical activity through social interactions	328
Table 20.1	Key areas for successful implementation of physical activity programmes	414
Table 21.1	Global trends and typical situations relevant to outdoor PA	429
Table 25.1	Designing streets for older people based on CABE (2011) principles (Musselwhite 2014)	514
Table 26.1	Characteristics of three studies presented in this chapter	537
Table 30.1	Key considerations for evaluating evidence for physical activity interventions	609
Table 30.2	"HARDWIRED" criteria for successful physical activity policy	611
Table 31.1	Strengths and limitations of subjective and objective methodologies measuring physical activity (compiled from Strath et al. 2013; Swank 2012; Neuman et al. 2000; Ainslie et al. 2003)	632

1

A Multidisciplinary Approach to Promoting Physical Activity Among Older People

Samuel R. Nyman

1.1 Introduction

It has been known since the 1950s that physical activity is linked with physical and mental health benefits for people of all ages (Kohl III et al. 2012). For example, leisure time physical activity is associated with a reduction in risk of 13 types of cancer, regardless of body size or smoking history (Moore et al. 2016). Further, participation in physical activity in mid-life can reduce the risk of poor health in later life, such as developing dementia, disability, and frailty (National Institute for Health and Care Excellence 2015). It seems that older people would like to live for many years in later life on the condition that they live a 'healthy old age', that is, with continued independence (Karppinenm et al. 2016). Thus, physical activity is key to helping people achieve 'healthy ageing' (World Health Organization [WHO] 2015).

However, we also know that many people are not as physically active as they could be, and thus their potential to maximise their health and well-being is not realised. For example, an estimated 9% of worldwide premature mortality is caused by lack of physical activity (Lee et al. 2012). As adults grow older, they are less likely to be physically active, and this decline in physical activity continues so that older people are the least likely to be physically active of all age groups (Hallal et al. 2012; McKee et al. 2015). This is

---

S. R. Nyman (✉)
Department of Psychology, Bournemouth University, Poole, UK

© The Author(s) 2018
S. R. Nyman et al. (eds.), *The Palgrave Handbook of Ageing and Physical Activity Promotion*, https://doi.org/10.1007/978-3-319-71291-8_1

why physical activity is a key component of policies aimed at improving the health and well-being of older people, such as 'successful ageing' in the USA and 'active ageing' in Europe. Successful ageing refers to the avoidance of disability and disease to enable continued activity in later life (Foster and Walker 2015). Active ageing, similarly, refers to facilitating older people to remain active—in terms of physical activity, employment, and social, economic, cultural, spiritual, and civic participation—to enable continued quality of life in later life (WHO 2002). While successful and active ageing policies are broader in scope, the focus of this handbook will solely be on physical activity promotion, a central element to any ageing well strategy. In response to current low levels of physical activity participation among older people, this handbook seeks to comprehensively answer the question, 'How can we best promote physical activity among older people?'

1.2 An Outline of the Rationale, Scope, and Contents of the Handbook

This handbook is for researchers, practitioners, postgraduates, and final year undergraduate students. It is to meet the need for a text on the best evidence about how to achieve physical activity promotion among older people. Our handbook meets this need by providing a multidisciplinary text co-edited by a panel of experts from the relevant disciplines. The chapters provide a series of overviews from experts in the field to give the reader an understanding of the current evidence base and associated key theoretical concepts. Each chapter covers what is known about the topic, what is unknown, and the practical implications of current theory and empirical evidence.

1.2.1 The Book's Unique Contribution to the Literature

Despite advances in the fields of gerontology and geriatrics, sports and exercise science, sociology, health psychology, and public health, knowledge is largely contained within disciplines as reflected in the current provision of academic texts on this subject. However, to address the present and substantial societal challenges such as population ageing, a multidisciplinary and collaborative approach is required. This edited volume will review the current evidence for what physical activities need to be promoted among older people and how these physical activities can be implemented to maximise engagement. The unique feature of this handbook is the team of editors and authors who represent a variety of disciplines and countries that have collaborated to produce for the first time a multidisciplinary handbook on this subject.

1.2.2 Scope of the Book

In accordance with ecological approaches to health promotion, the book will be divided into sections that follow a gradual progression from focusing on determinants of physical activity at the individual level, to the community level, and then finally to the structural level (Dahlgren and Whitehead 1991). The first section of the book will highlight the importance of promoting physical activity among older people from an epidemiological perspective. The second and third sections of the book will focus on the individual level in terms of what physical activities to promote (physiology) and how to maximise participation in physical activity (psychology). The fourth section will focus on the social and community network level (implementation of physical activities in different settings). The fifth and sixth sections will focus on the general socio-economic, cultural, and environmental conditions level in relation to both the physical (landscape and built environment architecture) and social environment (sociology). The final section will provide a discussion of current issues and debates in promoting physical activity among older people. From this handbook, the reader will benefit from the scientific knowledge of the following: why we need to promote physical activity in later life, which activities to promote and how to maximise participation, how the physical, social, and cultural environment facilitates/hinders activity, and future developments in this thriving field.

In the sections that follow, the focus of the handbook is introduced, and in particular, definitions are given for the terms 'physical activity' and 'older people'. An ecological approach is then provided as the framework for the handbook, along with a brief explanation of how this maps on to the handbook's different sections. The chapter then concludes with some applications of the material covered for practitioners working with older people.

1.3 What Do We Mean by Physical Activity?

Terms such as 'physical activity' and 'exercise' are often used interchangeably, but they actually refer to distinct concepts. 'Physical activity refers to body movement that is produced by the contraction of skeletal muscles and that increases energy expenditure' (Chodzko-Zajko et al. 2009, p. 1511).

In contrast, 'exercise refers to planned, structured, and repetitive movement to improve or maintain one or more components of physical fitness' (Chodzko-Zajko et al. 2009, p. 1511), with physical fitness defined as a set of measurable health- or skill-related attributes (Caspersen et al. 1985). Exercise is therefore a subcategory of physical activity and is planned, structured, and repetitive, whereas physical activity can be spontaneous and fluid. Exercise has the express purpose of improving/maintaining physical fitness, whereas physical activity could be conducted with a different intention. For example, someone may walk home because it is a sunny day and to enjoy the weather. They have been walking for 30 minutes, but not for the purpose of getting fit, and they decided to do this spontaneously. Likewise, some physical activities such as playing in the park with grandchildren may be for fun, and while they meet the criteria for physical activity, they would not meet the criteria for exercise.

1.3.1 Rationale for This Handbook's Focus on Physical Activity

While some chapters may focus more on exercise, for example, specific prescribed body movements for the purpose of rehabilitation and to recover strength in a certain area of the body, the handbook has an overall focus on physical activity. Physical activity encompasses a broader range of activity and so has been adopted for this handbook to encompass activities such as sports, activities of moderate intensity, vigorous intensity, muscle training, and lifestyle-based strategies for increasing physical activity. Moderate intensity activities include for example brisk walking, bike riding, dancing, swimming, and active travel (Department of Health, Physical Activity, Health Improvement, & Protection 2011). Vigorous intensity activities include for example running, playing sport, taking part in aerobic exercise classes, and using cardiovascular gym equipment (Department of Health et al. 2011). Muscle strengthening includes for example, weight training, working with resistance bands, carrying heavy loads, heavy gardening, push ups, and sit ups (Department of Health et al. 2011). In contrast to prescriptive exercise, lifestyle-based strategies for increasing physical activity are attempts to incorporate physical activity into people's everyday routines, such as encouraging people to walk to the shops rather than drive and to use the stairs rather than escalators in public buildings (Kerr et al. 2001).

There are different levels by which physical activity and exercise can be described (Chodzko-Zajko et al. 2009). People can carry out physical activity of different types (the activity being undertaken, e.g. brisk walking or swimming), frequency (how often they do the activity, e.g. weekly), duration (for how long they do the activity, e.g. for 30 minutes), and intensity (how strenuous, e.g. light, moderate, or vigorous). There are also other ways to categorise physical activity, for example, planned vs. unplanned, leisure vs. occupational (Caspersen et al. 1985), and various exercise categories, for example, aerobic exercise training, resistance exercise training, flexibility exercise, and balance training (Chodzko-Zajko et al. 2009).

There is also the issue of fidelity; are people carrying out the activity in the manner prescribed? This is important when a specific exercise intervention is being prescribed and deviation from the programme may either pose a risk to the participant or reduce its benefit. Therefore, fidelity is required when designing programmes to ensure they are congruent with any underlying theory or principles (Keller et al. 2009) and that they are delivered in the way intended (Moore et al. 2015).

1.3.2 Physical Activity Participation as Adherence

There is a debate on which term we should use when we are referring to the extent that an older person is following recommendations (e.g. by national governments) to be physically active, that is, the degree of 'adherence' or 'compliance' (e.g. Kyngäs et al. 2000). In this handbook different terms may be used interchangeably. Furthermore, there is a debate as to how we classify whether or not someone is currently adhering to physical activity recommendations (Hawley-Hague et al. 2016). Despite these debates, the approach taken in this handbook is one that considers older people's participation in physical activity as a voluntary choice and not one imposed upon them. Further, non-adherence or non-participation in physical activity is not perceived as deviant behaviour but can be considered as 'reasoned decision-making' (Donovan and Blake 1992). Both the motivations to be or not to be physically active are important to the study of the promotion of physical activity among older people, and decisions not to be physically active often represent complex situations that cannot be easily reduced to lack of will power (see the ecological approach adopted in this handbook described below). A stance that dictates to older people that they should be physically active and blames people for not being physically active fails to respect both the individual's autonomy and the complex interaction of factors at the individual level, social and community network level, and general socio-economic, cultural, and environmental conditions level (Dahlgren and Whitehead 1991; Michie et al. 2011; WHO 2002). The approach taken in this handbook is not to dictate to older people what they should do. Rather, this handbook seeks to aid the promotion of physical activity in a variety of ways to make physical activity more useful, convenient, relevant, and fun for older people to enjoy.

1.4 What Do We Mean by Older People?

There are several ways in which we might decide what constitutes an 'older person' (Victor 2006). Chronological age is often used as the criterion by which one is categorised as either 'old' or not. For example, one might deem older people to be aged 65 years or above. While this may seem straightforward, it is however more complex to apply. For example, why should the age be set at 65 and not say 60 or 70? Some researchers have set the bar as low as 50 years of age when including older people (Aalbers et al. 2011; van Stralen et al. 2009). Others argue that people aged in their 60s in say the 1900s and 1950s would have different life expectancies than in current times. Contextually then, in today's age, we might better categorise old age in respect of how many years one might expect to have left, which would be more like 75 years and above for an individual in France up from 58 years in 1900 and 65 years in 1956 (Sanderson and Scherbov 2015). Life expectancy also varies markedly within and between countries. If being 'old' is in relation to how long one has left to live, this will then mean someone could be 'old' much younger in less affluent areas. There are at least two reasons why age has often been set at around 65 years: retirement and illness. In industrialised nations, the age of retirement has been around the age of 65. However, there is no uniform age of retirement across countries, and the custom age to retire differs by professions. Therefore, employment status is not a satisfactory criterion to categorise whether someone is 'old' or not.

In regard to illness, it is undeniable that as we grow older we become more at risk of developing chronic (long-term) illnesses, such as diabetes, arthritis, and heart disease (Hart 1990; Hoffman et al. 1996; Jacobs et al. 2012). Not only that, we are also more at risk of developing more than one chronic illness, that is, comorbidity (Hughes et al. 2013; Marengoni et al. 2009; Sadanand et al. 2013). In later life, this occurs because of senescence, the breakdown of the maintenance function of the body, which is observable in gradual declines of biological and psychological functioning (Seifert et al. 1997; Stuart-Hamilton 1991). From this pattern we might be inclined to suggest that people could be categorised as being older by deterioration in health status, for example, through the development of a debilitating chronic illness or development of comorbidity. However, in taking a lifespan perspective, from the outset, people's rate of deterioration in health progresses at different rates. By old age, the heterogeneity of health status is far more pronounced than in younger decades and is larger than in any younger generation (Brody et al. 1987; Day 1985; Schaie 1988; Shephard 1997). Simply knowing the age of someone will actually tell you very little about the health status of an individual and vice versa (Ward 1984; WHO 2015).

1.4.1 Is Subjective Age a Viable Alternative?

Given the above unsatisfactory nature of using chronological age as an indicator of whether or not someone is 'old', some have suggested that subjective age is a viable alternative. One's subjective age—their perception of how old they are—is founded and continually moulded through the perceptions of ageing in one's culture and those around them (Settersten Jr. and Hagestad 2015). Part of the credence for using perceived age is that it is a better predictor than chronological age of an older person's health, independence, engagement in social activities, self-efficacy, and quality of life (Bowling et al. 2005). It appears that most adults perceive themselves to be younger than their chronological age, which is predictive of a slower decline in cognitive functioning (Stephan et al. 2016). Further, one's perceived age appears to be based on social comparisons and one feels younger if they have better functioning on age-relevant domains such as health and memory than their peers (Hughes and Lachman 2016).

However, this subjective approach will be difficult for some to accept who would much rather prefer more objective means of categorising if someone is old or not (e.g. by chronological age). Furthermore, subjective age is domain specific. For example, someone may feel physically younger than their chronological age, but older in terms of their social relationships (e.g. because of early grandparenthood). Also, information on someone's perceived age will not be readily available and will likely change with time and circumstances, and so one will not be able to fathom an individual's subjective age unless they use some form of validated questioning to obtain this information. One can foresee that this process and continual need for updating will be impractical and pose ethical dilemmas in circumstances where services are to be provided or not to people by age category.

1.4.2 Should We Categorise Older People into Young-Old, Middle-Old, and Old-Old?

To segment the older adult population into more meaningful categories, authors have distinguished between 'young', 'middle', and 'old' older adults. Young older adults are deemed to be aged 65–74 years and are generally free from physical limitations; middle older adults are aged 75–84 years, and many have some physical limitations; while old older adults are aged 85 years and above and are often dependent on carers for everyday tasks (Shephard 1994, 1997). These categories are of course not widely endorsed, because of the issues noted above. For example, some suggest the age categories should have different start and end points, and others question the categories because of the implied strong correlation between age and health status. It does stand to reason though to challenge the notion that all older people are alike and to consider the generational differences that may arise when promoting physical activity among individuals who are all aged 65 and above but differ in age by a decade or more.

Given the above, it is therefore not as straightforward to define old age as one may first imagine. The approach taken in this handbook is to define older people as broadly those aged 65 years and above. This is because the evidence base broadly draws on research conducted with adults aged 65 and above. However, this definition is used with the recognition of the heterogeneity of older people (some aged in their 60s will be very fit and healthy and others relatively frail), that it encompasses people of different generations (aged in their 60s, 70s, 80s, etc.), and the different contexts in which older people live (e.g. the number of years lived in good health will vary markedly within and between countries).

1.5 A Multidisciplinary Approach to Promoting Physical Activity Among Older People

An existing theoretical model is used in this handbook to incorporate the various relevant disciplines to the study of promoting physical activity among older people (see Fig. 1.1) (Dahlgren and Whitehead 1991). While the model was originally developed in regard to the determinants of health in general, its three layers can be applied to the determinants of physical activity participation among older people: (1) individual lifestyle factors, (2) social and community networks, and (3) general socio-economic, cultural, and environmental

A Multidisciplinary Approach to Promoting Physical Activity...

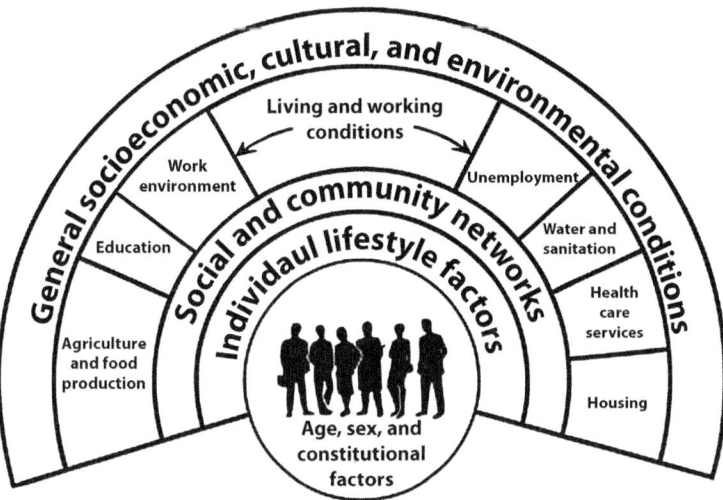

Fig. 1.1 The main determinants of health (Dahlgren and Whitehead 1991)

conditions (Dahlgren and Whitehead 1991). This model shows how the different factors that determine physical activity participation are all important and related. Strategies to promote physical activity participation among older people at one level may work either in concert or in discord to efforts at another level (Dahlgren and Whitehead 1991). Clearly, strategies that seek to promote health at all levels in concert will be more effective. For example, recreational parks could be provided at the community level, motivational and educational strategies could be employed to encourage people to use them at the individual level, and mass media campaigns could be used to change cultural norms at the generic socio-economic, cultural, and environmental conditions level (Sallis et al. 2006).

Similar models have been developed since the one described above. For example, in the WHO's (2002) model of the determinants of active ageing, they included the following determinants that can be categorised into the Dahlgren and Whitehead's (1991) layers, with gender and culture threaded throughout: (1) individual lifestyle factors: behavioural determinants and personal determinants; (2) social and community networks: social determinants; and (3) general socio-economic, cultural, and environmental conditions: physical environment, economic determinants, and health and social services. The WHO (2015) has now turned its focus to functional ability in later life. However, this still retains the incorporation of individual and societal elements to bring about maximising health among older people, the combination of intrinsic capacity within individuals, environmental features, and their interaction (Beard et al. 2016). Likewise, the potential for strategies at different layers to negatively impact on each other are encompassed in more recent complex systems perspectives, that take account of delays, unintended consequences, competing interests, and so on that may negatively affect a strategy to increase physical activity participation (Kohl III et al. 2012).

A more recent example of an ecological approach is the COM-B (Michie et al. 2011, 2014). It theorises that behaviour (B) is determined by the combination of three broad categories of determinants: Capability (C, the individual's psychological and physical ability to be physically active), Opportunity (O, the availability of facilities and culturally appropriate places to be physically active), and Motivation (M, the individual's habitual and planned patterns of physical activity). The COM-B has an associated Behaviour Change Wheel with nine interventions designed to address one or more deficits in the COM-B model (e.g. an area that if addressed would increase physical activity) and seven policies that if implemented would facilitate the provision of such interventions (Michie et al. 2011, 2014).

Such theoretical models that include not only individual-level factors but those of the wider environment and policy levels are known as ecological models (Sallis et al. 2006; Spence and Lee 2003). Ecological models like the one in Fig. 1.1 emphasise the importance of different levels of influence on health and their interconnection (Bauman et al. 2012). They draw attention to the combination and interaction of factors—individual, interpersonal, environmental, regional or national policy, and global determinants—and acknowledge these factors across the lifespan (Bauman et al. 2012). These models can become complex as they are specified to particular domains of active living, such as active recreation, household activities, active transport, and occupational activities (Sallis et al. 2006). Yet at the root of these more specific models is the one illustrated in Fig. 1.1, that multiple levels are at work in determining the physical activity of people of all ages and that these levels can interact to either promote or hinder physical activity (Spence and Lee 2003).

1.5.1 Ecological Model Adopted for This Handbook

This handbook will focus on each section of the levels of the model as illustrated in Fig. 1.1 as they apply to the promotion of physical activity among older people. While ecological models require testing, current evidence supports the inclusion of each level in a comprehensive model of determinants of physical activity promotion rather than one level in isolation (Sallis et al. 2006).

It is not the purpose of this handbook to provide an exposition of how exactly the different levels of an ecological model interact. Most models leave this open, largely due to the dependence on specific contexts to answer this question. Some have suggested that factors within each layer can influence physical activity participation individually and through interaction between layers. Some evidence supports this view with an American study finding an interaction effect: community-dwelling older people were more likely to be physically active if they were living in a supportive environment (conducive to physical activity), but much more so among older people with positive psychological attributes towards participating in physical activity (Carlson et al. 2012). Others have posited that the levels beyond the individual are mediated by the individual level, that is, biological and psychological variables (Spence and Lee 2003). Partial support for this approach has been found in a survey study of older people, where psychological variables (intention and self-efficacy) mediated the relationship between several factors and physical activity. However, this result was weaker among those with poorer health and of a lower socioeconomic status (Sniehotta et al. 2013).

For the purpose of this handbook, Sections 2–6 inclusively provide details on some of the key aspects of one of the three layers of the ecological model illustrated in Fig. 1.1. This serves to provide an understanding of how each layer can contribute to physical activity participation among older people. While each section is presented individually representing a different discipline, nonetheless, one acknowledges that the layers do not operate in isolation and will in reality often interact with at least one other layer if not all the other layers at any given time. The purpose of this handbook is to bring these different disciplines together into one volume. Such an ecological approach is theorised to be superior to working within separate disciplines and appears to be a core ingredient to the sustained impact of community-based physical activity interventions with older people (Haggis et al. 2013).

1.6 Sections of the Handbook

Below, the layers of the ecological model in Fig. 1.1 are briefly mapped to the seven sections of this handbook, with an example to illustrate the importance of each one.

1.6.1 Section 1: Epidemiology: The Need for Promoting Physical Activity Among Older People

Epidemiology is concerned with the incidence of disease in certain populations and the reasons for them (Coggon et al. 2016). Expertise in the area of population statistics is required to understand the scale of the problem of physical inactivity and its association with risks to health and well-being. Observational studies at more local levels are also required to understand what inhibits people participating in physical activity. For example, fear of falling, as well as age and severe mobility impairment, has been associated with being homebound or infrequently outdoors in an American survey (Smith et al. 2016).

1.6.2 Sections 2–3: Individual Level

1.6.2.1 Section 2: Physiology: Selection of What Physical Activity to Promote Among Older People

Physiology is concerned with how all aspects of a biological being interact to form a whole (Physiological Society 2016), and so exercise physiology is concerned with how the whole body responds to exercise and physical activity (British Association of Sport and Exercise Sciences 2016). Physiotherapists use this knowledge to help rehabilitate people who wish to recover movement and physical functioning, for example, due to increasing frailty (Chartered Society of Physiotherapy 2016). These sciences of the human body are important as they help us to understand *what* specific physical activities should be promoted to older people. For example, if we wish to prevent falls among older people, then we should promote physical activities that challenge balance (i.e. activity while standing), use a higher dose (50 hours or more), and do not include a walking programme (Sherrington et al. 2008).

1.6.2.2 Section 3: Psychology: How to Maximise Participation in Physical Activity Among Older People

Psychology is the scientific study of mind and behaviour (British Psychological Society 2016). This field is important for understanding what helps or hinders people at the individual level to initiate and maintain a physically active lifestyle. From this, behaviour change techniques can be applied to help maximise older people's participation in physical activity (Greaves et al. 2011; Uphill, on behalf of the Behaviour Change Advisory Group 2014). For example, helping people set goals for how much walking they will do that day and to monitor how much walking they have actually done can increase walking activity for some individuals (Nyman et al. 2016).

1.6.3 Section 4: Social and Community Network Level: Implementation of Physical Activities for Older People in Different Settings

Implementation science is the study of methods for applying research evidence in policy and practice, with a focus on the role of staff and other stakeholders in the provision of evidence-based healthcare (Fogarty International Center, National Institutes of Health 2016). It is important to broaden our understanding from the individual factors that can act as barriers and facilitators of physical activity promotion to the broader levels (social and community network level). For example, a Canadian mobilisation strategy was introduced in acute care settings for vulnerable older people (Moore et al. 2014). The investigators found that barriers to implementing the programme of mobilising the older patients concerned several areas: the healthcare professionals (e.g. time constraints), the patients (perceived need to play the 'sick role'), and the hospital unit (e.g. if the equipment was readily available). Thus, this approach recognises that barriers to implementation of physical activity promotion initiatives can thwart the good intentions of older people. If such barriers are identified, then strategies can be put in place to try to overcome them and for the programme to be more widely adopted.

1.6.4 Sections 5–6: General Socio-economic, Cultural, and Environmental Conditions Level

1.6.4.1 Section 5: Landscape and Built Environment Architecture: Physical Environmental Factors and Physical Activity Among Older People

Architecture is a design profession where people use both science and the arts to create effective private and shared spaces for people for a variety of uses. The landscape refers to an area of land, whereas the built environment is in relation to man-made structures, and so is typically used to refer to urban environments. It is important to understand the influential role of the physical environment on physical activity patterns among older people. For example, people with access to public transport and public parks are more likely to be physically active, as this encourages walking to bus stops and train stations for travel and the use of parks for recreational physical activity (Sallis et al. 2016). If neighbourhoods that are not 'activity friendly' were altered to encourage physical activity, then this could increase physical activity among individuals by an estimated 68–89 minutes per week (Sallis et al. 2016).

1.6.4.2 Section 6: Sociological Factors and Physical Activity Among Older People

Sociology is the scientific study of human social behaviour, with the aim of identifying underlying meanings through examination of cultural and societal systems (British Sociological Association 2016). An understanding of the social environment is important for identifying how the social context can influence older people's physical activity. For example, by analysing the social context of gymnasiums, a study showed that expectations of ageing as a period of decline in physical ability and traditional approaches to exercise to obtain fitness used by their younger instructors could constrain older people's physical activity participation (Tulle and Dorrer 2012).

1.6.5 Section 7: Current Issues and Debates in Promoting Physical Activity Among Older People

The last section of the handbook explores some current issues and debates around promoting physical activity among older people. This provides an opportunity to explore the more emergent areas of knowledge relevant to physical activity promotion, such as the use of technology to promote physical activity. For example, exercise performed through playing video games or 'exergames' shows promise as a safe and effective alternative means of increasing physical function among older people (Skjæret et al. 2016). People then associate exercise with a fun game, something that they may be more likely to do than other forms of traditional exercise that may be less appealing.

1.7 Conclusion

For the first time, this handbook brings together current knowledge from several disciplines in the hope that it will advance understanding in promoting physical activity among older people. An existing ecological approach is put forward that combines the relevant and varied disciplines in the promotion of physical activity to older people. Practitioners would do well to consider all the layers in this model (see Fig. 1.1) or similar when promoting physical activity to older people. They will then be able to identify if any determinants are present in the layers that may hinder physical activity and how these might be addressed. In addition, strategies that seek to promote physical activity using multiple layers in concert are likely to have greater impact than one layer in isolation.

Suggested Further Reading

- Ecological models of physical activity: Sallis et al. (2006).
- The benefits of physical activity for older people and the terms 'physical activity' and 'exercise': Chodzko-Zajko et al. (2009).
- The COM-B model and Behaviour Change Wheel: Michie et al. (2011).

References

Aalbers, T., Baars, M. A. E., & Olde Rikkert, M. G. M. (2011). Characteristics of effective internet-mediated interventions to change lifestyle in people aged 50 and older: A systematic review. *Ageing Research Reviews, 10*, 487–497.

Bauman, A. E., Reis, R. S., Sallis, J. F., Wells, J. C., Loos, R. J. F., Martin, B. W., et al. (2012). Correlates of physical activity: Why are some people physically active and others not? *Lancet, 380*, 258–271.

Beard, J. R., Officer, A., Araujo de Carvalho, I., Sadana, R., Pot, A. M., Michel, J.-P., et al. (2016). The world report on ageing and health: A policy framework for healthy ageing. *Lancet, 387*, 2145–2154.

Bowling, A., See-Tai, S., Ebrahim, S., Gabriel, Z., & Solanki, P. (2005). Attributes of age-identity. *Ageing & Society, 25*, 479–500.

British Association of Sport and Exercise Sciences. (2016). http://www.bases.org.uk/Physiology

British Psychological Society. (2016). *Discover psychology*. Retrieved June 21, 2016, from [On-line].

British Sociological Association. (2016). *Discover sociology*. Durham: British Sociological Association.

Brody, J. A., Brock, D. B., & Williams, T. F. (1987). Trends in the health of the elderly population. *Annual Review of Public Health, 8*, 211–234.

Carlson, J. A., Sallis, J. F., Saelens, B. E., Frank, L. D., Kerr, J., Cain, K. L., et al. (2012). Interactions between psychosocial and built environment factors in explaining older adults' physical activity. *Preventive Medicine, 54*, 68–73.

Caspersen, C. J., Powell, K. E., & Christenson, G. M. (1985). Physical activity, exercise, and physical fitness: Definitions and distinctions for health-related research. *Public Health Reports, 100*, 126–131.

Chartered Society of Physiotherapy. (2016). *What is physiotherapy?* Retrieved June 21, 2016, from [On-line].

Chodzko-Zajko, W. J., Proctor, D. N., Fiatarone Sing, M. A., Minson, C. T., Nigg, C. R., Salem, G. J., et al. (2009). Exercise and physical activity for older adults. *Medicine & Science in Sports & Exercise, 41*, 1510–1530.

Coggon, D., Rose, G., & Barker, D. J. P. (2016). *Epidemiology for the uninitiated* (4th ed.). London: BMJ.

Dahlgren, G., & Whitehead, M. (1991). *Policies and strategies to promote social equity in health: Background document to WHO – Strategy paper for Europe*. Stockholm: Institute for Futures Studies.

Day, A. T. (1985). *'We can manage': Expectations about care and varieties of family support among people 75 years and over, Institute of Family Studies Monograph* (Vol. 5). Melbourne: Institute of Family Studies.

Department of Health, Physical Activity, Health Improvement, & Protection. (2011). *Start active, stay active: A report on physical activity for health from the four home countries' chief medical officers*. London: Department of Health, Physical Activity, Health Improvement and Protection.

Donovan, J. L., & Blake, D. R. (1992). Patient non-compliance: Deviance or reasoned decision-making? *Social Science & Medicine, 34*, 507–513.

Fogarty International Center, National Institutes of Health. (2016). *Implementation science information and resources*. Retrieved June 21, 2016, from [On-line].

Foster, L., & Walker, A. (2015). Active and successful aging: A European policy perspective. *Gerontologist, 55*, 83–90.

Greaves, C. J., Sheppard, K. E., Abraham, C., Hardeman, W., Roden, M., Evans, P. H., et al. (2011). Systematic review of reviews of intervention components associated with increased effectiveness in dietary and physical activity interventions. *BMC Public Health, 11*, e119. https://doi.org/10.1186/1471-2458-11-119

Haggis, C., Sims-Gould, J., Winters, M., Gutteridge, K., & McKay, H. A. (2013). Sustained impact of community-based physical activity interventions: Key elements for success. *BMC Public Health, 27*, e892. https://doi.org/10.1186/1471-2458-13-892.

Hallal, P. C., Andersen, L. B., Bull, F. C., Guthold, R., Haskell, W., & Ekelund, U. (2012). Global physical activity levels: Surveillance progress, pitfalls, and prospects. *Lancet, 380*, 247–257.

Hart, S. (1990). Psychology and the health of elderly people. In P. Bennett, J. Weinman, & P. Spurgeon (Eds.), *Current developments in health psychology* (pp. 247–275). London: Harwood Academic.

Hawley-Hague, H., Horne, M., Skelton, D. A., & Todd, C. (2016). Review of how we should define (and measure) adherence in studies examining older adults' participation in exercise classes. *BMJ Open, 6*, e011560. https://doi.org/10.1136/bmjopen-2016-011560

Hoffman, C., Rice, D., & Sung, H.-Y. (1996). Persons with chronic conditions: Their prevalence and costs. *Journal of the American Medical Association, 276*, 1473–1479.

Hughes, M. L., & Lachman, M. E. (2016). Social comparisons of health and cognitive functioning contribute to changes in subjective age. *Journals of Gerontology Series B: Psychological Sciences and Social Sciences*. https://doi.org/10.1093/geronb/gbw044. Published online 25 April.

Hughes, L. D., McMurdo, M. E. T., & Guthrie, B. (2013). Guidelines for people not for diseases: The challenges of applying UK clinical guidelines to people with multimorbidity. *Age and Ageing, 42*, 62–69.

Jacobs, J. M., Maaravi, Y., Cohen, A., Bursztyn, M., Ein-Mor, E., & Stessman, J. (2012). Changing profile of health and function from age 70 to 85 years. *Gerontology, 58*, 313–321.

Karppinenm, H., Laakkonen, M.-L., Strandberg, T. E., Huohvanainen, E. A., & Pitkala, K. H. (2016). Do you want to live to be 100? Answers from older people. *Age and Ageing, 45*, 543–549.

Keller, C., Fleury, J., Sidani, S., & Ainsworth, B. (2009). Fidelity to theory in PA intervention research. *Western Journal of Nursing Research, 31*, 289–311.

Kerr, J., Eves, F. F., & Carroll, D. (2001). The influence of poster prompts on stair use: The effects of setting, poster size and content. *British Journal of Health Psychology, 6*, 397–405.

Kohl, H. W., III, Craig, C. L., Lambert, E. V., Inoue, S., Alkandari, J. R., Leetongin, G., et al. (2012). The pandemic of physical inactivity: Global action for public health. *Lancet, 380*, 294–305.

Kyngäs, H., Duffy, M. E., & Kroll, T. (2000). Conceptual analysis of compliance. *Journal of Clinical Nursing, 9*, 5–12.

Lee, I.-M., Shiroma, E. J., Lobelo, F., Puska, P., Blair, S. N., & Katzmarzyk, P. T. (2012). Effect of physical inactivity on major non-communicable diseases worldwide: An analysis of burden of disease and life expectancy. *Lancet, 380*, 219–229.

Marengoni, A., Rizzuto, D., Wang, H. X., Winblad, B., & Fratiglioni, L. (2009). Patterns of chronic multimorbidity in the elderly population. *Journal of the American Geriatrics Society, 57*, 225–230.

McKee, G., Kearney, P. M., & Kenny, R. A. (2015). The factors associated with self-reported physical activity in older adults living in the community. *Age and Ageing, 44*, 586–592.

Michie, S., van Stralen, M. M., & West, R. (2011). The behaviour change wheel: A new method for characterising and designing behaviour change interventions. *Implementation Science, 6*, e42. https://doi.org/10.1186/1748-5908-6-42

Michie, S., Atkins, L., & West, R. (2014). *The behaviour change wheel: A guide to designing interventions.* Great Britain: Silverback.

Moore, J. E., Mascarenhas, A., Marquez, C., Almaawiy, U., Chan, W.-H., D'Souza, J., et al. (2014). Mapping barriers and intervention activities to behaviour change theory for Mobilization of Vulnerable Elders in Ontario (MOVE ON), a multi-site implementation intervention in acute care hospitals. *Implementation Science, 9*, e160. https://doi.org/10.1186/s13012-014-0160-6.

Moore, G. F., Audrey, S., Barker, M., Bond, L., Bonell, C., Hardeman, W., et al. (2015). Process evaluation of complex interventions: Medical Research Council guidance. *BMJ, 350*, h1258. https://doi.org/10.1136/bmj.h1258.

Moore, S. C., Lee, I.-M., Weiderpass, E., Campbell, P. T., Sampson, J. N., Kitahara, C. M., et al. (2016). Association of leisure-time physical activity with risk of 26 types of cancer in 1.44 million adults. *JAMA Internal Medicine, 176*, 816–825.

National Institute for Health and Care Excellence. (2015). *Dementia, disability and frailty in later life – Mid-life approaches to delay or prevent onset.* London: National Institute for Health and Care Excellence.

Nyman, S. R., Goodwin, K., Kwasnicka, D., & Callaway, A. (2016). Increasing walking among older people: A test of behaviour change techniques using factorial randomised N-of-1 trials. *Psychology & Health, 31*, 313–330.

Physiological Society. (2016). *What is physiology?* Retrieved June 21, 2016, from [On-line].

Sadanand, S., Shivakumar, P., Girish, N., Loganathan, S., Bagepally, B. S., Kota, L. N., et al. (2013). Identifying elders with neuropsychiatric problems in a clinical setting. *Journal of Neurosciences in Rural Practice, 4*, S24–S30.

Sallis, J. F., Cervero, R. B., Ascher, W., Henderson, K. A., Kraft, M. K., & Kerr, J. (2006). An ecological approach to creating active living communities. *Annual Review of Public Health, 27*, 297–322.

Sallis, J. F., Cerin, E., Conway, T. L., Adams, M. A., Frank, L. D., Pratt, M., et al. (2016). Physical activity in relation to urban environments in 14 cities worldwide: A cross-sectional study. *Lancet, 387*, 2207–2217.

Sanderson, W. C., & Scherbov, S. (2015). Faster increases in human life expectancy could lead to slower population aging. *PLoS One, 10*, e0121922. https://doi.org/10.1371/journal.pone.0121922.

Schaie, K. W. (1988). Methodological issues in ageing research: An introduction. In K. W. Schaie, R. T. Campbell, W. Meredith, & S. C. Rawlings (Eds.), *Methodological issues in ageing research* (pp. 1–11). New York: Springer.

Seifert, K. L., Hoffnung, R. J., & Hoffnung, M. (1997). *Lifespan development.* Boston: Houghton Mifflin Company.

Settersten Jr, R. A., & Hagestad, G. O. (2015). Subjective aging and new complexities of the life course. *Annual Review of Gerontology and Geriatrics, 35*, 29–53.

Shephard, R. J. (1994). Determinants of exercise in people aged 65 years and older. In R. K. Dishman (Ed.), *Advances in exercise adherence* (pp. 343–360). Leeds: Human Kinetics.

Shephard, R. J. (1997). *Aging, physical activity, and health*. Leeds: Human Kinetics.

Sherrington, C., Whitney, J. C., Lord, S. R., Herbert, R. D., Cumming, R. G., & Close, J. C. T. (2008). Effective exercise for the prevention of falls: A systematic review and meta-analysis. *Journal of the American Geriatrics Society, 56*, 2234–2243.

Skjæret, N., Nawaz, A., Morat, T., Schoene, D., Helbostad, J. L., & Vereijken, B. (2016). Exercise and rehabilitation delivered through exergames in older adults: An integrative review of technologies, safety and efficacy. *International Journal of Medical Informatics, 85*, 1–16.

Smith, A. R., Chen, C., Clarke, P., & Gallagher, N. A. (2016). Trajectories of outdoor mobility in vulnerable community-dwelling elderly: The role of individual and environmental factors. *Journal of Aging and Health, 28*, 796–811.

Sniehotta, F. F., Gellert, P., Witham, M. D., Donnan, P. T., Crombie, I. K., & Mcmurdo, M. E. T. (2013). Psychological theory in an interdisciplinary context: Psychological, demographic, health-related, social, and environmental correlates of physical activity in a representative cohort of community-dwelling older adults. *International Journal of Behavioral Nutrition and Physical Activity, 10*, e106. https://doi.org/10.1186/1479-5868-10-106.

Spence, J. C., & Lee, R. E. (2003). Toward a comprehensive model of physical activity. *Psychology of Sport and Exercise, 4*, 7–24.

Stephan, Y., Sutin, A. R., Caudroit, J., & Terracciano, A. (2016). Subjective age and changes in memory in older adults. *Journals of Gerontology Series B: Psychological Sciences and Social Sciences, 71*, 675–683.

Stuart-Hamilton, I. (1991). *The psychology of ageing: An introduction*. London: Jessica Kingsley.

Tulle, E., & Dorrer, N. (2012). Back from the brink: Ageing, exercise and health in a small gym. *Ageing & Society, 32*, 1106–1127.

Uphill, M., & on behalf of the Behaviour Change Advisory Group. (2014). *Behaviour change: Physical (in)activity*. London: British Psychological Society.

van Stralen, M. M., De Vries, H., Mudde, A. N., Bolman, C., & Lechner, L. (2009). Determinants of initiation and maintenance of physical activity among older adults: A literature review. *Health Psychology Review, 3*, 147–207.

Victor, C. R. (2006). What is old age? In S. J. Redfern & F. M. Ross (Eds.), *Nursing older people* (4th ed., pp. 7–21). London: Churchill Livingstone.

Ward, R. A. (1984). *The ageing experience: An introduction to social gerontology* (2nd ed.). London: Harper & Row.

World Health Organization [WHO]. (2002). *Active ageing: A policy framework*. Geneva: World Health Organization.

World Health Organization [WHO]. (2015). *World report on ageing and health*. Geneva: World Health Organization.

Section 1

The Need for Promoting Physical Activity Among Older People

Geeske Peeters

In epidemiology, the health and wellbeing of a population are described in numbers. These numbers come to life when they tell a story. In this section, we tell the story of the benefits of a physically active lifestyle on the health and wellbeing of older people.

In Chap. 2, the authors set the scene by describing what we mean when we label people as being 'physically active' or 'physically inactive'. It also describes how many people are considered physically active or inactive and how this is influenced by gender and culture. Understanding these definitions and the volume of people who are active or inactive is important to understand the scale of the health problems on a societal level that may be attributable to inactivity. It also helps us to understand the size of the group of people who may benefit from physical activity programs.

In Chap. 3, the authors describe the main health problems that are known to be linked with physical inactivity. The health problems that are discussed include cardiovascular disease, type 2 diabetes, musculoskeletal disorders, cancer, obesity, and mental health problems. The associations between physical activity and cognitive and physical functioning are also discussed. The varied range of health problems linked with physical activity demonstrates the wide-ranging effects that physical activity has on the body and brain. It also shows

---

G. Peeters (✉)
Global Brain Health Institute, University of California San Francisco, San Francisco, CA, USA / Trinity College Dublin, Dublin, Ireland

the potential gain in health if programs can effectively encourage people to maintain an active lifestyle.

In Chap. 4, the impact of physical inactivity on the society is described. Via its effects on health, physical activity also influences our wellbeing. In research, wellbeing is referred to as *quality of life*. Another important outcome is health services use and the related economical costs. Information about the effects of physical activity on wellbeing and costs is used by policymakers to decide whether government funding of physical activity programs can be justified.

The information described in these chapters is based on data from epidemiological studies. Two types of study design are particularly important in this context: observational studies and experimental studies. In observational studies, the emphasis is on observing the natural course of health and disease and factors that may influence health and disease. Observational studies typically measure a wide range of factors such as socio-demographic factors (such as age and gender), lifestyle, symptoms, diagnoses, functioning, wellbeing or health services use. Information from observational studies is important to describe how many people in the population display a given behaviour, such as being physically active, or how many people have a given health problem, such as cardiovascular disease. The information can also be used to examine whether relationships exist between factors and health outcomes. Information from observational studies is used to inform policy documents and clinical guidelines about the magnitude of a given health problem. The information is also used to inform the development of intervention programs. More specifically, observational studies provide insight into whom to target with health promotion programs and the content of these programs. For example, if more people are physically inactive in disadvantaged neighbourhoods than in affluent neighbourhoods, the effectiveness of the promotion programs may be better when offered in disadvantaged neighbourhoods and tailored to local needs and preferences. It is important to understand that information from observational studies alone is insufficient to draw conclusions about the causality of a relationship. Following on from the previous example, the finding that people in disadvantaged neighbourhoods are less active than people in affluent neighbourhoods may be explained by other factors than living in that neighbourhood, such as differences between the neighbourhoods in age or availability of sports facilities.

In experimental studies, researchers intend to evaluate the effect of a given experiment or intervention on one or more health outcomes of interest. The effect is measured by comparing two or more groups who are offered alternative programs. The most common design is a two-group comparison, whereby one group is offered the intervention and the other group serves as the control group. Ideally, participants are assigned to the intervention or control group at random. If a random group allocation occurs, this study design is called a 'randomised controlled trial'. The random group allocation reduces the risk of bias from differences between the groups at the start of the study. For example, to evaluate the effectiveness of a physical activity program on daily functioning in frail older adults, half the participants will be offered the program. Their daily functioning before and after the program will be compared with the other half of the participants who were not offered the program. The control group typically receives 'care as usual', but may sometimes be offered an alternative program that is not considered to influence the outcome of interest. This type of study design allows us to examine the direct effect of the intervention on the outcome. This study design also allows us to draw conclusions about the causality of a relationship. If in the previous example the daily functioning improved in the intervention group, but declined in the control group, and all other factors remained stable, it can be concluded that the physical activity program *caused* the improvement in daily functioning.

A type of study that the authors frequently refer to in this section is a systematic review of previous studies. In a review of the literature, researchers systematically collect and compare the findings from all the relevant previous studies on a specific topic. A systematic review often includes a *meta-analysis*. In a meta-analysis, the findings from previous studies are pooled to form one aggregate estimate. This technique can be applied to results from both observational studies (e.g. prevalence rates or associations) and experimental studies (e.g. effect of an intervention). The more studies that find the same results, the stronger the evidence for a given relationship or the effectiveness of an intervention.

In conclusion, epidemiological data provide information on the size of a given health problem and help identify and evaluate preventive, curative, or management strategies. Observational studies inform how components of each layer of the ecological model are associated with the natural course of health and disease. Experimental studies inform how manipulation of any or multiple of the components of the layers of the ecological model can *change* the natural course of health and disease.

2

The Problem of Physical Inactivity Worldwide Among Older People

Robert L. Hill and Kristiann C. Heesch

2.1 Introduction

At its simplest, physical activity is any bodily movement that results from the use of skeletal muscles (those attached to bone). Young children on playgrounds seem to delight in movement, walking sometimes, running often. As we grow older, however, we tend to move with joy and energy less frequently. Even as teenagers and young adults, many of us find it difficult to move about enough each week to stay as healthy as we could. For adults, reaching the recommended minimum level of physical activity each week becomes more and more difficult at and beyond middle age (Bijnen et al. 1998; Sims et al. 2014; Sun et al. 2013). The consequences of failing to be sufficiently physically active, though, are usually negative for the individual (Warburton et al. 2006), and they are a matter of concern for healthcare systems of countries around the world (Kohl et al. 2012).

Systematic research into the effects of physical activity on health began with the recognition that heart disease was less common among people working in occupations that required movement than among those in sedentary occupations (Blair and Morris 2009). More recently, researchers have called for a war on inactivity because of epidemiological evidence linking chronic diseases to

---

R. L. Hill (✉)
School of Public Health and Social Work, Queensland University of Technology, Kelvin Grove, QLD, Australia

K. C. Heesch
School of Public Health and Social Work and Institute of Health and Biomedical Innovation, Queensland University of Technology, Kelvin Grove, Australia

insufficient amounts of regular physical movement (Booth et al. 2002). These are reasons enough for researchers to seek what are often referred to as physical activity prevalence estimates, evidence-based calculations of how much physical activity people are engaging in regularly. Because of two tendencies associated with age, a decline in physical activity and an increase in the likelihood of chronic disease, the category 'older adults' is of particular interest to those concerned about public health. Although researchers sometimes select other starting points for inclusion in their studies, the 65th birthday is often chosen as the threshold for entry into this cohort. This is despite the fact that '65 years of age and above' places under a single umbrella people living through decades—as many as four in some instances—of physical and mental change.

2.2 Surveillance of Physical Activity

The editors of a recent handbook on surveillance studies (Lyon et al. 2012) recognised that surveillance is often heard or read as a 'loaded term', calling to mind spying, police work, and threats to privacy. And, indeed, the *Routledge Handbook of Surveillance Studies* is about the collection of personal data by governments, corporations, and individuals, not about physical activity or health. Those new to public health research, then, may be surprised to see 'physical activity surveillance' in academic papers until it becomes clear that nothing more sinister than 'monitoring' is intended. Surveillance of physical activity involves researchers asking individuals to voluntarily and anonymously provide information about their physical activity patterns. The data from one person are collated with data from other persons who agree to provide information about their physical activity patterns. The accumulation of data over time allows for trends in physical activity levels to be calculated and monitored for whole populations or smaller sub-groups of people (Bull and Bauman 2011), thereby contributing to the primary goal of PA measurement: better understanding of how individuals and their circumstances influence the physical activity they do on a regular basis (Bauman et al. 2006). Clear progress in physical activity surveillance has come about since the start of this century because people from all over the world have freely provided information about their behaviour (Hallal et al. 2012).

2.3 Levels of Physical Activity

Physical activity prevalence studies seek information about the degree to which populations within countries and groups of countries are 'meeting guidelines', which means attaining at least the minimum levels of physical activity recommended for health benefits. Since the release in 1995 of a report by a panel of experts convened in the United States (Pate et al. 1995), the recommended minimum level of physical activity for adults 18–64 years of age and also for adults 65 years old and above in the US has been 150 minutes per week of moderate-intensity physical activity in bouts of 10 minutes or more. This guideline, now recommended by the World Health Organization (WHO) and often expressed as 30 minutes of physical activity at least the intensity of brisk walking, 5 days per week, has been adopted by other developed countries (Sparling et al. 2015) and, in spite of many variations, is still the basis of most national physical activity guidelines in Europe (Kahlmeier et al. 2015).

Subsequent US government recommendations allow the guideline to be met by 75 minutes of vigorous-intensity physical activity (such as swimming laps or jogging) over a week or a combination of vigorous- and moderate-intensity physical activities (Haskell et al. 2007). Further, these recommendations state that adults over 65 years of age who cannot meet the guideline should be as physically active as abilities and conditions allow and that they should do exercises to improve balance. Adults of all ages are urged to do muscle-strengthening exercises, such as lifting weights or using resistance bands, on two or more days of each week.

2.3.1 Prevalence: How Many People Are Meeting Guidelines?

Definitive answers to questions about adherence to physical activity guidelines, despite many published papers about this topic, are difficult to find. A large gap between highest and lowest estimates of the percentage of people meeting physical activity guidelines was reported in an international systematic review of papers about the physical activity of adults 60 years of age and above (Sun et al. 2013). The 53 papers reviewed came from 13 predominately English-speaking countries. Forty-seven papers reported estimates derived from self-reported data from surveys. These gave prevalence estimates that ranged from 11% to 83%. Of the six papers that drew upon objectively measured data, prevalence estimates reported were as low as 2% and as high as 87%. The span of estimates recorded by most (41) of the 53 studies was smaller, from 20% to 60%, but this is still a difference of 40 percentage points in physical activity prevalence estimates. A large gap between highest and lowest estimates of the percentage of people meeting physical activity guidelines was also reported in an Australia-focused study published a year earlier (Hill and Brown 2012). The researchers reported a 30 percentage point difference in prevalence estimates across studies, from 25% to 55%. This systematic review of papers about Australians 65 years of age and older included 22 studies published between 2000 and 2010 that had included at least 500 participants. All but two of the studies had collected self-reported physical activity data, and the two studies that collected objectively measured physical activity data (by pedometer) were not included in prevalence estimates because their physical activity outcome (steps) was not comparable to the estimates derived from the self-report measures. Two reviews of published reports on prevalence estimates for older adults, then, one drawing on estimates from many countries and the other on estimates within a single country, show differences of 40 percentage points and 30 percentage points, respectively, in estimates of how many older adults are regularly meeting guidelines for maintaining or enhancing health.

Prevalence estimates from the US also lack consistency. Data collected between 1999 and 2013 for the three leading national surveys in the US showed a 13 percentage point difference in the proportion of persons 65 years of age and above who were reported to be meeting the US physical activity guideline (Keadle et al. 2016). The lowest adherence rate, from the 2011–2012 National Health and Nutrition Examination Survey (NHANES), was 27% of adults interviewed (Centers for Disease Control and Prevention [CDC] 2017a). The highest was 44% of adults interviewed as part of the 2013 Behavioral Risk Factor Surveillance System (BRFSS) (CDC 2017b). In the middle of this range was the estimate that of adults who completed the 2013 National Health Interview Survey (NHIS) (CDC 2017), 36% met the guidelines.

Why so much difference, study to study, in prevalence estimates? Physical activity participation can be calculated in varying ways. Some studies follow the WHO physical activity recommendation that only physical activities that last ten minutes or longer be counted in physical activity prevalence estimates. Others include all physical activity, regardless of duration. To account for the health effects of higher-intensity physical activities, some studies multiply by two all minutes judged to have been spent in vigorous-intensity physical activity; others do not. Also, the studies use a variety of recall periods, the lengths of time for which each respondent is asked to remember and report their physical activities: the previous 7 days, 2 weeks, or even the previous 12 months. Some studies ask for daily physical activity amounts rather than just weekly totals, while others do not. Formulas used to calculate physical activity vary. Most studies focus on leisure-time physical activity, which is usually defined as all physical activity other than that associated with occupations, housework, or transportation (Lin et al. 2011), but some include these activities. Given these limitations and given the widely varying prevalence estimates that result, caution is warranted in interpreting statements about the proportions of populations adhering to physical activity guidelines, especially when comparing physical activity prevalence estimates across countries or regions. In short: many estimates, little consistency.

2.4 Sources of Variation in Prevalence Rates

2.4.1 Country-to-Country Differences: Culture, Practices

The difficulties inherent in collecting physical activity data vary greatly from country to country. In some, physical activity prevalence estimates can be derived from nationwide sources of data. Canadian researchers, for example, can draw upon information from an ongoing, population-wide surveillance system that began in 1934 after the importance of physical activity to health and fitness was recognised (Craig et al. 2017). A 2008 report on leisure-time activity data from the Canadian Community Health Survey (CCHS) Cycle 1.1 provided telephone survey data from Canadians 65 years of age and older (Ashe et al. 2009). Selection of participants for surveys is made easier in Sweden by the fact that Swedes have registered personal identification numbers that can be used to track individuals (Sundquist et al. 2004). The Longitudinal Aging Study Amsterdam (LASA) recruited participants from three regions of the Netherlands (Amsterdam and vicinity, Oss and vicinity, and Zwolle and vicinity) and has collected physical activity data from older adults since 1992 (Stel et al. 2004). The large-scale NHANES, BRFSS, and NHIS in the US are conducted routinely by the CDC (see http://www.cdc.gov/): NHANES since 1959, BRFSS since 1984, and NHIS since 1957. A recent analysis of physical activity data that was conducted as part of the UK Biobank study allowed for the analysis of objectively measured physical activity data from a large cohort (Doherty et al. 2017). In Australia the National Health Survey has been collecting data on moderate- to vigorous-intensity exercise of persons aged 15 years and older since 1989 (Australian Bureau of Statistics 2015), and a number of cohort studies have collected physical activity data on national samples of adults over time (e.g., the Australian Longitudinal Study of Women's Health [see http://www.alswh.org.au/] and the Australian Diabetes, Obesity, and Lifestyle Study [see http://www.baker.edu.au/ausdiab/]). Large or long-term studies such as these can be especially valuable for calculating within-country prevalence estimates.

Comparisons of physical activity data among countries are more complex, however, particularly when they include nations with low-, middle-, and high-income populations. Hallal et al. (2012) reviewed physical activity surveillance studies from 122 countries with various levels of development. Self-report data from these countries, which contained nearly nine-tenths of the world's population, indicated that 31% of those 15 years of age or older were not meeting guidelines. The authors, however, suggested that this estimate should be read with caution because perceptions about what constitutes physical activity can vary across countries, genders, and age groups.

Variations among countries in the sorts of data available can have a significant impact on prevalence estimates. Due to differences in the data collected, Macniven, Bauman, and Abouzeid (2012) said, country-level prevalence estimates calculated from responses to 56 surveys from 29 Asia-Pacific nations represented only a loose collection of estimates of the percentages of people meeting physical activity guidelines. These ranged from 7% in the Maldives to 93% in the Philippines. It was not possible to produce a broadly applicable prevalence estimate across countries. Among the issues that the authors noted were incompatibilities in surveillance systems and differences in what was counted as physical activity. They also noted that housework and garden work, particularly important to the physical activity levels of people in developing countries, were assessed in some studies but not in others. Variations in the types of physical activities measured were also evident across 13 studies included in a meta-analysis (Tak et al. 2013). The meta-analysis included data from older participants from nine countries on four continents. The authors stressed the need for greater consistency in how moderate- and vigorous-intensity physical activity for older adults is defined.

Some Western countries have also included housework and garden work in their surveillance of physical activity, while some have not. Analysis of Dutch data from the 1999/2000 LASA Physical Activity Questionnaire indicated that large proportions of Dutch people performed light housework (96%), heavy housework (75%), and gardening (43%) (Stel et al. 2004). Physical activities examined among older Canadians included gardening (32%), but activities of daily living such as housework, cleaning, and being a carer, were not assessed (Ashe et al. 2009). Gardening and housework were not assessed in a large Swedish study (Sundquist et al. 2004). For the UK Biobank study (Doherty et al. 2017), an objective measure of physical activity that could not assess the types of activities performed was used. In the US, some surveys include questions about housework and gardening and others do not. Self-report data from the 2003–2004 NHANES survey, for example, included housework, and as a result, researchers estimated that 51% of respondents adhered to the 150-minute per week moderate-intensity physical activity recommendation (Troiano et al. 2008). The omission of housework and garden activities can be a source of inaccuracy, particularly in calculating physical activity prevalence estimates for women (Brown et al. 2012).

Findings from studies across the world show that active travel—walking and riding a bicycle to get from place to place—is a type of physical activity that is important to include in physical activity prevalence study, although it is not always specifically captured in surveillance efforts. A study of older Chinese men, which did take note of active travel, reported that 56% of the men in Shanghai usually walked or rode a bicycle daily, including for transportation (Lee et al. 2012). Travel-related physical activity was found to be similarly significant in Uganda, a largely rural country in sub-Saharan Africa. A majority of Ugandans relied on either walking or bike riding for transportation, activities that account for 25% of Ugandans' weekly physical activity in total (Guwatudde et al. 2016). The median amount of time spent in moderate-intensity physical activity was 1470 minutes a week, and 94% of these Ugandans met the WHO physical activity guideline. The percentage of trips taken by bicycle in the windy but delightfully flat Netherlands was 17% in 2005 (Pucher and Buehler 2008). In Sweden, bicycles were used for 9% of trips in 2001–2002 (Hagströmer et al. 2010). The comparable percentage around that same time in the US, the UK, and Australia was about 1% (Pucher and Buehler 2008). Being able to make these comparisons requires the assessment of active travel specifically. Surveys that ask respondents to report only on leisure-time physical activity would not capture active travel unless a respondent considered active travel to be part of their leisure-time activity.

In short, country-to-country comparisons of the physical activity prevalence estimates of adults are made difficult by differences in the quality of resources available to researchers, differences in economic conditions, and variations in measures used to assess physical activity.

2.4.2 Age-Group Differences

Both men and women in the US become less physically active beyond age 65: adherence to the US physical activity guidelines was recently shown to have declined from 42% for those 65–74 years of age to 31% for those 75–84 years of age, and to 18% for those 85 years and older (Keadle et al. 2016). Thirty percent of Canadians 65 years old and older met their country's guideline when they were surveyed in 2000 and 2001, but the proportion of older adults meeting the guideline declined with increasing age (Ashe et al. 2009). Doherty and colleagues, in their UK Biobank study that categorised participants above the age of 45 in decade bands, found that total physical activity declined, on average, by 7.5% in each decade of age difference (Doherty et al. 2017). The evidence indicates, in short, that population-level physical activity levels generally decline as people age. However, data from the Netherlands shows that travel by walking or riding a bicycle contributes significantly to the fact that the average Dutch adult aged 65 years or older exceeds the WHO physical activity guideline by a greater amount than do younger Dutch adults (Fishman et al. 2015). Therefore, declines in physical activity are not seen everywhere.

2.4.3 Gender Differences

Gender differences in physical activity participation are indicated from data collected in the US, Canada, Australia, and some European countries (Ashe et al. 2009; Caspersen et al. 2000; Hagströmer et al. 2010; Sims et al. 2014). Men in these countries tend to be more physically active than women. A 51-country, worldwide survey in 2008 found that more women than men aged 60–69 years were not meeting physical activity guidelines except in seven Eastern European countries, and that inactivity is 'worrisome' for some countries and subgroups, particularly for women in this age range (Guthold et al. 2008). The evidence to date suggests that in many countries population-level physical activity generally decreases with age and that the decrease is greater for women than for men. However, these gender differences are not observed everywhere.

Women are reported to be more physically active than men in the Netherlands, for example. Data from the Dutch National Travel Survey (2010–2012) indicate that Dutch women cycle farther per day on average than Dutch men (Fishman et al. 2015). Women have been shown to be more physically active in Shanghai, China, as well. A cohort of Chinese men between the ages of 40 and 74 years reported more moderate- to vigorous-intensity physical activity on a regular basis and spent more time engaged in sport and leisure-time physical activities than the women (Lee et al. 2007). However, Chinese women in the same age range and living in the same area, because of greater participation in active travel and housework, had a total physical activity level 1.8 times greater than that of their male counterparts. The men made 33% of their trips by automobile. The women? Three percent. As these findings indicate, the types of physical activity normally engaged in by men and women can vary. When all physical activity, including activities more often performed by women than by men, is included in physical activity prevalence estimates (and sometimes, as in the case of the Netherlands study, when they are not), older women can be shown to be getting as much physical activity as older men, or more.

Indeed, some published observations of gender differences may not be correct, given that walking, housework, and childcare—more often women's activities—are not normally included in physical activity totals from self-report measures (Brown et al. 2012; Hansen et al. 2012). Reflecting on two large, single-gender Australian studies that did not assess light-intensity physical activities, Brown et al. (2012) reasoned that some observed gender differences in physical activity levels may have been due to women having had a 'background' level of not-counted light-intensity physical activities, such as shopping, preparing meals, doing laundry, and handling carer responsibilities. Sundquist et al. (2004) concur, noting that bias is introduced into self-reported physical activity data if surveys do not assess gardening or household-related activities. In a Norwegian study, Hansen et al. (2012) reported that women accumulated more objectively measured minutes of light-intensity physical activity than men and that a higher percentage of women than men accumulated at least 10,000 objectively measured steps per day. Therefore, physical activities that are, in most cultures, regularly undertaken more often by women than by men need to be considered in calculations of physical activity prevalence.

2.5 The Different Measures Used for Calculating Prevalence Estimates

Most prevalence estimates in this chapter were derived from responses to survey questions about physical activity. Such self-report data are and have been for some time the most common source of information for the calculation of physical activity prevalence estimates. Some prevalence estimates, however, were calculated from data collected from pedometers and accelerometers. The use of these devices to obtain objective measurements of physical activity has, in recent years, become more frequent. Worn on a wrist or the hip, pedometers are electronic or electromechanical devices that count the steps a wearer takes. Accelerometers, which may incorporate the functions of the pedometer, are more complicated devices that measure changes in the velocity (i.e., acceleration) of the wearer's movement.

Asking respondents to recall their previous physical activities for surveys is usually the least costly option for collecting the data needed to estimate the prevalence of physical activity. Therefore, surveys are usually the most feasible tools for collecting information about physical activity levels although survey data have well-known limitations (Mâsse et al. 2005; Washburn 2000). These limitations include 'social-desirability bias', which happens when respondents allow their recollections to be influenced by the need for approval or affirmation, and 'recall bias', which results from inaccurate recollection of details about past behaviour. Australians between 65 and 85 years of age were shown to experience difficulties with accurately recalling and reporting on the duration and intensity of physical activities that they had performed over the previous week (Heesch et al. 2010). The duration of a walk, for example, was sometimes reported as the number of minutes from the beginning of the walk period to its end even when some of those minutes were spent standing still and conversing with a neighbour. Another issue identified by Heesch and colleagues was the previously mentioned problem of whether to include activities that had not lasted for at least ten minutes; some respondents ignored instructions to include only bouts of physical activity lasting that long. This problem, however, is not limited to studies that rely on surveys for the collection of physical activity data.

Some researchers collecting and tabulating accelerometer data include only physical activity undertaken for at least ten minutes and some do not. In the seminal 1995 set of public health recommendations, the CDC and the American College of Sports Medicine advocated for daily amounts of physical activity totalling 30 minutes and indicated that this total could be attained by the accumulation of intermittent bouts of physical activity lasting as little as 8–10 minutes (Pate et al. 1995). The authors of an update of this report, published in 2007, said something similar: that short bouts of moderate- to vigorous-intensity physical activity 'usually lasting ten minutes' may be effective in reducing chronic disease risk (Haskell et al. 2007).

Decisions to include all physical activity or only bouts of physical activity that last at least ten minutes have significant consequences on physical activity estimates. Accelerometer data from participants, who were part of five cross-sectional studies in England, Portugal, Norway, and Sweden, showed that only 32% of men and women between the ages of 20 and 75 years failed to meet the physical activity guideline of at least 150 minutes per week of moderate- to vigorous-intensity physical activity (Loyen et al. 2016). However, when bouts of physical activity lasting less than ten minutes were removed from the totals, the proportion that failed to meet the guideline jumped 40 percentage points to 72%. A recent accelerometer study of Europeans and South Asians found differences of as much as 43 percentage points in estimates of physical activity guideline adherence depending on whether or not the ten-minute minimum duration threshold was used in calculations (Iliodromiti et al. 2016).

These problems are, of course, about how data are collected and analysed. The raw data collected by accelerometers, while limited in some ways, are not subject to the biases that can diminish the accuracy of self-report information about physical activity. Therefore, some researchers now view accelerometry as the minimum standard for physical activity assessment in epidemiologic research (Corder and van Sluijs 2010), and the incorporation of accelerometer functions into mass-marketed mobile phones (known as cell phones in some countries) suggests the possibility of additional ways of obtaining objectively measured physical activity for scientific study (Kwapisz et al. 2011).

Accelerometers, however, cannot provide information about all types of physical activities (Gennuso et al. 2013). The possibility of underestimating physical activity levels because of accelerometer limitations may be less for older persons since walking is the preferred physical activity of persons 65 years of age and over (Hansen et al. 2012). Further details about accelerometers and other physical activity measures are presented in Chap. 31.

Whether self-report or objective measures are used for the collection of data for estimating physical activity prevalence, then, the evaluation of the accuracy and usefulness of those estimates must be judged in light of the methods and analyses of each study.

2.6 Implications

Current evidence indicates that in almost all countries in which physical activity has been assessed, physical activity prevalence is not high in older adults and that it may be lower in older women than in men, depending on the inclusion or exclusion of activities more commonly engaged in by women. These findings indicate that strategies to increase physical activity levels in older people are needed.

Further research is needed on the prevalence of physical activity in older adults, 65 years of age and older, in separate age groups. Current research usually lumps together all older adults, although health conditions and behaviours can change rapidly during the latter decades of life. With the proportion of older persons increasing in populations worldwide, differences in prevalence of physical activity across the older age ranges will become increasingly significant. More studies of the prevalence and health effects of light-intensity physical activity in older people are also needed.

2.7 Conclusions

Those of us who live in highly developed nations are not forced by circumstances to engage regularly in the levels of physical activity common in pre-industrial times. Strong evidence now tells us that the relative ease of modern life comes with negative health consequences. Since near the end of the previous century, health professionals and public officials of many nations have been advising people to engage in regular physical activity. Recognising the costs, both to individuals and to society, of not being sufficiently physically active, researchers have sought to learn how well their advice has been accepted and put into practice. Physical activity prevalence estimates have not been consistent and definitive, but in spite of their variations, they have generally pointed in the same direction: too few older adults are reaching levels of physical activity that offer maximum health benefit.

The basis of most national physical activity recommendations for adults, including those over 65 years of age, is the attainment of a minimum of 150 minutes of moderate-intensity physical activity per week, 75 minutes of vigorous-intensity physical activity or a combination of moderate- and vigorous-intensity physical activity. Light-intensity physical activity is encouraged for those unable or unwilling to engage in those intensities of physical activity because there is strong evidence in the literature that doing some physical activity is better for one's health and future well-being than doing none.

Currently, although it is sometimes included in the physical activity data of some countries, light-intensity physical activity is generally excluded from physical activity prevalence assessments. Where it is included, women are often shown to be closer to their male counterparts in being physically active. This is likely to be the case elsewhere because many women in many cultures, more often than men, expend energy doing housework, being caretakers, gardening, and shopping.

Age-related declines in physical activity occur throughout adulthood and become more acute in the later decades of life, so it is important to assess what physical activity men and women, especially older ones, are doing. Surveillance over time of physical activity allows policymakers to learn what population-level strategies are effective at increasing physical activity levels and to plan for potential demands on healthcare services. This much we know: while training for a marathon may be beyond the capabilities of most of older adults, engaging in physical activity at levels that can maintain or even enhance our health is not.

Suggested Further Reading

- Sun, F., Norman, I. J., & While, A. E. (2013). Physical activity in older people: A systematic review. *BMC Public Health, 13*(1), 449.
- Guthold, R., Ono, T., Strong, K. L., Chatterji, S., & Morabia, A. (2008). Worldwide variability in physical inactivity. *American Journal of Preventive Medicine, 34*(6), 486–494. https://doi.org/10.1016/j.amepre.2008.02.013.

References

Ashe, M. C., Miller, W. C., Eng, J. J., & Noreau, L. (2009). Older adults, chronic disease and leisure-time physical activity. *Gerontology, 55*(1), 64–72. https://doi.org/10.1159/000141518.

Australian Bureau of Statistics. (2015). Australian demographic statistics, Sept 2014 (No. 3101.0). Retrieved May 30, 2017, from http://www.abs.gov.au/AUSSTATS/abs@.nsf/Lookup/3101.0Main+Features1Sep%202014

Bauman, A., Phongsavan, P., Schoeppe, S., & Owen, N. (2006). Physical activity measurement – A primer for health promotion. *Promotion & Education, 13*(2), 92–103. https://doi.org/10.1177/10253823060130020103.

Bijnen, F. C., Feskens, E. J., Caspersen, C. J., Mosterd, W. L., & Kromhout, D. (1998). Age, period, and cohort effects on physical activity among elderly men during 10 years of follow-up: The Zutphen elderly study. *The Journals of Gerontology, Series A: Biological Sciences and Medical Sciences, 53A*(3), M235–M241. https://doi.org/10.1093/gerona/53A.3.M235.

Blair, S. N., & Morris, J. N. (2009). Healthy hearts—And the universal benefits of being physically active: Physical activity and health. *Annals of Epidemiology, 19*(4), 253–256. https://doi.org/10.1016/j.annepidem.2009.01.019.

Booth, F. W., Chakravarthy, M. V., Gordon, S. E., & Spangenburg, E. E. (2002). Waging war on physical inactivity: Using modern molecular ammunition against an ancient enemy. *Journal of Applied Physiology, 93*(1), 3–30.

Brown, W. J., McLaughlin, D., Leung, J., McCaul, K. A., Flicker, L., Almeida, O. P., et al. (2012). Physical activity and all-cause mortality in older women and men. *British Journal of Sports Medicine, 46*(9), 664–668. https://doi.org/10.1136/bjsports-2011-090529.

Bull, F. C., & Bauman, A. E. (2011). Physical inactivity: The "Cinderella" risk factor for noncommunicable disease prevention. *Journal of Health Communication, 16*(Suppl 2), 13–26.

Caspersen, C. J., Pereira, M. A., & Curran, K. M. (2000). Changes in physical activity patterns in the United States, by sex and cross-sectional age. *Medicine & Science in Sports & Exercise, 32*(9), 1601–1609.

Centers for Disease Control and Prevention, National Center for Chronic Disease Prevention and Health Promotion. (2017). Behavioral risk factor surveillance system. Retrieved May 30, 2017, from https://www.cdc.gov/brfss/

Centers for Disease Control and Prevention, National Center for Health Statistics. (2017a). National health and nutrition examination survey. Retrieved May 30, 2017, from https://www.cdc.gov/nchs/nhanes/

Centers for Disease Control and Prevention, National Center for Health Statistics. (2017b). National health interview survey. Retrieved May 30, 2017, from https://www.cdc.gov/nchs/nhis/

Corder, K., & van Sluijs, E. M. (2010). Comparing physical activity across countries—Current strengths and weaknesses. *American Journal of Epidemiology, 171*(10), 1065–1068. https://doi.org/10.1093/aje/kwq068.

Craig, C. L., Cameron, C. A., & Bauman, A. (2017). Utility of surveillance research to inform physical activity policy: An exemplar from Canada. *Journal of Physical Activity and Health, 14*, 229–239. https://doi.org/10.1123/jpah.2015-0698.

Doherty, A., Jackson, D., Hammerla, N., Plötz, T., Olivier, P., Granat, M. H., et al. (2017). Large scale population assessment of physical activity using wrist worn accelerometers: The UK Biobank study. *PLoS One, 12*(2), e0169649. https://doi.org/10.1371/journal.pone.0169649.

Fishman, E., Böcker, L., & Helbich, M. (2015). Adult active transport in the Netherlands: An analysis of its contribution to physical activity requirements. *PLoS One, 10*(4), e0121871. https://doi.org/10.1371/journal.pone.0121871.

Gennuso, K. P., Gangnon, R. E., Matthews, C. E., Thraen-Borowski, K. M., & Colbert, L. H. (2013). Sedentary behavior, physical activity, and markers of health in older adults. *Medicine & Science in Sports & Exercise, 45*(8), 1493–1500. https://doi.org/10.1249/MSS.0b013e318288a1e5.

Guthold, R., Ono, T., Strong, K. L., Chatterji, S., & Morabia, A. (2008). Worldwide variability in physical inactivity: A 51-country survey. *American Journal of Preventive Medicine, 34*(6), 486–494. https://doi.org/10.1016/j.amepre.2008.02.013.

Guwatudde, D., Kirunda, B. E., Wesonga, R., Mutungi, G., Kajjura, R., Kasule, H., et al. (2016). Physical activity levels among adults in Uganda: Findings from a countrywide cross-sectional survey. *Journal of Physical Activity and Health, 13*(9), 938–945. https://doi.org/10.1123/jpah.2015-0631.

Hagströmer, M., Troiano, R. P., Sjostrom, M., & Berrigan, D. (2010). Levels and patterns of objectively assessed physical activity—A comparison between Sweden and the United States. *American Journal of Epidemiology, 171*(10), 1055–1064. https://doi.org/10.1093/aje/kwq069.

Hallal, P. C., Andersen, L. B., Bull, F. C., Guthold, R., Haskell, W., & Ekelund, U. (2012). Global physical activity levels: Surveillance progress, pitfalls, and prospects. *The Lancet, 380*(9838), 247–257. https://doi.org/10.1016/S0140-6736(12)60646-1.

Hansen, B. H., Kolle, E., Dyrstad, S. M., Holme, I., & Anderssen, S. A. (2012). Accelerometer-determined physical activity in adults and older people. *Medicine & Science in Sports & Exercise, 44*(2), 266–272. https://doi.org/10.1249/MSS.0b013e31822cb354.

Haskell, W. L., Lee, I.-M., Pate, R. R., Powell, K. E., Blair, S. N., Franklin, B. A., et al. (2007). Physical activity and public health: Updated recommendation for adults from the American College of Sports Medicine and the American Heart Association. *Circulation, 116*(9), 1081–1093. https://doi.org/10.1161/CIRCULATIONAHA.107.185649.

Heesch, K. C., van Uffelen, J. G. Z., Hill, R. L., & Brown, W. (2010). What do IPAQ questions mean to older adults? Lessons from cognitive interviews. *International Journal of Behavioral Nutrition and Physical Activity, 7*(1), 35. https://doi.org/10.1186/1479-5868-7-35.

Hill, R. L., & Brown, W. J. (2012). Older Australians and physical activity levels: Do we know how many are meeting guidelines? *Australasian Journal on Ageing, 31*(4), 208–217. https://doi.org/10.1111/j.1741-6612.2011.00582.x.

Iliodromiti, S., Ghouri, N., Celis-Morales, C. A., Sattar, N., Lumsden, M. A., & Gill, J. M. (2016). Should physical activity recommendations for South Asian adults be ethnicity-specific? Evidence from a cross-sectional study of South Asian and White European men and women. *PLoS One, 11*(8), e0160024. https://doi.org/10.1371/journal.pone.0160024.

Kahlmeier, S., Wijnhoven, T. M. A., Alpiger, P., Schweizer, C., Breda, J., & Martin, B. W. (2015). National physical activity recommendations: Systematic overview and analysis of the situation in European countries. *BMC Public Health, 15*(1), 133. https://doi.org/10.1186/s12889-015-1412-3.

Keadle, S. K., McKinnon, R., Graubard, B. I., & Troiano, R. P. (2016). Prevalence and trends in physical activity among older adults in the United States: A comparison across three national surveys. *Preventive Medicine, 89*, 37–43. https://doi.org/10.1016/j.ypmed.2016.05.009.

Kohl, H. W., Craig, C. L., Lambert, E. V., Inoue, S., Alkandari, J. R., Leetongin, G., & Kahlmeier, S. (2012). The pandemic of physical inactivity: Global action for public health. *The Lancet, 380*(9838), 294–305. https://doi.org/10.1016/S0140-6736(12)60898-8.

Kwapisz, J. R., Weiss, G. M., & Moore, S. A. (2011). Activity recognition using cell phone accelerometers. *ACM SIGKDD Explorations Newsletter, 12*(2), 74–82. https://doi.org/10.1145/1964897.1964918.

Lee, S.-A., Xu, W. H., Zheng, W., Li, H., Yang, G., Xiang, Y.-B., & Shu, X. O. (2007). Physical activity patterns and their correlates among Chinese men in Shanghai. *Medicine & Science in Sports & Exercise, 39*(10), 1700–1707. https://doi.org/10.1249/mss.0b013e3181238a52.

Lee, I.-M., Shiroma, E. J., Lobelo, F., Puska, P., Blair, S. N., & Katzmarzyk, P. T. (2012). Effect of physical inactivity on major non-communicable diseases worldwide: An analysis of burden of disease and life expectancy. *The Lancet, 380*(9838), 219–229. https://doi.org/10.1016/S0140-6736(12)61031-9.

Lin, Y.-P., Huang, Y.-H., Lu, F.-H., Wu, J.-S., Chang, C.-J., & Yang, Y.-C. (2011). Non-leisure time physical activity is an independent predictor of longevity for a Taiwanese elderly population: An eight-year follow-up study. *BMC Public Health, 11*(1), 428. https://doi.org/10.1186/1471-2458-11-428.

Loyen, A., Clarke-Cornwell, A. M., Anderssen, S. A., Hagströmer, M., Sardinha, L. B., Sundquist, K., et al. (2016). Sedentary time and physical activity surveillance through accelerometer: Pooling in four European countries. *Sports Medicine*. https://doi.org/10.1007/s40279-016-0658-y.

Lyon, D., Haggerty, K. D., & Ball, K. (2012). Introducing surveillance studies. In K. Ball, K. Haggerty, & D. Lyon (Eds.), *Routledge handbook of surveillance studies* (pp. 15–18). New York: Routledge.

Macniven, R., Bauman, A., & Abouzeid, M. (2012). A review of population-based prevalence studies of physical activity in adults in the Asia-Pacific region. *BMC Public Health, 12*, 41. https://doi.org/10.1186/1471-2458-12-41.

Mâsse, L. C., Fuemmeler, B. F., Anderson, C. B., Matthews, C. E., Trost, S. G., Catellier, D. J., & Treuth, M. (2005). Accelerometer data reduction: A comparison of four reduction algorithms on select outcome variables. *Medicine and Science in Sports and Exercise, 37*(11), S544–S554.

Pate, R. R., Pratt, M., Blair, S. N., Haskell, W. L., Macera, C. A., Bouchard, C., et al. (1995). Physical activity and public health. *JAMA, 273*(5), 402–407. https://doi.org/10.1001/jama.1995.03520290054029.

Pucher, J., & Buehler, R. (2008). Making cycling irresistible: Lessons from the Netherlands, Denmark and Germany. *Transport Reviews, 28*(4), 495–528. https://doi.org/10.1080/01441640701806612.

Sims, J., Birrell, C. L., Hunt, S., Browning, C., Burns, R. A., & Mitchell, P. (2014). Prevalence of physical activity behaviour in older people: Findings from the dynamic analyses to optimise ageing (DYNOPTA) project and Australian national survey data. *Australasian Journal on Ageing, 33*(2), 105–113. https://doi.org/10.1111/j.1741-6612.2012.00648.x.

Sparling, P. B., Howard, B. J., Dunstan, D. W., & Owen, N. (2015). Recommendations for physical activity in older adults. *BMJ, 350*, h100. https://doi.org/10.1136/bmj.h100.

Stel, V. S., Smit, J. H., Pluijm, S. M., Visser, M., Deeg, D. J., & Lips, P. (2004). Comparison of the LASA physical activity questionnaire with a 7-day diary and pedometer. *Journal of Clinical Epidemiology, 57*(3), 252–258. https://doi.org/10.1016/j.jclinepi.2003.07.008.

Sun, F., Norman, I. J., & While, A. E. (2013). Physical activity in older people: A systematic review. *BMC Public Health, 13*, 449. https://doi.org/10.1186/1471-2458-13-449.

Sundquist, K., Qvist, J., Sundquist, J., & Johansson, S.-E. (2004). Frequent and occasional physical activity in the elderly. *American Journal of Preventive Medicine, 27*(1), 22–27. https://doi.org/10.1016/j.amepre.2004.03.011.

Tak, E., Kuiper, R., Chorus, A., & Hopman-Rock, M. (2013). Prevention of onset and progression of basic ADL disability by physical activity in community dwelling older adults: A meta-analysis. *Ageing Research Reviews, 12*(1), 329–338. https://doi.org/10.1016/j.arr.2012.10.001.

Troiano, R. P., Berrigan, D., Dodd, K. W., Mâsse, L. C., Tilert, T., & McDowell, M. (2008). Physical activity in the United States measured by accelerometer. *Medicine and Science in Sports and Exercise, 40*(1), 181–188.

Warburton, D. E. R., Nicol, C. W., & Bredin, S. S. D. (2006). Health benefits of physical activity: The evidence. *Canadian Medical Association Journal, 174*(6), 801–809. https://doi.org/10.1503/cmaj.051351.

Washburn, R. A. (2000). Assessment of physical activity in older adults. *Research Quarterly for Exercise and Sport, 71*(2), 79–88. https://doi.org/10.1080/02701367.2000.11082790.

3

The Benefits of Physical Activity for Older People

Annemarie Koster, Sari Stenholm, and Jennifer A. Schrack

3.1 Introduction

Engaging in physical activity yields important benefits throughout the lifespan. This chapter focuses on the health benefits of physical activity among older adults. The evidence of physical activity in relation to mortality, major non-communicable diseases, and important health outcomes in old age including physical and cognitive function is presented. This chapter also touches upon the mechanisms underlying the health effects of physical activity, including the molecular and epigenetic effects.

3.1.1 Overall Mortality

According to the World Health Organization (WHO), physical inactivity is among the ten leading causes of death worldwide (WHO 2009). Physical inactivity, high blood pressure, smoking, high blood glucose, and obesity

---

A. Koster (✉)
Department of Social Medicine, CAPHRI Care and Public Health Research Institute, Maastricht University, Maastricht, The Netherlands

S. Stenholm
Department of Public Health, University of Turku, Turku, Finland

J. A. Schrack
Department of Epidemiology & Core Faculty, Center on Aging and Health, Johns Hopkins Bloomberg School of Public Health, Baltimore, MD, USA

form the five leading risk factors. Together, these five risk factors are responsible for a quarter of all deaths in the world (WHO 2009).

Physical inactivity, defined as not meeting physical activity recommendations, causes 9% of premature death worldwide which is more than 5.3 million of the 57 million deaths that occurred worldwide in 2008 (Lee et al. 2012). While the health benefits of higher levels of physical activity are convincing, lower levels of physical activity also have important health benefits. Analyses of data from over 600,000 individuals 21–90 years of age show that even a low level of leisure time in moderate-to-vigorous-intensity physical activity was associated with reduced mortality (Arem et al. 2015). A meta-analysis of prospective cohort studies of older adults shows that even those who participate in moderate-to-vigorous-intensity physical activity for shorter durations of time per week than recommended reduce their mortality by 22% (Hupin et al. 2015). Taken together, these studies suggest that even low doses of moderate-to-vigorous-intensity physical activity lower mortality risk in older adults.

Findings from recent studies measuring physical activity with objective measures such as accelerometers confirm earlier studies in which physical activity was measured with self-reported measures. These findings further strengthen the evidence for an association between physical activity and mortality. Data from the American National Health and Nutrition Survey showed that both light-intensity physical activity and moderate-to-vigorous physical activity are associated with a lower all-cause mortality risk (Fishman et al. 2016). Further, in a German cohort, walking duration was clearly associated with overall mortality in community-dwelling older people (Klenk et al. 2016).

3.1.2 Cardiorespiratory Health

Cardiorespiratory diseases are the number one cause of death worldwide. In 2012 it was estimated that 31% of all global deaths were from cardiovascular diseases and 11% from respiratory diseases (WHO 2014). Of note, most of these diseases could be prevented by adopting a healthy lifestyle, including physical activity.

Physical activity is an important modifiable risk factor of cardiovascular disease, and increased physical activity has been shown to positively impact cardiorespiratory health. There is strong evidence that supports a dose-response relationship between physical activity and cardiovascular disease outcomes including coronary heart disease (CHD), peripheral vascular disease, and stroke as summarized in the 2012 report for the Australian physical activity guidelines (Brown et al. 2012). Moreover, regular physical activity has been linked to superior lung function and capacity in older adults (Berry et al. 2003) and to curb risk of chronic obstructive pulmonary disease with ageing (Garcia-Aymerich et al. 2007).

A meta-analysis that quantified the relationship between physical activity and coronary heart disease showed that meeting the physical activity guidelines of 150 minutes per week of moderate-to-vigorous-intensity physical activity lowered the risk of coronary heart disease by 14% (Sattelmair et al. 2011). Additional health benefits were found in those with physical activity levels above the recommended levels. Importantly, lower risks were also found among persons who were physically active below the recommended level supporting the statement that more is better than none. Another meta-analysis of prospective cohort studies examined the association between physical activity and risk of heart failure (Pandey et al. 2015). The study concludes that physical activity is associated in a dose-response manner with lower risk for heart failure, although results were more modest compared to that reported for CHD.

3.1.3 Type 2 Diabetes

Worldwide the prevalence of type 2 diabetes is rapidly increasing. In 2013 an estimated 382 million people had diabetes, and this number is expected to rise to 592 million by 2035 (Guariguata et al. 2014).

Physical activity is a key element and modifiable risk factor in the prevention and management of type 2 diabetes. There is robust evidence that increasing physical activity reduces the risk of type 2 diabetes (Colberg et al. 2010; Warburton et al. 2010). A meta-analysis shows that all types of activity, including light, moderate, and vigorous physical activity as well as resistance training, occupational activity, and walking, reduced the risk of type 2 diabetes (Aune et al. 2015).

Physical activity has also shown to be important in those at risk for type 2 diabetes. For example, physical activity can prevent the onset of type 2 diabetes in people who are at risk for developing such disease (Warburton et al. 2010). Exercise and/or lifestyle intervention trials have clearly shown a positive effect of exercise or physical activity in the prevention of type 2 diabetes. Diabetes prevention programmes in different countries including the US, Finland, China, and India have shown that a lifestyle intervention in which physical activity plays a key role is effective in preventing type 2 diabetes in high-risk individuals (Diabetes Prevention Program Research et al. 2009; Li et al. 2008; Lindström et al. 2006; Ramachandran et al. 2006).

Furthermore, intervention studies have shown that physical activity in persons with type 2 diabetes is important in diabetes management; it can enhance insulin action and may prevent or delay the onset of diabetes-related complications (Haskell et al. 2007). A systematic review and meta-analysis of randomized controlled trials on the effect of exercise on glycaemic control in type 2 diabetes patients show that structured exercise that consists of aerobic exercise, resistance training, or both improved glucose control (Umpierre et al. 2011).

3.1.4 Musculoskeletal Health

Musculoskeletal disorders are common among older adults, and they cause more functional limitations in the adult population in most welfare states than any other group of disorders. Low back and neck pain are among the five leading diseases that cause disability worldwide (Murray et al. 2015). Another common disease is osteoarthritis, which is characterized by loss of joint cartilage that leads to pain and loss of function primarily in the knees and hips. Physical activity positively influences most structural components of the musculoskeletal system that are related to functional capabilities and the risk of degenerative diseases. Physical activity also has the potential to postpone or prevent prevalent musculoskeletal disorders, such as low back pain, neck and shoulder pain, and osteoarthritis. Furthermore, exercise can contribute to the rehabilitation of musculoskeletal disorders and recovery from orthopaedic surgery. Evidence from exercise intervention studies recommends strength, flexibility and aerobic training for rehabilitation of non-specific chronic low back pain (Gordon and Bloxham 2016). Similarly, water- and land-based exercises can reduce pain and improve physical function among persons with symptomatic knee and hip osteoarthritis (Fransen et al. 2014, 2015).

Fractures are frequent among older adults and result mainly due to falls and osteoporosis. Falling is a multifactorial problem including both external (e.g., environmental and housing conditions) and internal risk factors (e.g., low muscle strength, poor vision, impaired mobility, and medication). Osteoporosis is characterized by reduced bone mass and micro-architectural deterioration of bone tissues, leading to enhanced bone fragility and increased risk of fractures. Regular physical activity can reduce the risk of fractures by increasing bone strength and by improving balance and mobility to prevent older persons from falling (Kohrt et al. 2004). Meta-analyses on exercise interventions suggest that exercise programmes for older adults should include not only weight-bearing endurance and resistance activities aimed at preserving bone mass (Kelley et al. 2001; Martyn-St James and Carroll 2010) but also activities designed to improve balance and prevent falls (Kohrt et al. 2004). For fall prevention, group and home-based exercise programmes containing balance and strength training exercises or Tai Chi effectively reduce the risk of falls (Gillespie et al. 2012).

3.1.5 Cancer

Cancer is a disease often associated with ageing and a leading cause of mortality worldwide. In 2012, there were 14.1 million reported new cancer cases and 8.2 million cancer deaths (*Global Cancer Facts & Figures* 2015). There are currently over 32 million cancer survivors worldwide, with an expected 19.3 million new cases diagnosed each year ("Global Cancer Statistics" 2016). The majority of these survivors are over the age of 65 years.

Given the worldwide incidence and prevalence of cancer, there is increasing interest in physical activity as a non-pharmacological intervention and prevention method (Speck et al. 2010). The World Cancer Research Fund estimates that 20–25% of cancers are related to overweight/obesity, poor nutrition, and/or physical inactivity (*Global Cancer Facts & Figures* 2015). Given the high prevalence of physical inactivity in developed countries, any decrease in risk of cancer associated with physical activity may be highly relevant to prevention efforts. Since the early 1990s, accumulating evidence has suggested that regular, sustained participation in physical activity protects against cancers of some sites (*Food, Nutrition, Physical Activity, and the Prevention of Cancer: a Global Perspective* 2007), with up to a 10–40% reduction in lung, breast, prostate, endometrium, and colon/rectum cancers (Moore et al. 2016). This evidence is consistent across age groups, with the strongest evidence for protection from breast cancer in post-menopausal women (*Food, Nutrition, Physical Activity, and the Prevention of Cancer: a Global Perspective* 2007).

In an analysis examining the association between leisure time physical activity and 26 different types of cancer across 12 large cohort studies (Moore et al. 2016), increasing levels of leisure time physical activity were associated with lower risk of 13 out of 26 cancers, including: oesophageal, gallbladder, liver, lung, small intestine, endometrial, leukaemia, myeloma, colon, rectum, bladder, and breast. In general, for those reporting participation in regular sustained physical activity, the risk reduction was generally greater than 20%, with higher levels of activity providing greater protection (Moore et al. 2016). Moreover, these results appear to be generalizable to those who are overweight or obese, or with a history of smoking. Mechanistically, these results may indicate that regular physical activity invokes its protective effects through healthier levels of circulating hormones and curbing excessive weight gain.

Given the large number of cancer patients and survivors (e.g., those who have either been cured or are in remission) worldwide, there is also great interest in the potential health benefits of physical activity during and after cancer treatments. Specifically, the role of physical activity in combating the physiologic (nausea, decreased muscle mass and quality, pain management, loss of appetite) and psychological effects of treatment (anxiety, quality of life, self-esteem) and in improving body strength and curbing fatigue is of great interest to many clinicians and researchers (Hurria et al. 2012; Speck et al. 2010). Although the potentially debilitating effects of cancer treatment make this type of research challenging, there are several studies that have shown a positive effect during treatment, with an even greater effect in survivors (Speck et al. 2010).

3.1.6 Obesity

Obesity is one of the major global public health challenges of our times. The prevalence of overweight and obesity has increased significantly over the past three decades and concerns about the health risks associated with obesity have become nearly universal (Ng et al. 2014). Physical inactivity is an important risk factor for weight gain. Body fat accumulates when the energy content of the food and drinks consumed exceeds the energy expended by an individual's metabolism and physical activity. Further, as obesity imposes higher cardiovascular and respiratory demands, as well as causes backache, joint pain due to arthritis, and sweating when exercising, weight gain itself may lead to less activity.

Strong scientific evidence based on long-term epidemiological studies shows that physical activity helps people to maintain a stable weight over time (Wareham et al. 2005). On the other hand, physical activity alone is not very effective in reducing weight, because a high amount of physical activity is needed unless the person also reduces his/her calorie intake (Church et al. 2009; Kallings et al. 2009; Street et al. 2015). In general, weight loss among older adults is under dispute, since weight loss may have harmful effects by promoting sarcopenia and bone loss. Therefore, it has been suggested that weight management for older obese adults should focus more on maintaining weight and improving physical function than promoting weight loss. Physical activity has an important role herein. Randomized controlled trials conducted among older obese adults suggest that the combination of controlled weight loss through dietary changes and exercise produce the most beneficial effects on physical functioning and quality of life and reduced the pain (Rejeski et al. 2010). In addition, they also report positive changes in body composition, that is, decreased weight and fat mass, and improved glycaemic control (Dunstan et al. 2002; Miller et al. 2006; Rejeski et al. 2010).

Without external support, substantial weight reduction and long-term maintenance of the reduced body weight is very difficult for many obese individuals. Therefore the good news is that obesity-related increased risk for mortality, cardiovascular diseases, type 2 diabetes, and functional decline can be reduced considerably, although not completely eliminated, by increasing physical activity, and even more if aerobic fitness improves simultaneously (Fogelholm 2010; Koster et al. 2008). Thus, promoting physical activity among obese older persons is highly recommended.

3.1.7 Sleep

Accounting for a third of daily hours, sleep is an essential physiological process with restorative functions. Short and long sleep duration, sleep-related disturbances, and their daytime consequences are common in older adults, and they are associated with decreased health and increased mortality (Covassin and Singh 2016; Gallicchio and Kalesan 2009; Youngstedt and Kripke 2004).

Results from systematic reviews and meta-analyses indicate that physical exercise can alleviate sleep problems (Montgomery and Dennis 2002; Yang et al. 2012). Findings from randomized controlled trials suggest that regular aerobic or resistance exercise training improves total sleep duration and global sleep quality in older adults (Montgomery and Dennis 2002; Yang et al. 2012). Those who exercised perceived significantly shorter time to fall asleep after going to bed and reduced medication use for insomnia (Yang et al. 2012). In addition, Tai Chi exercise, a form of traditional Chinese low- to moderate-intensity mind-body exercise, has shown to improve self-reported sleep quality and sleep duration and reduce daytime dysfunction in older adults (Du et al. 2015). These results suggest that physical activity could be viewed as a complementary and alternative approach for treating sleep problems.

3.1.8 Mental Health

Poor mental health is an important public health concern in old age. There is evidence that physical activity and exercise can be effective in improving mental health and mental well-being in old age (Windle 2014; Windle et al.

2010). Depression is the most common mental health condition in old age. A recent study shows that physical activity in midlife was associated with lower depressive symptoms in old age (Chang et al. 2016). A systematic review and meta-analysis of randomized controlled trials of exercise for depression in older people shows that for people with symptoms of depression, structured exercise will likely reduce the severity of depression (Bridle et al. 2012). Further, a recent umbrella review of meta-analyses assessed the impact of exercise on depression in old age and concluded that exercise significantly reduces depressive symptoms and would therefore play a central role in the treatment of older adults with depression (Catalan-Matamoros et al. 2016).

3.1.9 Physical Functioning

Physical inactivity is a major independent risk factor for functional limitations and disability (Koster et al. 2008; Warburton et al. 2006, 2010). Long-term follow-up studies have shown that engagement in physical activity throughout adulthood is associated with reduced decline in physical functioning and lower rate of mobility problems (Stenholm et al. 2016). On the other hand, initiating physical activity even at very old ages is associated with better survival and functioning (Stessman et al. 2009).

According to a large systematic review based on 66 studies among healthy adults aged 65 years and older (Paterson and Warburton 2010), aerobic exercise training (such as walking and cycling) have shown to be effective in preventing functional limitations and potentially delaying mobility disability with advancing age. In adjunct to the aerobic exercise, diverse training including strength and balance training helps to counteract the age-related loss of muscle mass and maintain muscle strength and functioning (Cruz-Jentoft et al. 2014; Liu and Latham 2009). All these features are needed in daily activities and they also help to prevent falls.

So far the largest randomized controlled trial aiming at preventing mobility disability is the Lifestyle Interventions and Independence for Elders (LIFE) in the USA. This study showed that structured moderate-intensity physical activity programme including aerobic, resistance, and flexibility training activities reduced major mobility disability among older adults at risk of disability compared with a health education programme (Pahor et al. 2014). These findings suggest that even the most vulnerable older adults can benefit from physical activity.

3.1.10 Cognitive Functioning

As people live longer worldwide, there is a substantial increase in age-related conditions including cognitive impairment (e.g., problems with memory). Epidemiological evidence suggests that physical activity is associated with lower risk of cognitive decline in old age (Bauman et al. 2016; Paterson and Warburton 2010). A review and meta-analysis of longitudinal observational studies summarized the evidence on physical activity and cognitive decline and dementia (Blondell et al. 2014). The study shows that compared with people with lower levels of physical activity, those with higher levels of physical activity have reduced risks of cognitive decline and dementia.

Results from randomized trials are mixed (Carvalho et al. 2014). A review examined the effect of aerobic physical activity on improving cognitive function in healthy adults without known cognitive impairment (Young et al. 2015). Based on the available data from randomized controlled trials, physical activity did not improve cognitive function in older adults. Results from the Lifestyle Interventions and Independence for Elders (LIFE) study also reported that a 24-month moderate-intensity activity programme did not result in improvements in cognitive function among sedentary older adults (Sink et al. 2015). Results from the randomized controlled trials in older adults and the short-term nature of most trials may suggest that earlier initiation of physical activity in midlife may be necessary to maintain and improve cognitive function in old age. A meta-analysis of randomized controlled trials that evaluated the effect of physical activity on cognitive function in patients with dementia shows that participating in physical activity has beneficial effects on cognitive function in patients with dementia (Groot et al. 2016). There is also evidence that, instead of focusing only on physical activity, multi-domain interventions including dietary counselling, cognitive training, and vascular risk monitoring could improve or maintain cognitive functioning in at-risk elderly people (Ngandu et al. 2015).

3.2 Mechanisms

Regular engagement in physical activity has well-established benefits on cardiovascular and metabolic health beyond weight loss (Thyfault and Wright 2016). There is increasing evidence that physical activity has favourable effects on metabolic and inflammatory processes, including liver function and insulin action (Thyfault and Wright 2016).

The potential "epigenetic" pathways (or the interactions between genes and environmental influences and exposures) of physical activity in ageing are just beginning to be understood. Specifically, how does lifelong physical activity affect health and longevity with ageing? It is well established that those who engage in regular physical activity later in life tend to have lower rates of disability and mortality, even when physical activity is initiated at older ages (Pahor et al. 2014), yet the lifelong benefits of physical activity are not fully understood due to difficulties with following participants for life and/or recall bias associated with late-life questionnaires (Schrack et al. 2014). One study that followed more than 650,000 participants aged 40 and older for an average of ten years found that those who engaged in 75 minutes of brisk walking per week lived 1.8 years longer, and those who engaged in a minimum of 150 minutes per week of moderate-intensity exercise lived 3.4 years longer than those who reported no regular exercise (Janssen et al. 2013). This provides strong evidence for the benefits of mid-to-late-life activity, even if limited to regular walking, and emphasizes the need for a greater understanding of the associations between intensity, duration, and frequency of physical activity and health outcomes across the life course.

There are multiple mechanisms through which physical activity imposes health benefits, some of which are only recently beginning to be understood. It has long been recognized that skeletal muscle contraction during physical activity stimulates increases in skeletal muscle mitochondrial content (the "power houses" of the cells that regulate metabolism and energy supply), oxygen consumption, and glucose uptake and increases the sensitivity of the muscle to insulin (Holloszy and Narahara 1967). Beyond the skeletal-muscular effects, there is evidence that other tissues, such as liver and fat tissues, also benefit from physical activity and may play a role in improvements in metabolism by improving sensitivity to insulin and reducing inflammatory burden (Fealy et al. 2012; Thyfault and Wright 2016).

Ageing is characterized by both short-term and sustained increases in inflammation, which may be the result of infectious or chronic diseases or ageing itself (Ferrucci and Guralnik 2003; Ferrucci et al. 1999). This persistent low-grade inflammatory state has been linked to loss of muscle function and a greater risk of fatigue and disability with ageing (Barbieri et al. 2003; Cesari et al. 2004; Ferrucci et al. 1999; Nicklas et al. 2016). Physical activity has been shown to reduce inflammation and corresponding health risks, independent of—and combined with—weight loss (Nicklas et al. 2016). Given the detrimental role of inflammation in multiple chronic diseases and conditions of ageing (diabetes, kidney and liver disease, cardiovascular disease, fatigue, and physical function), optimizing opportunities to intervene to protect against and reduce inflammatory burden are of utmost importance. This further emphasizes the importance of initiating or sustaining physical activity later in life to improve the risk of developing disease and disability over and above the benefits of drug treatment.

3.3 Implications for Practice

This chapter highlights the important health benefits of physical activity in old age. Despite the clear evidence, only a small proportion of older adults meet the recommended physical activity levels (Bauman et al. 2016). Therefore, developing and implementing physical activity interventions that combine aerobic activity with strength and balance training is key to improving health, preventing non-communicable diseases, maintaining functioning, and promoting active ageing. Next to exercise programmes which clearly have important health benefits, also alternative strategies to increase physical activity in daily life should be emphasized more. Especially in those who have led a sedentary lifestyle for decades, increasing physical activity in daily life by, for example, adopting strategies to decrease sedentary behaviour may be a more feasible approach for older adults to become more active.

The current evidence of the health benefits of physical activity in old age as presented in this chapter mainly rely on subjective physical activity data (e.g., questionnaires) which are often limited to certain activities and are prone to bias. The use of objective monitoring of physical activity will give the opportunity to assess physical activity across the entire movement intensity spectrum and throughout the day. Thereby, future studies will provide more insight about, for example, light-intensity physical activity and its contribution to health outcomes. Moreover, dose-response studies will obtain insight into the amount of physical activity in different intensity levels that provide health benefits. Further, objective physical activity data collected over a longer time period will also give the chance to examine patterns of activity over time, that is, over the course of the day, week, or year (seasonal variation). Taken together, future studies with objective physical activity data will provide more detailed information on the health benefits of physical activity in different intensity levels which will also be important for the development of successful interventions to increase physical activity in older adults.

3.4 Conclusion

Engaging in physical activity lowers mortality risk and reduces the risk of major chronic diseases in old age including cardiovascular disease, type 2 diabetes, musculoskeletal disorders, different types of cancer, and obesity. Moreover, physical activity has been associated with better sleep, more favourable mental health, and better cognitive function and is important in lowering the risk of functional limitations and disability. In a society where the proportion of older people is growing faster than any other age group and where people are living longer, improving the health and well-being of older adults is a major societal challenge. Promoting physical activity is an important target to maintain and improve health and functioning in old age.

Suggested Further Reading

- Bauman, A., Merom, D., Bull, F. C., Buchner, D. M., & Fiatarone Singh, M. A. (2016). Updating the evidence for physical activity: Summative reviews of the epidemiological evidence, prevalence, and interventions to promote "active aging". *Gerontologist, 56*(Suppl 2), S268–S280.
- McArdle, W. D., Katch, F. I., & Katch, V. L. (2015). *Exercise physiology: Nutrition, energy, and human performance* (8th ed.). Baltimore: Wolters Kluwer Health/Philadelphia: Lippincott Williams & Wilkins.

References

AICR. (2007). *Food, nutrition, physical activity, and the prevention of cancer: A global perspective*. Washington, DC: AICR.

American Cancer Society. (2015). *Global cancer facts & figures* (3rd ed.). Atlanta: American Cancer Society.

Arem, H., Moore, S. C., Patel, A., Hartge, P., Berrington de Gonzalez, A., Visvanathan, K., et al. (2015). Leisure time physical activity and mortality: A detailed pooled analysis of the dose-response relationship. *Journal of the American Medical Association Internal Medicine, 175*(6), 959–967.

Aune, D., Norat, T., Leitzmann, M., Tonstad, S., & Vatten, L. J. (2015). Physical activity and the risk of type 2 diabetes: A systematic review and dose-response meta-analysis. *European Journal of Epidemiology, 30*(7), 529–542.

Barbieri, M., Ferrucci, L., Ragno, E., Corsi, A., Bandinelli, S., Bonafe, M., et al. (2003). Chronic inflammation and the effect of IGF-I on muscle strength and power in older persons. *American Journal of Physiology. Endocrinology and Metabolism, 284*(3), E481–E487.

Bauman, A., Merom, D., Bull, F. C., Buchner, D. M., & Fiatarone Singh, M. A. (2016). Updating the evidence for physical activity: Summative reviews of the epidemiological evidence, prevalence, and interventions to promote "active aging". *The Gerontologist, 56*(Suppl 2), S268–S280.

Berry, M. J., Rejeski, W. J., Adair, N. E., Ettinger, W. H., Jr., Zaccaro, D. J., & Sevick, M. A. (2003). A randomized, controlled trial comparing long-term and short-term exercise in patients with chronic obstructive pulmonary disease. *Journal of Cardiopulmonary Rehabilitation and Prevention, 23*(1), 60–68.

Blondell, S. J., Hammersley-Mather, R., & Veerman, J. L. (2014). Does physical activity prevent cognitive decline and dementia?: A systematic review and meta-analysis of longitudinal studies. *BMC Public Health, 14*, 510.

Bridle, C., Spanjers, K., Patel, S., Atherton, N. M., & Lamb, S. E. (2012). Effect of exercise on depression severity in older people: Systematic review and meta-analysis of randomised controlled trials. *British Journal of Psychiatry, 201*(3), 180–185.

Brown, W. J., Bauman, A. E., Bull, F. C., & Burton, N. W. (2012). Development of evidence-based physical activity recommendations for adults (18–64 years). Report prepared for the Australian Government Department of Health.

Carvalho, A., Rea, I. M., Parimon, T., & Cusack, B. J. (2014). Physical activity and cognitive function in individuals over 60 years of age: A systematic review. *Journal of Clinical Intervention in Aging, 9*, 661–682.

Catalan-Matamoros, D., Gomez-Conesa, A., Stubbs, B., & Vancampfort, D. (2016). Exercise improves depressive symptoms in older adults: An umbrella review of systematic reviews and meta-analyses. *Psychiatry Research, 244*, 202–209.

Cesari, M., Penninx, B. W., Pahor, M., Lauretani, F., Corsi, A. M., Rhys Williams, G., et al. (2004). Inflammatory markers and physical performance in older persons: The InCHIANTI study. *Journals of Gerontology Series A: Biological Sciences and Medical Sciences, 59*(3), 242–248.

Chang, M., Snaedal, J., Einarsson, B., Bjornsson, S., Saczynski, J. S., Aspelund, T., et al. (2016). The association between midlife physical activity and depressive symptoms in late life: Age gene/environment susceptibility-Reykjavik study. *Journals of Gerontology Series A: Biological Sciences and Medical Sciences, 71*(4), 502–507.

Church, T. S., Martin, C. K., Thompson, A. M., Earnest, C. P., Mikus, C. R., & Blair, S. N. (2009). Changes in weight, waist circumference and compensatory responses with different doses of exercise among sedentary, overweight postmenopausal women. *PLoS One, 4*(2), e4515.

Colberg, S. R., Sigal, R. J., Fernhall, B., Regensteiner, J. G., Blissmer, B. J., Rubin, R. R., et al. (2010). Exercise and type 2 diabetes: The American College of Sports Medicine and the American Diabetes Association: Joint position statement. *Diabetes Care, 33*(12), e147–e167.

Covassin, N., & Singh, P. (2016). Sleep duration and cardiovascular disease risk: Epidemiologic and experimental evidence. *Sleep Medicine Clinics, 11*(1), 81–89.

Cruz-Jentoft, A. J., Landi, F., Schneider, S. M., Zuniga, C., Arai, H., Boirie, Y., et al. (2014). Prevalence of and interventions for sarcopenia in ageing adults: A systematic review. Report of the International Sarcopenia Initiative (EWGSOP and IWGS). *Age and Ageing, 43*(6), 748–759.

Diabetes Prevention Program Research Group, Knowler, W. C., Fowler, S. E., Hamman, R. F., Christophi, C. A., Hoffman, H. J., et al. (2009). 10-year follow-up of diabetes incidence and weight loss in the diabetes prevention program outcomes study. *The Lancet, 374*(9702), 1677–1686.

Du, S., Dong, J., Zhang, H., Jin, S., Xu, G., Liu, Z., et al. (2015). Taichi exercise for self-rated sleep quality in older people: A systematic review and meta-analysis. *International Journal Nursing Studies, 52*(1), 368–379.

Dunstan, D. W., Daly, R. M., Owen, N., Jolley, D., De Courten, M., Shaw, J., & Zimmet, P. (2002). High-intensity resistance training improves glycemic control in older patients with type 2 diabetes. *Diabetes Care, 25*(10), 1729–1736.

Fealy, C. E., Haus, J. M., Solomon, T. P., Pagadala, M., Flask, C. A., McCullough, A. J., & Kirwan, J. P. (2012). Short-term exercise reduces markers of hepatocyte apoptosis in nonalcoholic fatty liver disease. *Journal Applied Physiology (1985), 113*(1), 1–6.

Ferrucci, L., & Guralnik, J. M. (2003). Inflammation, hormones, and body composition at a crossroad. *The American Journal of Medicine, 115*(6), 501–502.

Ferrucci, L., Harris, T. B., Guralnik, J. M., Tracy, R. P., Corti, M. C., Cohen, H. J., et al. (1999). Serum IL-6 level and the development of disability in older persons. *Journal of the American Geriatrics Society, 47*(6), 639–646.

Fishman, E. I., Steeves, J. A., Zipunnikov, V., Koster, A., Berrigan, D., Harris, T. A., & Murphy, R. (2016). Association between objectively measured physical activity and mortality in NHANES. *Medicine & Science in Sports and Exercise, 48*(7), 1303–1311.

Fogelholm, M. (2010). Physical activity, fitness and fatness: Relations to mortality, morbidity and disease risk factors. A systematic review. *Obesity Reviews, 11*, 202–221.

Fransen, M., McConnell, S., Hernandez-Molina, G., & Reichenbach, S. (2014). Exercise for osteoarthritis of the hip. *The Cochrane Database of Systematic Reviews, 4*, Cd007912.

Fransen, M., McConnell, S., Harmer, A. R., Van der Esch, M., Simic, M., & Bennell, K. L. (2015). Exercise for osteoarthritis of the knee. *The Cochrane Database of Systematic Review, 1*, Cd004376.

Gallicchio, L., & Kalesan, B. (2009). Sleep duration and mortality: A systematic review and meta-analysis. *Journal Sleep Research, 18*(2), 148–158.

Garcia-Aymerich, J., Lange, P., Benet, M., Schnohr, P., & Anto, J. M. (2007). Regular physical activity modifies smoking-related lung function decline and reduces risk of chronic obstructive pulmonary disease: A population-based cohort study. *American Journal of Respiratory and Critical Care Medicine, 175*(5), 458–463.

Gillespie, L. D., Robertson, M. C., Gillespie, W. J., Sherrington, C., Gates, S., Clemson, L. M., & Lamb, S. E. (2012). Interventions for preventing falls in older people living in the community. *The Cochrane Database of Systematic Reviews, 9*, Cd007146.

Global Cancer Statistics. (2016, August 31). Retrieved from http://www.cdc.gov/cancer/international/statistics.htm

Gordon, R., & Bloxham, S. (2016). A systematic review of the effects of exercise and physical activity on non-specific chronic low back pain. *Healthcare, 4*(2), 1–19.

Groot, C., Hooghiemstra, A. M., Raijmakers, P. G., van Berckel, B. N., Scheltens, P., Scherder, E. J., et al. (2016). The effect of physical activity on cognitive function in patients with dementia: A meta-analysis of randomized control trials. *Ageing Research Reviews, 25*, 13–23.

Guariguata, L., Whiting, D. R., Hambleton, I., Beagley, J., Linnenkamp, U., & Shaw, J. E. (2014). Global estimates of diabetes prevalence for 2013 and projections for 2035. *Diabetes Research and Clinical Practice, 103*(2), 137–149.

Haskell, W. L., Lee, I. M., Pate, R. R., Powell, K. E., Blair, S. N., Franklin, B. A., et al. (2007). Physical activity and public health: Updated recommendation for adults from the American College of Sports Medicine and the American Heart Association. *Medicine & Science in Sports and Exercise, 39*(8), 1423–1434.

Holloszy, J. O., & Narahara, H. T. (1967). Nitrate ions: Potentiation of increased permeability to sugar associated with muscle contraction. *Science, 155*(3762), 573–575.

Hupin, D., Roche, F., Gremeaux, V., Chatard, J. C., Oriol, M., Gaspoz, J. M., et al. (2015). Even a low-dose of moderate-to-vigorous physical activity reduces mortality by 22% in adults aged >/=60 years: A systematic review and meta-analysis. *British Journal Sports Medicine, 49*(19), 1262–1267.

Hurria, A., Mohile, S. G., & Dale, W. (2012). Research priorities in geriatric oncology: Addressing the needs of an aging population. *Journal of the National Comprehensive Cancer Network, 10*(2), 286–288.

Janssen, I., Carson, V., Lee, I. M., Katzmarzyk, P. T., & Blair, S. N. (2013). Years of life gained due to leisure-time physical activity in the U.S. *American Journal of Preventive Medicine, 44*(1), 23–29.

Kallings, L. V., Sierra Johnson, J., Fisher, R. M., Faire, U., Stahle, A., Hemmingsson, E., & Hellenius, M. L. (2009). Beneficial effects of individualized physical activity on prescription on body composition and cardiometabolic risk factors: Results from a randomized controlled trial. *European Journal of Cardiovascular Prevention and Rehabilitation, 16*(1), 80–84.

Kelley, G. A., Kelley, K. S., & Tran, Z. V. (2001). Resistance training and bone mineral density in women: A meta-analysis of controlled trials. *American Journal of Physical Medicine and Rehabilitation, 80*(1), 65–77.

Klenk, J., Dallmeier, D., Denkinger, M. D., Rapp, K., Koenig, W., Rothenbacher, D., & Acti, F. E. S. G. (2016). Objectively measured walking duration and sedentary behaviour and four-year mortality in older people. *PLoS One, 11*(4), e0153779.

Kohrt, W. M., Bloomfield, S. A., Little, K. D., Nelson, M. E., & Yingling, V. R. (2004). American College of Sports Medicine position stand: Physical activity and bone health. *Medicine & Science in Sports and Exercise, 36*(11), 1985–1996.

Koster, A., Patel, K. V., Visser, M., van Eijk, J. T. M., Kanaya, A. M., de Rekeneire, N., et al. (2008). Joint effects of adiposity and physical activity on incident mobility limitation in older adults. *Journal of the American Geriatrics Society, 56*(4), 636–643.

Lee, I. M., Shiroma, E. J., Lobelo, F., Puska, P., Blair, S. N., & Katzmarzyk, P. T. (2012). Effect of physical inactivity on major non-communicable diseases worldwide: An analysis of burden of disease and life expectancy. *The Lancet, 380*(9838), 219–229.

Li, G., Zhang, P., Wang, J., Gregg, E. W., Yang, W., Gong, Q., et al. (2008). The long-term effect of lifestyle interventions to prevent diabetes in the China Da Qing diabetes prevention study: A 20-year follow-up study. *The Lancet, 371*(9626), 1783–1789.

Lindström, J., Ilanne-Parikka, P., Peltonen, M., Aunola, S., Eriksson, J. G., Hemiö, K., et al. (2006). Sustained reduction in the incidence of type 2 diabetes by lifestyle intervention: Follow-up of the Finnish Diabetes Prevention Study. *The Lancet, 368*(9548), 1673–1679.

Liu, C. J., & Latham, N. K. (2009). Progressive resistance strength training for improving physical function in older adults. *The Cochrane Database of Systematic Reviews, 3*, CD002759.

Martyn-St James, M., & Carroll, S. (2010). Effects of different impact exercise modalities on bone mineral density in premenopausal women: A meta-analysis. *Journal of Bone and Mineral Metabolism, 28*(3), 251–267.

Miller, G. D., Nicklas, B. J., Davis, C., Loeser, R. F., Lenchik, L., & Messier, S. P. (2006). Intensive weight loss program improves physical function in older obese adults with knee osteoarthritis. *Obesity (Silver Spring), 14*(7), 1219–1230.

Montgomery, P., & Dennis, J. (2002). Physical exercise for sleep problems in adults aged 60+. *The Cochrane Database of Systematic Reviews, 4*, Cd003404.

Moore, S. C., Lee, I. M., Weiderpass, E., Campbell, P. T., Sampson, J. N., Kitahara, C. M., et al. (2016). Association of leisure-time physical activity with risk of 26 types of cancer in 1.44 million adults. *Journal of the American Medical Association Internal Medicine, 176*(6), 816–825.

Murray, C. J., Barber, R. M., Foreman, K. J., Ozgoren, A. A., Abd-Allah, F., Abera, S. F., et al. (2015). Global, regional, and national disability-adjusted life years (DALYs) for 306 diseases and injuries and healthy life expectancy (HALE) for 188 countries, 1990–2013: Quantifying the epidemiological transition. *The Lancet, 368*(10009), 2145–2191.

Ng, M., Fleming, T., Robinson, M., Thomson, B., Graetz, N., Margono, C., et al. (2014). Global, regional, and national prevalence of overweight and obesity in children and adults during 1980–2013: A systematic analysis for the Global Burden of Disease Study 2013. *The Lancet, 384*(9945), 766–781.

Ngandu, T., Lehtisalo, J., Solomon, A., Levalahti, E., Ahtiluoto, S., Antikainen, R., et al. (2015). A 2 year multidomain intervention of diet, exercise, cognitive training, and vascular risk monitoring versus control to prevent cognitive decline in at-risk elderly people (FINGER): A randomised controlled trial. *The Lancet, 385*(9984), 2255–2263.

Nicklas, B. J., Beavers, D. P., Mihalko, S. L., Miller, G. D., Loeser, R. F., & Messier, S. P. (2016). Relationship of objectively-measured habitual physical activity to chronic inflammation and fatigue in middle-aged and older adults. *Journals of Gerontology Series A: Biological Sciences and Medical Sciences, 71*, 1437–1443.

Pahor, M., Guralnik, J. M., Ambrosius, W. T., Blair, S., Bonds, D. E., Church, T. S., et al. (2014). Effect of structured physical activity on prevention of major mobility disability in older adults: The LIFE study randomized clinical trial. *Journal American Medical Association, 311*(23), 2387–2396.

Pandey, A., Garg, S., Khunger, M., Darden, D., Ayers, C., Kumbhani, D. J., et al. (2015). Dose-response relationship between physical activity and risk of heart failure: A meta-analysis. *Circulation, 132*(19), 1786–1794.

Paterson, D. H., & Warburton, D. E. (2010). Physical activity and functional limitations in older adults: A systematic review related to Canada's physical activity guidelines. *International Journal of Behavioural Nutrition and Physical Activity, 7*, 38.

Ramachandran, A., Snehalatha, C., Mary, S., Mukesh, B., Bhaskar, A. D., Vijay, V., & Indian Diabetes Prevention, P. (2006). The Indian diabetes prevention programme shows that lifestyle modification and metformin prevent type 2 diabetes in Asian Indian subjects with impaired glucose tolerance (IDPP-1). *Diabetologia, 49*(2), 289–297.

Rejeski, W. J., Marsh, A. P., Chmelo, E., & Rejeski, J. J. (2010). Obesity, intentional weight loss and physical disability in older adults. *Obesity Reviews, 11*(9), 671–685.

Sattelmair, J., Pertman, J., Ding, E. L., Kohl, H. W., Haskell, W., & Lee, I. M. (2011). Dose response between physical activity and risk of coronary heart disease: A meta-analysis. *Circulation, 124*(7), 789–795.

Schrack, J. A., Zipunnikov, V., Goldsmith, J., Bai, J., Simonsick, E. M., Crainiceanu, C., & Ferrucci, L. (2014). Assessing the "physical cliff": Detailed quantification of age-related differences in daily patterns of physical activity. *Journals of Gerontology Series A: Biological Sciences and Medical Sciences, 69*(8), 973–979.

Sink, K. M., Espeland, M. A., Castro, C. M., Church, T., Cohen, R., Dodson, J. A., et al. (2015). Effect of a 24-month physical activity intervention vs health education on cognitive outcomes in sedentary older adults: The LIFE randomized trial. *Journal of the American Medical Association, 314*(8), 781–790.

Speck, R. M., Courneya, K. S., Masse, L. C., Duval, S., & Schmitz, K. H. (2010). An update of controlled physical activity trials in cancer survivors: A systematic review and meta-analysis. *Journal of Cancer Survivorship, 4*(2), 87–100.

Stenholm, S., Koster, A., Valkeinen, H., Patel, K. V., Bandinelli, S., Guralnik, J. M., & Ferrucci, L. (2016). Association of physical activity history with physical function and mortality in old age. *Journals of Gerontology Series A: Biological Sciences and Medical Sciences, 71*(4), 496–501.

Stessman, J., Hammerman-Rozenberg, R., Cohen, A., Ein-Mor, E., & Jacobs, J. M. (2009). Physical activity, function, and longevity among the very old. *Archives of Internal Medicine, 169*(16), 1476–1483.

Street, S. J., Wells, J. C., & Hills, A. P. (2015). Windows of opportunity for physical activity in the prevention of obesity. *Obesity Reviews, 16*(10), 857–870.

Thyfault, J. P., & Wright, D. C. (2016). "Weighing" the effects of exercise and intrinsic aerobic capacity: Are there beneficial effects independent of changes in weight? *Applied Physiology, Nutrition, and Metabolism, 41*(9), 911–916. https://doi.org/10.1139/apnm-2016-0122

Umpierre, D., Ribeiro, P. A., Kramer, C. K., Leitao, C. B., Zucatti, A. T., Azevedo, M. J., et al. (2011). Physical activity advice only or structured exercise training and association with HbA1c levels in type 2 diabetes: A systematic review and meta-analysis. *Journal of the American Medical Association, 305*(17), 1790–1799.

Warburton, D. E., Nicol, C. W., & Bredin, S. S. (2006). Health benefits of physical activity: The evidence. *Canadian Medical Association Journal, 174*(6), 801–809.

Warburton, D. E., Charlesworth, S., Ivey, A., Nettlefold, L., & Bredin, S. S. (2010). A systematic review of the evidence for Canada's physical activity guidelines for adults. *International Journal of Behavioral Nutrition and Physical Activity, 7*, 39.

Wareham, N. J., van Sluijs, E. M., & Ekelund, U. (2005). Physical activity and obesity prevention: A review of the current evidence. *Proceedings of the Nutrition Society, 64*(2), 229–247.

WHO. (2009). *Global health risks: Mortality and burden of disease attributable to selected major risks*. Geneva: WHO.

WHO. (2014). *Global status report on noncommunicable diseases 2014*. Geneva: WHO.

Windle, G. (2014). Exercise, physical activity and mental well-being in later life. *Reviews in Clinical Gerontology, 24*(04), 319–325.

Windle, G., Hughes, D., Linck, P., Russell, I., & Woods, B. (2010). Is exercise effective in promoting mental well-being in older age? A systematic review. *Aging & Mental Health, 14*(6), 652–669.

Yang, P. Y., Ho, K. H., Chen, H. C., & Chien, M. Y. (2012). Exercise training improves sleep quality in middle-aged and older adults with sleep problems: A systematic review. *Journal of Physiotherapy, 58*(3), 157–163.

Young, J., Angevaren, M., Rusted, J., & Tabet, N. (2015). Aerobic exercise to improve cognitive function in older people without known cognitive impairment. *The Cochrane Database of Systematic Reviews, 4*, CD005381.

Youngstedt, S. D., & Kripke, D. F. (2004). Long sleep and mortality: Rationale for sleep restriction. *Sleep Medicine Reviews, 8*(3), 159–174.

4

The Benefits of Physical Activity in Later Life for Society

Geeske Peeters, Sheila Tribess, and Jair S. Virtuoso-Junior

4.1 Introduction

This health economics chapter discusses the evidence for the consequences of physical inactivity and benefits of physical activity for the individual and society. The consequences and benefits will be discussed in terms of quality of life and participation on the individual level, and in terms of the burden on the health care system and their associated costs to economies on the societal level. These outcomes are discussed first for community-dwelling older adults and later for those living in long-term residential accommodation and older adults with dementia. In the previous chapter, a wide range of health problems was described that are, at least in part, attributable to insufficient levels of physical activity. Through its effects on health problems, physical inactivity is also believed to affect quality of life, health care utilisation and the consequent health care expenditures. This pathway is illustrated in Fig. 4.1.

G. Peeters (✉)
Global Brain Health Institute, University of California San Francisco, San Francisco, CA, USA / Trinity College Dublin, Dublin, Ireland

S. Tribess • J. S. Virtuoso-Junior
Department of Sports Science, Institute of Health Sciences, Federal University of Triangulo Mineiro, Uberaba, MG, Brazil

© The Author(s) 2018
S. R. Nyman et al. (eds.), *The Palgrave Handbook of Ageing and Physical Activity Promotion*, https://doi.org/10.1007/978-3-319-71291-8_4

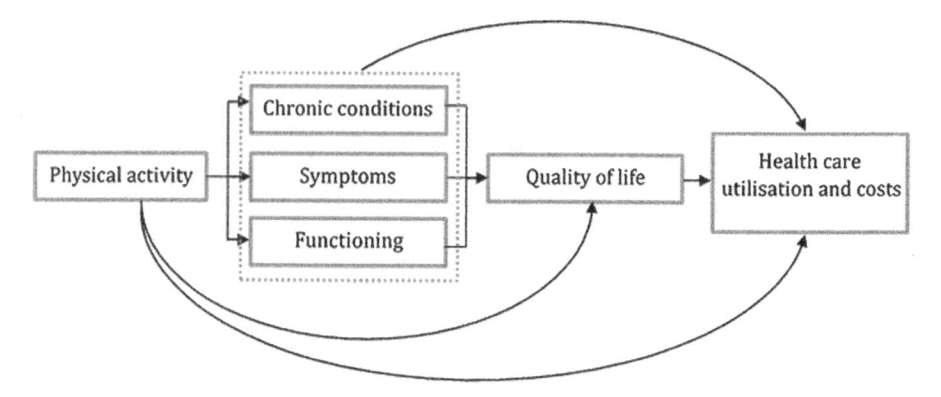

Fig. 4.1 Theoretical pathway of how physical activity may influence quality of life, health care utilisation and health care costs

4.2 Burden of Disease

The burden of a causal factor, in this case physical inactivity, on a health condition can be expressed as the *population attributable risk* (PAR). PAR reflects the proportion of the condition's burden that could in theory be avoided if the entire population would become sufficiently physically active. For example, a PAR of 6% for coronary heart disease means that 6% of disease burden from coronary heart disease can be attributed to physical inactivity and could potentially be avoided if all those inactive would become active. In this context, the term "burden" refers to the impact of the condition on the morbidity, disability, quality of life, mortality and financial costs. It is calculated based on the prevalence of the condition and the relative risk of the given condition associated with physical inactivity. PARs are usually calculated for the entire (adult) population and are not age specific. Based on data collected by the World Health Organization, globally physical inactivity has been estimated to account for 6% of the burden of disease from coronary heart disease, 7% of the burden of disease from type II diabetes, 10% of the burden of disease from breast cancer and 10% of the burden of disease from colon cancer (Lee et al. 2012). PARs for physical inactivity vary across countries and tend to be higher in South and Latin American, Caribbean, Eastern Mediterranean and Western Pacific countries than in European and Northern American countries, and even lower in African and South-East Asian countries (Lee et al. 2012). Based on the information used to calculate these PARs, the costs associated with physical inactivity for health care systems worldwide in 2013 have been estimated at US$53.8 billion (equivalent to €48.0 billion and £41.9 billion), of which US$31.2 billion was paid by the public sector, US$12.9

billion by the private sector and US$9.7 billion by households (Ding et al. 2016). A study in over 40,000 Australian women showed that the PAR for ischemic heart disease was higher for physical inactivity than for other risk factors such as smoking and being overweight (Brown et al. 2015). These findings suggest that, at least in theory, greater health gains may be achieved by promoting physical activity than through the promotion of other health behaviours.

4.3 Health Care Utilisation and Costs

By multiplying the PAR for physical inactivity with the total costs associated with a given condition, the costs of that condition attributable to inactivity can be estimated. Note however, that this reflects the estimated *theoretical* costs, which is based on a number of assumptions and may deviate from the *actual* costs associated with physical inactivity. Another way of estimating the costs of inactivity is by comparing the costs of inactive people with the costs of active people. Information collected in observational cohort studies and administrative records are particularly useful in this context. Observational cohort studies are studies that either take a "snapshot" of the health and behaviour of a large group of people at a particular time, or that take series of snapshots of the same group of people over time to monitor how health and behaviour change as people grow older. Examples of administrative records are hospital discharge records and health insurance claims records.

Observational studies consistently show that those who are more active use fewer health services. More active older adults are less likely to require hospital admissions and spend fewer days in a hospital. They also pay fewer visits to their family physicians and outpatient clinics. The hypothesis that these associations are explained by health problems is confirmed in studies which show that associations with number of hospital admissions and days spent in hospital were no longer statistically significant when health problems were accounted for (Li et al. 2011; Perkins and Clark 2001). However, even among people with chronic conditions, those who are physically active use less health services than those who are inactive (Sari 2014). Compared with being inactive, low levels of physical activity may be sufficient to lower the need for health services, but those who do higher levels of physical activity are likely to achieve greater benefits (Peeters et al. 2017).

The association between physical activity and health services use also translates to health-related costs. Higher levels of physical activity are associated with lower costs for health services. However, there is great variation in the magnitude of effects between studies. For example, the difference in mean annual costs between the highest and lowest levels of physical activity was as high as US$3445 (equivalent to €1947 and £2320) in a 2001 US study (Perkins and Clark 2001) and as low as US$152 (equivalent to €134 and £105) in a 2011 Japanese study (Yang et al. 2011). These findings should be interpreted in the context of the specific details of the studies. Compared with the US study, the Japanese study included an older sample (100% vs. 41% aged over 70 years) and did not include costs of emergency room visits. Also, the Japanese study excluded people with health problems that limited them in participating in physical activity and so included a healthier group of people than the US study. Because of these differences between studies, it is not possible to provide an accurate global estimate of the average difference in costs between active and inactive older adults.

The evidence for the associations between physical activity and health care utilisation and costs comes from a limited number of studies conducted in Australia, Canada, Japan, Taiwan and the USA. While one can reasonably assume that these associations also exist in other countries, this has yet to be supported with evidence, particularly in developing countries. The organisational structure and funding of health services have a great impact on the total health care utilisation and costs in a country. This also influences the magnitude of the effect of physical activity on the outcomes. In other words, the actual difference in health care utilisation and costs between active and inactive people is likely to vary between countries with different health care systems. It is therefore difficult to extrapolate findings across countries.

The results from the observational studies described above tell us that those who are physically active have lower needs for health services and therefore lower health care costs. However, these studies do not tell us whether these findings reflect a *causal* relationship. A causal relationship exists if changes in health services and costs are a direct or indirect result of a change in physical activity. The findings may also be explained by the fact that healthier people are in a better position to be physically active than less healthy people. If the latter is true, then a change in physical activity would not lead to a change in health services use or costs. Also, these studies do not tell us whether physical activity programs can effectively contribute to reducing health care use and costs, which is beneficial from the health economic perspective. To answer these questions, we need to look at the results of randomised controlled trials. Such trials are studies in which the effectiveness of an intervention (e.g. a physical activity program) is estimated by comparing a group receiving the intervention with a control group not receiving the intervention. Participants in the study are randomly allocated to either the intervention group or the control group. Randomisation is done to ensure the groups are similar at the start of the intervention in terms of demographic, health and lifestyle factors, so that the effect of the intervention can be examined without potential masking effects of these factors.

There is sufficient evidence that physical activity programs can indeed improve older people's physical activity levels (Hobbs et al. 2013; Richards et al. 2013). But do the improved physical activity levels also lead to cost savings?

The few randomised controlled trials conducted in older populations that have measured health services costs found that participants in the physical activity programs had higher health care costs than those in the non-exercise control groups (Chen et al. 2008; Farag et al. 2015; Groessl et al. 2009; Hagberg and Lindholm 2006). The higher costs in the physical activity groups compared with control groups are partly explained by cost of the physical activity program itself, which need to be included in the calculation of the total costs. Moreover, the majority of trials measured the costs of the intervention and health services use during 12 months. However, the preventive effects of physical activity on health outcomes and subsequently health services use may not become evident until years after starting a physical activity program. For example, it has been estimated that the time needed to achieve 50% of the effect of active travel interventions in the general population was 2 years for cardiovascular disease and depression, 3 years for diabetes and 17 years for cancer and dementia (Jarrett et al. 2012). Prolonged exposure to physical activity is required to achieve health benefits. Reviews of the literature have shown that physical activity programs are effective at increasing physical activity at 12 months, but the longer-term effectiveness is unclear. This is mainly due to lack of studies that included a longer-term follow-up (Hobbs et al. 2013; Richards et al. 2013). Studies with longer follow-up durations are required to establish the complete net cost impact of physical activity programs among older adults.

4.4 Quality of Life and Quality-Adjusted Life Years

The constant expansion of life expectancy and the high burden of non-communicable diseases in the population mean that people are living longer, but not necessarily in good health. Particularly in the care of older adults, a shift has occurred from a focus on reducing morbidity and mortality to a focus on increasing quality of life. Along with morbidity and mortality, quality of life is an important outcome to consider when evaluating the impact of physical activity on health. The World Health Organization defines quality of life as "the individual's perception of their position in life in the context of the culture and value systems in which they live and in relation to their goals, expectations, standards, and concerns. It is a broad ranging concept affected in a complex way by the person's physical health, psychological state, level of independence, social relationships and their relationship to salient features of their environment" (The WHOQOL group 1998, p. 1570). To quantify quality of life, we measure the components that are believed to influence it. A variety of quality of life questionnaires are available that measure different combinations of components. This needs to be kept in mind when interpreting the research findings.

A review of the literature that included 27 cross-sectional studies showed that older adults who are more active report better quality of life (Vagetti et al. 2014). The same review included four longitudinal cohort studies, which showed that being active now is associated with better quality of life up to four years later. These findings seem to be consistent across studies regardless of what instrument was used to measure quality of life. The findings are also similar in men and women and across countries.

Randomised controlled trials that evaluated the effects of specific physical activity or exercise programs showed that these programs can indeed contribute to modest improvements in people's quality of life (Vagetti et al. 2014). Programs that have been found to improve quality of life in older adults living in the community typically include a combination of supervised/group exercises and home exercises. The programs offer a mix of endurance, strength, balance and flexibility exercises, sometimes complimented with walking (Figueira et al. 2012), Tai Chi (Fox et al. 2007) or with the goal to achieve 150 minutes of physical activity per week (Groessl et al. 2016). Positive effects on wellbeing have been found after as little as 12 weeks of participation (Figueira et al. 2012). However, one study found that, while wellbeing improved during the 6 months of the physical activity program, it declined during the 6 months after the program finished (McAuley et al. 2000). A study in which the program continued for 2.6 years showed that quality of life was higher at the end of the 2.6 years in the exercise group compared with the control group (Groessl et al. 2016). These findings suggest that the benefits of physical activity for wellbeing over time can only be sustained if an active lifestyle is maintained.

So far, we have discussed the effects of physical activity on quality of life as if quality of life is a single concept. But as explained earlier, quality of life is measured by measuring the components that are known to influence it. Physical activity may have a stronger effect on certain components of quality of life than others. Looking at the findings from cohort studies and randomised controlled trials combined, there is strong evidence that physical activity has a positive impact on the components of quality of life related to functional capacity, activity, autonomy, death/dying, intimacy and mental wellbeing (Vagetti et al. 2014; Windle et al. 2010). It also seems likely that physical activity has a positive impact on physical functioning, social relationships, emotional wellbeing, overall health, pain and environment (Vagetti et al. 2014). In contrast, the association between physical activity and sensory function is unclear (Vagetti et al. 2014). Interestingly, one trial showed that walking improved mental aspects of wellbeing more than non-aerobic exercises (Awick et al. 2015). Another trial showed that after three months of exercise, physical functioning was better in the resistance training group than in the functional task training group, while there were no group differences in any of the other components (de Vreede et al. 2007). These findings suggest that different programs have different effects on each of the components of quality of life. However, given the countless different physical activity programs and numerous quality of life questionnaires that are available, it is understandable that not all combinations of programs have been compared using each of these questionnaires. It is therefore not possible to give a definite answer as to which program improves what component of quality of life.

In the introduction of this chapter, we suggested that physical activity would impact quality of life via its effects on physical, mental, social and emotional functioning (Sawatzky et al. 2007). But even among people with chronic conditions, an active lifestyle can contribute to better quality of life due to its positive effects on symptoms and functioning. Also, psychological factors such as self-efficacy (confidence in their ability to carry out the activity), self-esteem and positive affect (mood) seem to play a role in this pathway. That is, those who are more physically active have better self-efficacy, self-esteem and positive affect (Elavsky et al. 2005; McAuley et al. 2006). In turn, those with better self-efficacy have fewer functional limitations, higher self-worth and higher life satisfaction (McAuley et al. 2006). These positive effects subsequently accumulate into a better quality of life (Elavsky et al. 2005).

Earlier in this chapter, the focus was on *the net cost impact*, that is, the costs of moving one person from an inactive to an active lifestyle. Here, we move on to a different aspect of health economics, namely *cost-utility*. A cost-utility ratio expresses the costs of achieving the equivalent of an additional year of life lived in perfect health. Net health gains within the cost-utility ratio are expressed in *quality-adjusted life years* (QALYs). The QALY is a measure that combines improvement in quality of life with reductions in mortality in a single measure of health gain. The cost-utility of 13 trials of primary care and general public delivered physical activity interventions in adults (of any age) has been estimated to range from £275 to £68,898 per QALY gained (equivalent to €348–86,877 and US$520–129,862 based on 2008 exchange rates) (Garrett et al. 2011). Studies among older adults are scarce but tend to report cost-utility rates towards the high end of the range reported for adults. An Australian study that compared the effectiveness of a physiotherapist-led home exercise program during one year with usual care in adults over the age of 60 years after hospital admission found that costs per QALY gained were £50,170 in the exercise group relative to usual care (equivalent to €62,402 and US$80,465 based on 2012 exchange rates) (Farag et al. 2015). A US study that compared the effectiveness of a physical activity promotion program with a health education program among older adults at risk of mobility limitations found that costs per QALY gained were £31,453 in the physical activity group relative to the education group (equivalent to €36,956 and US$49,167 based on 2013 exchange rates) (Groessl et al. 2016). A literature review of exercise programs offered for falls prevention estimated the cost per QALY gained to be £44,764 (€54,933 or US$70,834) for group-based exercise, £27,936 (€34,540 or US$44,205) for Tai Chi and £59,045 (€73,004 or US$93,432) for home exercise (Church et al. 2012).

In nearly all studies that evaluated physical activity programs in older adults, the cost-utility ratios were above the *willingness-to-pay thresholds* of £20,000–30,000 reported by the UK National Institute for Health and Clinical Excellence (National Institute for Health and Care Excellence 2013) and the generally accepted thresholds of US$20,000–50,000 (Ubel et al. 2003). *Willingness-to-pay* is the hypothetical limit to resources that the society is willing to allocate to medical interventions. It reflects how much a society is willing to pay to increase a person's life lived in good health by one year. Thus, if the cost-utility ratio falls under the willingness-to-pay threshold, then the intervention is considered cost effective, because the costs of improving the quality of life is lower than the threshold that the society is willing to pay to extend a person's life lived in good quality by one year. Only the cost-utility ratio for Tai Chi fell under the willingness-to-pay threshold, suggesting that Tai Chi may be a cost-effective program to improve quality of life. For all other programs, the cost-utility ratios were at or above the willingness-to-pay thresholds. This means that the costs of running these interventions are not justified given the modest improvements in quality of life.

The costs-utility gained tend to be lower for programs that do not require supervision, such as walking programs and brief tailored advice (Garrett et al.

2011). This is understandable as supervision by a qualified professional is usually the largest contributor to the costs of the program. However, in older adults, walking programs are not recommended for those with a high falls risk, and supervision may be required to ensure safety. Cost-utility gained also tends to be lower for group-based exercise than individual exercise, even when delivered at home (Church et al. 2012). Programs with higher frequency and longer duration of exercise may be more effective in improving the components that make up quality of life, but are also more expensive. The challenge is to find the optimal balance between the program's costs and its potential benefits. It is uncertain what the required minimum level is of supervision, frequency and duration to achieve sustainable improvements in physical activity, health outcomes and quality of life.

4.5 Participation

Another aspect of how physical activity may influence society is through its effects on *participation*. The term participation refers to "involvement in a life situation" (World Health Organization 2002). Examples of what participation involves include engaging in social relationships and social roles such as caring for grandchildren, engaging in paid or voluntary work and being a member of a club.

Findings from observational studies show that those who are more physically active have higher levels of participation than those who are inactive (Levasseur et al. 2010). They also feel more satisfied with their level of social participation and have better social networks (Levasseur et al. 2010; Loke et al. 2016). Findings from 19 randomised controlled trials further suggest that programs originally developed to prevent falls that included an exercise component may also improve participation in life roles in older adults living in the community (Fairhall et al. 2011). However, the effect of these programs on participation is small. It is unclear what proportion of that small effect can be attributed to the exercise component of the programs rather than the social components of the programs such as being in a group and receiving attention from supervisors.

4.6 Older Adults Living in Residential Aged Care

The evidence supporting the relationships between physical activity and quality of life, health services use and costs described in this chapter so far is mainly based on studies conducted among older adults living in the community.

To date, little research has been done among older adults living in residential aged care. However, the few studies that have been done suggest that older adults living in residential aged care may also benefit from physical activity.

Observational studies have shown that the average level of physical activity among aged care residents is low. However, those who do participate in physical activities tend to have better cognitive and physical functioning than those who do not. They are also more socially active and report better self-perceived health and quality of life (Edvardsson et al. 2014; Fernandez-Mayoralas et al., 2015).

Randomised controlled trials that have looked at the effectiveness of exercise programs in residents of long-term care accommodation found mixed results; some found positive effects on measures of quality of life (Bruyere et al. 2005; Cakar et al. 2010; Dechamps et al. 2010; Rolland et al. 2007), whereas others did not (Chin et al. 2004; Kerse et al. 2008; MacRae et al. 1996). Interestingly, one study found that a high-intensity exercise program successfully improved psychological wellbeing in residents with dementia, but not in the total group including residents with and without dementia (Conradsson et al. 2010). As there were many differences between the studies and only a few studies in total, it is still unclear whether only certain types of programs can effectively improve quality of life or whether programs are effective in specific subgroups. It is thus not yet possible to conclude which programs may be beneficial for quality of life in which circumstances. However, the studies with positive effects showed that participants in the exercise groups were able to maintain their level of daily functioning and neuropsychological functioning, while participants in the (non-exercise) control groups showed a decline over the same period (Dechamps et al. 2010; Rolland et al. 2007; Underwood et al. 2013). As may be expected, residents who attend more exercise classes are more likely to maintain their level of functioning (Rolland et al. 2007). The exercise-related maintenance of daily functioning and neuropsychological functioning also translates to maintenance of quality of life (Deschamps et al. 2009). While in community-dwelling older adults physical activity is believed to have the potential to *improve* quality of life, in long-term care residents physical activity may have the potential to *prevent or delay decline* in quality of life.

While the above supports the idea that physical activity can contribute to maintaining or improving the quality of life of residents of long-term care accommodation, the relationship between physical activity and residents' health care utilisation and costs are less clear. The findings from community-dwelling older adults cannot be extrapolated to those living in long-term care accommodation as the level of physical activity is much lower, while health care needs are high. In these frail older adults, small improvements or delays in decline in functioning are unlikely to result in changes in their need for care. Unless physical activity can contribute to reducing events such as fractures or infections that require hospital admission, physical activity is unlikely to make substantial contributions to cost savings in this population. Indeed, one large-scale study that evaluated a physical activity program to reduce depression across 78 care homes in the United Kingdom found no differences between the intervention and control groups in QALYs or costs (Underwood et al. 2013). However, participating in physical activities may be important for maintaining participation in social activities and through that contribute to maintaining quality of life.

4.7 Older Adults with Dementia

One group of older adults that warrants specific attention in this paragraph is the group of older adults with dementia. In absence of an effective cure for dementia, there is a strong emphasis on maintaining quality of life and reducing caregiver burden, and physical activity has been put forward as a promising method to achieve this. Unfortunately, strong evidence supporting the benefits of physical activity in people with dementia is still lacking. A recent extensive Cochrane review identified 17 randomised controlled trials that examined the effectiveness of physical activity programs in community-dwelling people with dementia, but none of these trials presented results for quality of life or health care costs (Forbes et al. 2015). The review further pointed out that there was emerging evidence that participation in physical activity programs may have beneficial effects on performing daily activities, but not on neuropsychological functioning, depression, cognitive functioning or caregiver burden. In contrast, another literature review concluded that there is evidence supporting a positive effect of physical activity on caregiver burden (Orgeta and Miranda-Castillo 2014). The conclusions from these reviews were based on a small number of studies that examined each of the outcomes and there were many differences between trials hampering a meaningful comparison of the studies. The results of a randomised controlled trial published after these two literature reviews suggest that exercise programs in community-dwelling older adults with dementia may result in cost savings when considering behavioural and psychological symptoms but not when considering gains in QALYs (D'Amico et al. 2016). However, as dementia is climbing on the political agenda and more money is becoming available for research in this area, the evidence base will rapidly increase over the coming years. Indeed, a number of randomised controlled trials are currently underway, which will give insight into the role that physical activity has to play in improving the quality of life for people with dementia and their carers.

4.8 Indications for Future Research

No studies have evaluated the full sequence of the hypothesised causal pathway in older adults (Fig. 4.1). In particular health economic evaluations of physical activity promotion programs in older adults are lacking. Randomised controlled trials with longer-term follow-up of behaviour, health outcomes, health services use and costs are required to evaluate whether physical activity programs can indeed contribute to cost savings through preventing chronic conditions and functional decline in older adults. To increase the cost-utility of physical activity programs, strategies should be explored to reduce the costs of the physical activity programs and to improve the effectiveness of the programs in terms of quality of life. Moreover, verification of these relationships in older adults living in residential aged care and in people with dementia is warranted.

4.9 Key Practical Implications for Physical Activity Promotion

- The burden of disease attributable to physical inactivity is substantial and ranges from 6% for coronary heart disease to 10% for breast and colon cancer.
- There is currently insufficient evidence that physical activity programs can contribute to reducing health services use and costs in older adults in the community and in residents of long-term care accommodation.
- Participation in physical activity programs can contribute to modest improvements in wellbeing in community-dwelling older adults. Once an active lifestyle is achieved, it needs to be maintained to continue to experience the benefits. These benefits in wellbeing appear to exist for any type of physical activity, which means that promotion programs can be tailored to the person's preferences and abilities.
- In residents of long-term care accommodation, participation in physical activity programs may contribute to preventing or delaying decline in quality of life.
- In older adults living with dementia, participation in physical activity programs is likely to contribute to maintaining or improving daily functioning, but its benefits in terms of quality of life and health care utilisation are still unclear.

4.10 Conclusion

A substantial part of the burden associated with chronic health conditions common in later life can be attributed to physical inactivity. Inactive older adults have higher health care needs with poorer quality of life and subsequently higher health care costs than those who are physically active. While physical activity programs have the potential to improve people's quality of life and participation in the community, effects are modest. Moreover, this comes with a financial cost, at least in the short term. Longer-term follow-up studies are required to demonstrate whether physical activity promotion programs can contribute to reducing the need for and costs of health services in older adults. As the political focus is moving from health care to maintaining quality of life in older adults with dementia and/or those living in long-term care accommodation, there is a strong need for high-quality studies to strengthen the evidence for the role that physical activity programs can play in these populations.

Suggested Further Reading

- 2015 WHO Report on Aging and Health – for a broad perspective on policy implications of ageing for society.
- Lee, S., Lobelo, P., Blair, K., & Lancet Physical Activity Series Working Group. (2012). Effect of physical inactivity on major non-communicable diseases worldwide: An analysis of burden of disease and life expectancy. *Lancet, 380*, 219–229. (For country specific estimates of PARs for five major conditions associated with physical activity).

References

Awick, E. A., Wojcicki, T. R., Olson, E. A., Fanning, J., Chung, H. D., Zuniga, K., et al. (2015). Differential exercise effects on quality of life and health-related quality of life in older adults: A randomized controlled trial. *Quality of Life Research, 24*(2), 455–462. https://doi.org/10.1007/s11136-014-0762-0.

Brown, W. J., Pavey, T., & Bauman, A. E. (2015). Comparing population attributable risks for heart disease across the adult lifespan in women. *British Journal of Sports Medicine, 49*(16), 1069–1076. https://doi.org/10.1136/bjsports-2013-093090.

Bruyere, O., Wuidart, M. A., Di Palma, E., Gourlay, M., Ethgen, O., Richy, F., & Reginster, J. Y. (2005). Controlled whole body vibration to decrease fall risk and improve health-related quality of life of nursing home residents. *Archives of Physical Medicine and Rehabilitation, 86*(2), 303–307. https://doi.org/10.1016/j.apmr.2004.05.019.

Cakar, E., Dincer, U., Kiralp, M. Z., Cakar, D. B., Durmus, O., Kilac, H., et al. (2010). Jumping combined exercise programs reduce fall risk and improve balance and life quality of elderly people who live in a long-term care facility. *European Journal of Physical and Rehabilitation Medicine, 46*(1), 59–67.

Chen, I. J., Chou, C.-L., Yu, S., & Cheng, S.-P. (2008). Health services utilization and cost utility analysis of a walking program for residential community elderly. *Nursing Economics, 26*(4), 263–269.

Chin, A. P. M. J., van Poppel, M. N., Twisk, J. W., & van Mechelen, W. (2004). Effects of resistance and all-round, functional training on quality of life, vitality and depression of older adults living in long-term care facilities: A 'randomized' controlled trial [ISRCTN87177281]. *BMC Geriatrics, 4*, 5. https://doi.org/10.1186/1471-2318-4-5.

Church, J., Goodall, S., Norman, R., & Haas, M. (2012). The cost-effectiveness of falls prevention interventions for older community-dwelling Australians. *Australian and New Zealand Journal of Public Health, 36*(3), 241–248. https://doi.org/10.1111/j.1753-6405.2011.00811.x.

Conradsson, M., Littbrand, H., Lindelof, N., Gustafson, Y., & Rosendahl, E. (2010). Effects of a high-intensity functional exercise programme on depressive symptoms and psychological well-being among older people living in residential care facilities: A cluster-randomized controlled trial. *Aging and Mental Health, 14*(5), 565–576. https://doi.org/10.1080/13607860903483078.

D'Amico, F., Rehill, A., Knapp, M., Lowery, D., Cerga-Pashoja, A., Griffin, M., et al. (2016). Cost-effectiveness of exercise as a therapy for behavioural and psychological symptoms of dementia within the EVIDEM-E randomised controlled trial. *International Journal of Geriatric Psychiatry, 31*(6), 656–665. https://doi.org/10.1002/gps.4376.

de Vreede, P. L., van Meeteren, N. L., Samson, M. M., Wittink, H. M., Duursma, S. A., & Verhaar, H. J. (2007). The effect of functional tasks exercise and resistance exercise on health-related quality of life and physical activity. A randomised controlled trial. *Gerontology, 53*(1), 12–20. https://doi.org/10.1159/000095387.

Dechamps, A., Diolez, P., Thiaudiere, E., Tulon, A., Onifade, C., Vuong, T., et al. (2010). Effects of exercise programs to prevent decline in health-related quality of life in highly deconditioned institutionalized elderly persons: A randomized controlled trial. *Archives of Internal Medicine, 170*(2), 162–169. https://doi.org/10.1001/archinternmed.2009.489.

Deschamps, A., Onifade, C., Decamps, A., & Bourdel-Marchasson, I. (2009). Health-related quality of life in frail institutionalized elderly: Effects of a cognition-action intervention and Tai Chi. *Journal of Aging and Physical Activity, 17*(2), 236–248.

Ding, D., Lawson, K. D., Kolbe-Alexander, T. L., Finkelstein, E. A., Katzmarzyk, P. T., van Mechelen, W., & Pratt, M. (2016). The economic burden of physical inactivity: A global analysis of major non-communicable diseases. *The Lancet, 388*(10051), 1311–1324. https://doi.org/10.1016/S0140-6736(16)30383-X.

Edvardsson, D., Petersson, L., Sjogren, K., Lindkvist, M., & Sandman, P. O. (2014). Everyday activities for people with dementia in residential aged care: Associations with person-centredness and quality of life. *International Journal of Older People Nursing, 9*(4), 269–276. https://doi.org/10.1111/opn.12030.

Elavsky, S., McAuley, E., Motl, R. W., Konopack, J. F., Marquez, D. X., Hu, L., et al. (2005). Physical activity enhances long-term quality of life in older adults: Efficacy, esteem, and affective influences. *Annals of Behavioral Medicine, 30*(2), 138–145. https://doi.org/10.1207/s15324796abm3002_6.

Fairhall, N., Sherrington, C., Clemson, L., & Cameron, I. D. (2011). Do exercise interventions designed to prevent falls affect participation in life roles? A systematic review and meta-analysis. *Age and Ageing, 40*(6), 666–674. https://doi.org/10.1093/ageing/afr077.

Farag, I., Howard, K., Hayes, A. J., Ferreira, M. L., Lord, S. R., Close, J. T., et al. (2015). Cost-effectiveness of a home-exercise program among older people after hospitalization. *Journal of the American Medical Directors Association, 16*(6), 490–496. https://doi.org/10.1016/j.jamda.2015.01.075.

Fernandez-Mayoralas, G., Rojo-Perez, F., Martinez-Martin, P., Prieto-Flores, M. E., Rodriguez-Blazquez, C., Martin-Garcia, S., et al. (2015). Active ageing and quality of life: Factors associated with participation in leisure activities among institutionalized older adults, with and without dementia. *Aging and Mental Health, 19*(11), 1031–1041. https://doi.org/10.1080/13607863.2014.996734.

Figueira, H. A., Figueira, A. A., Cader, S. A., Guimaraes, A. C., De Oliveira, R. J., Figueira, J. A., et al. (2012). Effects of a physical activity governmental health programme on the quality of life of elderly people. *Scandinavian Journal of Public Health, 40*(5), 418–422. https://doi.org/10.1177/1403494812453885.

Forbes, D., Forbes, S. C., Blake, C. M., Thiessen, E. J., & Forbes, S. (2015). Exercise programs for people with dementia. *Cochrane Database of Systematic Reviews, 4*, Cd006489. https://doi.org/10.1002/14651858.CD006489.pub4.

Fox, K. R., Stathi, A., McKenna, J., & Davis, M. G. (2007). Physical activity and mental well-being in older people participating in the better ageing project. *European Journal of Applied Physiology, 100*(5), 591–602. https://doi.org/10.1007/s00421-007-0392-0.

Garrett, S., Elley, C. R., Rose, S. B., O'Dea, D., Lawton, B. A., & Dowell, A. C. (2011). Are physical activity interventions in primary care and the community cost-effective? A systematic review of the evidence. *British Journal of General Practice, 61*(584), e125–e133. https://doi.org/10.3399/bjgp11X561249.

Groessl, E. J., Kaplan, R. M., Blair, S. N., Rejeski, W. J., Katula, J. A., King, A. C., et al. (2009). A cost analysis of a physical activity intervention for older adults. *Journal of Physical Activity and Health, 6*(6), 767–774.

Groessl, E. J., Kaplan, R. M., Castro Sweet, C. M., Church, T., Espeland, M. A., Gill, T. M., et al. (2016). Cost-effectiveness of the LIFE physical activity intervention for older adults at increased risk for mobility disability. *Journals of Gerontology. Series A, Biological Sciences and Medical Sciences, 71*(5), 656–662. https://doi.org/10.1093/gerona/glw001.

Hagberg, L. A., & Lindholm, L. (2006). Cost-effectiveness of healthcare-based interventions aimed at improving physical activity. *Scandinavian Journal of Public Health, 34*(6), 641–653.

Hobbs, N., Godfrey, A., Lara, J., Errington, L., Meyer, T. D., Rochester, L., et al. (2013). Are behavioral interventions effective in increasing physical activity at 12 to 36 months in adults aged 55 to 70 years? A systematic review and meta-analysis. *BMC Medicine, 11*(1), 75. https://doi.org/10.1186/1741-7015-11-75.

Jarrett, J., Woodcock, J., Griffiths, U. K., Chalabi, Z., Edwards, P., Roberts, I., & Haines, A. (2012). Effect of increasing active travel in urban England and Wales on costs to the National Health Service. *Lancet, 379*(9832), 2198–2205.

Kerse, N., Peri, K., Robinson, E., Wilkinson, T., von Randow, M., Kiata, L., et al. (2008). Does a functional activity programme improve function, quality of life, and falls for residents in long term care? Cluster randomised controlled trial. *BMJ (Clinical Research Ed.), 337*, a1445. https://doi.org/10.1136/bmj.a1445.

Lee, I. M., Shiroma, E. J., Lobelo, F., Puska, P., Blair, S. N., & Katzmarzyk, P. T. (2012). Effect of physical inactivity on major non-communicable diseases worldwide: An analysis of burden of disease and life expectancy. *Lancet, 380*(9838), 219–229. https://doi.org/10.1016/s0140-6736(12)61031-9.

Levasseur, M., Desrosiers, J., & Whiteneck, G. (2010). Accomplishment level and satisfaction with social participation of older adults: Association with quality of life and best correlates. *Quality of Life Research, 19*(5), 665–675. https://doi.org/10.1007/s11136-010-9633-5.

Li, C. L., Chu, S. J., Sheu, J. T., & Huang, L. Y. (2011). Impact of physical activity on hospitalization in older adults: A nationwide cohort from Taiwan. *Archives of Gerontology and Geriatrics, 53*(2), 141–145. https://doi.org/10.1016/j.archger.2010.09.014.

Loke, S. C., Lim, W. S., Someya, Y., Hamid, T. A., & Nudin, S. S. (2016). Examining the disability model from the international classification of functioning, disability, and health using a large data set of community-dwelling Malaysian older adults. *Journal of Aging and Health, 28*(4), 704–725. https://doi.org/10.1177/0898264315609907.

MacRae, P. G., Asplund, L. A., Schnelle, J. F., Ouslander, J. G., Abrahamse, A., & Morris, C. (1996). A walking program for nursing home residents: Effects on walk endurance, physical activity, mobility, and quality of life. *Journal of the American Geriatrics Society, 44*(2), 175–180.

McAuley, E., Blissmer, B., Marquez, D. X., Jerome, G. J., Kramer, A. F., & Katula, J. (2000). Social relations, physical activity, and well-being in older adults. *Preventive Medicine, 31*(5), 608–617. https://doi.org/10.1006/pmed.2000.0740.

McAuley, E., Konopack, J. F., Motl, R. W., Morris, K. S., Doerksen, S. E., & Rosengren, K. R. (2006). Physical activity and quality of life in older adults: Influence of health status and self-efficacy. *Annals of Behavioral Medicine, 31*(1), 99–103. https://doi.org/10.1207/s15324796abm3101_14.

National Institute for Health and Care Excellence. (2013, April). Guide to the methods of technology appraisal 2013. Retrieved April 10, 2016, from https://www.nice.org.uk/article/pmg9/chapter/Foreword

Orgeta, V., & Miranda-Castillo, C. (2014). Does physical activity reduce burden in carers of people with dementia? A literature review. *International Journal of Geriatric Psychiatry, 29*(8), 771–783.

Peeters, G. M., Gardiner, P. A., Dobson, A. J., & Brown, W. J. (2017). Associations between physical activity, medical costs and hospitalisations in older Australian women: Results from the Australian longitudinal study on Women's health. *Journal of Science and Medicine in Sport*. https://doi.org/10.1016/j.jsams.2017.10.022.

Perkins, A. J., & Clark, D. O. (2001). Assessing the association of walking with health services use and costs among socioeconomically disadvantaged older adults. *Preventive Medicine, 32*(6), 492–501. https://doi.org/10.1006/pmed.2001.0832.

Richards, J., Hillsdon, M., Thorogood, M., & Foster, C. (2013). Face-to-face interventions for promoting physical activity. *Cochrane Database of Systematic Reviews, 9*, Cd010392. https://doi.org/10.1002/14651858.CD010392.pub2.

Rolland, Y., Pillard, F., Klapouszczak, A., Reynish, E., Thomas, D., Andrieu, S., et al. (2007). Exercise program for nursing home residents with Alzheimer's disease: A 1-year randomized, controlled trial. *Journal of the American Geriatrics Society, 55*(2), 158–165. https://doi.org/10.1111/j.1532-5415.2007.01035.x.

Sari, N. (2014). Sports, exercise, and length of stay in hospitals: Is there a differential effect for the chronically ill people? *Contemporary Economic Policy, 32*(2), 247–260. https://doi.org/10.1111/coep.12028.

Sawatzky, R., Liu-Ambrose, T., Miller, W. C., & Marra, C. A. (2007). Physical activity as a mediator of the impact of chronic conditions on quality of life in older adults. *Health and Quality of Life Outcomes, 5*, 68. https://doi.org/10.1186/1477-7525-5-68.

The WHOQOL group. (1998). The World Health Organization Quality of Life Assessment (WHOQOL): Development and general psychometric properties. *Social Science and Medicine, 46*(12), 1569–1585.

Ubel, P. A., Hirth, R. A., Chernew, M. E., & Fendrick, A. M. (2003). What is the price of life and why doesn't it increase at the rate of inflation? *Archives of Internal Medicine, 163*(14), 1637–1641. https://doi.org/10.1001/archinte.163.14.1637.

Underwood, M., Lamb, S. E., Eldridge, S., Sheehan, B., Slowther, A., Spencer, A., et al. (2013). Exercise for depression in care home residents: A randomised controlled trial with cost-effectiveness analysis (OPERA). *Health Technology Assessment, 17*(2046–4924 (Electronic)), 1–281.

Vagetti, G. C., Barbosa Filho, V. C., Moreira, N. B., Oliveira, V., Mazzardo, O., & Campos, W. (2014). Association between physical activity and quality of life in the elderly: A systematic review, 2000–2012. *Revista Brasileira de Psiquiatria, 36*(1), 76–88. https://doi.org/10.1590/1516-4446-2012-0895.

Windle, G., Hughes, D., Linck, P., Russell, I., & Woods, B. (2010). Is exercise effective in promoting mental well-being in older age? A systematic review. *Aging and Mental Health, 14*(6), 652–669. https://doi.org/10.1080/13607861003713232.

World Health Organization. (2002). *Towards a common language for functioning, disability and health: ICF, the international classification of functioning, disability and health*. Geneva: World Health Organization.

Yang, G., Niu, K., Fujita, K., Hozawa, A., Ohmori-Matsuda, K., Kuriyama, S., et al. (2011). Impact of physical activity and performance on medical care costs among the Japanese elderly. *Geriatrics & Gerontology International, 11*(2), 157–165. https://doi.org/10.1111/j.1447-0594.2010.00651.x.

Section 2

Selection of What Physical Activity to Promote Among Older People

Terry Haines

Physical activity is putatively held as being beneficial for people of all ages. This is particularly the case for older adults as a means for protecting against age-related decline in physical and mental function, or as a means of rehabilitation following a period of ill health or surgery. The problem that confronts health professionals seeking to use physical activity as a means of enhancing the health and well-being of older adults is heterogeneity. If one takes a global perspective, it has previously been identified that physical activity in low- and middle-income countries is primarily driven by occupational, household, and transportation requirements (Macniven et al. 2012). However, in high-income countries, physical activity is more likely to take place in the context of leisure-time activities. These differences at the level of international sociodemographics point towards a raft of variations across communities, clinical conditions, treatment settings, and inter-individual preferences that will need to be accounted for. It is important that health professionals have a well-rounded understanding of the basic principles of exercise prescription and how to vary these to meet the needs of individuals or groups. This section seeks to lay the foundations of the basic requirements of exercise prescription and explain how these can be varied across a range of different contexts that health professionals may seek to use exercise and physical activity-based interventions in a clinical setting.

T. Haines (✉)
School of Primary and Allied Health Care, Monash University

People seeking to help older adults to attain health benefits through physical activity face two essential problems. First, knowing what form of physical activity is going to best help older adults obtain the desired health benefits. This includes understanding which components of the musculoskeletal, cardiopulmonary, and neurological systems are being targeted, how to localise the targeted systems, and how to induce enough stimulus to elicit the desired physiological response while minimising the risk of injury and harm. For each problem, one could argue that there is a theoretically 'optimal' physical activity or exercise programme that could be designed for that individual older adult. However, identification of the optimal must be balanced against the second essential problem; knowing how to promote participation in the physical activity or exercise programme by the subject older adult. The optimal programme may be an idealised goal, yet unobtainable reality. There are many factors—medical, physical, attitudinal, cognitive, emotional, social, and environmental—that create a complex tapestry restricting participation in the optimal programme. Thus, the health professional is confronted with a balancing act, attempting to mix the ideal with the realistic so that they can best be of assistance to the older adult.

There are many factors that can influence how health professionals conceptualise what is likely to be an optimal physical activity or exercise programme and how to adapt this to make it a reality. This section has been divided into chapters focused on the basic principles of exercise and physical activity prescription and builds upon this through the prism of clinical contexts in which encounters with older adults take place, be that the body system primarily affected by the disorder afflicting the older adult or the stage of the healthcare journey.

Chapter 5 describes the frequency, intensity, type, and time (FITT) principle framework for exercise prescription, highlights some of the current limitations we face in using this approach, and then discusses the principles of specificity, overload, and recovery. Chapter 6 discusses use of a bio-psychosocial approach to assessment of an older adult prior to commencing an exercise programme before discussing a range of physical activity options that may be of interest to the general older adult population and strategies to promote participation in them. The focus then narrows in the following chapters to examine physical activity and exercise prescription in specific clinical areas. Chapter 7 examines the health benefits of physical activity for older adults with cardiorespiratory conditions, strategies to promote physical activity in this population, and changes in physical activity behaviour (including telemedicine applications). Chapter 8 explores factors impacting on declining physical activity in older adults with neurological disorders, enhanced neuroplasticity (the brain's ability to adapt from learning or injury) from physical activity, and important considerations when prescribing exercise and physical activity programmes for common neurological disorders. Chapter 9 moves the clinical context to disorders of the musculoskeletal system, adapting principles of exercise prescription to conditions including osteoporosis and fracture, osteoarthritis, rheumatic diseases, and other musculoskeletal disorders. Finally, Chap. 10 transports the reader to the management of older adults who are acutely unwell and may be experiencing combinations of cardiorespiratory, neurological, and musculoskeletal disorders superimposed on the additional risks of being hospitalised. This chapter includes important information about safety and monitoring of acutely unwell older adults who are participating in physical activity.

This section will equip readers with a thorough understanding of physical activity and exercise programme prescription necessary for effectively enhancing the health and well-being of older adults in a range of clinical and health service delivery contexts.

Reference

Macniven, R., Bauman, A., & Abouzeid, M. (2012). A review of population-based prevalence studies of physical activity in adults in the Asia-Pacific region. *BMC Public Health, 12*, e41.

5

Principles of Physical Activity Promotion Among Older People

Melanie K. Farlie, David A. Ganz, and Terry P. Haines

5.1 Introduction

Physical inactivity has long been held to have a deleterious effect on muscle strength, size, and function. This has been observed in younger and older adults alike. There is a difference between physiological changes in response to disuse (atrophy), disease (cachexia), and the physiological effects of aging (sarcopenia) (Evans 2010). The functional capacity of an older adult may be limited by all three processes simultaneously and present as a difficult picture to remedy for health practitioners and those seeking to promote the health, independence, and well-being of this population. Promotion of physical activity is now seen as a front-line approach to supporting people with these problems. It may be used as an adjunct or complete alternative to medication for disease management (Australian and New Zealand Society of Geriatric Medicine 2014; Phillips and Kennedy 2012). However, this has not always been the case.

Several "myths" about physical activity in older adults have crept into the public consciousness (Sell and Frierman 2010). Among them is the concern that older adults may not benefit from physical activity because the functional

---

M. K. Farlie (✉) • T. P. Haines
Allied Health Research Unit, Monash Health, and Faculty of Medicine, Nursing and Health Sciences, Monash University, Cheltenham, VIC, Australia

D. A. Ganz
US Department of Veterans Affairs Greater Los Angeles Healthcare System, University of California at Los Angeles, Los Angeles, CA, USA

decline due to ageing is inevitable and that participation in some forms of exercise (particularly strength training) may not be safe. Indeed, the physiological response of older adults to physical activity has not always been considered to follow the same pathway as that of younger people. Formative work in this field indicated that an eight-week progressive resistance training program resulted in comparable percentage increases in strength between younger and older men, yet via different mechanisms (Moritani and Devries 1980). Older subjects were observed to have increased muscle activation via neural mechanisms throughout this period. Young subjects showed strength gains due to neural factors only at the initial stage, with increase in muscle size (hypertrophy) becoming the dominant factor after some four weeks of training. However, work published in the late 1980s observed increase in muscle size in response to strength training in adults 60–72 years (Frontera et al. 1988).

In the early 1990s, Fiatarone and colleagues investigated high-intensity strength training for ten frail older adults (six females, four males) residing in long-term care, ranging in age from 86 to 96 years (Fiatarone et al. 1990). This study investigated the feasibility (was it well tolerated, safe, nonmaleficent) and the physiological adaptations (strength, muscle size, functional mobility) of strength training in this population. The program trained the major leg muscle groups for eight weeks. Results of this study indicated that the program was feasible for nine subjects who were able to complete the program with a 98.8% attendance rate and no adverse events. Physiologically, average strength gains were 174% ± 31% ($p < 0.0001$) and the size of quadriceps and hamstring muscles increased in participants who maintained body weight during the study (total change 11.7% ± 5%, $p < 0.05$). Mobility improved for those who could complete tandem walk at baseline ($n = 5$), two participants no longer required a gait aid and one participant was newly able to sit-to-stand without using his/her arms. These improvements indicate that functional improvements had been attained in the "very old" following a high-intensity strength training regimen.

5.2 The FITT Principle: An Exercise Prescription Framework

Health professionals are increasingly recognising the primary treatment benefits of exercise in the promotion of health and the prevention of disease in adults. Increases in physical activity have been directly linked to a reduction in all-cause mortality (Wen et al. 2011). Health professionals are well positioned to educate older adults about recommended physical activity levels, and prescribe physical activities that are currently achievable based on current physical activity levels and fitness, and to guide older adults towards achieving recommended levels of physical activity for optimal health (Costello et al. 2011; Day et al. 2011; Phillips and Kennedy 2012; Walters et al. 2015). The inclusion of exercise prescription in health consultations has been described as analogous to medication prescription (Phillips and Kennedy 2012; Vuori et al. 2013). Some have recommended primary care physicians write "exercise prescriptions" like pharmaceutical scripts (Phillips and Kennedy 2012), and recommendations are available to guide healthcare professionals in the prescription of exercises for different therapeutic aims and older adult sub-populations, as shown in Table 5.1 (Australian and New Zealand Society of Geriatric Medicine 2014; de Souto Barreto et al. 2016; Hordern et al. 2012; Nelson et al. 2007; Shubert 2011; Tiedemann et al. 2011; Weening-Dijksterhuis et al. 2011).

The FITT principle is an acronym commonly used to describe the four key variables underpinning any exercise prescription: frequency, intensity, type, and time. Depending on the type of exercise, different application of these variables determines the physiological responses to exercise that are anticipated. Laboratory and clinical research in both animals and humans have been used to identify the different combinations within these parameters that are likely to lead to differential improvements in muscular strength, power, endurance, and flexibility. Consequently, there are a number of exercise and physical activity recommendations that have been published by expert consensus groups, such as the American College of Sports Medicine. These are presented in Table 5.1, along with relevant information regarding the FITT parameters expected to induce differential exercise effects in older adult populations (Australian and New Zealand Society of Geriatric Medicine 2014; Bauman et al. 2016; Chodzko-zajko et al. 2009; de Souto Barreto et al. 2016; Hordern et al. 2012; Tiedemann et al. 2011) .

5.2.1 Types of Exercise

Training programs for older adults include exercises that target muscle strength, cardiorespiratory fitness, balance training and falls prevention, flexibility, and functional activities for maintenance or improvement of mobility independence, including walking, sit-to-stand, and transfers (e.g., from bed to chair). The type of exercise prescribed can be individualised within the recommended guidelines depending on the needs and interests of an individual. For example, cardiorespiratory fitness can be trained by walking, running, cycling, hiking, or swimming.

Table 5.1 Exercise prescription guidelines for older adults from position statements and recommendation reports

Recommending organisation/group	Target population	Muscle strength	Cardiorespiratory/aerobic fitness	Balance training and falls prevention	Flexibility	Functional mobility
World Health Organisation (2010)	Adults 65 years+	Major muscle groups ≥2 days per week	150 minutes moderate or 75 minutes vigorous intensity per week	Balance exercises at least 3 days per week if poor mobility		As much as possible for adults not meeting minimum recommendations Encourage incidental activity
International Association of Gerontology and Geriatrics (de Souto Barreto et al. 2016)	Adults in care able to rise from chair and walk	1–2 sets, high intensity. 2 days per week, ≥48 hours between sessions	Increase heart rate without undue fatigue ≤45 minutes 2 days per week			
American College of Sports Medicine (Nelson et al. 2007)	Adults 65 years+	8–10 exercises, 10–15 repetitions ≥2 days per week, moderate to high intensity	Moderate intensity 30 minutes, 5 days per week, or vigorous intensity 20 minutes, 3 days per week		10 minutes, ≥2 days per week	
Australian and New Zealand Society for Geriatric Medicine (2014)	Older adults			Exercise to maintain or improve balance in those with increased falls risk ≥2 hours per week, ≥6 months, challenging		
Exercise and Sports Science Australia (Tiedemann et al. 2011)	Adults ± history of falls			≥2 hours per week, ≥6 months, challenging		
Exercise and Sports Science Australia (Hordern et al. 2012)	Adults with type 2 diabetes or pre-diabetes	2–4 sets of 8–10 repetitions, ≥2 days per week, 60 minutes within weekly total	Moderate intensity ≤210 minutes or vigorous ≤125 minutes per week			

The type of exercise program prescribed may be chosen on the basis of the intended physiological gain, such as selection of a resistance training program to improve strength. Programs that target multiple physiological gains may be selected and may prove to be a more efficient means to attain improvements in multiple physiological areas. Holviala et al. (2011), for example, randomised 26 men with an average age of 56 years to a 21-week combined strength (whole body machine weights 2x/week) and cardiorespiratory (stationary cycle 2x/week) fitness program and reported significant improvements in strength, balance, and walking outcomes compared to the 26 men doing cardiorespiratory fitness exercises alone.

The exercise prescribed may also be chosen depending on the preferences of the older adult for exercise types that they enjoy more or perceive benefit from. Honouring preferences is important, as long-term participation in exercise and physical activity programs is frequently found to be sub-optimal (Costello et al. 2011). The proportion of older adults not meeting recommended physical activity guidelines has ranged globally from 18.8% to 58.8% (Bauman et al. 2016). Hence, strategies to improve rates of participation in exercise and physical activity programs are required. Studies investigating exercise type selection and participation have found improved adherence if older adults are interested in the type of activity, perceive the benefits of performing that type of activity outweigh the costs (financial and non-financial) of participating, and have confidence (self-efficacy) they can engage in the activity safely (Australian and New Zealand Society of Geriatric Medicine 2014; Haines et al. 2016; Merom et al. 2012).

Exercise programs can include several different types of activity to attain the same physiological benefit. Strength training programs can comprise body weight resistance exercises (i.e., sit-to-stand, squats, step-ups for quadriceps and gluteal strength) for relatively frail adults or be performed with added resistance in the form of exercise bands, free weights, or machine weights depending on the strength of the individual. Aerobic exercise can progress from walking to jogging to running but also include other types of continuous motion exercise that increases heart rate, for example, swimming, cycling, dancing, and hiking. Balance training programs can include static (standing in place) or dynamic (weight shift from one space to another) exercises and may be multidimensional, for example, Tai Chi or dance, or use equipment such as computerised force platforms or gaming systems, balance boards, or foam mats. Balance exercises may also include practice of agility such as obstacle negotiation or additional complexity of dual tasks that may be either motor (e.g., carrying a glass of water while walking without spilling) or cognitive (e.g., counting backwards from 100 in 3's). Flexibility programs include stretching, which may be simple extension of limbs through full range of motion, or more dynamic, such as some forms of yoga practice. Functional mobility programs are usually prescribed for frailer older adults who are dependent on activities of daily living and commonly involve practice of bed and chair transfer activities, walking, and negotiation of stairs. Engaging in multiple types of exercise or rotating between them to achieve the same physiological or functional benefit can be a useful way to prevent boredom from interfering with participation in the long term.

5.2.2 Frequency of Exercise

Frequency of exercise relates to the number of times an exercise is performed over a given time period (e.g., a week or a day). Shorter, more frequent bouts of exercise spread across a day or a week may be one strategy that can be used to assist older adults to achieve recommended exercise targets. For example, 30 minutes of continuous walking may not be possible for an individual in the early stages of establishing an exercise program, but a 10-minute walk 3 times a day or a 5-minute walk every 2 hours up to 6 times a day may be achievable. Some exercises, such as strength training, can be performed most days of the week if different parts of the body are targeted. For example, an older adult may perform upper-limb strength training 2 days a week and lower-limb strength training on 2 other days of the week, as long as there is 48 hours of rest for each muscle group between exercise sessions. There are no clear guidelines on how frequently balance exercises need to be performed; however, given that the recommended duration of balance exercise training to prevent falls is 120 minutes per week, this would equate to 20 minutes on 6 days a week or 17 minutes 7 days a week.

5.2.3 Intensity of Exercise

Of all the exercise variables, intensity is the variable that is most difficult to describe. The construct of intensity is different for each form of exercise, and most exercise types have more than one validated method of measuring intensity. Other exercise types, such as balance exercise, have no validated method of measuring intensity (Farlie et al. 2013). Regardless of how exercise intensity is measured, the construct is measured relative to the individual's physical capacity.

One approach to measuring exercise intensity is to look at the energy expended by an individual to perform that activity relative to how much energy expended during sedentary activities. The term metabolic equivalents, or METs, is used for this purpose (Kisner and Colby 2007; Norton et al. 2010). The lower the MET level of an activity, the lower the energy expenditure required. 1 MET is equivalent to 3.5 ml of oxygen consumed per kilogram of body weight per minute and is the energy required while sitting at rest (Brown et al. 2005; Kisner and Colby 2007). Maximal MET thresholds range from 9 up to 20 METs for elite athletes (Kisner and Colby 2007; Norton et al. 2010). Care should be taken in prescribing the intensity of an activity program based on tables of "average" METs for different activities. A table of MET values for different household activities was previously published by Jetté, Sidney, and Blümchen (1990) where undertaking weeding in the garden was ascribed a value of 3.5 METs. Although this tells a health professional how many METs people who perform this activity expend on average, it does not mean that an older adult who is encouraged to weed her garden will work at an intensity of 3.5 METs just because she is performing this activity.

Intensity of physical activity is measured relative to numerous physiological responses (i.e., respiratory rate, oxygen uptake, circulating lactate, and adrenaline levels), and the increase in those responses is usually exponential as exercise intensity increases (Norton et al. 2010). One of the most common methods of measuring exercise intensity in research and clinical practice is the rating of perceived exertion measure (Borg 1974; Norton et al. 2010). Initially, Borg developed the Borg rating of perceived exertion scale in the 1960s to measure the intensity of cardiorespiratory exercise (Borg 1973; Noble 1982; Pandolf 1983). Unlike some physiological responses to exercise, a linear relationship between heart rate and work during exercise has been reported in studies of the rating of perceived exertion scale (Borg 1973, 1982a, b; Skinner et al. 1973). The Borg rating of perceived exertion scale uses a scale of 6–20, which corresponds with the normal adult heart rate range of 60–200 beats per minute (Borg 1970), where the score is relative to the heart rate of the individual (i.e., a rating of perceived exertion of 6/20 generally corresponds to a heart rate of 60 beats per minute, while a rating of perceived exertion of 15/20 generally corresponds to a heart rate of 150 beats per minute) (Borg 1982a, b). The Borg rating of perceived exertion scale is recommended for monitoring physical activity in cardiac and pulmonary rehabilitation programs (Mezzani et al. 2013; Nici et al. 2006) and has been shown to be a valid measure in clinical studies of cardiovascular exercise such as monitoring of treadmill running and cycling (Dunbar 1993).

The "1-repetition maximum" (1-RM) method is the gold standard for determining the appropriate level of resistance for strength training programs; however, a number of "repetition to fatigue" formulae have also been published (American College Sports Medicine 2014; Wood et al. 2002). With concerns about potential harm to older adults performing a 1-repetition maximum test, repetitions to fatigue methods, also known as sub-maximal testing, to predict 1-repetition maximum have popular appeal. Though the 1-repetition maximum method has been used without adverse event in numerous studies of older adults undergoing strength training programs (Fiatarone et al. 1990, 1993, 1994; Fiatarone Singh 2002; Frontera et al. 1988), a large empirical study of older adults demonstrated that the predictive value of repetition to fatigue measures correlate poorly with the 1-repetition maximum (Wood et al. 2002). This study recommended that repetition to fatigue measures are most accurate when fatigue occurs at less than ten repetitions, and the calculation method proposed by Mayhew and colleagues (1992) was most accurate at predicting the 1-repetition maximum from repetition to fatigue methods in older adults. Recommended protocols to maximise the safety of the 1-repetition maximum assessment in older adults included limiting the number of attempts within sessions and incremental increases in weight lifted to the 1-repetition maximum point with close attention to correct technique and avoidance of compensatory movements or use of momentum (American College Sports Medicine 2014; Chodzko-zajko et al. 2009; Fiatarone et al. 1994; Rogers et al. 2003). A 10-point rating of perceived exertion has also been validated for use for measuring the intensity of strength training programs (Sweet et al. 2004). When using a rating of perceived exertion scale for strength training, a score of 10 is equivalent to the effort required to lift a weight once, or the "1-repetition maximum" (1-RM), while an 8/10 is equivalent to 80% of the 1-RM and so on (Sweet et al. 2004). High-intensity strength training generally corresponds to 8–10 repetitions to fatigue (Kisner and Colby 2007) or 5–6/10 on the rating of perceived exertion (Sweet et al. 2004), while moderate-intensity strength training is 13–15 repetitions to fatigue (Kisner and Colby 2007) or 3–4/10 on the rating of perceived exertion (Sweet et al. 2004).

With regard to flexibility exercises, or stretching, the intensity is "determined by the load placed on soft tissue to elongate it" (Kisner and Colby 2007, p. 79). Conventionally, a low-load stretch over a long duration has been advocated as safe and effective for improvement of flexibility (Kisner and Colby 2007); however, a recent systematic review identified that there are few studies that examine the intensity of stretching in older adults, and the intensity of stretching is poorly described. When the intensity of stretching is described, it is usually relative to either the end of passive range or rated on a pain scale where the pain induced is proportional to the load of the stretch (Apostolopoulos et al. 2015). This is an area that requires further research and development of validated intensity scales to better understand intensity of flexibility exercises.

Similarly, there is currently no validated method of measuring balance exercise intensity (Farlie et al. 2013); however, one observational study has described verbal and non-verbal markers of balance exercise intensity (Farlie et al. 2016) and defined balance exercise intensity as "the degree of challenge to the balance control system relative to the capacity of the individual to maintain balance" (Farlie et al. 2016, p. 314). The American College of Sports Medicine defines high-intensity balance exercise as "the highest level that can be tolerated without inducing a fall or a near-fall" (2014, p. 589). Other researchers have used taxonomies of task difficulty (Tiedemann et al. 2011) or recommendations around training volume (frequency × duration) (Sherrington et al. 2011) as proxies for balance exercise intensity; however, both of these approaches have their limitations (Farlie et al. 2013). Recommendations arising from systematic reviews and meta-analyses (Gillespie et al. 2012; Howe et al. 2011; Sherrington et al. 2011) as well as expert opinion from falls and balance clinicians (Haas et al. 2012) indicate that balance exercises need to be of an intensity that is "challenging" to the individual, but more research and development of a validated balance exercise intensity scale is required before this can be quantified.

5.2.4 Time Exercising

Time spent exercising can be prescribed in as small a unit as seconds up to minutes or hours. Flexibility and balance exercises are more likely to be prescribed in bouts lasting several seconds to minutes, while extremely weak or deconditioned older adults may only be able to perform muscle strengthening or cardiorespiratory exercises for less than one minute, before building up exercise tolerance and endurance. Healthy older adults are likely to be able to perform strength and aerobic training for extended periods of time, up to many hours for some cardiorespiratory exercises such as jogging, dancing, or other sports.

The most recent global physical activity recommendations, released by the World Health Organization in 2010, were developed by an international advisory group, followed by peer review, and are primarily based on evidence reviews used to update the physical activity recommendations of the US

Centers for Disease Control and Prevention (Physical Activity Guidelines Advisory Committee 2008) and the Canadian Physical Activity Guidelines (Paterson et al. 2007). A search of Chinese and Russian language scientific literature, using the same search strategy, was also performed and found no additional recommendations beyond those found in the English language studies reviewed (World Health Organisation 2010). These recommendations advise older adults to perform aerobic exercise bouts in minimal sets of 10-minutes duration (World Health Organisation 2010), however, exercise duration less than 10-minutes and below the recommended 150-minutes per week still conveys health benefits and should be encouraged (Sparling et al. 2015). The ideal recommended physical activity duration is at least 75 minutes a week of vigorous or 150 minutes a week of moderate-intensity aerobic exercise, in minimum bouts of 10 minutes at a time to maintain physical fitness. This equates to just over 10 minutes a day of vigorous exercise or 20 minutes a day of moderate-intensity exercise. For additional health benefits, these exercise durations are recommended to be doubled (World Health Organisation 2010). At least six months of aerobic exercise is recommended to achieve reductions in inflammatory markers, and this is also linked to reduction in truncal fat stores (Woods et al. 2012). Ten minutes of stretching two times a week (Nelson et al. 2007) and up to two hours a week of balance training (Sherrington et al. 2011) are the current recommendations for those forms of exercise; however, with neither of these forms of exercise having a validated measure of intensity (Apostolopoulos et al. 2015; Farlie et al. 2013), ideal exercise duration at any intensity is yet to be determined. Such investigations may reveal that lesser or greater amounts of exercise are needed to have a therapeutic effect if the intensity variable can be controlled at a low, moderate, or high level.

5.3 Specificity

The specificity principle applies to all forms of exercise (Kisner and Colby 2007) and to sub-categories of exercise such as balance (Giboin et al. 2015; Kummel et al. 2016) and strength training (Morrissey et al. 1995). Specificity describes the phenomenon that for improvements in a certain physiological outcome, exercise needs to target that physiological system. So for improvements in the cardiorespiratory system to occur, cardiorespiratory exercise needs to be performed at an adequate intensity for an adequate duration. Balance performance will not improve if balance ability is not challenged during balance exercise programs and so on. Equally so, some forms of exercise target multiple physiological systems at once; for example, Tai Chi can convey strength, cardiorespiratory, and balance improvements from one program due to the multifaceted nature of the exercise that stimulates all three physiological systems (Kuramoto 2006; Takeshima et al. 2007).

5.4 Overload

Closely related to the principle of specificity is the principle of overload. To induce a training effect, the system being exercised needs to be stimulated by taking it beyond the current capacity of the system. To induce an increase in muscle cross-sectional area, micro-trauma from skeletal muscle overload through appropriate levels of resistance is required and has been shown to occur in older adults in similar fashion to younger adults (American College Sports Medicine 2014; Fiatarone et al. 1994; Kisner and Colby 2007). Care needs to be taken however with overloading and the potential functional consequences in older adults. Delayed onset muscle soreness (DOMS) (Clarkson and Hubal 2002), which may be a nuisance in a younger adult, may incapacitate frail older adults if they were barely able to perform everyday activities of daily living, such as sit-to-stand, prior to the exercise program. Exercise may cause inflammation; however, repeated active overload leads to adaptation and attenuation of the inflammatory response with continuous exercise programs (Woods et al. 2012). Another form of overload that is potentially harmful to older adults might be the risk of injury from falls performing a vigorous walking program or dance routine. This would be an example of overload of the balance system that induces a fall.

5.5 Exercise Recovery in Older Adults

Conventional phases of exercise recovery are the immediate post-exercise period (acute) and 24–72-hour period (chronic) (Borges et al. 2016). The acute recovery phase is characterised by return of cardiorespiratory function to resting levels (Borges et al. 2016; Daanen et al. 2012) as well as return of hormonal and biochemical homeostasis, protein resynthesis, and replenishment of glycogen stores (Borges et al. 2016; Hausswirth and Meur 2011). The chronic recovery period is characterised by "time it takes to restore physical performance back to pre-exercise values" (Borges et al. 2016, p. 152) represented by full physiological recovery from the exercise session (Borges et al.

2016). Given the multifaceted nature of exercise recovery at a macro- and micro-level, there does not appear to be clear evidence as yet as to which recovery factors may specifically be affected by age; however, the recovery time in between exercise sessions is considered a key factor in prevention of injury and reduction of risk of over-training (Borges et al. 2016; Kreher and Schwartz 2012). A recent narrative review of exercise recovery in older adults concludes that there is little research that compares exercise recovery of younger and older adults (Borges et al. 2016). Other reviewers note that knowledge in this area is lacking due to a predominance of hypotheses drawn from rodent studies and a paucity of research into recovery of older adult humans performing typical exercise loads, and heterogeneity in how exercise induced damage, fatigue, and recovery is measured (Barker et al. 2015). More research is needed before any definitive claims can be made regarding the impact of age on exercise recovery.

5.6 Implications

The practical implications of the principles of physical activity promotion in older adults are illustrated through the following case study. Consider Mrs X, a 78-year-old lady who has fallen over twice in the past month while in her house and is now fearful of further falls. She describes that on both occasions she was carrying objects around her house (the washing and shopping) when she felt her right knee give way beneath her. Upon questioning, Mrs X reveals that she has some osteoarthritis in her knees and has previously had a transient ischaemic attack (mini-stroke). She was a one-pack-per-week smoker for 20 years before quitting 35 years ago. She does not participate in a formal exercise program, and her physical activity has become increasingly limited over the past five years. She completes most household activities independently, with assistance from her daughter to do the vacuuming and collect her shopping.

The sensation that her knees are giving way indicates that she may have weakness in her quadriceps muscles, which function to straighten the knee. The cause of this weakness may be related to her knee osteoarthritis (pain inhibition of muscle contraction), transient ischaemic attack, progressive disuse over recent years (atrophy), or a combination of these and other factors. Regardless of the cause, it is likely that a strength training program will need to be prescribed, along with plans to reverse her gradually decreasing physical activity levels. An exercise as simple as standing up and sitting down from a chair is a **type** of exercise that can be used to strengthen the quadriceps muscles. You ask Mrs X to stand up and down from a chair as many times as she can. She is able to do this 20 times, but you notice she is using her arms to push up and down on the arms of the chair. You give Mrs X a rest for a few minutes and then ask her to stand up and down from the chair again, but this time with her arms folded in front of her. This time she can manage only seven repetitions, and she reports that she is worried her knee will start feeling sore soon. You decide that performing the exercise in this way makes Mrs X work at a good **intensity** to elicit the strengthening physiological response that is desired. You tell her to perform this exercise seven **times** in the morning and seven times in the evening (a **frequency** of twice per day). You deliberately instruct her to perform this exercise in the morning and the evening, rather than performing two sets close together, so that her knee joint would have sufficient time to **recover** between sets in case some pain is provoked. After a couple of weeks, she is able to perform this exercise more easily and can perform 15 repetitions before needing to rest. You decide to make the exercise a little harder (**overload**) by making her stand up and sit down from a slightly lower chair so that she is again only able to complete seven or eight repetitions before needing to rest.

Increasing Mrs X's physical activity levels may be a difficult task. Beyond her muscular weakness around her knee, she now has a fear of falling, and may be fearful of provoking pain in her knee if she uses it too much. A key action here may be to discuss with Mrs X her **preferences** for physical activity that she feels capable (or near capable) of participating in and encourage her to gradually increase her exposure to her preferred physical activity as the strength in the muscles around her right knee improves. It may also be useful to enlist the support of her daughter when returning to perform an activity she has not been able to for a while (e.g., vacuuming) to provide reassurance and encouragement, boosting her sense of **self-efficacy**.

5.7 Conclusion

A key health promotion message for older adults involves pursuing exercise and physical activity. A large number of clinical trials have shown that even high-intensity physical activity can be safe and lead to physiological and health benefits in the short and long term even in the oldest old. The therapeutic principles of exercise prescription (FITT) can be used by health professionals alongside a number of physical activity recommendations available from scientific and expert consensus groups to guide activity recommendations for older adults. More research is needed particularly in the areas of balance and flexibility exercise intensity measurement and dosage, and human studies of exercise recovery in older adults.

Suggested Further Reading

- American College of Sports Medicine. (2014). *ACSM's resource manual of guidelines for exercise testing and prescription* (7th ed.). Philadelphia: Wolters Kluwer Lippincott Williams and Wilkins.
- Bauman, A., Merom, D., Bull, F. C., Buchner, D. M., & Fiatarone-Singh, M. A. (2016). Updating the evidence for physical activity: Summative reviews of the epidemiological evidence, prevalence, and interventions to promote "active aging". *The Gerontologist, 56*(Supp2), S268–S280.

References

American College Sports Medicine. (2014). *ACSM's resource manual of guidelines for exercise testing and prescription* (7th ed.). Philadelphia: Wolters Kluwer Lippincott Williams and Wilkins.

Apostolopoulos, N., Metsios, G. S., Flouris, A. D., Koutedakis, Y., & Wyon, M. A. (2015). The relevance of stretch intensity and position—A systematic review. *Frontiers in Psychology, 6*, 1128. https://doi.org/10.3389/fpsyg.2015.01128.

Australian and New Zealand Society of Geriatric Medicine. (2014). Position statement – Exercise guidelines for older adults. *Australasian Journal on Ageing, 33*(4), 287–294. https://doi.org/10.1111/ajag.12194.

Barker, A. L., Bird, M. L., & Talevski, J. (2015). Effect of pilates exercise for improving balance in older adults: A systematic review with meta-analysis. *Archives of Physical Medicine and Rehabilitation, 96*(4), 715–723. https://doi.org/10.1016/j.apmr.2014.11.021.

Bauman, A., Merom, D., Bull, F. C., Buchner, D. M., & Fiatarone Singh, M. A. (2016). Updating the evidence for physical activity: Summative reviews of the epidemiological evidence, prevalence, and interventions to promote "active aging". *The Gerontologist, 56*(Suppl 2), S268–S280. https://doi.org/10.1093/geront/gnw031.

Borg, G. (1970). Perceived exertion as an indicator of somatic stress. *Scandinavian Journal of Rehabilitation Medicine, 2*(2), 92–98.

Borg, G. (1973). Perceived exertion: A note on "history" and methods. *Medicine and Science in Sports, 5*(2), 90.

Borg, G. (1974). Perceived exertion. *Exercise and Sport Sciences Reviews, 2*(1), 131–154.

Borg, G. (1982a). Ratings of perceived exertion and heart rates during short-term cycle exercise and their use in a new cycling strength test. *International Journal of Sports Medicine, 3*(3), 153–158.

Borg, G. (1982b). Psychophysical bases of perceived exertion. *Medicine and Science in Sports and Exercise, 14*(5), 377–381.

Borges, N., Reaburn, P., Driller, M., & Argus, C. (2016). Age-related changes in performance and recovery kinetics in masters athletes: A narrative review. *Journal of Aging & Physical Activity, 24*(1), 149–157.

Brown, C. J., Gottschalk, M., Van Ness, P. H., Fortinsky, R. H., & Tinetti, M. E. (2005). Changes in physical therapy providers' use of fall prevention strategies following a multicomponent behavioral change intervention. *Physical Therapy, 85*(5), 394–403.

Chodzko-Zajko, W. J., Proctor, D. N., Fiatarone Singh, M. A., Minson, C. T., Nigg, C. R., Salem, G. J., & Sinner, J. S. (2009). American College of Sports Medicine position stand. Exercise and physical activity for older adults. *Medicine and Science in Sports and Exercise, 41*(7), 1510–1530. https://doi.org/10.1249/MSS.0b013e3181a0c95c.

Clarkson, P., & Hubal, M. (2002). Exercise-induced muscle damage in humans. *American Journal of Physical Medicine and Rehabilitation, 81*(Suppl), S52–S69.

Costello, E., Kafchinski, M., Vrazel, J., & Sullivan, P. (2011). Motivators, barriers, and beliefs regarding physical activity in an older adult population. *Journal of Geriatric Physical Therapy, 34*(3), 138–147. https://doi.org/10.1519/JPT.0b013e31820e0e71.

Daanen, H. A., Lamberts, R. P., Kallen, V. L., Jin, A., & Van Meeteren, N. L. (2012). A systematic review on heart-rate recovery to monitor changes in training status in athletes. *International Journal of Sports Physiology and Performance, 7*(3), 251–260.

Day, L., Finch, C. F., Hill, K. D., Haines, T. P., Clemson, L., Thomas, M., & Thompson, C. (2011). A protocol for evidence-based targeting and evaluation of statewide strategies for preventing falls among community-dwelling older people in Victoria, Australia. *Injury Prevention, 17*(2), e3. https://doi.org/10.1002/14651858.

de Souto Barreto, P., Morley, J. E., Chodzko-Zajko, W., Pitkala, K. H., Weening-Djiksterhuis, E., Rodriguez-Mañas, L., et al. (2016). Recommendations on physical activity and exercise for older adults living in long-term care facilities: A taskforce report. *Journal of the American Medical Directors Association, 17*(5), 381–392. https://doi.org/10.1016/j.jamda.2016.01.021.

Dunbar, C. (1993). Practical use of ratings of perceived exertion in a clinical setting. *Sports Medicine, 16*(4), 221–224.

Evans, W. J. (2010). Skeletal muscle loss: Cachexia, sarcopenia, and inactivity. *The American Journal of Clinical Nutrition, 91*(4), 1123S–1127S. https://doi.org/10.3945/ajcn.2010.28608A.

Farlie, M. K., Robins, L., Keating, J. L., Molloy, E., & Haines, T. P. (2013). An absence of intensity reporting in the prescription of balance exercises in randomised controlled trials: A systematic review. *Journal of Physiotherapy, 59*(4), 227–235.

Farlie, M. K., Molloy, E., Keating, J. L., & Haines, T. P. (2016). Clinical markers of the intensity of balance challenge: Observational study of older adult responses to balance tasks. *Physical Therapy, 96*(3), 313–323. https://doi.org/10.2522/ptj.20140524.

Fiatarone Singh, M. A. (2002). Exercise comes of age: Rationale and recommendations for a geriatric exercise prescription. *The Journals of Gerontology, 57A*(5), M262–M282.

Fiatarone, M., Marks, E. C., Ryan, N. D., Meredith, C. N., Lipsitz, L. A., & Evans, W. J. (1990). High-intensity strength training in nonagenarians. *JAMA, 263*(22), 3029–3034.

Fiatarone, M. A., O'Neill, E. F., Doyle, N., Clements, K. M., Roberts, S. B., Kehayias, J. J., et al. (1993). The Boston FICSIT study: The effects of resistance training and nutritional supplementation on physical frailty in the oldest old. *Journal of the American Geriatrics Society, 41*(3), 333–337.

Fiatarone, M. A., O'Neill, E. F., Ryan, N. D., Clements, K. M., Solares, G. R., Nelson, M. E., et al. (1994). Exercise training and nutritional supplementation for physical frailty in very elderly people. *New England Journal of Medicine, 330*(25), 1769–1775.

Frontera, W. R., Meredith, C. N., Reilly, K. P., Knuttgen, H. G., & Evans, W. J. (1988). Strength conditioning in older men: Skeletal muscle hypertrophy and improved function. *Journal of Applied Physiology, 64*(3), 1038–1044.

Giboin, L.-S., Gruber, M., & Kramer, A. (2015). Task-specificity of balance training. *Human Movement Science, 44*, 22–31. https://doi.org/10.1016/j.humov.2015.08.012.

Gillespie, L., Robertson, M., Gillespie, W., Sherrington, C., Gates, S., Clemson, L., & Lamb, S. (2012). Interventions for preventing falls in older people living in the community. *Cochrane Database of Systematic Reviews, 9*, CD007146.

Haas, R., Maloney, S., Pausenberger, E., Keating, J., Sims, J., Molloy, E., et al. (2012). Clinical decision making in exercise prescription for fall prevention. *Physical Therapy, 92*(5), 666–679.

Haines, T. P., Hill, K. D., Vu, T., Clemson, L., Finch, C. F., & Day, L. (2016). Does action follow intention with participation in home and group-based falls prevention exercise programs? An exploratory, prospective, observational study. *Archives of Gerontology and Geriatrics, 64*, 151–161. https://doi.org/10.1016/j.archger.2016.02.003.

Hausswirth, C., & Meur, Y. L. (2011). Physiological and nutritional aspects of post-exercise recovery specific recommendations for female athletes. *Sports Medicine, 41*(10), 861–882.

Holviala, J., Kraemer, W., Sillanpää, E., Karppenen, H., Avela, J., Kauhanen, A., et al. (2011). Effects of strength, endurance and combined training on muscle strength, walking speed and dynamic balance in aging men. *European Journal of Applied Physiology, 112*(4), 1335–1347.

Hordern, M. D., Dunstan, D. W., Prins, J. B., Baker, M. K., Singh, M. A. F., & Coombes, J. S. (2012). Exercise prescription for patients with type 2 diabetes and pre-diabetes: A position statement from exercise and sport science Australia.

Journal of Science and Medicine in Sport, 15(1), 25–31. https://doi.org/10.1016/j.jsams.2011.04.005.

Howe, T. E., Rochester, L., Jackson, A., Banks, P. M. H., & Blair, V. A. (2011). Exercise for improving balance in older people. *Cochrane Database of Systematic Reviews, 4*, CD004963.

Jetté, M., Sidney, K., & Blümchen, G. (1990). Metabolic equivalents (METS) in exercise testing, exercise prescription, and evaluation of functional capacity. *Clinical Cardiology, 13*(8), 555–565. https://doi.org/10.1002/clc.4960130809.

Kisner, C., & Colby, L. A. (2007). *Therapeutic exercise: Foundation and techniques* (5th ed.). Philadelphia: F.A Davis Company.

Kreher, J. B., & Schwartz, J. B. (2012). Overtraining syndrome: A practical guide. *Sports Health, 4*(2), 128–138. https://doi.org/10.1177/1941738111434406.

Kummel, J., Kramer, A., Giboin, L.-S., & Gruber, M. (2016). Specificity of balance training in healthy individuals: A systematic review and meta-analysis. *Sports Medicine, 46*, 1261–1271. https://doi.org/10.1007/s40279-016-0515-z.

Kuramoto, A. (2006). Therapeutic benefits of tai chi exercise: Research review. *Wisconsin Medical Journal, 105*(7), 42–46.

Mayhew, J. L., Ball, T. E., Arnold, M. D., & Bowen, J. C. (1992). Relative muscular endurance performance as a predictor of bench press strength in college men and women. *Journal of Strength and Conditioning Research, 6*(4), 200–206.

Merom, D., Pye, V., Macniven, R., van der Ploeg, H., Milat, A., Sherrington, C., et al. (2012). Prevalence and correlates of participation in fall prevention exercise/physical activity by older adults. *Preventive Medicine, 55*(6), 613–617. https://doi.org/10.1016/j.ypmed.2012.10.001.

Mezzani, A., Hamm, L. F., Jones, A. M., McBride, P. E., Moholdt, T., Stone, J. A., et al. (2013). Aerobic exercise intensity assessment and prescription in cardiac rehabilitation: A joint position statement of the European Association for Cardiovascular Prevention and Rehabilitation, the American Association of Cardiovascular and Pulmonary Rehabilitation and the Canadian Association of Cardiac Rehabilitation. *European Journal of Preventive Cardiology, 20*(3), 442–467. https://doi.org/10.1177/2047487312460484.

Moritani, T., & Devries, H. A. (1980). Potential for gross muscle hypertrophy in older men. *Journal of Gerontology, 35*(5), 672–682. https://doi.org/10.1093/geronj/35.5.672.

Morrissey, M. C., Harman, E. A., & Johnson, M. J. (1995). Resistance training modes: Specificity and effectiveness. *Medicine & Science in Sports & Exercise, 27*(5), 648–660.

Nelson, M. E., Rejeski, W. J., Blair, S. N., Duncan, P., Judge, J. O., King, A., et al. (2007). Physical activity and public health in older adults: Recommendations from the American College of Sports Medicine and the American Heart Association. *Medicine and Science in Sports and Exercise, 39*(8), 1435–1445.

Nici, L., Donner, C., Wouters, E., Zuwallack, R., Ambrosino, N., Bourbeau, J., et al. (2006). American Thoracic Society/European Respiratory Society statement on pulmonary rehabilitation. *American Journal of Respiratory and Critical Care Medicine, 173*(12), 1390–1413. https://doi.org/10.1164/rccm.200508-1211ST.

Noble, B. (1982). Clinical applications of perceived exertion. *Medicine and Science in Sports and Exercise, 14*(5), 406–411.

Norton, K., Norton, L., & Sadgrove, D. (2010). Position statement on physical activity and exercise intensity terminology. *Journal of Science and Medicine in Sport, 13,* 496–502.

Pandolf, K. B. (1983). Advances in the study and application of perceived exertion. *Exercise and Sports Sciences Reviews, 11,* 118–158.

Paterson, D. H., Jones, G., & Rice, C. (2007). Ageing and physical activity: Evidence to develop exercise recommendations for older adults. *Applied Physiology, Nutrition and Metabolism, 32,* S69–S108.

Phillips, E. M., & Kennedy, M. A. (2012). The exercise prescription: A tool to improve physical activity. *PM&R, 4*(11), 818–825. https://doi.org/10.1016/j.pmrj.2012.09.582.

Physical Activity Guidelines Advisory Committee. (2008). *Physical activity guidelines advisory committee report.* Washington, DC: Department of Health and Human Services.

Rogers, M. E., Rogers, N. L., Takeshima, N., & Islam, M. M. (2003). Methods to assess and improve the physical parameters associated with fall risk in older adults. *Preventive Medicine, 36*(3), 255–264. https://doi.org/10.1016/S0091-7435(02)00028-2.

Sell, K., & Frierman, S. (2010). Debunking the myths surrounding exercise and older individuals. Paper presented at the *new directions in American health care conference,* Hofstra University, Hampstead, New York.

Sherrington, C., Tiedmann, A., Fairhall, N., Close, J., & Lord, S. (2011). Exercise to prevent falls in older adults: An updated meta-analysis and best practice recommendations. *NSW Public Health Bulletin, 22*(3–4), 78–83.

Shubert, T. (2011). Evidence-based exercise prescription for balance and falls prevention: A current review of the literature. *Journal of Geriatric Physical Therapy, 34*(3), 100–108. https://doi.org/10.1002/14651858.

Skinner, J., Hustler, R., Bergsteinova, V., & Buskirk, E. (1973). The validity and reliability of a rating scale of perceived exertion. *Medicine and Science in Sports, 5*(2), 94–96.

Sparling, P. B., Howard, B. J., Dunstan, D. W., et al. (2015). Recommendations for physical activity in older adults. *BMJ, 350,* h100. https://doi.org/10.1136/bmj.h100

Sweet, T. W., Foster, C., McGuigan, M. R., & Brice, G. (2004). Quantification of resistance training using the session rating of perceived exertion method. *Journal of Strength and Conditioning Research, 18*(4), 796–802.

Takeshima, N., Rogers, N. L., Rogers, M. E., Islam, M. M., Koizumi, D., & Lee, S. (2007). Functional fitness gain varies in older adults depending on exercise mode. *Medicine & Science in Sports & Exercise, 39*(11), 2036–2043.

Tiedemann, A., Sherrington, C., Close, J. C. T., & Lord, S. R. (2011). Exercise and sports science Australia position statement on exercise and falls prevention in older people. *Journal of Science and Medicine in Sport, 14*(6), 489–495. https://doi.org/10.1016/j.jsams.2011.04.001.

Vuori, I. M., Lavie, C. J., & Blair, S. N. (2013). Physical activity promotion in the health care system. *Mayo Clinic Proceedings, 88*(12), 1446–1461. https://doi.org/10.1016/j.mayocp.2013.08.020.

Walters, M. E., Dijkstra, A., de Winter, A. F., & Reijneveld, S. A. (2015). Development of a training programme for home health care workers to promote preventive activities focused on a healthy lifestyle: An intervention mapping approach. *BMC Health Services Research, 15*(263). https://doi.org/10.1186/s12913-015-0936-7

Weening-Dijksterhuis, E., de Greef, M., Scherder, E., Slaets, J., & van der Schans, C. (2011). Frail institutionalized older persons: A comprehensive review on physical exercise, physical fitness, activities of daily living, and quality-of-life. *American Journal of Physical Medicine and Rehabilitation, 90*(2), 156–168.

Wen, C. P., Wai, J. P., Tsai, M. K., Yang, Y. C., Cheng, T. Y., Lee, M. C., et al. (2011). Minimum amount of physical activity for reduced mortality and extended life expectancy: A prospective cohort study. *Lancet, 378*, 1244–1253. https://doi.org/10.1016/s0140-6736(11)60749-6.

Wood, T. M., Maddalozzo, G. F., & Harter, R. A. (2002). Accuracy of seven equations for predicting 1-RM performance of apparently healthy, sedentary older adults. *Measurement in Physical Education and Exercise Science, 6*(2), 67–94. https://doi.org/10.1207/S15327841MPEE0602_1.

Woods, J. A., Wilund, K. R., Martin, S. A., & Kistler, B. M. (2012). Exercise, inflammation and aging. *Aging and Disease, 3*(1), 130–140.

World Health Organisation. (2010). *Global recommendations on physical activity for health*. Geneva: World Health Organization.

6

Promotion of Physical Activity for the General Older Population

Anne-Marie Hill

6.1 Introduction

As described in Chap. 5, multiple national and international best practice guidelines recommend that older people of all ages engage in exercise. Exercise is a predictor of successful ageing, which has been defined as including independent living, active engagement in life as well as high health-related quality of life (Depp and Jeste 2006; Peel et al. 2005). However, older people report barriers to engaging in exercise including low self-efficacy, chronic medical conditions, and pain and fears about injury, as well as financial cost of programmes and no adaptation of the programme for older adults (Baert et al. 2011; Bunn et al. 2008; Burton et al. 2016; Hill et al. 2011; Korkiakangas et al. 2011). Therefore, all health professionals need to understand how to address these barriers when they prescribe exercise or encourage older people to participate in regular physical activity. Facilitating older people to engage in physical activity requires health professionals to adopt evidence-based behaviour change approaches (Michie et al. 2011, 2013) (see Section 3).

A.-M. Hill (✉)
School of Physiotherapy and Exercise Science, Curtin University, Bentley, WA, Australia

6.2 Prescribing an Exercise Programme for an Older Person

All older people, 60 years and over in good health, can be encouraged to commence exercise programmes immediately with suitable initial prescription. However, if the older person has been inactive for some time, and since over 50% of older people are known to have at least one chronic health condition (Australian Bureau of Statistics, 2015a), it is good clinical practice to recommend that the older person undergo a medical check-up prior to commencing an exercise programme. This is also important as a health practitioner's positive recommendation to participate in exercise is likely to enhance the likelihood that the older person will engage in offered programmes (Bethancourt et al. 2014; Hill et al. 2011; Kerse et al. 2005; Orrow et al. 2012; Snodgrass et al. 2005).

6.2.1 Assessment and Initial Prescription

The underpinning rational when conducting an initial assessment for an older person is to use a comprehensive bio-psycho-social approach. Older people are more likely to have chronic disease and comorbid conditions; hence, it is important to assess the older person using functional tests, as well as assessing mood, cognition, and social support (Lewis and Bottomley 2008). Functional measures may include a walking test and a Timed up and Go test (Podsiadlo and Richardson 1991), the older person should be asked if they have fallen in the past year, if they have had their vision checked recently, and the therapist should also assess physical function of joints and muscles and the cardiorespiratory system. Medications and chronic health conditions should be discussed and further advice from the doctor should be sought as required, prior to commencing the exercise programme. Additionally, enquiring about social supports and whether the older person reports any depressed mood should be routinely undertaken by all health professionals and if any further support is required the older person should be referred to local health or social services to receive appropriate care and services.

In sum, for general exercise prescription for older sedentary people, a tailored approach should be used which "fits" the exercise to the older person. Key components can be summarised as:

(1) *Ensure programme adherence to national exercise guidelines for people aged 60 years and over*
(2) *Adapt and tailor the prescription for the presence of acute or chronic health conditions*

(3) *Tailor the programme to fit the older person's preferences for what type and amount of exercise to undertake*
(4) *Provide ongoing social and behavioural supports for undertaking the programme*
(5) *Ensure the programme is enjoyable*

6.3 Cardiovascular Training

Cardiovascular activities which could be undertaken by people aged 60 years and over include walking, swimming, skiing, running, bicycle riding, dancing, and other forms of group activities where sustained movement is undertaken. Organised sports such as basketball, tennis, and golf also provide strong cardiovascular benefits. The health practitioner should determine if the older person has a past history of engagement in any of these activities, as this could inform their recommendations.

Older people should ideally aim to meet guidelines for cardiovascular activity by engaging in moderate-intensity, aerobic physical activity for a minimum of 30 minutes 5 days a week or vigorous intensity aerobic activity for a minimum of 20 minutes 3 days each week (Chodzko-Zajko et al. 2009). Combinations of moderate- and vigorous-intensity activity can be performed to meet this recommendation. The intensity of the activity should be tailored appropriately, as each older person's individual level of fitness will vary. The health practitioner should explain to the older person how to assess their intensity of activity: given the heterogeneity of fitness levels in older adults, for some older adults, a moderate-intensity walk is a slow walk, and for others, it is a brisk walk (Chodzko-Zajko et al. 2009).

6.3.1 Walking

Walking is a key component of cardiovascular exercise prescription for older people as it is simple, requires no special equipment, and can be performed either alone or in company, and most usually in older person's local environment. Additionally, it incurs a low risk of injury and can be undertaken by older people who are frail or those who have moderate to serious health conditions such as cardiovascular disease or stroke. In these cases, support and tailoring from a health professional is recommended. Walking is currently the most popular form of physical activity in the United States (Simpson et al. 2003). Among people aged 55–64 years and 45–54 years in Australia, walking for exercise was the also most popular activity (34 and

30%, respectively), compared to golf (7.2% for 55–64 year olds) and lawn bowls (4.7% for people aged 65 years and over) (Australian Bureau of Statistics 2015b). Walking improves functional capacity as well as aerobic fitness and lowers the risk of cardiovascular disease (Albright and Thompson 2006; Boone-Heinonen et al. 2009; Murtagh et al. 2010).

Various strategies can be employed to increase and sustain the older person's participation in walking programmes. The use of pedometers and smart devices to record walking activity among older adults is now popular (Cavanaugh et al. 2007; Strath et al. 2009), although the acceptability will vary among older adults, who may or may not use these types of technology. Monitoring steps taken is only one way to track physical activity and some older adults may prefer to count minutes of activity or record the distance that they walk, rather than wear any type of step-counting device (Tudor-Locke et al. 2011).

Treadmill walking is another form of walking that some older adults may prefer and a home treadmill can be a comparable option for an older adult who does not have the capacity, for health or other reasons, to go outside (Watt et al. 2010). It offers balance support and graduated levels of intensity that allows an older person to undertake their walking in a safe, climate-controlled environment. Conversely for those older adults who would like to socialise through exercise but in a safe and climate controlled environment, mall walking could be a good option. Mall walking programmes are increasingly popular such as programmes run in Australia, the United States, and Canada (Cardiac Health Foundation of Canada 2017; Farren et al. 2015; COTA 2016), and many programmes are free. Malls have been found to provide safe, accessible, and affordable exercise environments for middle-aged and older adults. Mall walking programmes include features such as programme leaders, blood pressure checks, and warm-up exercises which facilitate participation (Farren et al. 2015). They also have a strong social component, which enhances adherence to the programme and the social and emotional benefits of undertaking this exercise. Walking in groups has been shown to increase levels of physical activity which indicates that walking groups could be a useful means of assisting an older client to sustain their activity over time as well as incur social benefits from participating in a regular group activity (Kassavou et al. 2013).

6.3.2 Cycling

Cycling is another option for cardiovascular activity. While cycling may require some level of previous experience, it could be excellent if the older person enjoys this mode of exercise. After walking, aerobics or fitness programmes, and swimming, recreational cycling is the fourth most popular adult physical recreation in Australia (Titze et al. 2014). The health benefits of cycling have been shown to outweigh the injury risks (de Hartog et al. 2010). Moreover, stationary cycling like treadmill training can be a safe alternative for older people who have other limitations, such as those older people with dementia, low vision, or poor balance. Systematic reviews demonstrate a positive relationship between cycling and improvements in cardiorespiratory fitness and disease risk factors as well as significant risk reduction for all-cause and cancer mortality and for cardiovascular, cancer, and obesity morbidity in middle-aged and older men and women (Oja et al. 2011). A large national Australian survey reported that one-third of cyclists met the physical activity guidelines of at least 150 minutes of moderate to vigorous intensity physical activity through cycling and half of cyclists accumulate 90 cycling minutes or more per week (Titze et al. 2014).

6.4 Strength Training

Strength or resistance training has been established as highly beneficial for older people to undertake and should be an essential component of all exercise programmes for older populations with necessary adaptation where required for chronic or acute illness. Strength training is known to cause a substantial increase muscle mass and motor activity in older populations, including among older people and even frailer older people (Fielding et al. 2002; Lee et al. 2015; Seynnes et al. 2004; Stewart et al. 2014).

Benefits for strength training are established as both physical and psychological. Physical benefits include reducing the risk of falls, improving bone strength, improvement in glycaemic control, muscle mass, and power (Chodzko-Zajko et al. 2009; Folland and Williams 2007; Liu and Latham 2009). Psychological improvements including improvement in quality of life and improved mood have also been shown to result from strength training (Seguin and Nelson 2003). Importantly, strength training results in functional benefits for older people including improvement in gait speed, ability to get out of a chair, and ability to undertake activities of daily living (Liu and Latham Nancy 2009; Seguin and Nelson 2003; Wilhelm et al. 2012). This means that strength training is an important component in programmes prescribed for older people who may have limitations in functional capacity resulting from chronic health conditions, as they can make important functional gains (see Chaps. 8 and 34).

Strength training programmes should include variation, gradual progressive overload, careful attention to recovery and stress, and specificity (American College of Sports Medicine 2009). Exercises should be prescribed after a baseline assessment, and for those older people who have not completed strength training, a gradual programme should commence with exercises that use body weight only, for example, small squats and sit-to-stand exercises, with subsequent gradual introduction of weights, which can include elastic resistance (Martins et al. 2013; Yang et al. 2015). Consideration should be given to using small weights and elastic bands as equipment for prescribing a home programme, as many older people may prefer this mode of training rather than using a gym. Home programmes also demonstrate good outcomes for older people, especially frailer older people (Clemson et al. 2010; Seguin and Nelson 2003). Strength-training guidelines suggest that two to three sessions of strength training per week should be undertaken (Petrella and Chudyk 2008; Seguin and Nelson 2003; American College of Sport Medicine 2009), while other researchers recommend even higher intensities (Mayer et al. 2011), but one session per week can still confer benefits, especially functional benefits (Liu and Latham 2009).

A systematic review synthesised studies that evaluated what barriers and enablers older people report to engaging in strength training. Enablers included preventing disability, reducing risk of falls, building or toning muscles, feeling more alert, and better concentration. Looking too muscular and thinking participation increased the risk of having a heart attack, stroke, or death, despite the minimal likelihood of these occurring, were barriers (Burton et al. 2017; Burton et al. 2016). Since injury is known to be a barrier to commencing and a reason for stopping exercise (Baert et al. 2011; Burton et al. 2017), careful monitoring should be undertaken to ensure the patient or client increases the dose and intensity of the exercises carefully.

6.5 Balance Training

Balance training should be a critical and ongoing component of all older peoples' general exercise programmes, regardless of age, comorbidity, or social situation. It is well known that one in three older adults fall each year and that this rises to one in two adults over 80 years (Campbell et al. 1990; Milat et al. 2011). Falls are a major cause of injury among older people, with over 90% of hip fractures caused by falls (Kreisfield and Newson 2006). Falls are also the cause of the rising incidence of traumatic brain injury among older people (Helps et al. 2008). There is established evidence that exercise reduces both falls and the risk of falls among older community-dwelling adults (Gillespie et al. 2012). The effectiveness of the exercise is strongly associated with the balance components that are in the programme. A meta-analysis of exercise programmes that targeted falls reduction demonstrated that those programmes that included balance training, which provided a moderate or high challenge to balance and did not include walking training, had the greatest effect on reducing falls (Sherrington et al. 2008). Therefore, it is important that exercise which targets balance is performed by all older people. A large meta-analysis of over 94 studies which evaluated various forms of exercise interventions found that "3-dimensional" exercises (which included Tai Chi, qi gong, dance, and yoga) were effective in improving balance. Gait, balance, coordination, and functional tasks also had some positive effects on balance (Howe et al. 2011).

6.6 Benefits of Specific Modes of Exercise

Some modes of exercise offer a blend of cardiovascular, strength, flexibility, and balance exercises. These types of programmes can be beneficial for an older person and if the chosen programme does not include all forms of exercise, then a specific, additional activity can be undertaken. For example, Tai Chi may offer balance, strength, and flexibility but less cardiovascular benefits. However, a brisk walking programme, performed in addition to regular Tai Chi classes, would ensure a comprehensive programme for the individual concerned.

6.6.1 Swimming

Swimming or aquatic exercises can include lane/lap swimming but also water classes, hydrotherapy, and water walking and can suit a wide variety of older adults. Swimming is a low-impact sport and as such can be a regular general exercise for even frailer older people, as well as for condition-specific therapy such as osteoarthritis. Swimming has been found to improve blood pressure among older people (Nualnim et al. 2012). Although a systematic review in 2009 suggested that the cardiovascular benefits of swimming on cardiovascular health are not well understood (Tanaka 2009), a systematic review, which included swimming among other cardiovascular activities, found that engaging in moderate to vigorous physical activity, even below the guideline recommendations, improved cardiovascular markers and survival benefits (Loprinzi 2015).

While swimming does offer some resistance to muscles when activities are undertaken, a systematic review indicated that the inadequate application of resistance in the water is a significant contributor to the limited effectiveness of aquatic exercises in improving hip and knee muscle strength in people with musculoskeletal conditions (Heywood et al. 2016). The effect of the low-gravity environment means that swimming is not an exercise that should be prescribed in isolation. Balance may also not be improved to sufficient levels to reduce falls risk by swimming when compared to balance-specific land-based activities, such as Tai Chi (Wong et al. 2011).

While the benefits of swimming may be less comprehensive than other exercise modalities for the general older population, older adults who have chronic medical conditions, such as chronic pain, joint problems such as arthritic conditions or a very high risk of falls, should be encouraged to incorporate swimming into their exercise programme if safe to do so. Swimming can play an important role in ensuring that at least some physical activity is undertaken and that cardiovascular components of the programme reach sufficient intensity (Loprinzi 2015). A systematic review found that aquatic exercise may have small, short-term but clinically relevant effects on patient-reported pain, disability, and quality of life in people with knee and hip osteoarthritis (Bartels et al. 2016).

6.6.2 Dancing

Dancing takes many forms, and there is evidence for its use as a therapeutic modality for older people, including in Parkinson's disease, mental health, and for physical health and functional benefits (Hui et al. 2009; McNeely et al. 2015; Vankova et al. 2014). The enjoyment of dancing makes it an activity that promotes engagement and adherence and it can be done by a wide range of older people. Dancing requires minimal equipment, although structured dance benefits by having a trained instructor to provide the older person with guidelines and routines to follow. A systematic review of 18 studies conducted among older populations found evidence to suggest that dance, regardless of its style, can significantly improve muscular strength and endurance, balance, and other aspects of functional fitness in older adults (Hwang and Braun 2015). There is evidence that dancing can significantly improve older peoples' aerobic capacity, lower body muscle endurance, strength and flexibility, and, in particular, static and dynamic balance and gait performance (Keogh et al. 2009).

6.6.3 Tai Chi

Tai Chi is described as an ancient form of Chinese exercise which uses slow sustained movements as its key exercise parameter (Hackney and Wolf 2014). This form of exercise has been investigated in multiple randomised trials and found to significantly improve balance, with meta-analyses supporting these individual trials (Low et al. 2009). As with other exercise, the intensity of the intervention has been found to be a factor in whether it is effective with trials showing no effect when the intervention intensity is low (Hackney and Wolf 2014; Logghe et al. 2011). Intensity of balance exercises has been discussed in Chap. 5. Meta-analyses have also found that Tai Chi significantly reduces falls and the risk of falling among older people (Gillespie et al. 2012; Low et al. 2009) (see Chap. 8).

6.6.4 Other Modes of Exercise

Other modes of exercise, including formal sports such as tennis, aerobic classes, and gym-based programmes such as Pilates programmes can also offer enjoyable alternatives for older adults and therefore assist them to engage in sustained and broad types of exercise. Pilates has been found to have both physical benefits such as improving muscle strength and balance and also some psychological benefits such as improving mood (Bullo et al. 2015; Roh 2016; Tolnai et al. 2016). Yoga is also another programme that shows both physical and psychological outcomes in small trials and could be a feasible and appropriate activity for older people (Tiedemann et al. 2013; Gothe and McAuley 2016; Wertman et al. 2016). As with other forms of exercise though, this requires an experienced instructor who can tailor the programme to be safe but of sufficient intensity for the older person to obtain benefits. There is also limited evidence that suggests yoga improves strength or cardiovascular fitness.

An associated barrier identified with older peoples' engagement in these types of exercises is that qualitative findings report that participation in activities that use complex motor skills is low (Kraft et al. 2015). Modifying activities to suit the older persons' ability and age and increasing exposure prior to older age may help maintain participation into old age. These researchers further suggested that existing and new sports should be modified for older age groups and made available (Kraft et al. 2015). The feasibility of engaging in these types of activities should be discussed with the older person. Social, financial, and environmental factors will influence whether these programmes are a long-term option for the individual.

6.7 Promoting Adherence and Enjoyment of Exercise Programmes

Regardless of modality chosen, one of the key problems for the health professional is to address the multiple barriers that older people report prevent them from exercising. Health professional advice in offering feedback, choice of programme and strategies such as exercise diaries will assist in maintaining participation (Cress et al. 2005; McDermott and Mernitz 2006; McPhate et al. 2013) (see Section 3).

6.8 Implications

A case study illustrates how health professionals can translate these principles into practice.

Case Study Jim is a retired bank manager who is widowed and lives alone in the community. He volunteers one day a week at a local library but does no formal exercise. Jim has osteoarthritis of knees and hypertension controlled by medication. He still drives. Jim currently has some mild knee pain and visits the therapist to get treatment for this on the advice of his doctor.

What would be good advice to give Jim regarding exercise and how would you go about assessing and encouraging him to undertake an exercise programme?
Answer: Taking a history from Jim about his previous likes/dislikes and exercise habits is critical, along with a falls screen and a cardiovascular fitness test such as a six-minute walk test (Steffen et al. 2002). Jim could also be asked to fill a pre-prepared questionnaire which gathers details about his usual physical activity and exercise. Jim could be advised to schedule a checkup with his doctor about taking up the suggested activities as affirmation from his doctor will be important in promoting uptake of the suggested programme.

Elements to consider in a programme are: Jim is currently doing no activity, so a gradual increase in activity is important and the programme will first and foremost be enjoyable. It should include a range of cardiovascular, balance, strength, and flexibility exercises. Some focus on exercises that are suitable for knee strength in particular would be useful. Regular walking could be suggested initially and, depending on Jim's motivation and social connections, Tai Chi or a dancing class could offer regular balance and cardiovascular and some strength components. Jim may enjoy swimming or bowling which offers a range of balance and cardiovascular and flexibility modes of exercise. He could attend a community programme that offers a range of strength, balance, and flexibility all in one-class setting. This could be a gym or other health setting. Alternatively, he could be given a home programme, either one prescribed via a health website or a written home programme which includes a full range of exercises. Jim could be given small weights to use by the therapist initially and then advised on the right sort of weights to purchase. Stationary cycling at home, if he is able to purchase a stationary bike, would be a good cardiovascular option, if he prefers not to take long outdoor walks.

The therapist should offer a broad choice of programmes and specifically enquire about possible barriers to engagement, including Jim's ability to pay for associated costs of the exercise programme that is planned, as well as his intentions and motivation to engage in such a programme. Barriers should be specifically addressed and the programme tailored by the therapist. For example, since Jim has painful knees, the first element of the cardiovascular programme could be hydrotherapy with land-based adjuvant walking. Jim should be given specific advice regarding any onset of knee pain while completing his programme, as this would be a barrier to continued engagement. Motivational cues should be sought and discussed by Jim and the therapist. Jim volunteers at the library, therefore, he could ask his co-volunteers if they participate in a programme that he can also join. Prompts and cues such as affirmation, advice, and an exercise diary should be issued by the therapist. Therapists can access a range of high-quality resources which provide older people with instruction, resources, and support to complete exercise such as those available on the British Heart Foundation National Centre website (Townsend et al. 2015) and the US government exercise guidelines for older adults and their implementation (2008 Physical Activity Guidelines for Americans: Be Active, Healthy, and Happy! 2008). Since Jim lives alone, it will also be important to discuss where he could obtain formal or informal social support. If Jim uses devices such as a smartphone then text reminders and communication could be useful and online exercise sites where Jim can interact and record his programme should be considered.

6.8.1 Advice for Health Professionals

Health professionals such as therapists have high levels of expertise in prescribing exercises and as such are a key facilitator for older people to undertake exercise. Professional guidance and support has been demonstrated to be a facilitator of older people engaging in exercise programmes (Bethancourt et al. 2014; Burton et al. 2017; Picorelli et al. 2014). Therefore, all health professionals should seek training and information on how to communicate with older people regarding physical activity and how to use sound behaviour change guidelines when prescribing exercises (Cress et al. 2005; Michie et al. 2011). The interaction between the health professional and the client is vital as it can be a barrier or motivator to older people gaining access to suitable programmes and undertaking the recommended exercises (Dickinson et al. 2011; Korkiakangas et al. 2011; Lee et al. 2013). Detailed guidance about what activities older people should undertake and how to successfully engage with older people can also be found in national exercise guidelines, such as those on the British Heart Foundation National Centre website (Townsend et al. 2015).

6.9 Conclusion

Physical activity and exercise are known to have established benefits in the broad population, and this includes people aged 60 years and older. However, low levels of exercise among this population remains a problem, therefore, it is important that health professionals are aware of the barriers and enablers to exercise for older people and take these into consideration when prescribing a programme. Programmes should focus on developing the older person's self-efficacy and emphasising enjoyment of participation and be informed by best practice guidelines. Health professionals should incorporate effective behaviour change methods when engaging with the older person regarding physical activity, to maximise uptake, engagement, and adherence.

Suggested Reading

- Burton, E., Farrier, K., Lewin, G., Pettigrew, S., Hill, A. M., Airey, P., et al. (2017). Motivators and barriers for older people participating in resistance training: a systematic review. *Journal of Aging and Physical Activity, 25*(2), 1–41. doi:https://doi.org/10.1123/japa.2015-0289
- Chodzko-Zajko, W. J., Proctor, D. N., Fiatarone Singh, M. A., Minson, C. T., Nigg, C. R., Salem, G. J., & Skinner, J. S. (2009). American College of Sports Medicine position stand. Exercise and physical activity for older adults. *Medicine and Science in Sports and Exercise, 41*(7), 1510–1530. doi:https://doi.org/10.1249/MSS.0b013e3181a0c95c

References

Albright, C., & Thompson, D. L. (2006). The effectiveness of walking in preventing cardiovascular disease in women: A review of the current literature. *Journal of Womens Health, 15*(3), 271–280. https://doi.org/10.1089/jwh.2006.15.271.

American College of Sports Medicine. (2009). American College of Sports Medicine position stand. Progression models in resistance training for healthy adults. *Medicine and Science in Sports and Exercise, 41*(3), 687–708. https://doi.org/10.1249/MSS.0b013e3181915670.

Australian Bureau of Statistics. (2015a). Disability, ageing and carers, Australia: Summary of findings, 2015. Retrieved from Canberra http://www.abs.gov.au/ausstats/abs@.nsf/mf/4430.0

Australian Bureau of Statistics. (2015b). Australian Health Survey, participation in sport and physical recreation, Australia, 2013–14. Retrieved from Canberra http://www.abs.gov.au/AUSSTATS/abs@.nsf/Lookup/4177.0

Baert, V., Gorus, E., Mets, T., Geerts, C., & Bautmans, I. (2011). Motivators and barriers for physical activity in the oldest old: A systematic review. *Ageing Research Reviews, 10*(4), 464–474. https://doi.org/10.1016/j.arr.2011.04.001.

Bartels, E. M., Juhl, C. B., Christensen, R., Hagen, K. B., Danneskiold-Samsoe, B., Dagfinrud, H., & Lund, H. (2016). Aquatic exercise for the treatment of knee and hip osteoarthritis. *The Cochrane Database of Systematic Reviews, 3*, Cd005523. https://doi.org/10.1002/14651858.CD005523.pub3.

Bethancourt, H. J., Rosenberg, D. E., Beatty, T., & Arterburn, D. E. (2014). Barriers to and facilitators of physical activity program use among older adults. *Clinical Medicine & Research, 12*(1–2), 10–20. https://doi.org/10.3121/cmr.2013.1171.

Boone-Heinonen, J., Evenson, K. R., Taber, D. R., & Gordon-Larsen, P. (2009). Walking for prevention of cardiovascular disease in men and women: A systematic review of observational studies. *Obesity Reviews: An Official Journal of the International Association for the Study of Obesity, 10*(2), 204–217. https://doi.org/10.1111/j.1467-789X.2008.00533.x.

Bullo, V., Bergamin, M., Gobbo, S., Sieverdes, J. C., Zaccaria, M., Neunhaeuserer, D., & Ermolao, A. (2015). The effects of Pilates exercise training on physical fitness and wellbeing in the elderly: A systematic review for future exercise prescription. *Preventive Medicine, 75*, 1–11. https://doi.org/10.1016/j.ypmed.2015.03.002.

Bunn, F., Dickinson, A., Barnett-Page, E., McInnes, E., & Horton, K. (2008). A systematic review of older people's perceptions of facilitators and barriers to participation in falls-prevention interventions. *Ageing & Society, 28*(04), 449–472. https://doi.org/10.1017/S0144686X07006861.

Burton, E., Lewin, G., Pettigrew, S., Hill, A. M., Bainbridge, L., Farrier, K., et al. (2016). Identifying motivators and barriers to older community-dwelling people participating in resistance training: A cross-sectional study. *Journal of Sports Science*, 1–10. https://doi.org/10.1080/02640414.2016.1223334.

Burton, E., Farrier, K., Lewin, G., Pettigrew, S., Hill, A. M., Airey, P., et al. (2017). Motivators and barriers for older people participating in resistance training: A systematic review. *Journal of Aging and Physical Activity, 25*(2), 1–41. https://doi.org/10.1123/japa.2015-0289.

Campbell, A. J., Borrie, M. J., Spears, G. F., Jackson, S. L., Brown, J. S., & Fitzgerald, J. L. (1990). Circumstances and consequences of falls experienced by a community population 70 years and over during a prospective study. *Age and Ageing, 19*(2), 136–141. https://doi.org/10.1093/ageing/19.2.136.

Cardiac Health Foundation of Canada. (2017). *Mall walking programs.* Retrieved from http://www.cardiachealth.ca/

Cavanaugh, J. T., Coleman, K. L., Gaines, J. M., Laing, L., & Morey, M. C. (2007). Using step activity monitoring to characterize ambulatory activity in community-dwelling older adults. *Journal of the American Geriatrics Society, 55*(1), 120–124. https://doi.org/10.1111/j.1532-5415.2006.00997.x.

Chodzko-Zajko, W. J., Proctor, D. N., Fiatarone Singh, M. A., Minson, C. T., Nigg, C. R., Salem, G. J., & Skinner, J. S. (2009). American College of Sports Medicine position stand. Exercise and physical activity for older adults. *Medicine and Science in Sports and Exercise, 41*(7), 1510–1530. https://doi.org/10.1249/MSS.0b013e3181a0c95c.

Clemson, L., Singh, M. F., Bundy, A., Cumming, R. G., Weissel, E., Munro, J., et al. (2010). LiFE pilot study: A randomised trial of balance and strength training embedded in daily life activity to reduce falls in older adults. *Australian Occupational Therapy Journal, 57*(1), 42–50.

COTA, W. A. (2016). Active ageing – Mall walking. Retrieved from http://www.cotawa.org.au/activeageing/mall-walking

Cress, M. E., Buchner, D. M., Prohaska, T., Rimmer, J., Brown, M., Macera, C., et al. (2005). Best practices for physical activity programs and behavior counseling in older adult populations. *Journal of Aging and Physical Activity, 13*(1), 61–74.

de Hartog, J. J., Boogaard, H., Nijland, H., & Hoek, G. (2010). Do the health benefits of cycling outweigh the risks? *Environmental Health Perspectives, 118*(8), 1109–1116. https://doi.org/10.1289/ehp.0901747.

Depp, C. A., & Jeste, D. V. (2006). Definitions and predictors of successful aging: A comprehensive review of larger quantitative studies. *American Journal of Geriatric Psychiatry, 14*(1), 6–20. https://doi.org/10.1097/01.JGP.0000192501.03069.bc.

Dickinson, A., Horton, K., Machen, I., Bunn, F., Cove, J., Jain, D., & Maddex, T. (2011). The role of health professionals in promoting the uptake of fall prevention interventions: A qualitative study of older people's views. *Age and Ageing, 40*(6), 724–730. https://doi.org/10.1093/ageing/afr111.

Farren, L., Belza, B., Allen, P., Brolliar, S., Brown, D. R., Cormier, M. L., et al. (2015). Mall walking program environments, features, and participants: A scoping review. *Preventing Chronic Disease, 12*, E129. https://doi.org/10.5888/pcd12.150027.

Fielding, R. A., LeBrasseur, N. K., Cuoco, A., Bean, J., Mizer, K., & Fiatarone Singh, M. A. (2002). High-velocity resistance training increases skeletal muscle peak power in older women. *Journal of the American Geriatrics Society, 50*(4), 655–662.

Folland, J. P., & Williams, A. G. (2007). The adaptations to strength training: Morphological and neurological contributions to increased strength. *Sports Medicine, 37*(2), 145–168.

Gillespie Lesley, D., Robertson, M. C., Gillespie William, J., Sherrington, C., Gates, S., Clemson Lindy, M., & Lamb Sarah, E. (2012). Interventions for preventing falls in older people living in the community. *The Cochrane Database of Systematic Reviews, 9*. Retrieved from http://onlinelibrary.wiley.com/doi/10.1002/14651858.CD007146.pub3/abstract. doi:https://doi.org/10.1002/14651858.CD007146.pub3.

Gothe, N. P., & McAuley, E. (2016). Yoga is as good as stretching-strengthening exercises in improving functional fitness outcomes: Results from a randomized controlled trial. *The Journals of Gerontology. Series A, Biological Sciences and Medical Science, 71*(3), 406–411. https://doi.org/10.1093/gerona/glv127.

Hackney, M. E., & Wolf, S. L. (2014). Impact of Tai Chi Chu'an practice on balance and mobility in older adults: An integrative review of 20 years of research. *Journal of Geriatric Physical Therapy, 37*(3), 127–135. https://doi.org/10.1519/JPT.0b013e3182abe784.

Helps, Y., Henley, G., & Harrison, J. (2008). Hospital separations due to traumatic brain injury, Australia 2004–s05. Injury research and statistics series no. 45. Cat. no. INJCAT 116. Canberra: AIHW. Retrieved from http://www.aihw.gov.au/publication-detail/?id=6442468147

Heywood, S., McClelland, J., Mentiplay, B., Geigle, P., Rahmann, A., & Clark, R. (2016). The effectiveness of aquatic exercise in improving lower limb strength in musculoskeletal conditions: A systematic review and meta-analysis. *Archives of Physical Medicine and Rehabilitation., 98*(1), 173–186. https://doi.org/10.1016/j.apmr.2016.08.472.

Hill, A.-M., Hoffmann, T., McPhail, S., Beer, C., Hill, K. D., Brauer, S. G., & Haines, T. P. (2011). Factors associated with older patients' engagement in exercise after hospital discharge. *Archives of Physical Medicine and Rehabilitation, 92*(9), 1395–1403. https://doi.org/10.1016/j.apmr.2011.04.009.

Howe, T. E., Rochester, L., Neil, F., Skelton, D. A., & Ballinger, C. (2011). Exercise for improving balance in older people. *The Cochrane Database of Systematic Reviews, 11* Retrieved from http://onlinelibrary.wiley.com/doi/10.1002/14651858.CD004963.pub3/abstract.

Hui, E., Chui, B. T., & Woo, J. (2009). Effects of dance on physical and psychological well-being in older persons. *Archives of Gerontology and Geriatrics, 49*(1), e45–e50. https://doi.org/10.1016/j.archger.2008.08.006.

Hwang, P. W., & Braun, K. L. (2015). The effectiveness of dance interventions to improve older adults' health: A systematic literature review. *Alternative Therapies in Health and Medicine, 21*(5), 64–70.

Kassavou, A., Turner, A., & French, D. P. (2013). Do interventions to promote walking in groups increase physical activity? A meta-analysis. *The International Journal of Behavioral Nutrition and Physical Activity, 10*, 18–18. https://doi.org/10.1186/1479-5868-10-18.

Keogh, J. W., Kilding, A., Pidgeon, P., Ashley, L., & Gillis, D. (2009). Physical benefits of dancing for healthy older adults: A review. *Journal of Aging and Physical Activity, 17*(4), 479–500.

Kerse, N., Elley, C. R., Robinson, E., & Arroll, B. (2005). Is physical activity counseling effective for older people? A cluster randomized, controlled trial in primary care. *Journal of the American Geriatrics Society, 53*(11), 1951–1956. https://doi.org/10.1111/j.1532-5415.2005.00466.x.

Korkiakangas, E. E., Alahuhta, M. A., Husman, P. M., Keinanen-Kiukaanniemi, S., Taanila, A. M., & Laitinen, J. H. (2011). Motivators and barriers to exercise among adults with a high risk of type 2 diabetes—A qualitative study. *Scandinavian Journal of Caring Sciences, 25*(1), 62–69. https://doi.org/10.1111/j.1471-6712.2010.00791.x.

Kraft, K. P., Steel, K. A., Macmillan, F., Olson, R., & Merom, D. (2015). Why few older adults participate in complex motor skills: A qualitative study of older adults' perceptions of difficulty and challenge. *BMC Public Health, 15*(1), 1186. https://doi.org/10.1186/s12889-015-2501-z.

Kreisfield, R., Newson, R., & AIHW National Injury Surveillance Unit. (2006). Hip fracture injuries. Cat. no. INJ 93. Retrieved from Canberra http://www.aihw.gov.au/publication-detail/?id=6442467915

Lee, D.-C. A., McDermott, F., Hoffmann, T., & Haines, T. P. (2013). 'They will tell me if there is a problem': Limited discussion between health professionals, older adults and their caregivers on falls prevention during and after hospitalization. *Health Education Research, 28*(6), 1051–1066. https://doi.org/10.1093/her/cyt091.

Lee, J. S., Kim, C. G., Seo, T. B., Kim, H. G., & Yoon, S. J. (2015). Effects of 8-week combined training on body composition, isokinetic strength, and cardiovascular disease risk factors in older women. *Aging Clinical and Experimental Research, 27*(2), 179–186. https://doi.org/10.1007/s40520-014-0257-4.

Lewis, C. B., & Bottomley, J. M. (2008). *Geriatric rehabilitation: A clinical approach*. Prentice Hall: Pearson.

Liu, C.-j., & Latham Nancy, K. (2009). Progressive resistance strength training for improving physical function in older adults. *The Cochrane Database of Systematic Reviews, 3*. Retrieved from http://onlinelibrary.wiley.com/doi/10.1002/14651858.CD002759.pub2/abstract. doi:https://doi.org/10.1002/14651858.CD002759.pub2.

Logghe, I. H., Verhagen, A. P., Rademaker, A. C., Zeeuwe, P. E., Bierma-Zeinstra, S. M., Van Rossum, E., et al. (2011). Explaining the ineffectiveness of a Tai Chi fall prevention training for community-living older people: A process evaluation alongside a randomized clinical trial (RCT). *Archives of Gerontology and Geriatrics, 52*(3), 357–362. https://doi.org/10.1016/j.archger.2010.05.013.

Loprinzi, P. D. (2015). Dose-response association of moderate-to-vigorous physical activity with cardiovascular biomarkers and all-cause mortality: Considerations by individual sports, exercise and recreational physical activities. *Preventive Medicine, 81*, 73–77. https://doi.org/10.1016/j.ypmed.2015.08.014.

Low, S., Ang, L. W., Goh, K. S., & Chew, S. K. (2009). A systematic review of the effectiveness of Tai Chi on fall reduction among the elderly. *Archives of Gerontology and Geriatrics, 48*(3), 325–331. https://doi.org/10.1016/j.archger.2008.02.018.

Martins, W. R., de Oliveira, R. J., Carvalho, R. S., de Oliveira Damasceno, V., da Silva, V. Z. M., & Silva, M. S. (2013). Elastic resistance training to increase muscle strength in elderly: A systematic review with meta-analysis. *Archives of Gerontology and Geriatrics, 57*(1), 8–15. https://doi.org/10.1016/j.archger.2013.03.002.

Mayer, F., Scharhag-Rosenberger, F., Carlsohn, A., Cassel, M., Müller, S., & Scharhag, J. (2011). The intensity and effects of strength training in the elderly. *Deutsches Ärzteblatt International, 108*(21), 359–364. https://doi.org/10.3238/arztebl.2011.0359.

McDermott, A. Y., & Mernitz, H. (2006). Exercise and older patients: Prescribing guidelines. *American Family Physician, 74*(3), 437–444.

McNeely, M. E., Duncan, R. P., & Earhart, G. M. (2015). Impacts of dance on non-motor symptoms, participation, and quality of life in Parkinson disease and healthy older adults. *Maturitas, 82*(4), 336–341. https://doi.org/10.1016/j.maturitas.2015.08.002.

McPhate, L., Simek, E. M., & Haines, T. P. (2013). Program-related factors are associated with adherence to group exercise interventions for the prevention of falls: A systematic review. *Journal of Physiotherapy, 59*(2), 81–92. https://doi.org/10.1016/s1836-9553(13)70160-7.

Michie, S., van Stralen, M. M., & West, R. (2011). The behaviour change wheel: A new method for characterising and designing behaviour change interventions. *Implementation Science, 6*, 42. https://doi.org/10.1186/1748-5908-6-42.

Michie, S., Richardson, M., Johnston, M., Abraham, C., Francis, J., Hardeman, W., et al. (2013). The behavior change technique taxonomy (v1) of 93 hierarchically clustered techniques: Building an international consensus for the reporting of behavior change interventions. *Annals of Behavioral Medicine, 46*(1), 81–95. https://doi.org/10.1007/s12160-013-9486-6.

Milat, A. J., Watson, W. L., Monger, C., Barr, M., Giffin, M., & Reid, M. (2011). Prevalence, circumstances and consequences of falls among community-dwelling older people: Results of the 2009 NSW falls prevention baseline survey. *N S W Public Health Bulletin, 22*(4), 43–48. https://doi.org/10.1071/NB10065.

Murtagh, E. M., Murphy, M. H., & Boone-Heinonen, J. (2010). Walking: The first steps in cardiovascular disease prevention. *Current Opinion in Cardiology, 25*(5), 490–496. https://doi.org/10.1097/HCO.0b013e32833ce972.

Nualnim, N., Parkhurst, K., Dhindsa, M., Tarumi, T., Vavrek, J., & Tanaka, H. (2012). Effects of swimming training on blood pressure and vascular function in adults >50 years of age. *American Journal of Cardiology, 109*(7), 1005–1010. https://doi.org/10.1016/j.amjcard.2011.11.029.

Oja, P., Titze, S., Bauman, A., de Geus, B., Krenn, P., Reger-Nash, B., & Kohlberger, T. (2011). Health benefits of cycling: A systematic review. *Scandinavian Journal of Medicine & Science in Sports, 21*(4), 496–509. https://doi.org/10.1111/j.1600-0838.2011.01299.x.

Orrow, G., Kinmonth, A. L., Sanderson, S., & Sutton, S. (2012). Effectiveness of physical activity promotion based in primary care: Systematic review and meta-analysis of randomised controlled trials. *BMJ, 344*, e1389. https://doi.org/10.1136/bmj.e1389.

Peel, N. M., McClure, R. J., & Bartlett, H. P. (2005). Behavioral determinants of healthy aging. *American Journal of Preventive Medicine, 28*(3), 298–304. https://doi.org/10.1016/j.amepre.2004.12.002.

Petrella, R. J., & Chudyk, A. (2008). Exercise prescription in the older athlete as it applies to muscle, tendon, and arthroplasty. *Clinical Journal of Sport Medicine, 18*(6), 522–530. https://doi.org/10.1097/JSM.0b013e3181862a5e.

Picorelli, A. M., Pereira, L. S., Pereira, D. S., Felicio, D., & Sherrington, C. (2014). Adherence to exercise programs for older people is influenced by program characteristics and personal factors: A systematic review. *Journal of Physiotherapy, 60*(3), 151–156. https://doi.org/10.1016/j.jphys.2014.06.012.

Podsiadlo, D., & Richardson, S. (1991). The timed "up & go": A test of basic functional mobility for frail elderly persons. *Journal of the American Geriatrics Society, 39*(2), 142–148.

Roh, S. Y. (2016). The effect of 12-week Pilates exercises on wellness in the elderly. *Journal of Exercise Rehabilitation, 12*(2), 119–123. https://doi.org/10.12965/jer.1632590.295.

Seguin, R., & Nelson, M. E. (2003). The benefits of strength training for older adults. *American Journal of Preventive Medicine, 25*(3), 141–149. https://doi.org/10.1016/S0749-3797(03)00177-6.

Seynnes, O., Fiatarone Singh, M. A., Hue, O., Pras, P., Legros, P., & Bernard, P. L. (2004). Physiological and functional responses to low-moderate versus high-intensity progressive resistance training in frail elders. *The Journals of Gerontology. Series A, Biological Sciences and Medical Sciences, 59*(5), 503–509.

Sherrington, C., Whitney, J. C., Lord, S. R., Herbert, R. D., Cumming, R. G., & Close, J. C. T. (2008). Effective exercise for the prevention of falls: A systematic review and meta-analysis. *Journal of the American Geriatrics Society, 56*(12), 2234–2243.

Simpson, M. E., Serdula, M., Galuska, D. A., Gillespie, C., Donehoo, R., Macera, C., & Mack, K. (2003). Walking trends among U.S. adults: The behavioral risk factor surveillance system, 1987–2000. *American Journal of Preventive Medicine, 25*(2), 95–100.

Snodgrass, S., Rivett, D. A., & Mackenzie, L. A. (2005). Perceptions of older people about falls injury prevention and physical activity. *Australasian Journal on Ageing, 24*(2), 114–118.

Steffen, T. M., Hacker, T. A., & Mollinger, L. (2002). Age- and gender-related test performance in community-dwelling elderly people: Six-minute walk test, berg balance scale, timed up & go test, and gait speeds. *Physical Therapy, 82*, 128–137.

Stewart, V. H., Saunders, D. H., & Greig, C. A. (2014). Responsiveness of muscle size and strength to physical training in very elderly people: A systematic review. *Scandinavian Journal of Medicine & Science in Sports, 24*(1), e1–10. https://doi.org/10.1111/sms.12123.

Strath, S. J., Swartz, A. M., & Cashin, S. E. (2009). Ambulatory physical activity profiles of older adults. *Journal of Aging and Physical Activity, 17*(1), 46–56.

Tanaka, H. (2009). Swimming exercise: Impact of aquatic exercise on cardiovascular health. *Sports Medicine, 39*(5), 377–387. https://doi.org/10.2165/00007256-200939050-00004.

Tiedemann, A., O'Rourke, S., Sesto, R., & Sherrington, C. (2013). A 12-week Iyengar yoga program improved balance and mobility in older community-dwelling people: A pilot randomized controlled trial. *The Journals of Gerontology. Series A, Biological Sciences and Medical Sciences, 68*(9), 1068–1075. https://doi.org/10.1093/gerona/glt087.

Titze, S., Merom, D., Rissel, C., & Bauman, A. (2014). Epidemiology of cycling for exercise, recreation or sport in Australia and its contribution to health-enhancing physical activity. *Journal of Science and Medicine in Sport, 17*(5), 485–490. https://doi.org/10.1016/j.jsams.2013.09.008.

Tolnai, N., Szabo, Z., Koteles, F., & Szabo, A. (2016). Physical and psychological benefits of once-a-week Pilates exercises in young sedentary women: A 10-week longitudinal study. *Physiology & Behavior, 163*, 211–218. https://doi.org/10.1016/j.physbeh.2016.05.025.

Townsend, N., Wickramasinghe, K., Williams, J., Bhatnagar, P., & Rayner, M. (2015). Physical activity statistics. Retrieved from London http://www.bhfactive.org.uk/

Tudor-Locke, C., Craig, C. L., Aoyagi, Y., Bell, R. C., Croteau, K. A., De Bourdeaudhuij, I., et al. (2011). How many steps/day are enough? For older adults and special populations. *International Journal of Behavioral Nutrition and Physical Activity, 8*(1), 80. https://doi.org/10.1186/1479-5868-8-80.

US Department of Health and Human Services. (2008). *Physical activity guidelines for Americans. Be active, healthy and happy!* Washington, DC. Accessed at https://health.gov/paguidelines/pdf/paguide.pdf

Vankova, H., Holmerova, I., Machacova, K., Volicer, L., Veleta, P., & Celko, A. M. (2014). The effect of dance on depressive symptoms in nursing home residents. *Journal of the American Medical Directors Association, 15*(8), 582–587. https://doi.org/10.1016/j.jamda.2014.04.013.

Watt, J. R., Franz, J. R., Jackson, K., Dicharry, J., Riley, P. O., & Kerrigan, D. C. (2010). A three-dimensional kinematic and kinetic comparison of overground and treadmill walking in healthy elderly subjects. *Clinical Biomechanics (Bristol, Avon), 25*(5), 444–449. https://doi.org/10.1016/j.clinbiomech.2009.09.002.

Wertman, A., Wister, A. V., & Mitchell, B. A. (2016). On and off the mat: Yoga experiences of middle-aged and older adults. *Canadian Journal on Aging, 35*(2), 190–205. https://doi.org/10.1017/s0714980816000155.

Wilhelm, M., Roskovensky, G., Emery, K., Manno, C., Valek, K., & Cook, C. (2012). Effect of resistance exercises on function in older adults with osteoporosis or osteopenia: A systematic review. *Physiotherapy Canada, 64*(4), 386–394. https://doi.org/10.3138/ptc.2011-31BH.

Wong, A. M. K., Chou, S.-W., Huang, S.-C., Lan, C., Chen, H.-C., Hong, W.-H., et al. (2011). Does different exercise have the same effect of health promotion for the elderly? Comparison of training-specific effect of Tai Chi and swimming on motor control. *Archives of Gerontology and Geriatrics, 53*(2), e133–e137. https://doi.org/10.1016/j.archger.2010.07.009.

Yang, H.-J., Chen, K.-M., Chen, M.-D., Wu, H.-C., Chang, W.-J., Wang, Y.-C., & Huang, H.-T. (2015). Applying the transtheoretical model to promote functional fitness of community older adults participating in elastic band exercises. *Journal of Advanced Nursing, 71*(10), 2338–2349. https://doi.org/10.1111/jan.12705.

7

Promotion of Physical Activity for Older People with Cardiorespiratory Conditions

Narelle S. Cox, Jennifer M. Patrick, and Anne E. Holland

7.1 Introduction

Identifying acceptable, accessible, and effective means to promote the uptake and maintenance of regular physical activity participation by people with chronic cardiorespiratory disease is an ongoing challenge for clinicians, researchers, and policy makers alike. With regular exercise and physical activity participation, older adults who have chronic respiratory or cardiovascular disease are able to achieve improvements in functional capacity and quality of life (QOL) and reduce morbidity and mortality (Garcia-Aymerich et al. 2006; Taylor et al. 2004). Yet despite these clinical and lifestyle benefits, older adults with chronic respiratory or cardiovascular disease are noticeably inactive compared to their well peers (Pitta et al. 2005; Troosters et al. 2010). In addition,

---

N. S. Cox (✉)
Physiotherapy, La Trobe University, Melbourne, VIC, Australia

Institute for Breathing and Sleep, Melbourne, VIC, Australia

J. M. Patrick
Cardiac Rehabilitation Unit, Caulfield Hospital, Alfred Health, Melbourne, VIC, Australia

A. E. Holland
Physiotherapy, La Trobe University, Melbourne, VIC, Australia

Institute for Breathing and Sleep, Melbourne, VIC, Australia

Physiotherapy, Alfred Health, Melbourne, VIC, Australia

people with cardiorespiratory disease are less likely to report participation in moderate-vigorous physical activity compared to healthy populations (Marcus et al. 2000). Such data indicate a need to develop effective interventions to encourage increased physical activity participation in this group. While strategies to promote physical activity participation in the general population have been widely applied, the variety of targeted approaches for enhancing physical activity participation by those with chronic cardiorespiratory conditions remains somewhat limited. In this chapter, we will discuss current approaches to physical activity promotion for older adults with chronic cardiorespiratory conditions, highlight some of the barriers and facilitators to regular activity participation experienced by these patients, and identify potential new strategies for increasing physical activity participation including the use of telemedicine applications.

7.2 Health Benefits of Physical Activity for People with Chronic Cardiac and Respiratory Disease

Hundreds of millions of people suffer from chronic respiratory and cardiac diseases worldwide (Ferkol and Schraufnagel 2014; WHO 2010). Cardiac and respiratory diseases, in particular coronary heart disease (CHD) and chronic obstructive pulmonary disease (COPD), comprise four of the top five leading causes of death globally (Lozano et al. 2013). Their treatment and management contributes substantially to annual healthcare expenditure (Poulos et al. 2014; Townsend et al. 2014). Both disease classifications are slowly progressive and characterised by functional impairment, exacerbations which may require hospitalisation, and symptoms of breathlessness (dyspnea) and fatigue (Troosters et al. 2004). While the underlying cause of functional limitation differs, with people with COPD experiencing ventilatory insufficiency and individuals with CHD demonstrating inadequate cardiac output, both disease groups exhibit impaired skeletal muscle function, which is an important contributor to lack of exercise and functional limitations in these individuals (Gosker et al. 2000). The likely causes of skeletal muscle dysfunction in COPD and CHD are multifactorial and described in detail elsewhere (Gosker et al. 2000; Wüst and Degens 2007). Regular physical activity participation, including exercise training for endurance and strength capacity, aid in achieving peripheral muscle adaptations that improve functional capacity and reduce disability (Gosker et al. 2000).

7.2.1 Physical Activity and Chronic Respiratory Disease

COPD is commonly seen in people over the age of 40 years, with cigarette smoking being the most common cause. Low levels of physical activity participation are associated with increased morbidity and mortality in a variety of populations with chronic respiratory disease but particularly in people with COPD (Garcia-Aymerich et al. 2006; Pitta et al. 2005). Despite exhibiting breathlessness on exertion, reduced exercise tolerance, and marked disability (Waschki et al. 2011), people with moderate-severe COPD are able to achieve improvements in their physical and emotional well-being through exercise training and increased physical activity participation. Higher levels of activity participation can also help to limit extrapulmonary disease manifestations, such as systemic inflammation and cardiac dysfunction, commonly seen in people with COPD (Hill et al. 2015). In a prospective observational cohort of 170 people with COPD assessing the prognostic value of physical activity on survival, an increase in daily energy expenditure attributable to physical activity approximately equivalent to walking at a steady pace for around 30 minutes (Ainsworth et al. 2011) was associated with a 54% lower risk of death (Waschki et al. 2011). Reduced risk of mortality has also been found at 5–8 years' follow-up in people who made small increases in their daily physical activity (Garcia-Rio et al. 2012). Further, a number of studies have shown that volume and intensity of walking each day diminishes with worsening respiratory disease (Jehn et al. 2011; Troosters et al. 2010), with patients with severe COPD undertaking as little as 20% of the amount of physical activity that is completed by their healthy peers (Troosters et al. 2010). This association between decreasing physical activity and increasing disease severity may also influence need for hospitalisation, with those people who have very low physical activity levels being more likely to be admitted to a hospital (Garcia-Aymerich et al. 2006) and risk of hospital readmission being greater in those with ongoing low activity levels following hospital discharge (Borges and Carvalho 2012). However, it is not just those with established disease who struggle to undertake physical activity. Marked physical inactivity has also been identified in current smokers prior to a diagnosis (Furlanetto et al. 2014) and in people with newly diagnosed COPD in the absence of exercise intolerance (Van Remoortel et al. 2013). This evidence demonstrates that people with COPD and those at risk of chronic respiratory disease face numerous, specific challenges when trying to overcome the vicious cycle of breathlessness and physical inactivity (Wilson et al. 2015).

7.2.2 Physical Activity and Chronic Cardiovascular Disease

Regular physical activity participation helps to prevent the development of chronic cardiac disease and heart failure and can reduce symptoms in those with established disease (Thompson et al. 2003). Avoiding prolonged bouts of physical inactivity is also crucial in preventing insulin resistance and the development of type 2 diabetes (Healy et al. 2008) which when combined pose significant risk factors for the development of cardiovascular disease. Through exercise training and increased habitual physical activity, individuals can improve the physiological function of the heart (Thompson et al. 2003), which in turn can promote increased mobility and walking distance, less breathlessness associated with heart failure, and enhanced QOL (Briffa et al. 2006). Greater physical activity participation also creates improved coronary risk profile—specifically improved blood pressure, cholesterol, and insulin resistance (Ekblom-Bak et al. 2014).

In a systematic review of 48 trials including 8940 participants, participation in regular exercise and physical activity was associated with a 20% decrease in all-cause mortality and 26% reduction in cardiac mortality, independent of the type of heart disease diagnosis (Taylor et al. 2004). However, the dose-response relationship between physical activity and mortality in those with CHD is less clear. Two studies that used self-report measures of physical activity participation, each with at least a ten-year follow-up, report greater risk of cardiac and all-cause mortality in those who never or rarely undertake physical activity compared to regular light or moderate physical activity two to four times per week, along with a slight increase in risk for those who undertook vigorous or daily physical activity (Mons et al. 2014; Wannamethee et al. 2000). It is worth noting that the risk of mortality in those who undertook daily vigorous physical activity remained substantially lower than those never active (Mons et al. 2014; Wannamethee et al. 2000). Whether the same result would hold true for objectively measured physical activity has not been explored. Regardless of physical activity intensity, the benefits of physical activity participation on health in cardiac disease are transient, with a regression in gains made when activity is ceased (Briffa et al. 2006). Finding effective ways to sustain physical activity participation in this group is essential to maintaining the associated health benefits (Hardcastle et al. 2015).

7.3 Strategies to Promote Physical Activity in Older People with Chronic Cardiac and Respiratory Disease

A number of recent systematic reviews have investigated the relative merits of different interventions aimed to increase physical activity participation in people with chronic disease (Ng et al. 2012; Wilson et al. 2015). Solid conclusions as to the most effective intervention strategy remain elusive due to heterogeneity of outcomes, small sample sizes, limited studies of robust design, and a lack of comprehensive reporting of the frequency, intensity, type, and duration of intervention strategies (Wilson et al. 2015). In addition, it is difficult to interpret the magnitude of effect of any given intervention as there is no one best method for measuring or reporting physical activity outcomes, and these are reported inconsistently across studies.

Common strategies investigated to date include face-to-face exercise training—most often in the form of structured exercise rehabilitation classes; physical activity counselling; the use of a physical activity diary, or internet-mediated delivery (Martin and Woods 2012; Wilson et al. 2015). These strategies will be discussed in the following sections.

7.3.1 Exercise Rehabilitation

Exercise rehabilitation programmes that are multidisciplinary and comprise supervised exercise, evaluation, education, and maintenance, which draw upon goal-setting and self-monitoring skills (see Chap. 14), and are designed to optimise physical and social functioning (Spruit et al. 2013) and encourage adoption and maintenance of healthy lifestyle behaviours (Balady et al. 2007), are strongly supported by evidence for individuals with either chronic respiratory or cardiac conditions (Anderson et al. 2016; McCarthy et al. 2015). Exercise training principles employed in such programmes do not differ from those for the general population (see Fig. 7.1) and include endurance training, interval training, and the performance of resistance training to improve skeletal muscle function, enhance exercise capacity, reduce symptoms, and improve health-related QOL (Spruit et al. 2013).

Exercise		Details	Precautions	Potential outcome measures
Aerobic	Pulmonary rehabilitation	• Walking (treadmill or land) or cycling (stationary) • ≥ 30 minutes, can be achieved in multiple bouts of shorter duration • Initial intensity: 70–80% max speed on 6MWT or 60% Wmax from CPET. Borg scale 3-4. • 3-5 times/week	• Oxygen desaturation <88% • Heart rate >150 beats/minute • Evidence of exacerbation eg. Increased breathlessness or cough; fever.	• 6MWT • Incremental shuttle walk test • Endurance shuttle walk test • CPET • Endurance cycle test
	Cardiac Rehabilitation	• Walking (treadmill or land) or cycling (stationary) • 30-60 minutes, can be achieved in multiple bouts of ≥ 10 mins duration • Initial intensity: 70-80% max speed on Incremental shuttle walk test or 40-70% of heart rate reserve/VO2 reserve/VO2 peak from CPET. Borg RPE 11-14 (CHF patients 9 –13) • ≥5 times/week	• Chest pain • Sternal precautions post surgery • SBP >180, DBP > 100 • Resting heart rate > 100 • Symptomatic low BP • New arrhythmia	• Incremental shuttle walk test • CPET • 6MWT
Resistance	Pulmonary rehabilitation	• Functional activities • ≥ 2 upper and lower limb exercises • 8-12 repetitions for 1-3 sets of each exercise • 2-3 times/week	• Upper limb /shoulder pathology • Neck pain • Balance issues	• Hand held dynamometry • Grocery shelving test • 30-second sit-to-stand test
	Cardiac Rehabilitation	• Functional activities • 8-10 exercises for major upper and lower limb muscle groups • 8-15 repetitions for 2-3 sets of each exercise. Borg RPE 11-15 • ≥ 2 -3 times/week • Heavy resistance training where indicated e.g. return to sport/manual labour	• Commence >4 weeks post sternotomy, monitor for sternal instability • Pacemaker and /or Defibrillator – no above shoulder exercises on affected side until > 6 weeks post implant. Also no across body exercises	• Hand held dynamometry

Fig. 7.1 Components of exercise training in pulmonary rehabilitation (PR) and cardiac rehabilitation (CR). *6MWT* 6-minute walk test, *Wmax* work rate maximum, *CHF* congestive heart failure, *CPET* cardiopulmonary exercise test, *DBP* diastolic blood pressure, *RPE* rate of perceived exertion, *SBP* systolic blood pressure, *VO₂* oxygen consumption. (Sources: The pulmonary rehabilitation toolkit. Alison J et al., The Pulmonary Rehabilitation Toolkit on behalf of The Australian Lung Foundation (2009) www.pulmonaryrehab.com.au; The heart education assessment rehabilitation toolkit. National Heart Foundation of Australia. www.heartonline.org.au)

7.3.2 Pulmonary Rehabilitation

The effectiveness of pulmonary rehabilitation (PR) programmes has been widely reported, particularly for people with COPD, but more recent publications have highlighted that it also has benefits for people with interstitial lung disease, bronchiectasis, and asthma (Spruit et al. 2013), and even individuals with severe disease can exercise at sufficient training intensity to achieve musculoskeletal and cardiorespiratory adaptations (Spruit et al. 2013). A systematic review of 65 randomised controlled trials (RCTs) (involving 3822 participants) found that PR programmes of at least four weeks' duration achieve clinically and statistically significant improvements in all domains of the Chronic Respiratory Questionnaire (CRQ) as well as all domains of the St George's Respiratory Questionnaire (SGRQ) (McCarthy et al. 2015). Pulmonary rehabilitation was demonstrated to achieve superior outcomes for exercise capacity compared to usual care; with a clinically significant treatment effect on a six-minute-walk test distance (McCarthy et al. 2015). The common exercise elements of PR are summarised in Fig. 7.1.

Despite the effectiveness of PR programmes, the positive effects of PR on exercise capacity and QOL have consistently been shown to diminish over the 12 months following programme completion (Griffiths et al. 2000; Spruit et al. 2004). Furthermore, improvements in exercise capacity have largely failed to translate into improvements in habitual physical activity participation in this population (Ng et al. 2012). A systematic review of seven exercise training trials (two randomised, five single group interventions) in people with COPD found improvement in physical activity post-intervention was equivalent to no more than five minutes of walking per day (Ng et al. 2012). It is unlikely that this magnitude of improvement is clinically meaningful. Whether this inability to improve daily activity participation is a shortcoming of PR programmes, which typically do not include targeted behavioural change components specifically focused on physical activity participation (Hill et al. 2015; Ng et al. 2012), or a function of other barriers to participation in PR (Keating et al. 2011) is not clear. Barriers to referral, uptake, and participation in PR mean that fewer than 5% of eligible individuals attend PR annually (Brooks et al. 2007); therefore, even if there are small gains to be made in physical activity participation as a result of PR, most people with COPD are not in a position to attain them as they never complete a PR programme. This indicates that other models of service delivery may be required to increase uptake of PR and improve the impact on physical activity participation.

7.3.3 Cardiac Rehabilitation

The World Health Organization has identified cardiac rehabilitation (CR) as crucial in combating the global burden of cardiovascular disease. For people who have experienced a MI (myocardial infarction), completion of CR is associated with a 25% decrease in mortality (Turk-Adawi et al. 2014), and there is some evidence of a survival benefit in those with heart failure (O'Connor et al. 2009). Despite the nature of their disease, there are very few risks associated with CR participation (Turk-Adawi et al. 2014). A large observational study of more than 25,000 individuals participating in a CR programme reported just one cardiac event from a combined total of 50,000 hours of exercise training (Pavy et al. 2006), demonstrating that CR is a safe environment for exercise participation after a cardiac event or for those with chronic heart disease. The common exercise elements of CR are summarised in Fig. 7.1.

Yet, in spite of the benefits and relatively low risks associated with CR, similar to PR, referral rates remain low (Aragam et al. 2015; Johnston et al. 2013), and attendance and adherence to programmes is hampered by patient barriers including travel and transportation (Daly et al. 2002; Keating et al. 2011). Like PR programmes, effective CR programmes have been extensively studied. A recent systematic review of 63 RCTs, representing nearly 15,000 people with CHD, identified a 26% reduction in risk of cardiovascular mortality, an 18% reduction in hospitalisation risk, and an improvement in QOL in individuals who undertook exercise training compared to no exercise controls (Anderson et al. 2016).

In addition to supervised exercise training, people who attend CR are also encouraged to undertake at least 30 minutes of light-to-moderate intensity exercise on days when they don't attend CR (Woodruffe et al. 2015). However, similar to patients with chronic respiratory disease, the translation of exercise capacity gains made during CR into improvements in daily physical activity is inconsistent. A study of people attending supervised exercise rehabilitation (cardiac or pulmonary) found a significant improvement in exercise capacity at the completion of rehabilitation, but no change in moderate-vigorous physical activity time (Ramadi et al. 2015). Similarly, Jones et al. (2007) found cardiac rehabilitation participants to be noticeably inactive on non-CR days and that the majority of participants were insufficiently active to achieve recommended weekly step-count targets, even when attending twice weekly supervised exercise training (Jones et al. 2007). This highlights that rehabilitation strategies in isolation may not be sufficient to ensure ongoing, increased physical activity participation.

7.4 Changing Physical Activity Behaviour

Developing and implementing interventions that produce a demonstrable and lasting effect on physical activity participation, and clinical outcomes, is a complex challenge for healthcare researchers and clinicians. Key elements identified as contributing to effective physical activity promotions strategies are the exclusive targeting of physical activity (Conn et al. 2008); use of behavioural strategies, such as feedback and goal-setting (Conn et al. 2008; Kosma et al. 2005); and the capacity for self-monitoring (Conn et al. 2008). At present, there are relatively few prospective, randomised trials of such interventions, in populations with chronic cardiac or respiratory disease.

A meta-analysis of 168 studies of strategies to promote physical activity participation in adults with chronic illness found that although individual study outcomes were variable, overall physical activity behaviour scores improved from baseline as a result of intervention with a mean effect of 48 minutes per week (945 steps/day) increase in physical activity participation (Conn et al. 2008). Supervised exercise was identified as the most common intervention strategy employed (54%) and typically involved two 1-hour training sessions per week for approximately 12 weeks (Conn et al. 2008). However, supervised exercise training was no more effective than those interventions that relied solely on education or motivation sessions (Conn et al. 2008). The most effective strategies for promoting physical activity participation were those that had a singular focus on physical activity behaviour compared to strategies that addressed multiple aims, for example, physical activity participation and weight loss (Conn et al. 2008). Behavioural strategies that encouraged self-monitoring and goal-setting were also beneficial (Conn et al. 2008).

7.4.1 Activity Counselling, Motivational Interviewing, and Individually Tailored Physical Activity Promotion

Physical activity promotion interventions that are individually tailored are proposed to have the greatest long-term carryover of physical activity behaviour change; however, available results are variable. A six-month individually tailored, home-based exercise programme for people with CHD, using a heart rate recorder, diary, and follow-up phone calls, improved participation in high-intensity physical activity and exercise capacity (Karjalainen et al. 2012). However, a lack of reporting of control group outcomes and no follow-up beyond the conclusion of the intervention period make it difficult to ascertain the long-term uptake of activity participation. The complex nature of behaviour change relative to physical activity participation, and the potential difficulties patients may experience in maintaining activity programmes over a prolonged period, highlight some of the challenges in improving physical activity participation in people with chronic disease. The need for adequate and sustainable staffing and equipment resources to implement individually tailored health promotion programmes has been identified as a potential impediment to the success of such programmes (Kahn et al. 2002). Further, staff may require additional training in techniques such as motivational interviewing or health coaching in order to implement the behavioural strategies required for these types of programmes. For people living with chronic cardiorespiratory disease, the apparent need for repeated episodes of intervention or ongoing contact (such as phone calls) to encourage maintenance of physical activity promotion strategies may contribute to an unacceptable increase in therapeutic burden.

7.4.2 Interventions Using Self-Monitoring Devices

The use of a low-cost, easy-to-use monitoring device (Richardson 2010), such as a pedometer, enables individuals to self-monitor and set goals. This kind of behavioural strategy for improving physical activity participation has been found to produce greater improvement in daily activity participation in older adults attending hospital outpatient clinics compared to control (mean difference 2491 steps/day 95%CI: 1098 to 3885 step) (Bravata et al. 2007), particularly when combined with a daily step count goal (No step goal: mean change in steps/day 686, 95%CI: 1621 to 2994 steps, $p = 0.6$; step goal: mean change in steps/day 2998, 95%CI: 1646 to 4350 steps, $p < 0.001$)(Bravata et al. 2007).

In a large study of older veterans with COPD, the use of a pedometer and a web portal for monitoring step-count goals, was effective in achieving a significant increase in daily step count from baseline when compared to control participants at 4-months follow-up (adjusted difference of 779 steps (95%CI 241 to 1317 steps); $p = 0.005$) (Moy et al. 2015). In a similar group of patients, a three-month individualised programme utilising pedometer, activity diary, and physical activity counselling resulted in significantly greater improvement in daily step count compared to a control group receiving activity counselling and diary (Mendoza et al. 2015). A six-week pedometer feedback and activity counselling intervention following CR has also been effective at improving total activity time and QOL at six months post-intervention (Butler et al. 2009). The usefulness of pedometers in encouraging increased walking raises the question of whether the increasing accessibility of wearable activity monitoring devices, for example, Fitbits®, may be useful in promoting activity participation in these patient groups. In addition, activity interventions that do not require attendance at a healthcare centre may have an increased likelihood of being effective given they negate the need for transportation to a facility.

7.5 Promoting Physical Activity Using Telemedicine Applications

The use of technology to deliver healthcare consultations and health-related education has become increasingly feasible with advances in technological applications, without concomitant increases in cost (Bashshur 1995; Wootton 1996). Technologically assisted healthcare delivery is proposed to have benefits in terms of addressing inequalities in healthcare distribution (Bashshur 1995), particularly to rural and remote regions, as well as reducing travel time for both patients and caregivers (Wootton 1996). However, perceived need by those accessing the service may be crucial to the success of such healthcare delivery methods.

In both the COPD and cardiovascular disease populations, the use of telematic applications has gone beyond assessment, monitoring, and consultation to delivery of treatment or therapy (Brooks 2011; Neubeck et al. 2009). Pulmonary rehabilitation has been successfully delivered into the home (Holland et al. 2013; Tousignant et al. 2012) and remote healthcare centres (Stickland et al. 2011) using telerehabilitation with positive outcomes for adherence, QOL, and exercise capacity (Holland et al. 2013; Stickland et al. 2011). Also, the opportunity for virtual peer-to-peer interaction between participants could be useful in providing a therapeutic social network for people who may otherwise be isolated in their homes due to immobility associated with severe disease (Keating et al. 2011). While the feasibility of delivering PR remotely using telerehabilitation has been established, none of the programmes to date have evaluated their impact on physical activity participation.

Whether exercise rehabilitation undertaken in familiar surroundings allows for better translation into ongoing physical activity participation is an area for future exploration. In addition, the ability to access suitable data network infrastructure could have implications for the availability and success of such programmes (Holland et al. 2013).

Whilst not offering the remote supervision incorporated into telerehabilitation programmes, web-based CR programmes have also been trialled in people with angina. In a randomised controlled trial of six weeks of web-based rehabilitation, including education content, an online diary, and the ability to utilise web-based communication with care providers, compared to GP usual care, significant improvements in physical activity (step count), QOL, and angina frequency were found for the treatment group at the end of the intervention period (Devi et al. 2014). However, only improvements in QOL and angina frequency remained evident at the six-month follow-up (Devi et al. 2014). This further demonstrates the difficulties in eliciting behaviour change regarding physical activity participation in people with chronic disease.

Mobile phones, coupled with a device capable of recording and transmitting electrocardiograph (ECG) data, have been used in an 8-week randomised trial of home tele-CR comprising a home-based walking programme ($n = 77$) compared to standard, outpatient (cycle-based) CR ($n = 75$) (Piotrowicz et al. 2010). Adherence was greater in the home-based tele-CR group, with the individuals who did not complete the standard, outpatient (cycle-based) CR programme citing insufficient financial means to attend, particularly with respect to paying for transportation (Piotrowicz et al. 2010). With fewer than 5% of eligible people receiving PR annually (Brooks et al. 2007), and less than half of eligible people taking up a place in CR (Townsend et al. 2014), alternative models to deliver PR and CR, as well as interventions specifically focused on physical activity promotion, are required to improve both equity of access and patient-related outcomes.

Mobile phones have been used to promote physical activity participation or deliver maintenance PR programmes to people with COPD, with inconsistent outcomes. A randomised controlled trial conducted in 48 patients with moderate-to-severe COPD used mobile phones to deliver pacing music of an individualised tempo to guide walking speed (Liu et al. 2008). Participants in the intervention group undertook baseline assessment of exercise capacity, lung capacity, and QOL, attended monthly appointments during the three-month intervention period, and tri-monthly review appointments during the nine-month self-management phase (Liu et al. 2008). At the end of the intervention period, and at one-year follow-up, the intervention group demonstrated significant improvements in QOL and incremental shuttle walk test (ISWT) distance compared to control participants (Liu et al. 2008). In contrast, at the end of the intervention period and at 1 year, the control group reported significantly greater breathlessness following ISWT and recorded significantly more hospitalisations (22 vs. 2; $p < 0.01$)(Liu et al. 2008). A second RCT of 34 people with COPD implemented a virtual "activity coach", comprising accelerometer and smartphone, along with a symptom diary accessible via web portal for a period of 4 weeks as compared to a usual care control group (Tabak et al. 2014). There was no significant effect on physical activity participation (daily step count) ($p = 0.4$) or health status as measured by the Clinical COPD Questionnaire (mean difference: intervention group -0.34 ± 0.55, control group 0.02 ± 0.57; $p = 0.104$) (Tabak et al. 2014). However, compliance with the use of the "activity coach" was high, with 86% of participants complying with prescribed activity monitor wear (Tabak et al. 2014). The differences in outcomes achieved between these two physical activity promotion studies may be a function of the shorter intervention period in the study by Tabak et al. (2014) (four weeks vs. three months followed by a nine-month self-management programme (Liu et al. 2008)). Additionally, participants in the usual care control group in the study of Tabak et al. (2014) may have received physiotherapy comprising weekly group exercise training as a part of their usual care. The number of control group participants who received this supervised exercise training is unknown, but it may have served to obscure differences between the intervention and control groups as a result of the intervention alone.

Two studies have tested the feasibility of mobile phone-mediated coaching or self-monitoring to promote ongoing physical activity participation following a course of PR (Barberan-Garcia et al. 2014; Nguyen et al. 2009). In a small study of 17 people with COPD, all participants received a pedometer and sent symptom and activity participation monitoring data to the research team (Nguyen et al. 2009). Participants randomised to the intervention group (coaching) received individualised, positive feedback in response to their activity participation reports, while participants in the control group (self-monitoring) received standardised text responses encouraging them to continue with daily data input (Nguyen et al. 2009). Over 6-months' follow-up, there was no difference between groups in terms of maximum workload achieved during incremental cycle ergometry, exercise capacity (6MWD), or QOL ($p > 0.05$) (Nguyen et al. 2009). There was, however, a significant increase in daily step count recorded by the self-monitoring group compared to the participants receiving mobile coaching ($p = 0.04$) (Nguyen et al. 2009), although the small group sizes (intervention ($n = 9$) and control ($n = 8$)) limit the applicability of this finding. The largest trial of mobile phone technology to address the long-term maintenance of exercise training gains achieved during PR was a non-randomised controlled trial undertaken in 154 patients across 3 European sites (Barberan-Garcia et al. 2014). Following an eight-week programme of PR, participants were assigned to either a telehealth intervention using a mobile phone with wireless pulse oximetry, thrice weekly SMS reminders, and web access to a "personal health folder", or usual care control group (Barberan-Garcia et al. 2014). Two of the three study sites found no effect for the telehealth intervention on the primary outcome of exercise capacity (6MWT) due to technological and local organisational issues (Barberan-Garcia et al. 2014). A single study site ($n = 77$) reported a significant improvement in exercise capacity at the 12-month follow-up for participants in the telehealth group as compared to the usual care control group ($p = 0.01$) (Barberan-Garcia et al. 2014), as well as significant improvements in the activity domain of the St George's Respiratory Questionnaire ($p < 0.01$) (Barberan-Garcia et al. 2014). These studies indicate that using mobile phones to deliver activity-based interventions are feasible and that greater effect may be associated with longer intervention periods. However, access to technological support may be necessary to ensure the success of such programmes. The use of mobile devices to encourage physical activity participation may be considered minimally intrusive and be an approach that has more appeal over time, as a progressively ageing population has greater experience and familiarity with such devices (Fig. 7.2).

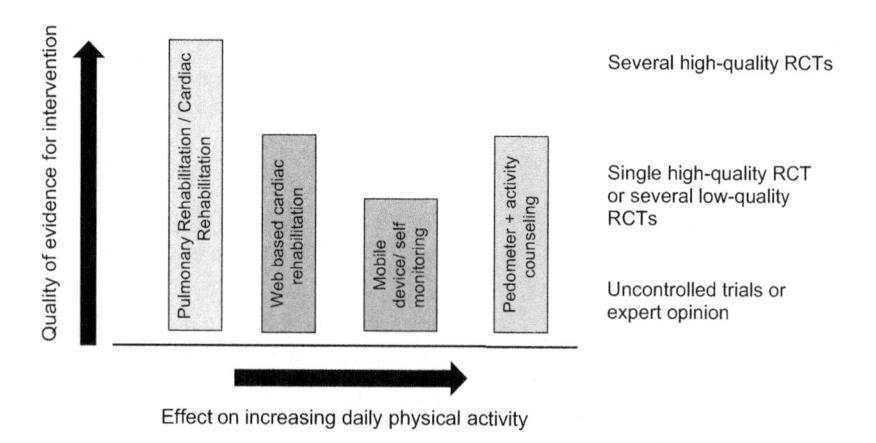

Fig. 7.2 Effect of interventions on increasing daily physical activity relative to quality of evidence

7.6 Implications

Participation in regular physical activity is a low-cost, effective strategy that produces meaningful health and patient-related outcomes for older people with chronic cardiorespiratory disease. However, accessing programmes and maintaining the gains achieved during supervised exercise programmes after completion remains challenging and their impact on physical activity participation on daily routines is limited. Identifying a suite of feasible, evidence-based methods to promote physical activity participation and address patient-related barriers to accessing both PR and CR are urgently needed. Accepting and implementing models of service delivery beyond traditional centre-based care, for example, home-based, self-monitored interventions are crucial to helping improve equity of access and service provision to older adults with chronic disease (Holland et al. 2017).

7.7 Conclusion

Presently, PR and CR programmes are the most effective means of improving functional capacity and QOL through exercise training and education in people with chronic cardiorespiratory disease. The use of mobile phone technology and other means of self-monitoring, particularly pedometers, provide accessible and promising means of supporting ongoing physical activity participation in this group.

Recommended Reading

- Ismail, H., McFarlane, J. R., Nojoumian, A. H., Dieberg, G., & Smart, N. A. (2013). Clinical outcomes and cardiovascular responses to different exercise training intensities in patients with heart failure: A systematic review and meta-analysis. *JACC: Heart Failure, 1*(6), 514–522. https://doi.org/10.1016/j.jchf.2013.08.006.
- Spruit, M. A., Singh, S. J., Garvey, C., ZuWallack, R., Nici, L., Rochester, C., et al. (2013). An official American Thoracic Society/European Respiratory Society statement: Key concepts and advances in pulmonary rehabilitation. *American Journal of Respiratory and Critical Care Medicine, 188*(8), e13–e64. https://doi.org/10.1164/rccm.201309-1634ST.

References

Ainsworth, B. E., Haskell, W. L., Herrmann, S. D., Bassett, D. R., Tudor-Locke, C., Greer, J. L., et al. (2011). 2011 compendium of physical activities: A second update of codes and MET values. *Medicine & Science in Sports & Exercise, 43*(8), 1575–1581.

Anderson, L., Thompson, D. R., Oldridge, N., Zwisler, A. D., Rees, K., Martin, N., & Taylor, R. S. (2016). Exercise-based cardiac rehabilitation for coronary heart disease. *Cochrane Database of Systematic Reviews*. https://doi.org/10.1002/14651858.CD001800.pub3.

Aragam, K. G., Dai, D., Neely, M. L., Bhatt, D. L., Roe, M. T., Rumsfeld, J. S., & Gurm, H. S. (2015). Gaps in referral to cardiac rehabilitation of patients undergoing percutaneous coronary intervention in the United States. *Journal of the American College of Cardiology, 65*(19), 2079–2088. https://doi.org/10.1016/j.jacc.2015.02.063.

Balady, G. J., Williams, M. A., Ades, P. A., Bittner, V., Comoss, P., Foody, J. M., et al. (2007). Core components of cardiac rehabilitation/secondary prevention programs: 2007 update: A scientific statement from the American Heart Association exercise, cardiac rehabilitation, and prevention committee, the council on clinical cardiology; the councils on cardiovascular nursing, epidemiology and prevention, and nutrition, physical activity, and metabolism; and the American Association of Cardiovascular and Pulmonary Rehabilitation. *Circulation, 115*(20), 2675–2682. Epub 2007 May 2618.

Barberan-Garcia, A., Vogiatzis, I., Solberg, H. S., Vilaró, J., Rodríguez, D. A., Garåsen, H. M., et al. (2014). Effects and barriers to deployment of telehealth wellness programs for chronic patients across 3 European countries. *Respiratory Medicine, 8*(4), 628–637. https://doi.org/10.1016/j.rmed.2013.12.006.

Bashshur, R. L. (1995). On the definition and evaluation of telemedicine. *Telemedicine Journal, 1*(1), 19–30.

Borges, R. C., & Carvalho, C. R. F. (2012). Physical activity in daily life in Brazilian COPD patients during and after exacerbation. *COPD: Journal of Chronic Obstructive Pulmonary Disease, 9*(6), 596–602. https://doi.org/10.3109/15412555.2012.705364.

Bravata, D. M., Smith-Spangler, C., Sundaram, V., Gienger, A. L., Lin, N., Lewis, R., et al. (2007). Using pedometers to increase physical activity and improve health: A systematic review. *JAMA, 298*(19), 2296–2304. https://doi.org/10.1001/jama.298.19.2296.

Briffa, T. G., Maiorana, A., Sheerin, N. J., Stubbs, A. G., Oldenburg, B. F., Sammel, N. L., & Allan, R. M. (2006). Physical activity for people with cardiovascular disease: Recommendations of the National Heart Foundation of Australia. *Medical Journal of Australia, 184*(2), 71–75.

Brooks, D. (2011). Telehealth technology: An emerging method of delivering pulmonary rehabilitation to patients with chronic obstructive pulmonary disease. *Canadian Respiratory Journal, 18*(4), 196.

Brooks, D., Sottana, R., Bell, B., Hanna, M., Laframboise, L., Selvanayagarajah, S., et al. (2007). Characterization of pulmonary rehabilitation programs in Canada in 2005. *Canadian Respiratory Journal: Journal of the Canadian Thoracic Society, 14*(2), 87–92.

Butler, L., Furber, S., Phongsavan, P., Mark, A., & Bauman, A. (2009). Effects of a pedometer-based intervention on physical activity levels after cardiac rehabilitation: A randomized controlled trial. *Journal of Cardiopulmonary Rehabilitation and Prevention, 29*(2), 105–114. https://doi.org/10.1097/HCR.0b013e31819a01ff.

Conn, V. S., Hafdahl, A. R., Brown, S. A., & Brown, L. M. (2008). Meta-analysis of patient education interventions to increase physical activity among chronically ill adults. *Patient Education and Counseling, 70*(2), 157–172.

Daly, J., Sindone, A. P., Thompson, D. R., Hancock, K., Chang, E., & Davidson, P. (2002). Barriers to participation in and adherence to cardiac rehabilitation programs: A critical literature review. *Progress in Cardiovascular Nursing, 17*(1), 8–17.

Devi, R., Powell, J., & Singh, S. (2014). A web-based program improves physical activity outcomes in a primary care angina population: Randomized controlled trial. *Journal of Medical Internet Research, 16*(9), e186. https://doi.org/10.2196/jmir.3340.

Ekblom-Bak, E., Ekblom, B., Vikstrom, M., de Faire, U., & Hellenius, M.-L. (2014). The importance of non-exercise physical activity for cardiovascular health and longevity. *British Journal of Sports Medicine, 48*, 233–238. https://doi.org/10.1136/bjsports-2012-092038.

Ferkol, T., & Schraufnagel, D. (2014). The global burden of respiratory disease. *Annals of the American Thoracic Society, 11*(3), 404–406. https://doi.org/10.1513/AnnalsATS.201311-405PS.

Furlanetto, K. C., Mantoani, L. C., Bisca, G., Morita, A. A., Zabatiero, J., Proenca, M., et al. (2014). Reduction of physical activity in daily life and its determinants in smokers without airflow obstruction. *Respirology, 19*(3), 369–375. https://doi.org/10.1111/resp.12236. Epub 12014 Feb 12232.

Garcia-Aymerich, J., Lange, P., Benet, M., Schnohr, P., & Anto, J. M. (2006). Regular physical activity reduces hospital admission and mortality in chronic obstructive pulmonary disease: A population based cohort study. *Thorax, 61*(9), 772–778.

Garcia-Rio, F., Rojo, B., Casitas, R., Lores, V., Madero, R., Romero, D., et al. (2012). Prognostic value of the objective measurement of daily physical activity in patients with COPD. *Chest, 142*(2), 338–346.

Gosker, H. R., Wouters, E., van der Vusse, G. J., & Schols, A. M. (2000). Skeletal muscle dysfunction in chronic obstructive pulmonary disease and chronic heart failure: Underlying mechanisms and therapy perspectives. *The American Journal of Clinical Nutrition, 71*, 1033–1047.

Griffiths, T. L., Burr, M. L., Campbell, I. A., Lewis-Jenkins, V., Mullins, J., Shiels, K., et al. (2000). Results at 1 year of outpatient multidisciplinary pulmonary rehabilitation: A randomised controlled trial. *Lancet, 355*, 362–368.

Hardcastle, S. J., McNamara, K., & Tritton, L. (2015). Using visual methods to understand physical activity maintenance following cardiac rehabilitation. *PLoS One, 10*(9), e0138218. https://doi.org/10.1371/journal.pone.0138218.

Healy, G. N., Wijndaele, K., Dunstan, D. W., Shaw, J. E., Salmon, J., Zimmet, P. Z., et al. (2008). Objectively measured sedentary time, physical activity and metabolic risk. *Diabetes Care, 31*(2), 369–371.

Hill, K., Gardiner, P. A., Cavalheri, V., Jenkins, S. C., & Healy, G. N. (2015). Physical activity and sedentary behaviour: Applying lessons to chronic obstructive pulmonary disease. *Internal Medicine Journal, 45*, 474–482.

Holland, A. E., Hill, C. J., Rochford, P., Fiore, J., Berlowitz, D. J., & McDonald, C. F. (2013). Telerehabilitation for people with chronic obstructive pulmonary disease: Feasibility of a simple, real time model of supervised exercise training. *Journal of Telemedicine and Telecare, 19*(4), 222–226. https://doi.org/10.1177/1357633X13487100.

Holland, A. E., Mahal, A., Hill, C. J., Lee, A. L., Burge, A. T., Cox, N. S., et al. (2017). Home-based rehabilitation for COPD using minimal resources: A randomised, controlled equivalence trial. *Thorax, 72*(1), 57–65.

Jehn, M., Schmidt-Trucksass, A., Meyer, A., Schindler, C., Tamm, M., & Stolz, D. (2011). Association of daily physical activity volume and intensity with COPD severity. *Respiratory Medicine, 105*(12), 1846–1852. https://doi.org/10.1016/j.rmed.2011.07.003.

Johnston, K. N., Young, M., Grimmer, K. A., Antic, R., & Frith, P. A. (2013). Barriers to, and facilitators for, referral to pulmonary rehabilitation in COPD patients from the perspective of Australian general practitioners: A qualitative study. *Primary Care Respiratory Journal, 22*, 319–324.

Jones, N. L., Schneider, P. L., Kaminsky, L. A., Riggin, K., & Taylor, A. M. (2007). An assessment of the total amount of physical activity of patients participating in a phase III cardiac rehabilitation program. *Journal of Cardiopulmonary Rehabilitation and Prevention, 27*(2), 81–85. https://doi.org/10.1097/01.hcr.0000265034.39404.07.

Kahn, E. B., Ramsey, L. T., Brownson, R. C., Heath, G. W., Howze, E. H., et al. (2002). The effectiveness of interventions to increase physical activity: A systematic review. *American Journal of Preventive Medicine, 22*(4S), 73–107.

Karjalainen, J. J., VKiviniemi, A. M., Hautala, A. J., Niva, J., Lepojarvi, S., Makikallio, T. H., et al. (2012). Effects of exercise prescription on daily physical activity and maximal exercise capacity in coronary artery disease patients with and without type 2 diabetes. *Clinical Physiology and Functional Imaging, 32*(6), 445–454.

Keating, A., Lee, A., & Holland, A. E. (2011). Lack of perceived benefit and inadequate transport influence uptake and completion of pulmonary rehabilitation in people with chronic obstructive pulmonary disease: A qualitative study. *Journal of Physiotherapy, 57*, 183–190.

Kosma, M., Cardinal, B. J., & McCubbin, J. A. (2005). A pilot study of a web-based physical activity motivational program for adults with physical disabilities. *Disability & Rehabilitation, 27*(23), 1435–1442. https://doi.org/10.1080/09638280500242713.

Liu, W. T., Wang, C. H., Lin, H. C., Lin, S. M., Lee, K. Y., Lo, Y. L., et al. (2008). Efficacy of a cell phone-based exercise programme for COPD. *European Respiratory Journal, 32*(3), 651–659.

Lozano, R., Naghavi, M., Foreman, K., Lim, S., Shibuya, K., Aboyans, V., et al. (2013). Global and regional mortality from 235 causes of death for 20 age groups in 1990 and 2010: A systematic analysis for the global burden of disease study 2010. *The Lancet, 380*(9859), 2095–2128.

Marcus, B. H., Forsyth, L. H., Stone, E. J., Dubbert, P. M., McKenzie, T. L., Dunn, A. L., et al. (2000). Physical activity behavior change: Issues in adoption and maintenance. *Health Psychology, 19*(1 Suppl), 32–41.

Martin, A. M., & Woods, C. B. (2012). What sustains long-term adherence to structured physical activity after a cardiac event? *Journal of Aging and Physical Activity, 20*, 135–147.

McCarthy, B., Casey, D., Devane, D., Murphy, K., Murphy, E., & Lacasse, Y. (2015). Pulmonary rehabilitation for chronic obstructive pulmonary disease. *Cochrane Database of Systematic Reviews*, CD003793.

Mendoza, L., Horta, P., Espinoza, J., Aguilera, M., Balmaceda, N., Castro, A., et al. (2015). Pedometers to enhance physical activity in COPD: A randomised controlled trial. *European Respiratory Journal, 45*, 347–354. https://doi.org/10.1183/09031936.00084514.

Mons, U., Hahmann, H., & Brenner, H. (2014). A reverse J-shaped association of leisure time physical activity with prognosis in patients with stable coronary heart disease: Evidence from a large cohort with repeated measurements. *Heart, 100*, 1043–1049.

Moy, M. L., Collins, R. J., Martinez, C. H., Kadri, R., Roman, P., Holleman, R. G., et al. (2015). An internet-mediated pedometer-based program improves health-related quality-of-life domains and daily step counts in COPD: A randomized controlled trial. *Chest, 148*(1), 128–137. https://doi.org/10.1378/chest.14-1466.

Neubeck, L., Redfern, J., Fernandez, R., Briffa, T., Bauman, A., & Freedman, S. B. (2009). Telehealth interventions for the secondary prevention of coronary heart disease: A systematic review. *European Journal of Cardiovascular Prevention & Rehabilitation, 16*(3), 281–289.

Ng, C. L. W., Mackney, J., Jenkins, S., & Hill, K. (2012). Does exercise training change physical activity in people with COPD? A systematic review and meta-analysis. *Chronic Respiratory Disease, 9*(1), 17–26. https://doi.org/10.1177/1479972311430335.

Nguyen, H. Q., Gill, D. P., Wolpin, S., Steele, B. G., & Benditt, J. O. (2009). Pilot study of a cell phone-based exercise persistence intervention post-rehabilitation for COPD. *International Journal of COPD, 4*, 301–313.

O'Connor, C. M., Whellan, D. J., Lee, K. L., Keteyian, S. J., Cooper, L. S., Ellis, S. J., et al. (2009). Efficacy and safety of exercise training in patients with chronic heart failure: HF-ACTION randomized controlled trial. *JAMA, 301*(14), 1439–1450. https://doi.org/10.1001/jama.2009.454.

Pavy, B., Iliou, M. C., Meurin, P., Tabet, J. Y., & Corone, S. (2006). Safety of exercise training for cardiac patients: Results of the French registry of complications during cardiac rehabilitation. *Archives of Internal Medicine, 166*, 2329–2334.

Piotrowicz, E., Baranowski, R., Bilinska, M., Stepnowska, M., Piotrowska, M., Wojcik, A., et al. (2010). A new model of home-based telemonitored cardiac rehabilitation in patients with heart failure: Effectiveness, quality of life, and adherence. *European Journal of Heart Failure, 12*, 164–171.

Pitta, F., Troosters, T., Spruit, M. A., Probst, V. S., Decramer, M., et al. (2005). Characteristics of physical activities in daily life in chronic obstructive pulmonary disease. *American Journal of Respiratory and Critical Care Medicine, 171*(9), 972–977.

Poulos, L. M., Correll, P. K., Toelle, B. G., Reddel, H. K., & Marks, G. B. (2014). *Lung disease in Australia*. Brisbane: Lung Foundation Australia.

Ramadi, A., Stickland, M. K., Rodgers, W., & Haennel, R. G. (2015). Impact of supervised exercise rehabilitation on daily physical activity of cardiopulmonary patients. *Heart & Lung, 44*, 9–14. https://doi.org/10.1016/j.hrtlng.2014.11.001.

Richardson, C. R. (2010). Objective monitoring and automated coaching: A powerful combination in physical activity interventions. *Physical Therapy Reviews, 15*(3), 154–162.

Spruit, M. A., Troosters, T., Trappenburg, J. C., Decramer, M., & Gosselink, R. (2004). Exercise training during rehabilitation of patients with COPD: A current perspective. *Patient Education and Counseling, 52*, 243–248.

Spruit, M. A., Singh, S. J., Garvey, C., ZuWallack, R., Nici, L., Rochester, C., et al. (2013). An official American Thoracic Society/European Respiratory Society statement: Key concepts and advances in pulmonary rehabilitation. *American Journal of Respiratory and Critical Care Medicine, 188*(8), e13–e64. https://doi.org/10.1164/rccm.201309-1634ST.

Stickland, M. K., Jourdain, T., Wong, E. Y. L., Rodgers, W. M., Jendzjowsky, N. G., & MacDonald, G. R. (2011). Using telehealth technology to deliver pulmonary rehabilitation to patients with chronic obstructive pulmonary disease. *Canadian Respiratory Journal, 18*(4), 216–220.

Tabak, M., et al. (2014). A telerehabilitation intervention for patients with chronic obstructive pulmonary disease: A randomized controlled pilot trial. *Clinical Rehabilitation, 28*(6), 582–591. https://doi.org/10.1177/0269215513512495. Epub 2013 Nov 29.

Taylor, R. S., Brown, A., Ebrahim, S., Jolliffe, J., Noorani, H., Rees, K., et al. (2004). Exercise-based rehabilitation for patients with coronary heart disease: Systematic review and meta-analysis of randomized controlled trials. *The American Journal of Medicine, 116*(10), 682–692. https://doi.org/10.1016/j.amjmed.2004.01.009.

Thompson, P. D., Buchner, D., Pina, I. L., Balady, G. J., Williams, M. A., Marcus, B. H., et al. (2003). Exercise and physical activity in the prevention and treatment of atherosclerotic cardiovascular disease: A statement from the council on clinical cardiology (subcommittee on exercise, rehabilitation, and prevention) and the council on nutrition, physical activity, and metabolism (subcommittee on physical activity). *Arteriosclerosis, Thrombosis, and Vascular Biology, 23*(8), e42–e49.

Tousignant, M., Marquis, N., Page, C., Imukuze, N., Metivier, A., St-Onge, V., et al. (2012). In-home telerehabilitation for older persons with chronic obstructive pulmonary disease: A pilot study. *International Journal of Telerehabilitation, 4*(1), 7–14.

Townsend, N., Williams, J., Bhatnagar, P., Wickramasinghe, K., & Raynor, M. (2014). In E. Dicks (Ed.), *Cardiovascular disease statistics 2014*. London: British Heart Foundation.

Troosters, T., Gosselink, R., & Decramer, M. (2004). Chronic obstructive pulmonary disease and chronic heart failure: Two muscle diseases? *Journal of Cardiopulmonary Rehabilitation, 24*, 137–145.

Troosters, T., Sciurba, F., Battaglia, S., Langer, D., Valluri, S. R., Martino, L., et al. (2010). Physical inactivity in patients with COPD, a controlled multi-center pilot-study. *Respiratory Medicine, 104*(7), 1005–1011. https://doi.org/10.1016/j.rmed.2010.01.012.

Turk-Adawi, K., Sarrafzadegan, N., & Grace, S. L. (2014). Global availability of cardiac rehabilitation. *Nature Reviews. Cardiology, 11*(10), 586–596. https://doi.org/10.1038/nrcardio.2014.98.

Van Remoortel, H., Hornikx, M., Demeyer, H., et al. (2013). Daily physical activity in subjects with newly diagnosed COPD. *Thorax, 68*, 962–963.

Wannamethee, S. G., Shaper, A. G., & Walker, M. (2000). Physical activity and mortality in older men with diagnosed coronary heart disease. *Circulation, 102*(12), 1358–1363.

Waschki, B., Kirsten, A., Holz, O., Muller, K.-C., Meyer, T., Watz, H., et al. (2011). Physical activity is the strongest predictor of all-cause mortality in patients with COPD: A prospective cohort study. *Chest, 140*(2), 331–342. https://doi.org/10.1378/chest.10-2521.

WHO. (2010). *Global status report on noncommunicable diseases*. Italy: WHO.

Wilson, J. J., O'Neill, B., Collins, E. G., & Bradley, J. (2015). Interventions to increase physical activity in patients with COPD: A comprehensive review. *COPD, 12*(3), 332–343. https://doi.org/10.3109/15412555.2014.948992.

Woodruffe, S., Neubeck, L., Clark, R. A., Gray, K., Ferry, C., Finan, J., et al. (2015). Australian cardiovascular health and rehabilitation association (ACRA) core components of cardiovascular disease secondary prevention and cardiac rehabilitation 2014. *Heart, Lung and Circulation, 24*(5), 430–441. https://doi.org/10.1016/j.hlc.2014.12.008.

Wootton, R. (1996). Telemedicine: A cautious welcome. *BMJ, 313*, 1375–1377.

Wüst, R. C. I., & Degens, H. (2007). Factors contributing to muscle wasting and dysfunction in COPD patients. *International Journal of Chronic Obstructive Pulmonary Disease, 2*(3), 289–300.

8

Promotion of Physical Activity for Older People with Neurological Conditions

Monica Rodrigues Perracini,
Sandra Maria Sbeghen Ferreira Freitas,
Raquel Simoni Pires, Janina Manzieri Prado Rico,
and Sandra Regina Alouche

8.1 Introduction

Older adults with neurological conditions may present with different levels of functional disability and deconditioning, which may result in low levels of physical activity (PA) and the adoption of sedentary behaviour over time (Benka Wallen et al. 2015; Moore et al. 2016a). However, despite the recognition of the benefits of PA in improving health and optimising function (Bauman et al. 2016), only about 30% of older people who have disabilities are engaged in PA programmes (Oguh et al. 2014).

Enhancing PA levels and decreasing sedentary behaviour may be particularly challenging for older people who suffer from neurological conditions. Usually, to a greater or lesser extent, these individuals experience a downward spiral of mobility disability, leading to low PA levels and increased sedentary behaviour (see Fig. 8.1). This scenario is commonly a consequence of the

---

M. R. Perracini (✉)
Master's and Doctoral Programs in Physical Therapy, Universidade Cidade de São Paulo, São Paulo, Brazil

Master's and Doctoral Programs in Gerontology, Universidade Estadual de Campinas, Campinas, Brazil

S. M. S. F. Freitas • R. S. Pires • J. M. P. Rico • S. R. Alouche
Master's and Doctoral Programs in Physical Therapy, Universidade Cidade de São Paulo, São Paulo, Brazil

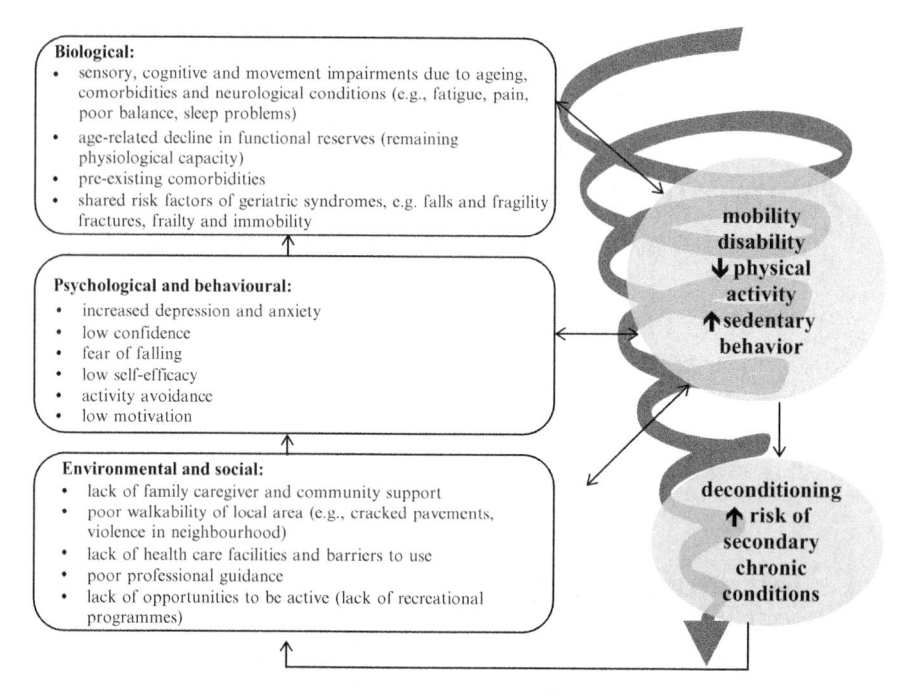

Fig. 8.1 Downward spiral of decreased physical activity and sedentary behaviour in older people with neurological conditions

negative and cumulative effect of the age-related changes in the physiological systems associated with impairments, either related to the neurological condition itself (Jones et al. 2012; Kunkel et al. 2015) or due to secondary chronic conditions such as obesity, depression, and physical inactivity (Paul et al. 2016; van Nimwegen et al. 2011). The difficulty in fulfilling family roles such as taking care of others and in maintaining work and social interactions might undermine an individual's experience of active ageing (Bauman et al. 2016).

Not surprisingly, many of these individuals may have difficulty incorporating PA into their daily activities, such as walking in the neighbourhood to go shopping instead of going by car, climbing stairs instead of using elevators, and helping with household tasks instead of depending on caregivers. As a consequence, their cardiovascular and neuromuscular systems often deteriorate (Tieges et al. 2015), leading to a vicious cycle of deconditioning, increased perceived physical effort needed to accomplish daily tasks, and personal discouragement about being active, which in turn may worsen overall conditioning (Anziska and Sternberg 2013). In particular, older adults with neurological conditions believe they should mainly increase their PA through exercise training, instead of by adopting a more active lifestyle (Koo et al. 2016). In this context, older adults perceive the lack of opportunities for and the inconvenience of using facilities and attending programmes, due to the individuals' poor physical function, as being important barriers (Koo et al. 2016).

Still, many factors contribute to the lack of recommendations and implementation of PA programmes for this population (Mulligan et al. 2012). Moreover, there is a gap in transferring the existing body of knowledge from evidence-based research to the effective implementation of PA programmes. In particular, many health care practitioners and patients have poor awareness about the effectiveness of PA in treating specific neurological conditions. In addition, health care professionals have insufficient training on evaluating and making appropriate prescriptions for exercise training and have limited experience regarding ongoing supervision and guidance (Billinger et al. 2014; Hoffmann et al. 2016).

8.2 Physical Activity and Neuroplasticity

Substantial evidence from basic research with animals (da Silva et al. 2016; Tennant et al. 2012) and from neuroimaging studies in humans (Heuninckx et al. 2005; Taniwaki et al. 2007) shows that PA promotes functional and structural adaptations in cognitive and motor pathways (Taniwaki et al. 2007), enhancing neuroplasticity (brain's capacity to change and adapt) both at old ages and following a brain lesion.

Treadmill training is one form of physical activity that has had a particular focus in literature seeking to understand the neurological impacts of physical activity. There is growing evidence to suggest that long-term treadmill training, generally based on 3 to 5 sessions per week for 4 or more weeks, lasting from 30 to 40 min, and of light-to-moderate intensity, results in motor improvement and the upregulation of neurotrophic factor expressions associated with an increase of the number of cells and with the process of creating functional neurons (neurogenesis) (Kim et al. 2004, 2010; van Praag et al. 2005) as well as preservation of neuronal structure and/or function and repair of neurological damage (Real et al. 2013; Tajiri et al. 2010; Tuon et al. 2012; Wu et al. 2011). In addition, aerobic exercise results in suppression of the programmed cell death (Kim et al. 2010), an increase in anti-inflammatory cytokine levels (e.g., preventing inflammatory process) (Gomes da Silva et al. 2013), and an increased vascularisation (Al-Jarrah et al. 2010; Wang et al. 2015). Finally, these effects induced by treadmill exercise have been shown to confer important structural protection against cognitive impairments (Al-Jarrah et al. 2010; Wang et al. 2015) due to the ability to maintain long-term potentiation, which is a critical physiological process involved in memory

Table 8.1 Exercise/PA recommendations for patients with neurological conditions

Type of exercise	Frequency	Duration	Intensity
Aerobic Large-muscle activities (e.g., walking, stationary cycle ergometry, treadmill, arm ergometry (arm cycle), functional activities)	3–4 days/week	20–60 min/session (or multiple 10-min sessions); 5–10 min of warm-up and cool-down activities; Neuromuscular diseases (NMD): 3–4 discontinuous trials with 15-min intervals	40–70% VO_2 reserve or heart rate (HR) reserve; 55–80% of max HR; NMD: Low intensity (e.g., 10 m distance) limited to 65% of VO_2 peak
Muscular strength/endurance Resistance training of upper and lower extremities and trunk using free weights, weight-bearing or partial weight-bearing activities, elastic bands, spring coils, pulleys Circuit training Functional mobility	2–3 days/week	1–3 sets of 10–15 repetitions of 8–10 exercises involving the major muscle groups	50–80% of 1 repetition maximum (RM); Resistance gradually increased over time as tolerance permits; NMD: Avoid eccentric contractions
Flexibility Stretching (trunk, upper and lower extremities)	2–3 days/week	Static stretches: Hold for 10–30 s; Before or after aerobic or strength training	Maintain stretch below discomfort; Within the normal range of movement
Neuromuscular Balance and coordination activities, tai chi, yoga Recreational activities Active-play video gaming and interactive computer games	2–3 days/week	Use as a complement to aerobic, muscular strength/endurance training, and stretching activities	Balance exercises should be of high intensity (progressively demanding)

consolidation. Table 8.1 summarises the recommendations regarding PA for older people with neurological conditions.

8.3 Stroke

After the first episode of stroke, a majority of survivors are physically inactive, and 40–60% of them engage in a range of sedentary behaviours (Baert et al. 2012; Butler and Evenson 2014; Kunkel et al. 2015; Moore et al. 2013;

Sjöholm et al. 2014; Tieges et al. 2015). Usually, stroke survivors spend 70–80% of their day engaged in sedentary behaviour (Sjöholm et al. 2014; Tieges et al. 2015). This scenario does not change within 3–12 months of the first stroke episode, independent of functional abilities (Moore et al. 2013; Tieges et al. 2015). Additionally, very little change in PA levels in stroke survivors was observed in the two or three years after a stroke. In a longitudinal study, in their third year after a stroke, the participants only spent 18% of their time standing, and only 10% was spent walking at a slow speed (5 steps/min) (Kunkel et al. 2015). Older stroke survivors are less active than older adults in general that spend around 20% of their non-sleeping time in low-light activities, such as walking (Arnardottir et al. 2013), suggesting that other factors other than age contribute to a low physical activity level in this population. Therefore, these individuals seem to reach a stable and very low PA level in a period up to 12 months after their stroke, but more longitudinal studies are needed to examine whether these improvements increase, decrease, or even stabilise thereafter, depending on the severity of neurological disease, functional ability, and other comorbidities.

PA programmes for stroke survivors should include regular aerobic exercise and strength and flexibility training (Billinger et al. 2014). The amount of PA recommended for this population is at least 40 min of moderate- to vigorous-intensity physical exercise 3 or 4 times a week (Kernan et al. 2014). The moderate-intensity exercises include activities such as walking briskly (three miles per hour), water aerobics, and bicycling (slower than ten miles per hour), while some examples of vigorous-intensity exercise include race walking, jogging, bicycling (ten miles per hour or faster), and aerobic dancing. The prescription of strength training should be cautious, including higher repetitions (10–15 repetitions) with reduced loads (Billinger et al. 2014). Furthermore, it is recommended that at the beginning of the PA programme, the exercise intensity should correspond to 40–50% of the patients' maximum heart rate (HR_{max}), with a progressive increment of 10% every four weeks up to 70–80% (Moore et al. 2016b).

An approach based on high-intensity aerobic treadmill exercise for stroke patients (60–80% of heart rate) (Gjellesvik et al. 2012; Globas et al. 2012) has been proposed as promoting significant effects on the cardiovascular system with increased oxygen consumption (measured by "peak VO_2") and decreased energetic cost during walking (Gjellesvik et al. 2012; Globas et al. 2012) to provide better physical fitness for stroke survivors, so that they can walk longer distances with less effort.

8.4 Parkinson's Disease

Parkinson's disease (PD) patients with mild to moderate disability present sedentary behaviour for 75–83% of the day (Benka Wallen et al. 2015; Jones et al. 2012). Regardless of the recommendations to be physically active, studies have shown that few PD individuals remain physically active through the years (Benka Wallen et al. 2015; Jones et al. 2012). However, despite the progression of the disease, PA has resulted in significant improvement in motor skills, functional mobility, and balance after a two-year PA intervention programme (Corcos et al. 2013).

Different types of exercise components have been recommended for PD, either as a single intervention or, more frequently, in combination. The most commonly recommended is treadmill training (Borrione et al. 2014; Earhart and Williams 2012; Frazzitta et al. 2015). Other exercise components include stretching exercises, aerobic and progressive resistance (Borrione et al. 2014; Corcos et al. 2013; Cruise et al. 2011), balance training (Frazzitta et al. 2015; Smania et al. 2010), and non-traditional approaches like tai chi (Li et al. 2012; Venglar 2013) and dancing (Duncan and Earhart 2012). Indeed, these interventions are effective in enhancing postural stability, increasing levels of confidence, facilitating postural transfers, and reducing the incidence of falls (Conradsson et al. 2015; Smania et al. 2010). In particular, treadmill training imposes a rhythm that reinforces the cyclic movement during walking, which contributes to minimising the inconsistency and variability of gait patterns (Frenkel-Toledo et al. 2005).

The prescription of progressive resistance training is also recommended to optimise motor skills and increase functional independence (Prodoehl et al. 2015). Moderately advanced PD individuals showed muscle adaptation to high-intensity exercise training involving strength, power, endurance, balance, and mobility functioning (Kelly et al. 2014). Evidence supports the recommendation of intensive resistance strength training with an intensity ranging from one to three sets of 5–20 repetitions at 40–80% of one-repetition maximum and shows that these interventions are feasible and safe. However, no effect has been observed for intensive endurance training (range of 60–90% of HR_{max}), and inconsistent results have been observed for balance and walking exercise programmes (Uhrbrand et al. 2015).

Exercise interventions targeting balance and mobility are very important to PD individuals to decrease the risk of falling and lessen the impact of movement dysfunctions (e.g., slow movement or bradykinesia, postural instability, and rigidity). Balance training is based on motor-learning principles (specificity, progression of level of difficulty, and variation), which involve the integration of sensorial cues and the adoption of different postural strategies (Conradsson et al. 2015; Smania et al. 2010). Virtual reality using exergames have been shown to be a very useful intervention to provide external cues and consequently facilitate movement and postural control in patients with PD (Gallagher et al. 2016).

8.5 Falls

Falls and fall-related injuries are strongly associated with age (Masud and Morris 2001). Around the world, between 20% and 45% of community-dwelling older individuals aged 60 and over fall each year (WHO 2007). About half of those who fall are recurrent fallers (two or more falls) (Masud and Morris 2001).

Falls are even more common among people with neurological-related disorders. Between 33% and 55% of stroke survivors fall within a year after their stroke (Ashburn et al. 2008; Nyberg and Gustafson 1995), and stroke survivors are more likely to fall recurrently than community-dwelling older adults (Mackintosh et al. 2005). Fall rates are substantially higher among PD individuals, of whom approximately 60% fall each year and 40% are recurrent fallers (Allen et al. 2013). Recurrent falls are very frequent even in PD individuals who are newly diagnosed and without previous falls, affecting 62% of them within 4 months of diagnosis (Lord et al. 2016).

Falls are a significant cause of injuries, fear, and loss of confidence, increased morbidity, restricted activities, institutionalisation, and mortality in all older people (WHO 2007) but particularly in those with neurological disorders (van Doorn et al. 2003). The risk of sustaining a hip fracture after a fall is doubled among older adults with Parkinson's disease (Benzinger et al. 2014) and tripled among those with dementia (Friedman et al. 2010).

For community-dwelling older adults in general, there is now substantial evidence that well-designed intervention strategies can reduce the risk of falls by around 30% (Gillespie et al. 2012). There is particularly strong evidence for the effectiveness of structured exercise in reducing falls among this population (Sherrington et al. 2011). The effects of exercise as a single intervention to prevent falls have been found to be similar to those of multifaceted interventions, therefore justifying the implementation of exercises as a fall-prevention strategy at the population level (Sherrington et al. 2011). A wide range of exercise programmes is available according to older people's abilities and limitations, and exercise should be prescribed based on the level of each person's capabilities and frailty status (Gillespie et al. 2012).

Overall, structured "multiple-component" exercise programmes delivered in a group or in a home-based format reduces falls among community-dwelling older adults by up to 42% (Gillespie et al. 2012). Different combinations of several exercise categories are included in multiple-component interventions, such as balance and gait, functional tasks, strength, flexibility, and endurance. The best exercise option to reduce falls is one that provides a high challenge to balance with a higher dose (more than 50 hours, which corresponds to at least 2 hours per week for 6 months) (Sherrington et al. 2011). However, most exercises that challenge balance need some degree of supervision, possibly making this particular recommendation not sustainable over time. Tai chi is a balance-based exercise that addresses key features to improve postural control and reduce falls, particularly among general populations of older people (excluding people in residential care facilities) (Gillespie et al. 2012) and among PD patients, such as weight shifting and ankle sway, changing the base of support, one-leg standing time, and training of rotational trunk movements with upright posture (Li et al. 2012).

There appear to be some populations where exercise programmes examined to date have not reduced the risk of falls, such as those who have recently been discharged from the hospital (Sherrington et al. 2014), older adults with severe visual impairment (Campbell et al. 2005), and long-term stroke survivors (Dean et al. 2012; Verheyden et al. 2013). Exercise interventions in these groups have resulted in enhanced mobility, but with no fall reduction. Particularly in the study with older adults recently discharged from hospital, the rate of falls increased in the group that received exercise as an intervention (Sherrington et al. 2014). During the rehabilitation process, some individuals increase their mobility skills and tend to rely more on their capabilities and adopt risk-taking behaviours during daily activities but lack good postural control to cope with highly demanding tasks, consequently increasing their risk of falling. This highlights the need for closer supervision and more intensive training associated with an educational programme for older people at high risk of falling (Sherrington et al. 2011).

Overall, the negative effects of inactivity and sedentary behaviour among older people as well as the well-known declining spiral that affects older people with activity avoidance induced by fear of falling make the recommendation of increasing physical activity levels to prevent falls in older people very plausible. However, increasing physical activity as a strategy to maintain or increase physical functioning and consequently prevent falls has not been formally investigated, and the poor quality of the available evidence limits this recommendation. Although walking is considered a natural exercise recommendation for older people, for the purpose of falls, prevention walking should only be prescribed as long as it is not at the expense of balance training. Walking training programmes being combined with balance training reduce their effect on fall prevention (Sherrington et al. 2011). Moreover, a 48-week walking programme was found to be ineffective in preventing falls in physically inactive older people (Voukelatos et al. 2015). Although brisk walking may enhance general fitness, it should be avoided for older people who are at high risk of falling (Sherrington and Tiedemann 2015; Sherrington et al. 2011).

8.6 Neuromuscular Diseases

Neuromuscular diseases (NMDs) are those hereditary and acquired diseases that affect the peripheral neuromuscular system, including those affecting the anterior horn cells of the spinal cord, peripheral nerves, neuromuscular junctions, and muscles. In particular, amyotrophic lateral sclerosis, post-polio syndrome, myasthenic syndrome in males, chronic idiopathic axonal polyneuropathy, and inclusion body myositis appear late in life and affect older people (Deenen et al. 2016). Primary patient impairments are a direct result of the pathophysiology of the diseases and are characterised by the progressive loss of muscle fibres, disuse, and overwork weakness. Concerns about muscle weakness, difficulties in exercising, and fatigue reduce PA and tend to increase the number of sedentary lifestyles. Other described factors that contribute to reduced PA in persons with NMDs include cardiopulmonary impairments; increased fat mass; abnormal shortening of muscle tissue (contractures); reduced mobility, motivation, and social reinforcement; and increased societal barriers (McDonald 2002). However, there is no evidence about the type, frequency, and intensity of exercise to be prescribed for dystrophies. Moderate-intensity strength training and aerobic exercise therapy show no harm in individuals with muscle disease, but there is insufficient evidence to conclude their benefits regarding muscle strength, aerobic capacity, pain, and fatigue (Voet et al. 2013).

Motor neuron diseases (MNDs) are neurodegenerative and progressive diseases with heterogeneous clinical manifestation but all involve the loss of upper and lower motor neurons. Structured exercise programmes may improve function and do not appear to be harmful (Simon et al. 2015). Specifically, in individuals with amyotrophic lateral sclerosis (ALS), stretching exercises can be used to maintain mobility by maintaining soft-tissue extensibility and preventing contractures, but no controlled studies are available to permit conclusions about its benefits. Moderate-intensity strengthening exercises can improve functioning and quality of life (for short-term or six-month-period comparisons), and aerobic and endurance exercises may be applied to patients with ALS even when respiratory insufficiency is present, with the support of non-invasive ventilation. All studies involving ALS are small due to its negative prognosis, leading to a premature death. But exercise seems to be more beneficial than harmful for these patients (Chen et al. 2008).

Peripheral neuropathies can compromise motor, sensory, or autonomic function or a combination of them according to the involvement of specific types of nerves. Neuropathic pain and loss of sensation often lead to tissue injuries and secondary complications like higher-impact forces on the foot joints, loss of joint alignment, and deformities besides skin ulcers. The most common peripheral neuropathy in older individuals, diabetic polyneuropathy, which is a progressive disability characterised by impaired balance, falls, skin injury, amputation, and pain, is a common consequence. Treadmill training improves vibration detection and nerve-conduction indices, and it also reduces pain interference in daily life activities, indicating benefits to peripheral nerve function. Although weight-bearing exercises have been previously discouraged to avoid foot skin injuries, there is currently evidence that these exercises are safe in individuals without foot deformities or vascular disease. Exercises do not increase fall incidence, pain, or neuropathic symptoms (Singleton et al. 2015).

In general, highly repetitive and heavy-resistance exercise can cause prolonged loss of muscle strength in weakened or denervated muscle. There is an abnormal balance between muscle injury and repair that could be harmful in patients with NMDs. Eccentric exercises (muscle contraction while it is lengthening under load) pose a risk of fibre damage (Anziska and Sternberg 2013). Muscle breakdown or cardiac events must be carefully monitored. Such complications are more frequent after eccentric exercise reaching the point of fatigue, which should be avoided (Moore et al. 2016a).

8.7 Implications for Practice

Clearly, the increase in PA levels is an important intervention that should be integrated into the whole pathway of care for older people with neurological conditions. Different programmes are to be delivered across all levels of health care and sites, including home-based exercises and exercises for older people living in long-term care facilities (WHO 2015). Particular attention should be given to those who become frail at some point during their life spans, since it is not uncommon that either older individuals themselves or their caregivers will believe that exercise is no longer suitable for their current functional status. Frail older people can benefit from PA programmes. Marked improvements have been observed from progressive resistance training and balance training in addition to aerobic exercises to address sarcopenia, immobility, and risk of falling. Furthermore, frailty should not be considered to be a contraindication to exercise (Bauman et al. 2016).

Prescriptions of PA to older people with neurological disorders will be better designed if based on a comprehensive geriatric assessment to accomplish specific needs, contraindications, and precautions regarding safety and monitoring of adverse outcomes as well as on individuals' and caregivers' preferences. Therefore, a comprehensive and behaviourally oriented PA programme should preferably be recommended by a multidisciplinary team and delivered using an older-person-centred and integrated care approach (Kernan et al. 2014; WHO 2015). Some older people will also benefit from the supervision of a physiotherapist or an occupational therapist to adapt the exercise practice to the individuals' capacities and disease progression and to facilitate their coping with the surrounding environment. Progressive increments in PA training are also recommended; otherwise, benefits will not occur. An emphasis on maximising function and on well-being and enabling autonomy may also ensure higher levels of adherence. However, one key action is to offer training to clinicians, rehabilitation professionals, and community health care providers about how to evaluate, prescribe, and deliver evidence-based PA programmes to this population (Anderson et al. 2017).

Research priorities should be driven to understand the best dose of exercise components, particularly balance and functional training exercises, along with the amount of exercise that should be recommended to avoid deconditioning without increasing the risk of falling. Furthermore, research in this area should incorporate more pragmatic clinical trials and assess the feasibility of delivering PA programmes in the community using different technologies, such as virtual reality, PA sensors, and mobile phone apps.

8.8 Conclusion

As the population ages, the prevalence of older people with neurological conditions who are increasingly physically inactive and have sedentary lifestyles is expected to increase worldwide. PA programmes are strongly recognised as a key intervention to overcome this scenario, yet they are generally under-prescribed. Evidence-based recommendations are available that should be tailored to older people's neurological conditions, needs, functional abilities, and preferences. However, the professionals involved in recommending and delivering PA must be well informed to overcome failures to implement sustainable PA programmes. Given the progression of the diseases and the secondary chronic conditions that may arise or preexist, PA programmes are to be of long duration and should be incorporated beyond the rehabilitation period, emphasising the need to implement behavioural and environmental strategies to encourage long-term adherence. In general, there is a lack of longitudinal studies to identify if an increase, stabilisation, or decrease in PA levels is related to the severity of the neurological disease, functional ability, or other comorbidities. Moreover, more research is needed to understand the interrelationships of the multifactorial nature of PA in this population regarding environmental and social barriers.

Suggested Further Reading

- Moore, G., Durstine, J., & Painter, P. (2016). *ACSM's exercise management for persons with chronic diseases and disabilities.* Champaign: Human Kinectics.
- Mackay-Lyons, M. (2013). *Cardiovascular and pulmonary system health in populations with neurological disorders.* In D. A. Umphred, R. T. Lazaro, M. L. Roller, G. U. Burton (Eds.), *Umphred neurological rehabilitation* (pp. 921–940). St. Louis: Elsevier Mosby.
- Hoffmann, T., Maher, C., Briffa, T., Sherrington, C., Bennell, K., Alison, J., et al. (2016). Prescribing exercise interventions for patients with chronic conditions. *The Canadian Medical Association Journal, 188*(7), 510–518. https://doi.org/10.1503/cmaj.150684.

References

Al-Jarrah, M., Jamous, M., Al Zailaey, K., & Bweir, S. O. (2010). Endurance exercise training promotes angiogenesis in the brain of chronic/progressive mouse model of Parkinson's disease. *NeuroRehabilitation, 26*(4), 369–373. https://doi.org/10.3233/NRE-2010-0574.

Allen, N., Schwarzel, A., & Canning, C. (2013). Recurrent falls in Parkinson's disease: A systematic review. *Parkinsons Disease, 2013*, 906274. https://doi.org/10.1155/2013/906274.

Anderson, C., Grant, R. L., & Hurley, M. V. (2017). Exercise facilities for neurologically disabled populations – Perceptions from the fitness industry. *Disability Health Journal, 10*(1), 157–162. https://doi.org/10.1016/j.dhjo.2016.09.006

Anziska, Y., & Sternberg, A. (2013). Exercise in neuromuscular disease. *Muscle & Nerve, 48*(1), 3–20. https://doi.org/10.1002/mus.23771.

Arnardottir, N. Y., Koster, A., Van Domelen, D. R., Brychta, R. J., Caserotti, P., Eiriksdottir, G., et al. (2013). Objective measurements of daily physical activity patterns and sedentary behaviour in older adults: Age, gene/environment susceptibility-Reykjavik study. *Age and Ageing, 42*(2), 222–229. https://doi.org/10.1093/ageing/afs160.

Ashburn, A., Hyndman, D., Pickering, R., Yardley, L., & Harris, S. (2008). Predicting people with stroke at risk of falls. *Age and Ageing, 37*(3), 270–276. https://doi.org/10.1093/ageing/afn066.

Baert, I., Feys, H., Daly, D., Troosters, T., & Vanlandewijck, Y. (2012). Are patients 1 year post-stroke active enough to improve their physical health? *Disability and Rehabilitation, 34*(7), 574–580. https://doi.org/10.3109/09638288.2011.613513.

Bauman, A., Merom, D., Bull, F., Buchner, D., & Fiatarone Singh, M. (2016). Updating the evidence for physical activity: Summative reviews of the epidemiological evidence, prevalence, and interventions to promote "active aging". *The Gerontologist, 56*(Suppl 2), S268–S280. https://doi.org/10.1093/geront/gnw031.

Benka Wallen, M., Franzen, E., Nero, H., & Hagstromer, M. (2015). Levels and patterns of physical activity and sedentary behavior in elderly people with mild to moderate Parkinson disease. *Physical Therapy, 95*(8), 1135–1141. https://doi.org/10.2522/ptj.20140374.

Benzinger, P., Rapp, K., Maetzler, W., Konig, H., Jaensch, A., Klenk, J., & Buchele, G. (2014). Risk for femoral fractures in Parkinson's disease patients with and without severe functional impairment. *PLoS One, 9*(5), e97073. https://doi.org/10.1371/journal.pone.0097073.

Billinger, S., Arena, R., Bernhardt, J., Eng, J., Franklin, B., Johnson, C., et al. (2014). Physical activity and exercise recommendations for stroke survivors: A statement for healthcare professionals from the American Heart Association/American Stroke Association. *Stroke, 45*(8), 2532–2553. https://doi.org/10.1161/STR.0000000000000022.

Borrione, P., Tranchita, E., Sansone, P., & Parisi, A. (2014). Effects of physical activity in Parkinson's disease: A new tool for rehabilitation. *World Journal of Methodology, 4*(3), 133–143. https://doi.org/10.5662/wjm.v4.i3.133.

Butler, E. N., & Evenson, K. R. (2014). Prevalence of physical activity and sedentary behavior among stroke survivors in the United States. *Top Stroke Rehabilitation, 21*(3), 246–255. https://doi.org/10.1310/tsr2103-246.

Campbell, A. J., Robertson, M. C., La Grow, S. J., Kerse, N. M., Sanderson, G. F., Jacobs, R. J., et al. (2005). Randomised controlled trial of prevention of falls in people aged > or =75 with severe visual impairment: The VIP trial. *The British Medical Journal, 331*(7520), 817. https://doi.org/10.1136/bmj.38601.447731.55.

Chen, A., Montes, J., & Mitsumoto, H. (2008). The role of exercise in amyotrophic lateral sclerosis. *Physical Medicine and Rehabilitation Clinics of North America, 19*(3), 545–557, ix–x. doi:https://doi.org/10.1016/j.pmr.2008.02.003.

Conradsson, D., Lofgren, N., Nero, H., Hagstromer, M., Stahle, A., Lokk, J., & Franzen, E. (2015). The effects of highly challenging balance training in elderly with Parkinson's disease: A randomized controlled trial. *Neurorehabilitation and Neural Repair, 29*(9), 827–836. https://doi.org/10.1177/1545968314567150.

Corcos, D. M., Robichaud, J. A., David, F. J., Leurgans, S. E., Vaillancourt, D. E., Poon, C., et al. (2013). A two-year randomized controlled trial of progressive resistance exercise for Parkinson's disease. *Movement Disorders, 28*(9), 1230–1240. https://doi.org/10.1002/mds.25380.

Cruise, K. E., Bucks, R. S., Loftus, A. M., Newton, R. U., Pegoraro, R., & Thomas, M. G. (2011). Exercise and Parkinson's: Benefits for cognition and quality of life. *Acta Neurologica Scandinavica, 123*(1), 13–19. https://doi.org/10.1111/j.1600-0404.2010.01338.x.

da Silva, P. G. C., Domingues, D. D., de Carvalho, L. A., Allodi, A., & Correa, C. L. (2016). Neurotrophic factors in Parkinson's disease are regulated by exercise: Evidence-based practice. *Journal of the Neurological Sciences, 363*, 5–15.

Dean, C., Rissel, C., Sherrington, C., Sharkey, M., Cumming, R., Lord, S., et al. (2012). Exercise to enhance mobility and prevent falls after stroke: The community stroke club randomized trial. *Neurorehabilitation and Neural Repair, 26*(9), 1046–1057. https://doi.org/10.1177/1545968312441711.

Deenen, J. C., van Doorn, P. A., Faber, C. G., van der Kooi, A. J., Kuks, J. B., Notermans, N. C., et al. (2016). The epidemiology of neuromuscular disorders: Age at onset and gender in the Netherlands. *Neuromusculae Disorders, 26*(7), 447–452. https://doi.org/10.1016/j.nmd.2016.04.011.

Duncan, R. P., & Earhart, G. M. (2012). Randomized controlled trial of community-based dancing to modify disease progression in Parkinson disease. *Neurorehabilitation and Neural Repair, 26*(2), 132–143. https://doi.org/10.1177/1545968311421614.

Earhart, G. M., & Williams, A. J. (2012). Treadmill training for individuals with Parkinson disease. *Physical Therapy, 92*(7), 893–897. https://doi.org/10.2522/ptj.20110471.

Frazzitta, G., Maestri, R., Bertotti, G., Riboldazzi, G., Boveri, N., Perini, M., et al. (2015). Intensive rehabilitation treatment in early Parkinson's disease: A randomized pilot study with a 2-year follow-up. *Neurorehabilitation and Neural Repair, 29*(2), 123–131. https://doi.org/10.1177/1545968314542981.

Frenkel-Toledo, S., Giladi, N., Peretz, C., Herman, T., Gruendlinger, L., & Hausdorff, J. M. (2005). Treadmill walking as an external pacemaker to improve gait rhythm and stability in Parkinson's disease. *Movement Disorders, 20*(9), 1109–1114. https://doi.org/10.1002/mds.20507.

Friedman, S., Menzies, I., Bukata, S., Mendelson, D., & Kates, S. (2010). Dementia and hip fractures: Development of a pathogenic framework for understanding and studying risk. *Geriatric Orthopaedic Surgery & Rehabilitation, 1*(2), 52–62. https://doi.org/10.1177/2151458510389463.

Gallagher, R., Damodaran, H., Werner, W. G., Powell, W., & Deutsch, J. E. (2016). Auditory and visual cueing modulate cycling speed of older adults and persons with Parkinson's disease in a virtual cycling (V-cycle) system. *Journal of Neuroengineering and Rehabilitation, 13*(1), 77. https://doi.org/10.1186/s12984-016-0184-z.

Gillespie, L., Robertson, M., Gillespie, W., Sherrington, C., Gates, S., Clemson, L., & Lamb, S. (2012). Interventions for preventing falls in older people living in the community. *The Cochrane Database of Systematic Reviews, 9*, 7146. https://doi.org/10.1002/14651858.CD007146.pub3.

Gjellesvik, T. I., Brurok, B., Hoff, J., Torhaug, T., & Helgerud, J. (2012). Effect of high aerobic intensity interval treadmill walking in people with chronic stroke: A pilot study with one year follow-up. *Top Stroke Rehabilitation, 19*(4), 353–360. https://doi.org/10.1310/tsr1904-353.

Globas, C., Becker, C., Cerny, J., Lam, J. M., Lindemann, U., Forrester, L. W., et al. (2012). Chronic stroke survivors benefit from high-intensity aerobic treadmill exercise: A randomized control trial. *Neurorehabilitation and Neural Repair, 26*(1), 85–95. https://doi.org/10.1177/1545968311418675.

Gomes da Silva, S., Simoes, P., Mortara, R., Scorza, F., Cavalheiro, E., da Graca Naffah-Mazzacoratti, M., & Arida, R. (2013). Exercise-induced hippocampal anti-inflammatory response in aged rats. *Journal of Neuroinflammation, 10*, 61. https://doi.org/10.1186/1742-2094-10-61.

Heuninckx, S., Wenderoth, N., Debaere, F., Peeters, R., & Swinnen, S. P. (2005). Neural basis of aging: The penetration of cognition into action control. *Journal of Neuroscience, 25*(29), 6787–6796. https://doi.org/10.1523/JNEUROSCI.1263-05.2005.

Hoffmann, T., Maher, C., Briffa, T., Sherrington, C., Bennell, K., Alison, J., et al. (2016). Prescribing exercise interventions for patients with chronic conditions. *The Canadian Medical Association Journal, 188*(7), 510–518. https://doi.org/10.1503/cmaj.150684.

Jones, C., Wieler, M., Carvajal, J., Lawrence, L., & Haennel, R. (2012). Physical activity in persons with Parkinson disease: A feasibility study. *Health, 04*(11), 1145–1152. https://doi.org/10.4236/health.2012.431173.

Kelly, N. A., Ford, M. P., Standaert, D. G., Watts, R. L., Bickel, C. S., Moellering, D. R., et al. (2014). Novel, high-intensity exercise prescription improves muscle mass, mitochondrial function, and physical capacity in individuals with Parkinson's disease. *Journal of Applied Physiology, 116*(5), 582–592. https://doi.org/10.1152/japplphysiol.01277.2013.

Kernan, W. N., Ovbiagele, B., Black, H. R., Bravata, D. M., Chimowitz, M. I., Ezekowitz, M. D., et al. (2014). Guidelines for the prevention of stroke in patients with stroke and transient ischemic attack: A guideline for healthcare professionals from the American Heart Association/American Stroke Association. *Stroke, 45*(7), 2160–2236. https://doi.org/10.1161/STR.0000000000000024.

Kim, Y., Kim, H., Shin, M., Chang, H., Jang, M., Shin, M., et al. (2004). Age-dependence of the effect of treadmill exercise on cell proliferation in the dentate gyrus of rats. *Neuroscience Letters, 355*(1–2), 152–154.

Kim, S., Ko, I., Kim, B., Shin, M., Cho, S., Kim, C., et al. (2010). Treadmill exercise prevents aging-induced failure of memory through an increase in neurogenesis and suppression of apoptosis in rat hippocampus. *Experimental Gerontology, 45*(5), 357–365. https://doi.org/10.1016/j.exger.2010.02.005.

Koo, K., Kim, C., Park, C., Byeun, J., & Seo, G. (2016). Restrictions of physical activity participation in older adults with disability: Employing keyword network analysis. *Journal of Exercise & Rehabilitation, 12*(4), 373–378. https://doi.org/10.12965/jer.1632690.345.

Kunkel, D., Fitton, C., Burnett, M., & Ashburn, A. (2015). Physical inactivity post-stroke: A 3-year longitudinal study. *Disability and Rehabilitation, 37*(4), 304–310. https://doi.org/10.3109/09638288.2014.918190.

Li, F., Harmer, P., Fitzgerald, K., Eckstrom, E., Stock, R., Galver, J., et al. (2012). Tai chi and postural stability in patients with Parkinson's disease. *The New England Journal of Medicine, 366*(6), 511–519. https://doi.org/10.1056/NEJMoa1107911.

Lord, S., Galna, B., Yarnall, A., Coleman, S., Burn, D., & Rochester, L. (2016). Predicting first fall in newly diagnosed Parkinson's disease: Insights from a fall-naive cohort. *Movement Disorders Journal, 31*(12), 1829–1836. https://doi.org/10.1002/mds.26742

Mackintosh, S., Goldie, P., & Hill, K. (2005). Falls incidence and factors associated with falling in older, community-dwelling, chronic stroke survivors (>1 year after stroke) and matched controls. *Aging Clinical Experimental Research, 17*(2), 74–81.

Masud, T., & Morris, R. (2001). Epidemiology of falls. *Age and Ageing, 30*(Suppl 4), 3–7.

McDonald, C. (2002). Physical activity, health impairments, and disability in neuromuscular disease. *American Journal of Physical Medicine & Rehabilitation, 81*(11 Suppl), S108–S120. https://doi.org/10.1097/01.PHM.0000029767.43578.3C.

Moore, S., Hallsworth, K., Plotz, T., Ford, G., Rochester, L., & Trenell, M. (2013). Physical activity, sedentary behaviour and metabolic control following stroke: A cross-sectional and longitudinal study. *PLoS One, 8*(1), e55263. https://doi.org/10.1371/journal.pone.0055263.

Moore, G., Durstine, J., & Painter, P. (2016a). *ACSM's exercise management for persons with chronic diseases and disabilities*. Champaign: Human Kinetics.

Moore, S. A., Jakovljevic, D. G., Ford, G. A., Rochester, L., & Trenell, M. I. (2016b). Exercise induces peripheral muscle but not cardiac adaptations after stroke: A randomized controlled pilot trial. *Archives of Physical Medicine & Rehabilitation, 97*(4), 596–603. https://doi.org/10.1016/j.apmr.2015.12.018.

Mulligan, H., Hale, L., Whitehead, L., & Baxter, G. (2012). Barriers to physical activity for people with long-term neurological conditions: A review study. *Adapted Physical Activity Quarterly, 29*(3), 243–265.

Nyberg, L., & Gustafson, Y. (1995). Patient falls in stroke rehabilitation. A challenge to rehabilitation strategies. *Stroke, 26*(5), 838–842.

Oguh, O., Eisenstein, A., Kwasny, M., & Simuni, T. (2014). Back to the basics: Regular exercise matters in Parkinson's disease: Results from the National Parkinson Foundation QII registry study. *Parkinsonism Related Disorders, 20*(11), 1221–1225. https://doi.org/10.1016/j.parkreldis.2014.09.008.

Paul, L., Brewster, S., Wyke, S., Gill, J., Alexander, G., Dybus, A., & Rafferty, D. (2016). Physical activity profiles and sedentary behaviour in people following stroke: A cross-sectional study. *Disability and Rehabilitation, 38*(4), 362–367. https://doi.org/10.3109/09638288.2015.1041615.

Prodoehl, J., Rafferty, M. R., David, F. J., Poon, C., Vaillancourt, D. E., Comella, C. L., et al. (2015). Two-year exercise program improves physical function in Parkinson's disease: The PRET-PD randomized clinical trial. *Neurorehabilitation and Neural Repair, 29*(2), 112–122. https://doi.org/10.1177/1545968314539732.

Real, C. C., Ferreira, A. F., Chaves-Kirsten, G. P., Torrao, A. S., Pires, R. S., & Britto, L. R. (2013). BDNF receptor blockade hinders the beneficial effects of exercise in a rat model of Parkinson's disease. *Neuroscience, 237*, 118–129. https://doi.org/10.1016/j.neuroscience.2013.01.060.

Sherrington, C., & Tiedemann, A. (2015). Physiotherapy in the prevention of falls in older people. *Journal of Physiotherapy, 61*(2), 54–60. https://doi.org/10.1016/j.jphys.2015.02.011.

Sherrington, C., Tiedemann, A., Fairhall, N., Close, J., & Lord, S. (2011). Exercise to prevent falls in older adults: An updated meta-analysis and best practice recommendations. *New South Wales Public Health Bulletin, 22*(3–4), 78–83. https://doi.org/10.1071/NB10056.

Sherrington, C., Lord, S., Vogler, C., Close, J., Howard, K., Dean, C., et al. (2014). A post-hospital home exercise program improved mobility but increased falls in older people: A randomised controlled trial. *PLoS One, 9*(9), e104412. https://doi.org/10.1371/journal.pone.0104412.

Simon, N., Huynh, W., Vucic, S., Talbot, K., & Kiernan, M. (2015). Motor neuron disease: Current management and future prospects. *Journal of Internal Medicine, 45*(10), 1005–1013. https://doi.org/10.1111/imj.12874.

Singleton, J., Smith, A., & Marcus, R. (2015). Exercise as therapy for diabetic and Prediabetic neuropathy. *Current Diabetes Reports, 15*(12), 120. https://doi.org/10.1007/s11892-015-0682-6.

Sjöholm, A., Skarin, M., Churilov, L., Nilsson, M., Bernhardt, J., & Lindén, T. (2014). Sedentary behaviour and physical activity of people with stroke in rehabilitation hospitals. *Stroke Research and Treatment, 2014*, 591897. https://doi.org/10.1155/2014/591897.

Smania, N., Corato, E., Tinazzi, M., Stanzani, C., Fiaschi, A., Girardi, P., & Gandolfi, M. (2010). Effect of balance training on postural instability in patients with idiopathic Parkinson's disease. *Neurorehabilitation and Neural Repair, 24*(9), 826–834. https://doi.org/10.1177/1545968310376057.

Tajiri, N., Yasuhara, T., Shingo, T., Kondo, A., Yuan, W., Kadota, T., et al. (2010). Exercise exerts neuroprotective effects on Parkinson's disease model of rats. *Brain Research, 1310*, 200–207. https://doi.org/10.1016/j.brainres.2009.10.075.

Taniwaki, T., Okayama, A., Yoshiura, T., Togao, O., Nakamura, Y., Yamasaki, T., et al. (2007). Age-related alterations of the functional interactions within the basal ganglia and cerebellar motor loops in vivo. *NeuroImage, 36*(4), 1263–1276. https://doi.org/10.1016/j.neuroimage.2007.04.027.

Tennant, K. A., Adkins, D. L., Scalco, M. D., Donlan, N. A., Asay, A. L., Thomas, N., et al. (2012). Skill learning induced plasticity of motor cortical representations is time and age-dependent. *Neurobiology of Learning and Memory, 98*(3), 291–302. https://doi.org/10.1016/j.nlm.2012.09.004.

Tieges, Z., Mead, G., Allerhand, M., Duncan, F., van Wijck, F., Fitzsimons, C., et al. (2015). Sedentary behavior in the first year after stroke: A longitudinal cohort study with objective measures. *Archives of Physical Medicine and Rehabilitation, 96*(1), 15–23. https://doi.org/10.1016/j.apmr.2014.08.015.

Tuon, T., Valvassori, S. S., Lopes-Borges, J., Luciano, T., Trom, C. B., Silva, L. A., et al. (2012). Physical training exerts neuroprotective effects in the regulation of neurochemical factors in an animal model of Parkinson's disease. *Neuroscience, 227*, 305–312. https://doi.org/10.1016/j.neuroscience.2012.09.063.

Uhrbrand, A., Stenager, E., Pedersen, M., & Dalgas, U. (2015). Parkinson's disease and intensive exercise therapy – A systematic review and meta-analysis of randomized controlled trials. *Journal of Neurology Science, 353*(1–2), 9–19. https://doi.org/10.1016/j.jns.2015.04.004.

van Doorn, C., Gruber-Baldini, A., Zimmerman, S., Hebel, J., Port, C., Baumgarten, M., et al. (2003). Dementia as a risk factor for falls and fall injuries among nursing home residents. *Journal of the American Geriatrics Society, 51*(9), 1213–1218.

van Nimwegen, M., Speelman, A., Hofman-van Rossum, E., Overeem, S., Deeg, D., Borm, G., et al. (2011). Physical inactivity in Parkinson's disease. *Journal of Neurology, 258*(12), 2214–2221. https://doi.org/10.1007/s00415-011-6097-7.

van Praag, H., Shubert, T., Zhao, C., & Gage, F. (2005). Exercise enhances learning and hippocampal neurogenesis in aged mice. *The Journal of Neuroscience, 25*(38), 8680–8685. https://doi.org/10.1523/JNEUROSCI.1731-05.2005.

Venglar, M. (2013). Tai chi improves balance in people with Parkinson's disease. *Evidence-Based Medicine Journal, 18*(1), e2. https://doi.org/10.1136/ebmed-2012-100664.

Verheyden, G., Weerdesteyn, V., Pickering, R., Kunkel, D., Lennon, S., Geurts, A., & Ashburn, A. (2013). Interventions for preventing falls in people after stroke. *The Cochrane Database of Systematic Reviews, 5*, CD008728. https://doi.org/10.1002/14651858.CD008728.pub2.

Voet, N., van der Kooi, E., Riphagen, I., Lindeman, E., van Engelen, B., & Geurts, A. (2013). Strength training and aerobic exercise training for muscle disease. *The Cochrane Database of Systematic Reviews, 7*, CD003907. https://doi.org/10.1002/14651858.CD003907.pub4.

Voukelatos, A., Merom, D., Sherrington, C., Rissel, C., Cumming, R., & Lord, S. (2015). The impact of a home-based walking programme on falls in older people: The easy steps randomised controlled trial. *Age and Ageing, 44*(3), 377–383. https://doi.org/10.1093/ageing/afu186.

Wang, S., Chen, L., Zhang, L., Huang, C., Xiu, Y., Wang, F., et al. (2015). Effects of long-term exercise on spatial learning, memory ability, and cortical capillaries in aged rats. *Medical Science Monitor: International Medical Journal of Experimental and Clinical Research, 21*, 945–954. https://doi.org/10.12659/MSM.893935.

WHO. (2007). WHO global report on falls prevention in older age. Retrieved from http://www.who.int/ageing/publications/Falls_prevention7March.pdf

WHO. (2015). World report on ageing and health. Retrieved from http://www.who.int/ageing/events/world-report-2015-launch/en

Wu, S. Y., Wang, T. F., Yu, L., Jen, C. J., Chuang, J. I., Wu, F. S., et al. (2011). Running exercise protects the substantia nigra dopaminergic neurons against inflammation-induced degeneration via the activation of BDNF signaling pathway. *Brain, Behavior, and Immunity, 25*(1), 135–146. https://doi.org/10.1016/j.bbi.2010.09.006.

9

Promotion of Physical Activity for Older People with Musculoskeletal Conditions

Steven M. McPhail

9.1 Introduction

A person's ability to undertake physical activity is indelibly linked to the functioning of their musculoskeletal system. Typically, the musculoskeletal system benefits from physical activity. Conversely, if the musculoskeletal system is hampered by injury or musculoskeletal dysfunction, this can create a substantial obstacle to undertaking physical activity (McPhail et al. 2014b). Unfortunately, deficits in the musculoskeletal system may increase with advancing age (Felson et al. 2000; McPhail et al. 2014a; US Department of Health Human Services 2004). Furthermore, the risk of injury from relatively minor forces may also increase with age-related frailty (Center et al. 2007; Gillespie et al. 2012; Wehren and Magaziner 2003). The concerns of health professionals wanting to uphold the principle of primum non nocere (first do no harm) may lead them to refrain from aggressive promotion of physical activity among older adults with musculoskeletal conditions, due to a fear of aggravating symptoms or causing further injury to the musculoskeletal system. However, the promotion of physical activity to older adults with musculoskeletal conditions need not necessarily carry undue risk. In contrast to the aforementioned perception, the risk of sedentary living to both the integrity of the musculoskeletal system and general health more broadly is likely to considerably outweigh any risk associated with appropriate promotion of

S. M. McPhail (✉)
Queensland University of Technology and Metro South Hospital and Health Service (Queensland), Brisbane, Australia

physical activity among people with musculoskeletal conditions (Howe et al. 2011; Marques et al. 2012).

A theoretical framework outlining potential interactions between body structures, lifestyle, chronic disease, ability (and desire) to undertake physical activity, and other factors in ongoing cycles of physical inactivity among people with musculoskeletal conditions is displayed in Fig. 9.1. This framework acknowledges that many factors may need to be considered to successfully promote physical activity among people with musculoskeletal conditions. It highlights the potential for a downward spiral of physical inactivity to contribute to worsening musculoskeletal health and subsequent musculoskeletal conditions, which in turn may contribute to further difficulty in undertaking physical activity. However, it also highlights the potential benefit of appropriate physical activity promotion that can break this cycle and perhaps even reverse it, whereby participating in physical activity may contribute to improved musculoskeletal health, physical function, and motivation to continue to be physically active.

This chapter addresses some of the key considerations when promoting physical activity among older people with deficits in their musculoskeletal system. The chapter will focus on some common groups of conditions that are prevalent among older adult populations, but the underpinning principles are likely to be applicable beyond the specific groups of conditions covered in this

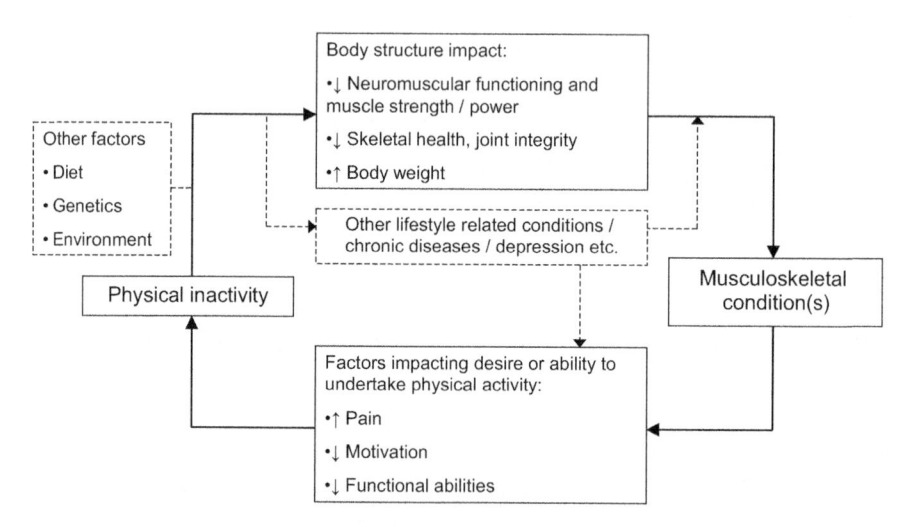

Fig. 9.1 Potential cycle of interactions between physical inactivity, body structures, lifestyle-related conditions and chronic diseases, musculoskeletal conditions, ability (and desire) to undertake physical activity. Note: downward (↓) and upward (↑) arrows represent decreased and increased, respectively.

chapter. A practical case study and questions for considering the practical implications of the concepts discussed in this chapter will be provided prior the conclusion of the chapter.

9.2 Osteopenia and Osteoporosis

Bone mineral density increases during childhood and adolescence before peaking in late adolescence or early adulthood (Sabatier et al. 1996). Throughout the remainder of the lifespan, bone mineral density plateaus somewhat and then begins to decline at a slow rate attributable to slight imbalances in the rates of mineral resorption and redeposition during normal inflammatory and bone remodelling processes (Talmage et al. 1986). It has been observed that physical activity, diet, and lifestyle factors can influence bone mineral density throughout adulthood (McLernon et al. 2012; Ruchan 2011). However, for many women and men, the loss of bone mineral density with age can lead to a weakening of the bones (osteopenia) which has been linked to an elevated risk of bone fractures (osteoporosis). It has been estimated that approximately two in five women (Melton et al. 1992; US Department of Health Human Services 2004) and one in five men (Kanis et al. 2000; Melton et al. 1992; US Department of Health Human Services 2004) will experience an osteoporotic fracture in their lifetime. The most common body regions affected by osteoporosis-related fractures may be the hip, spine, humerus (upper arm), and forearm (Johnell and Kanis 2006; Woltman and den Hoed 2010). The loss of bone mineral density associated with elevated fracture risk may often occur without any perceptible symptoms until the first fracture occurs (Jepsen et al. 2016). For this reason, the development of osteoporosis is often considered a silent disease process (Jepsen et al. 2016) and should be an important consideration for anyone seeking to promote physical activity among older adults. Physical activity can play an important role in reducing fracture risk among people with osteopenia and osteoporosis both by minimising further loss of bone mineral density (Howe et al. 2011) and also by reducing the risk of falling which is a frequent mechanism of injury among older adults (El-Khoury et al. 2013; Wehren and Magaziner 2003) (see Chap. 8).

In the context of people with or at risk of osteopenia or osteoporosis, there has been a substantial body of research examining whether physical activity interventions can help to minimise further bone mineral density loss (Howe et al. 2011; Marques et al. 2012). A Cochrane systematic review that examined the effectiveness of exercise-based interventions for preventing and treating osteoporosis among post-menopausal women assigned exercise interventions into one of six categories (Howe et al. 2011). These six categories are a useful way to conceptualise the types of exercise interventions that may be considered for the prevention or treatment of osteoporosis-related fractures in women and men. The first exercise category was static weight-bearing exercise and included static standing balance exercises. The second category was low-force dynamic weight-bearing exercise and included interventions like Tai Chi and walking. The third category was high-force dynamic weight-bearing exercises which comprised a large range of exercises including running, jumping, dancing, and use of vibration platforms. The fourth category was low-force non-weight-bearing exercises including low-load high-repetition strength training. The fifth category was high-force non-weight-bearing exercises including progressive resistance strength training. The sixth category comprised exercise interventions that included a combination of exercises from the other five categories (Howe et al. 2011).

The aforementioned Cochrane systematic review included 43 clinical trials of (a somewhat diverse range of) exercise interventions among post-menopausal women (Howe et al. 2011). With the exception of static weight-bearing exercise ($n = 1$), there were multiple studies (range $n = 6$ to $n = 12$) investigating exercise interventions in each of the other categories. An overarching conclusion was the effect of the exercise interventions on bone mineral density was typically of a small but clinically important and statistically significant magnitude (Howe et al. 2011). However, as one might expect, not all exercise types were equally effective for the prevention or treatment of osteoporosis. Non-weight-bearing high-force exercises were reported to be the most effective exercise intervention for neck of femur bone mineral density (Howe et al. 2011). This included high-force lower-limb progressive resistance strength training. However, for vertebral (small bones forming the backbone) bone mineral density, a combination of exercise types seemed to be the most effective intervention approach (Howe et al. 2011). For example, a combination of brisk walking and leg, abdominal, and back strengthening exercises have been reported to have a favourable effect on spine bone mineral density (Iwamoto et al. 2001). Evidence also generally supports a favourable effect of other weight-bearing exercises on bone mineral density (Howe et al. 2011). There is also some evidence to suggest that it may be possible to design and implement aquatic exercise programmes that exert sufficient force on the skeletal system for a beneficial effect on bone mineral density (Rotstein et al. 2008), although low-force aquatic exercise may be unlikely to yield a beneficial effect on bone mineral density.

Another important lesson from prior research examining exercise for people with osteoporosis was that fractures were relatively infrequent occurrences during the clinical trial observation periods (Howe et al. 2011). The Cochrane systematic review of exercise interventions among post-menopausal women estimated that approximately 7 out of every 100 women who exercised experienced a fracture, while 11 out of every 100 women who did not exercise experienced a fracture; although, this difference was not considered statistically significant (Howe et al. 2011). However, when it comes to promotion of physical activities for reducing fracture risk, bone mineral density is just one important risk factor that may be influenced by physical activity. Another key factor in the prevention of fractures among people with osteoporosis is reducing the risk of falling, for which there is a substantial and ever-expanding body of research (El-Khoury et al. 2013; Gillespie et al. 2012).

Systematic reviews of clinical trials have consistently highlighted the effectiveness of group-based and individual exercise interventions for reducing risk of falls and fall-related injuries among community-dwelling older adults at risk of falls and fracture (El-Khoury et al. 2013; Gillespie et al. 2012; Michael et al. 2010; Sherrington et al. 2011; Shier et al. 2016). The types of exercise interventions that have been investigated have varied but have typically included combinations of gait, balance, strength/progressive resistance training, and functional task training. Interventions that included a single exercise type seem to have been less effective than interventions that included more than one exercise type (Shier et al. 2016). The intensity, frequency, and duration of exercise also varied considerably across studies in the field. This may be partly explained by uncertainty that exists regarding optimal fall-prevention exercise parameters.

Although the promotion of exercise among older adults is important in the prevention and treatment of fractures, physical activities ought to be considered as one part of a multi-faceted intervention programme to optimise bone strength and reduce risk of fractures from falls among older adults. Other notable interventions that may be beneficial alongside participation in an appropriate exercise intervention for osteoporosis include medications to improve hormone and vitamin levels which have been linked to falls and fractures (Gillespie et al. 2012; Michael et al. 2010), and assessment and treatment of bone and falls risk factors including vitamin D deficiency, lifestyle factors, and comorbidities (Dumitrescu et al. 2008; Stenvall et al. 2007).

9.3 Recovery from Fragility Fractures

Fragility fractures are associated with osteoporosis and have broadly been defined as those that were susceptible to fracture from relatively minor forces (Turner 2002). Unfortunately, fragility fractures can occur quite frequently among people with osteoporosis despite best efforts to reduce risk. Even though advanced and timely surgical procedures to stabilise fractures are usually accessible and safely implemented, many older adults do not experience a full recovery and do not return to pre-morbid levels of daily functioning (Auais et al. 2012; Chudyk et al. 2009). Furthermore, those who have experienced an osteoporotic fracture are at an elevated risk of experiencing further osteoporotic fractures (Briggs et al. 2015; Center et al. 2007). The risk of undesirable outcomes following fragility fractures highlights the importance of appropriate post-fracture rehabilitation to improve physical functioning and help reduce risk of subsequent fractures. The overarching purposes of rehabilitative exercises following fractures are to restore function in the affected body regions, to prevent loss of function in non-effected body regions, and to try to reduce risk of falling and sustaining subsequent injuries. However, specific objectives of exercise prescription for people recovering from fragility fractures may be slightly different across each phase of the recovery.

Early acute fracture management and exercise commencement following a planned clinical pathway have been recommended for older adults who have sustained fragility fractures, particularly for hip fractures (Auais et al. 2012; Chudyk et al. 2009; Kanis et al. 2008). The acute management of fragility fractures may or may not involve surgical stabilisation dependent on the nature of the fracture (e.g., location, displacement, stability) and the patient's circumstances (e.g., age, other health-related risk factors). Regardless of whether or not surgical stabilisation of a fracture is required, exercise will usually be a key component of post-fracture rehabilitation protocols to facilitate recovery of function (Auais et al. 2012; Chudyk et al. 2009; Kanis et al. 2008). Clinical teams involved in the management of the fracture will typically provide specific instructions regarding the timing of commencement of exercise and any other salient points for consideration in the prescription of post-fracture rehabilitation exercises. This will usually include advice about whether (or when) it is safe to bear weight through the affected body region, and when active (or passive) range of motion and strengthening exercises can commence. Additionally, the treating clinical team may prescribe particular joint movements or resisted exercises to be avoided for a time to mitigate risk of re-injury or fracture malunion (faulty bone union). However, in general, some kind of early rehabilitative exercises for older people who have sustained a fracture will usually be permitted as soon as the fracture has been stabilised. In most cases, this will be in the hospital setting and often within the first 24 hours following surgical stabilisation (Chudyk et al. 2009).

Overarching objectives of early rehabilitation includes restoration of function while averting secondary complications associated with immobility and disuse. Earlier surgical stabilisation of fractures and earlier commencement of planned evidence-based rehabilitation activity have been associated with better clinical outcomes among older adults who have sustained fractures (Simunovic et al. 2010). The timing of exercise commencement, type, intensity, and duration of early rehabilitation exercises to be undertaken during the recovery period is likely to vary widely across fracture types and orthopaedic management of the injury. If there is doubt about the safety of a particular type of exercise for a specific patient, this should be discussed within the treating clinical team, including the surgical team involved in the fixation of the fracture, until consensus is reached. For lower limb and axial fractures, initial therapeutic exercise may focus on restoration of the ability to walk safely using gait re-training techniques and gait aids as necessary, as well as the commencement of joint range of motion and strengthening exercises. Early post-fracture exercise prescription following upper limb fractures may include range of motion and strengthening exercises, while also ensuring that the older person is able to walk safely. Pain levels experienced by the patient, concurrent injuries, and comorbid health conditions are also likely to be important considerations that will guide exercise prescription.

During the subacute phase of recovery following a fracture, exercises interventions ought to build on improvements made during the first week(s) of the recovery and aim to help the patient return to premorbid levels of functioning. Subacute rehabilitation exercises may occur while the older adults are still in an inpatient setting, as an outpatient visiting a hospital or rehabilitation centre, as supervised exercise in the home, or independent exercise in the home (Chudyk et al. 2009). Rehabilitation activities in the subacute phase for appendicular injuries will likely include progression of exercises to build strength and restore joint active range of motion, education, and gait re-training exercises (if indicated) (Chudyk et al. 2009). Older adults may also benefit from multidisciplinary intervention that addresses balance, home safety, polypharmacy, potential use of hip protectors (although hip protectors may have a detrimental influence on independence with toileting or cause discomfort), self-efficacy, and social support as well as exercise commencing in the post-acute period (Singh et al. 2012). Fall prevention exercise interventions may also be beneficial in the subacute phase of recovery (El-Khoury et al. 2013).

Research investigating the frequency, intensity, type, duration, and setting in which post-fracture rehabilitation exercises should be conducted has produced mixed findings that have not always been easy to interpret (Auais et al. 2012; Chudyk et al. 2009; Stenvall et al. 2007). However, there are some overarching principles which seem consistent both within the post-fracture rehabilitative exercise literature as well as literature in related fields (Ashworth et al. 2005; El-Khoury et al. 2013; Gillespie et al. 2012; Howe et al. 2011). First, the types of exercise to be carried out must be considered both safe and beneficial for assisting the patient to achieve meaningful outcomes (e.g., being able to complete tasks required for independent living). Second, many of the same exercise prescription principles that apply to any population are also important to consider for people recovering from fractures (e.g., frequency, intensity, type and time, overload, etc.). Third, the best kind of rehabilitation exercise programme is one that the patient will actually do. This third point may on first impression sound redundant, but prescription of a programme with physiologically appropriate types of exercise, at an appropriate frequency, intensity, and duration will be ineffective if the patient does not engage with the programme and undertake the prescribed exercises. It is perhaps for this reason that high-intensity centre-based supervised exercise programmes have sometimes yielded the greatest patient benefits (Ashworth et al. 2005). It is possible that older people may find it more challenging to complete exercises at the same intensity and frequency when unsupervised in their own home.

9.4 Osteoarthritis

Osteoarthritis is perhaps the most common painful musculoskeletal condition to affect older adults. The symptoms and signs of osteoarthritis include pain which is often described as activity related or mechanical in nature, joint stiffness, reduced physical function, local inflammation at the affected joints, crepitus (a grating sound or sensation in the joint), and potential joint deformity (Felson et al. 2000). Despite being colloquially known as the 'wear and tear' arthritis, the disease mechanisms underpinning osteoarthritis are complex. There is some debate as to whether osteoarthritis ought to be considered a single disease or several disorders that have a similar pathway and impact on joint structures (for a more detailed discussion of these points, see the review Felson et al. 2000). A range of risk factors for the development of osteoarthritis have been identified and include advancing age, bone density and hormonal factors, nutritional factors, genetics, and local biomechanical factors (including obesity) (Felson et al. 2000). It is noteworthy that some of these risk factors are modifiable, and there is scope for the inclusion of physical activity promotion in public health strategies to reduce risk of developing osteoarthritis. Nonetheless, this discussion will concentrate on physical activity promotion for older adults who have osteoarthritis rather than physical activity promotion at a population level. The discussion will focus on the two body regions most commonly affected by osteoarthritis: the knee and hip.

Cochrane systematic reviews have been conducted to examine land-based exercise interventions for people with knee and hip osteoarthritis. Clinical trial evidence supported the use of exercise interventions to reduce pain and increase function in people with knee osteoarthritis (Fransen et al. 2015). Specifically, high-quality evidence supported the use of exercise for reduction of pain, and medium quality evidence supported the use of exercise for improvement in physical function. Meta-analyses indicated that exercise interventions for knee osteoarthritis had a beneficial effect on pain comparable to the magnitude of non-steroidal anti-inflammatory medications (Fransen et al. 2015). Similarly, the review of land-based exercise interventions for people with hip osteoarthritis concluded that high-quality clinical trial evidence supports the use of exercise interventions for reducing pain and improving function among people with hip osteoarthritis (Fransen et al. 2014). For both hip and knee osteoarthritis, there was evidence to suggest that benefits can be maintained for six months after the cessation of the exercise interventions, although it was not possible to report on potential longer-term benefits beyond this time (Fransen et al. 2014, 2015).

Exercise interventions with clinical trial evidence to support their use with knee osteoarthritis included muscle strengthening, functional training, and aerobic fitness programmes. Although less common, evidence also supported the use of Tai Chi-based programmes for people with knee osteoarthritis (Fransen et al. 2015). There have been reports of exacerbations of knee osteoarthritis symptoms associated with exercise, but no serious adverse events have been reported in clinical trials to date. It is noteworthy that at the present time it is unclear whether higher-intensity exercise programmes or lower-intensity exercise programmes are the most beneficial for people with knee osteoarthritis. Similar to knee osteoarthritis, the exercise interventions supported by clinical trial evidence for people with hip osteoarthritis included muscle strength training, functional training, and aerobic fitness programmes, as well as Tai Chi (Fransen et al. 2014). These interventions were provided as part of individual exercise programmes or group-based exercise programmes. There is also moderate quality evidence to indicate that aquatic exercise may have clinically important beneficial effects on pain disability and quality of life among people with knee and hip arthritis (Bartels et al. 2016).

There are several overarching considerations for promoting exercise among people with osteoarthritis. It is important to understand which body regions are affected, as often older people may report pain bilaterally or in other body regions. This may influence exercise prescription choices so that benefits may be experienced in more than one body region while avoiding symptom exacerbations. It is important to consider the frequency, intensity, type, and duration of exercises that are likely to be beneficial for pain, function, and quality of life, while minimising the risk of symptom exacerbation more broadly. To this end, moderate- to high-impact exercises that may be appropriate in other clinical populations may not be suitable for people with osteoarthritis. It is also important to recognise that there is a known association between osteoporosis and osteoarthritis (Felson et al. 2000), meaning many of the principles that apply to exercise prescription for people with osteoarthritis will be applicable to people with osteoporosis and vice versa.

9.5 Rheumatic Diseases and Other Musculoskeletal Conditions

There are more than 100 different conditions that impact the musculoskeletal system that may be classified as rheumatic diseases (Gamez-Nava et al. 1998). This includes autoimmune and inflammatory conditions that affect soft tissues and the structural integrity of joints contributing to pain and dysfunction. There are also other musculoskeletal conditions that may not necessarily be attributed to a rheumatic disease but nonetheless cause pain and have adverse functional impacts among older adults, including localised acute soft tissue traumatic injuries (DeGrauw et al. 2016). Some of the most common types of musculoskeletal conditions present in an older adult population, in addition to those already discussed in this chapter, are spinal pain syndromes (including low back pain and neck pain syndromes), localised soft tissue rheumatism (localised clinical problems relating to tendons, ligaments, and other soft tissues), and fibromyalgia (a chronic condition that includes symptoms of widespread, pervasive pain and tenderness in the body, as well as other symptoms) (Gamez-Nava et al. 1998). The aetiology, symptoms, natural history of the condition, treatments, and prognosis vary widely across these types of conditions. Consequently, this section aims to highlight some overarching principles for consideration, including the structures and body regions affected, likely benefits from potential physical activity approaches (both condition-specific and broader health benefits), how potential benefits compare to the risks of the physical activities, and whether modifications to exercise programmes can be made to reduce risk while maintaining the potential for benefits to the older adult.

Autoimmune conditions that impact musculoskeletal structures are usually characterised by the body producing antibodies that attack the body's own soft tissues causing chronic inflammation, structural damage (e.g., to joints), pain, and immobility (Gamez-Nava et al. 1998). A reasonably common and useful case in point is rheumatoid arthritis. Rheumatoid arthritis is an autoimmune condition where antibodies attack the synovial membranes of joints (the lining of joints), typically causing inflammation, stiffness, pain, and eventual joint deformities (Gamez-Nava et al. 1998; Hurkmans et al. 2009). Rheumatoid arthritis is a systemic condition that can affect multiple joints, usually bilaterally. The most commonly affected joints in the early stages include the small joints of the hands and feet, but, as the disease progresses, wrist and ankle joints are also frequently affected (Gamez-Nava et al. 1998; Hurkmans et al. 2009). Among older adults who have had rheumatoid arthritis for many years, large joints like the elbows, knees, and shoulders (or other joints) may be affected.

A Cochrane systematic review concluded there is evidence to indicate that exercise prescription for people with rheumatoid arthritis can be beneficial (Hurkmans et al. 2009). In particular, the review focused on supervised intervention programmes with exercise sessions of at least 20 minutes occurring at least twice weekly for six or more weeks. The types of exercises included those targeted at improving aerobic capacity and/or muscle strength. It is noteworthy that among patients with rheumatoid arthritis, who may be considered to have a notable risk of symptom exacerbation, strengthening exercise loads may start as low as 30–50% of the patient's maximum (Hurkmans et al. 2009) (defined as either percentage of one repetition maximum, one maximum voluntary contraction, maximum speed, or subjective maximal exertion (Garber et al. 2011)). No serious adverse events were reported during trials of exercise interventions included in the aforementioned review. An important critique of the literature examining these exercise interventions is that older adults, and those with the most severe symptoms, may be under-represented on account of being less likely to volunteer for clinical trials of exercise interventions. It is plausible that 'drop outs' from exercise programmes, and symptom exacerbations with exercise, may be more common among frail older adults or those with the most severe symptoms than those included in clinical trials. Nonetheless, some exacerbations of symptoms, including joint pain and inflammation, have been reported in response to participation in exercises among people with rheumatoid arthritis during clinical trials, which highlights the importance of both tailoring exercises to the ability and exercise tolerance of the individual while closely monitoring for signs or symptoms of exacerbation (Hurkmans et al. 2009).

Rotator cuff conditions are another important group of conditions to consider when promoting physical activities among older adults as they may be either a person's primary source of concern or a comorbid condition that can impact on one's ability to participate in physical activities (Chard et al. 1991; Page et al. 2016). The rotator cuff is most commonly considered to include four scapular muscles and their tendons that work to provide stability to the shoulder. One or more rotator cuff tendons can be damaged, including partial tears, full-thickness tears, or complete tendon ruptures as a result of either a traumatic injury or 'wear and tear' associated with ongoing microtrauma that may be attributable to biomechanical factors (Chard et al. 1991; Kuhn 2009; Page et al. 2016). Rotator cuff conditions can be very painful and cause substantial functional impairment of the upper limb.

Some older adults with rotator cuff conditions will experience a reduction in pain and improvement in upper limb function with an appropriate exercise programme (e.g., shoulder range of motion, pain-free rotator cuff strengthening exercises, etc.) (Kuhn 2009; Page et al. 2016). Rotator cuff tears may also require surgical repair and implementation of a lengthy post-operative rehabilitation protocol that will usually be prescribed by the treating clinical team (Morris et al. 2015). The rehabilitation exercise protocol following rotator cuff surgical repairs will often include a period of immobilisation (e.g., in a sling), followed by passive movements only, then eventual introduction of active exercises, until finally strengthening exercises are introduced. It will often take up to 12 weeks or more before strengthening exercises are appropriate following rotator cuff surgery (Kuhn 2009; Morris et al. 2015); however, rehabilitation protocols will be dependent on surgical technique, tendons affected, as well as past experiences and personal preferences of the local treating clinical team.

9.6 Supporting and Monitoring

Prior research has indicated people with musculoskeletal disorders have reported a range of barriers to undertaking physical activity (McPhail et al. 2014b). This has included barriers related to their existing health conditions (including painful musculoskeletal conditions and other comorbidities);

being in poor physical condition; experiencing emotional, social, and psychological barriers (e.g., lack of motivation or fear and anxiety about potential for pain); difficulty accessing appropriate exercise facilities; and difficulty fitting exercise into existing (already busy) daily schedules (McPhail et al. 2014b). One of the most difficult challenges to effectively promoting physical activity among older adults may not be associated with mechanical or physiological deficits of the musculoskeletal system but rather challenges associated with facilitating sustained physical activity-related behaviour change among people who are fearful of exacerbating their condition. For this reason, access to appropriate monitoring and advice may be particularly important for older adults at risk of exacerbating an existing condition. In addition, sound behaviour change techniques for physical activity promotion may need to be considered (see Section 3).

Contemporary communication technologies (e.g., smartphones) offer great potential for both remote monitoring and behaviour change support to people with musculoskeletal conditions who are commencing or continuing exercise interventions. This may include an avenue to seek advice about how to modify, suspend, or cease an exercise programme if an exacerbation in symptoms occurs. While prior research has indicated older people with musculoskeletal disorders are not eager to receive physical activity supportive communications with health professionals via private messages on internet-based social media platforms, they are perhaps likely to engage with more traditional remote communication (e.g., speaking with a health professional via a telephone call) (McPhail et al. 2015). Remote communication for behaviour change support may not necessarily be burdensome on healthcare providers, in comparison to face-to-face clinic appointments, but potentially invaluable to older adults who are contemplating cessation of an exercise programme over (potentially unfounded) fears of it having deleterious effects on existing musculoskeletal (or other health) conditions (McPhail and Schippers 2012).

9.7 Case Study

The following case study is provided as an example to prompt consideration of the practical application of concepts raised in this chapter. This is followed by a broader list of questions for considering the implications for practice arising from the content discussed in this chapter.

9.7.1 Background

Mr. Jones is 72-year-old with a longstanding history of pain in both of his knees and has been diagnosed with bilateral knee osteoarthritis. He previously walked with his dog for 30 minutes in the morning most days of the week, but two years ago, Mr. Jones had an exacerbation of pain in his right leg (which he attributed to knee osteoarthritis). Subsequently, he has decided that he didn't want to risk hurting his knee again and has ceased his regular morning walking activity. He is currently sedentary most days. He is now having difficulty getting in and out of his car and walking up and down the supermarket isles when shopping. He is finding that he becomes increasingly fatigued when shopping and reports feeling like he needs to lean more and more on his shopping trolley as his legs feel increasingly weak and tired.

9.7.2 Upon Further Questioning

Mr. Jones indicates that he does not have any history of falling. He also indicates that his small dog is well trained (albeit not as fit as it used to be) and that he formerly walked the dog at a local park that does not require the dog to wear a leash. Together with further discussion with Mr. Jones, you conclude the dog is not likely to mechanically contribute to a fall by tripping or pulling Mr. Jones off balance.

9.7.3 Key Actions

You explain to Mr. Jones that keeping active and strengthening his leg muscles may actually minimise further knee pain rather than cause more knee pain. Furthermore, the difficulty that he is having with fatigue is likely being caused by physical deconditioning and muscle weakness (which is likely attributable to his sedentary lifestyle rather than directly to his osteoarthritis). Given he is coming from a low base level of fitness, you first prescribe some leg strengthening exercises that can be conducted safely in his home next to his kitchen bench (e.g., prescribing heel raises, repeated sit-to-stands, wall-squats, marching on the spot (using appropriate frequency, intensity, duration and overload principles discussed in Chap. 5)). As improvement in his strength and endurance occurs, you decide to expand his exercise programme to include intentional indoor walking tasks (e.g., perhaps walking at a safe and comfortable pace for five minutes inside the shopping centre, then resting on a chair, before repeating another five minutes of walking), with the goal of building up the comfortable and safe walking ability to permit 30 minutes of outdoor walking with his dog each morning again (which Mr. Jones believes will act as a positive incentive to participate in this exercise programme).

9.8 Implications

The presence of one or more musculoskeletal conditions may warrant careful consideration of which exercise programme(s) are appropriate in order to maximise potential benefits, while minimising risk of exacerbating underlying musculoskeletal conditions. Some or all of the following questions may be pertinent to consider when promoting physical activity among older adults:

- What health conditions are present (musculoskeletal and other health conditions)?
- What is the intended purpose of exercise or physical activity promotion?
- Which exercise strategies are likely to be the most beneficial?
- What is the risk profile of the individual in comparison to the potential exercise strategies under consideration?
- Can the exercise intervention(s) be modified to reduce risk while maintaining as much benefit as possible?
- What other barriers to being physically active are likely to be present (e.g., being anxious about pain)?
- Can you provide or are there any methods of support available to overcome barriers?
- What are the requirements for monitoring (e.g., for safety and symptom management) and progression of exercises?

9.9 Conclusions

There are a wide range of musculoskeletal conditions that can affect older adults. However, in the vast majority of cases, the presence of a musculoskeletal condition is not a contra-indication for participation in exercise and other physical activity. To the contrary, appropriate exercises can often reduce symptoms related to pain and dysfunction while also potentially reducing longer-term risks (e.g., of fall-related injuries). In addition, exercise has the potential to mitigate some underlying disease processes (e.g., minimising loss of bone mineral density). Nonetheless, there may be risk associated with some physical activities or exercise programmes and caution is warranted to avoid the recommendation of inappropriate exercises.

Suggested Reading

- Howe, T. E., Shea, B., Dawson, L. J., Downie, F., Murray, A., Ross, C., et al. (2011). Exercise for preventing and treating osteoporosis in postmenopausal women. *Cochrane Database of Systematic Reviews, 7*. https://doi.org/10.1002/14651858.CD000333.pub2.
- Fransen, M., McConnell, S., Hernandez-Molina, G., & Reichenbach, S. (2014). Exercise for osteoarthritis of the hip. *Cochrane Database of Systematic Reviews, 4*. https://doi.org/10.1002/14651858.CD007912.pub2.
- Fransen, M., McConnell, S., Harmer, A. R., Van der Esch, M., Simic, M., & Bennell, K. L. (2015). Exercise for osteoarthritis of the knee. *Cochrane Database of Systematic Reviews, 1*. https://doi.org/10.1002/14651858.CD004376.pub3.

References

Ashworth, N. L., Chad, K. E., Harrison, E. L., Reeder, B. A., & Marshall, S. C. (2005). Home versus center based physical activity programs in older adults. *Cochrane Database of Systematic Reviews, 1*, Cd004017. https://doi.org/10.1002/14651858.CD004017.pub2.

Auais, M. A., Eilayyan, O., & Mayo, N. E. (2012). Extended exercise rehabilitation after hip fracture improves patients' physical function: A systematic review and meta-analysis. *Physical Therapy, 92*, 1437+.

Bartels, E. M., Juhl, C. B., Christensen, R., Hagen, K. B., Danneskiold-Samsøe, B., Dagfinrud, H., & Lund, H. (2016). Aquatic exercise for the treatment of knee and hip osteoarthritis. *Cochrane Database of Systematic Reviews, 3*. https://doi.org/10.1002/14651858.CD005523.pub3.

Briggs, A. M., Sun, W., Miller, L. J., Geelhoed, E., Huska, A., & Inderjeeth, C. A. (2015). Hospitalisations, admission costs and re-fracture risk related to osteoporosis in Western Australia are substantial: A 10-year review. *Australian and New Zealand Journal of Public Health, 39*(6), 557–562. https://doi.org/10.1111/1753-6405.12381.

Center, J. R., Bliuc, D., Nguyen, T. V., & Eisman, J. A. (2007). Risk of subsequent fracture after low-trauma fracture in men and women. *JAMA, 297*(4), 387–394. https://doi.org/10.1001/jama.297.4.387.

Chard, M. D., Hazleman, R., Hazleman, B. L., King, R. H., & Reiss, B. B. (1991). Shoulder disorders in the elderly: A community survey. *Arthritis and Rheumatism, 34*(6), 766–769. https://doi.org/10.1002/art.1780340619.

Chudyk, A. M., Jutai, J. W., Petrella, R. J., & Speechley, M. (2009). Systematic review of hip fracture rehabilitation practices in the elderly. *Archives of Physical Medicine and Rehabilitation, 90*(2), 246–262. https://doi.org/10.1016/j.apmr.2008.06.036.

DeGrauw, X., Annest, J. L., Stevens, J. A., Xu, L., & Coronado, V. (2016). Unintentional injuries treated in hospital emergency departments among persons aged 65 years and older, United States, 2006–2011. *Journal of Safety Research, 56*, 105–109. https://doi.org/10.1016/j.jsr.2015.11.002.

Dumitrescu, B., van Helden, S., ten Broeke, R., Nieuwenhuijzen-Kruseman, A., Wyers, C., Udrea, G., et al. (2008). Evaluation of patients with a recent clinical fracture and osteoporosis, a multidisciplinary approach. *BMC Musculoskeletal Disorders, 9*(1), 109. https://doi.org/10.1186/1471-2474-9-109.

El-Khoury, F., Cassou, B., Charles, M. A., & Dargent-Molina, P. (2013). The effect of fall prevention exercise programmes on fall induced injuries in community dwelling older adults: Systematic review and meta-analysis of randomised controlled trials. *BMJ, 347*, f6234. https://doi.org/10.1136/bmj.f6234.

Felson, D. T., Lawrence, R. C., Dieppe, P. A., et al. (2000). Osteoarthritis: New insights. Part 1: The disease and its risk factors. *Annals of Internal Medicine, 133*(8), 635–646. https://doi.org/10.7326/0003-4819-133-8-200010170-00016.

Fransen, M., McConnell, S., Hernandez-Molina, G., & Reichenbach, S. (2014). Exercise for osteoarthritis of the hip. *Cochrane Database of Systematic Reviews, 4*. https://doi.org/10.1002/14651858.CD007912.pub2.

Fransen, M., McConnell, S., Harmer, A. R., Van der Esch, M., Simic, M., & Bennell, K. L. (2015). Exercise for osteoarthritis of the knee. *Cochrane Database of Systematic Reviews, 1*. https://doi.org/10.1002/14651858.CD004376.pub3.

Gamez-Nava, J. I., Gonzalez-Lopez, L., Davis, P., & Suarez-Almazor, M. E. (1998). Referral and diagnosis of common rheumatic diseases by primary care physicians. *Rheumatology, 37*(11), 1215–1219. https://doi.org/10.1093/rheumatology/37.11.1215.

Garber, C. E., Blissmer, B., Deschenes, M. R., Franklin, B. A., Lamonte, M. J., Lee, I.-M., et al. (2011). American College of Sports Medicine position stand. Quantity and quality of exercise for developing and maintaining cardiorespiratory, musculoskeletal, and neuromotor fitness in apparently healthy adults: Guidance for prescribing exercise. *Medicine and Science in Sports and Exercise, 43*(7), 1334–1359.

Gillespie, L. D., Robertson, M. C., Gillespie, W. J., Sherrington, C., Gates, S., Clemson, L. M., & Lamb, S. E. (2012). Interventions for preventing falls in older people living in the community. *Cochrane Database of Systematic Reviews, 9*, Cd007146. https://doi.org/10.1002/14651858.CD007146.pub3.

Howe, T. E., Shea, B., Dawson, L. J., Downie, F., Murray, A., Ross, C., et al. (2011). Exercise for preventing and treating osteoporosis in postmenopausal women.

Cochrane Database of Systematic Reviews, 7. https://doi.org/10.1002/14651858. CD000333.pub2.

Hurkmans, E., van der Giesen, F. J., Vliet Vlieland, T. P. M., Schoones, J., & Van den Ende, E. C. (2009). Dynamic exercise programs (aerobic capacity and/or muscle strength training) in patients with rheumatoid arthritis. Cochrane Database of Systematic Reviews, 4. https://doi.org/10.1002/14651858.CD006853.pub2.

Iwamoto, J., Takeda, T., & Ichimura, S. (2001). Effect of exercise training and detraining on bone mineral density in postmenopausal women with osteoporosis. Journal of Orthopaedic Science, 6(2), 128–132. https://doi.org/10.1007/s007760100059.

Jepsen, K. J., Bigelow, E. M. R., Ramcharan, M., Schlecht, S. H., & Karvonen-Gutierrez, C. A. (2016). Moving toward a prevention strategy for osteoporosis by giving a voice to a silent disease. Women's Midlife Health, 2(1), 3. https://doi.org/10.1186/s40695-016-0016-0.

Johnell, O., & Kanis, J. A. (2006). An estimate of the worldwide prevalence and disability associated with osteoporotic fractures. Osteoporosis International, 17(12), 1726–1733. https://doi.org/10.1007/s00198-006-0172-4.

Kanis, J. A., Johnell, O., Oden, A., Sembo, I., Redlund-Johnell, I., Dawson, A., et al. (2000). Long-term risk of osteoporotic fracture in Malmo. Osteoporosis International, 11(8), 669–674.

Kanis, J. A., Burlet, N., Cooper, C., Delmas, P. D., Reginster, J.-Y., Borgstrom, F., & Rizzoli, R. (2008). European guidance for the diagnosis and management of osteoporosis in postmenopausal women. Osteoporosis International, 19(4), 399–428. https://doi.org/10.1007/s00198-008-0560-z.

Kuhn, J. E. (2009). Exercise in the treatment of rotator cuff impingement: A systematic review and a synthesized evidence-based rehabilitation protocol. Journal of Shoulder and Elbow Surgery, 18(1), 138–160.

Marques, E. A., Mota, J., & Carvalho, J. (2012). Exercise effects on bone mineral density in older adults: A meta-analysis of randomized controlled trials. Age, 34(6), 1493–1515. https://doi.org/10.1007/s11357-011-9311-8.

McLernon, D. J., Powell, J. J., Jugdaohsingh, R., & Macdonald, H. M. (2012). Do lifestyle choices explain the effect of alcohol on bone mineral density in women around menopause? The American Journal of Clinical Nutrition, 95(5), 1261–1269. https://doi.org/10.3945/ajcn.111.021600.

McPhail, S., & Schippers, M. (2012). An evolving perspective on physical activity counselling by medical professionals. BMC Family Practice, 13(1), 1.

McPhail, S., Schippers, M., & Marshall, A. L. (2014a). Age, physical inactivity, obesity, health conditions, and health-related quality of life among patients receiving conservative management for musculoskeletal disorders. Clinical Interventions in Aging, 9, 1096–1080.

McPhail, S. M., Schippers, M., Marshall, A. L., Waite, M., & Kuipers, P. (2014b). Perceived barriers and facilitators to increasing physical activity among people with musculoskeletal disorders: A qualitative investigation to inform intervention development. *Clinical Interventions in Aging, 9*, 2113–2122. https://doi.org/10.2147/CIA.S72731.

McPhail, S. M., Schippers, M., Maher, C. A., & Marshall, A. L. (2015). Patient preferences for receiving remote communication support for lifestyle physical activity behaviour change: The perspective of patients with musculoskeletal disorders from three hospital services. *BioMed Research International, 2015*. http://dx.doi.org/10.1155/2015/390352.

Melton, L. J., Chrischilles, E. A., Cooper, C., Lane, A. W., & Riggs, B. L. (1992). Perspective. How many women have osteoporosis? *Journal of Bone and Mineral Research, 7*(9), 1005–1010. https://doi.org/10.1002/jbmr.5650070902.

Michael, Y. L., Whitlock, E. P., Lin, J. S., Fu, R., O'Connor, E. A., & Gold, R. (2010). Primary care-relevant interventions to prevent falling in older adults: A systematic evidence review for the U.S. preventive services task force. *Annals of Internal Medicine, 153*(12), 815–825. https://doi.org/10.7326/0003-4819-153-12-201012210-00008.

Morris, A. C., Singh, J. A., Bickel, C. S., & Ponce, B. A. (2015). Exercise therapy following surgical rotator cuff repair. *Cochrane Database of Systematic Reviews, 2*. https://doi.org/10.1002/14651858.CD011531.

Page, M. J., Green, S., McBain, B., Surace, S. J., Deitch, J., Lyttle, N., et al. (2016). Manual therapy and exercise for rotator cuff disease. *Cochrane Database of Systematic Reviews, 6*. https://doi.org/10.1002/14651858.CD012224.

Rotstein, A., Harush, M., & Vaisman, N. (2008). The effect of a water exercise program on bone density of postmenopausal women. *The Journal of Sports Medicine and Physical Fitness, 48*(3), 352–359.

Ruchan, I. (2011). The effect of physical activity on bone mineral density. *International Journal of Physical Sciences, 6*(16), 4097–4101.

Sabatier, J.-P., Guaydier-Souqui'eres, G., Laroche, D., Benmalek, A., Fournier, L., Guillon-Metz, F., et al. (1996). Bone mineral acquisition during adolescence and early adulthood: A study in 574 healthy females 10–24 years of age. *Osteoporosis International, 6*(2), 141–148. https://doi.org/10.1007/bf01623938.

Sherrington, C., Tiedemann, A., Fairhall, N., Close, J. C. T., & Lord, S. R. (2011). Exercise to prevent falls in older adults: An updated meta-analysis and best practice recommendations. *New South Wales Public Health Bulletin, 22*(4), 78–83. https://doi.org/10.1071/NB10056.

Shier, V., Trieu, E., & Ganz, D. A. (2016). Implementing exercise programs to prevent falls: Systematic descriptive review. *Injury Epidemiology, 3*(1), 16. https://doi.org/10.1186/s40621-016-0081-8.

Simunovic, N., Devereaux, P. J., Sprague, S., Guyatt, G. H., Schemitsch, E., DeBeer, J., & Bhandari, M. (2010). Effect of early surgery after hip fracture on mortality and complications: Systematic review and meta-analysis. *Canadian Medical Association Journal, 182*(15), 1609–1616. https://doi.org/10.1503/cmaj.092220.

Singh, N. A., Quine, S., Clemson, L. M., Williams, E. J., Williamson, D. A., Stavrinos, T. M., et al. (2012). Effects of high-intensity progressive resistance training and targeted multidisciplinary treatment of frailty on mortality and nursing home admissions after hip fracture: A randomized controlled trial. *Journal of the American Medical Directors Association, 13*(1), 24–30. https://doi.org/10.1016/j.jamda.2011.08.005.

Stenvall, M., Olofsson, B., Lundström, M., Englund, U., Borssén, B., Svensson, O., et al. (2007). A multidisciplinary, multifactorial intervention program reduces postoperative falls and injuries after femoral neck fracture. *Osteoporosis International, 18*(2), 167–175. https://doi.org/10.1007/s00198-006-0226-7.

Talmage, R., Stinnett, S., Landwehr, J., Vincent, L., & Mccartney, W. H. (1986). Age-related loss of bone mineral density in non-athletic and athletic women. *Bone and Mineral, 1*(2), 115–125.

Turner, C. H. (2002). Biomechanics of bone: Determinants of skeletal fragility and bone quality. *Osteoporosis International, 13*(2), 97–104. https://doi.org/10.1007/s001980200000.

US Department of Health Human Services. (2004). *Bone health and osteoporosis: A report of the surgeon general* (p. 87). Rockville: US Department of Health and Human Services, Office of the Surgeon General.

Wehren, L. E., & Magaziner, J. (2003). Hip fracture: Risk factors and outcomes. *Current Osteoporosis Reports, 1*(2), 78–85. https://doi.org/10.1007/s11914-003-0013-8.

Woltman, K., & den Hoed, P. T. (2010). Osteoporosis in patients with a low-energy fracture: 3 years of screening in an osteoporosis outpatient clinic. *The Journal of Trauma, 69*(1), 169–173. https://doi.org/10.1097/TA.0b013e3181ca081f.

10

Promotion of Physical Activity for Acutely Unwell Older People

Nina Beyer and Charlotte Suetta

10.1 Introduction

The life expectancy of older people is steadily increasing and consequently the number of older people with diseases and disabilities related to ageing (Manton et al. 1993). The number of older patients undergoing major surgical procedures is also growing, and this poses a major challenge for anaesthetists and surgeons due to the increased risk of postoperative complications in older patients. With ageing, there is decay in skeletal muscle function, and sarcopenia is now generally used to describe the age-related loss of muscle mass and strength, which is believed to play a major role in the pathogenesis (i.e. the origin and development of a disease) of frailty and disability at old age (Roubenoff 2000). Further, illness is associated with catabolic stress, an ametabolic process in which energy is released through the conversion of complex molecules into more simple ones, especially by degradation of the protein from skeletal muscle mass (catabolism, i.e. tissue breakdown). The catabolic stress combined with physical inactivity during hospital admission contribute to a number of negative outcomes in older adults, including loss of muscle

---

N. Beyer (✉)
Department of Clinical Medicine, Faculty of Health and Medical Sciences, University of Copenhagen, Copenhagen, Denmark

C. Suetta
Department of Clinical Physiology, Nuclear Medine & PET, Rigshospitalet and Faculty of Health and Medical Sciences, University of Copenhagen, Copenhagen, Denmark

mass and strength, reduction in the ability to perform activities of daily living, readmissions, and institutionalisation (Covinsky et al. 2003).

Traditionally, medical care of patients has focused on the treatment of disease, and expectations from health professionals, patients, and caregivers are often that care is provided to the patients rather than with the patient. In the last century, bed rest was an important part of the treatment for various diseases and part of post-surgery regimens. It was not until 1999 that a systematic review of 39 randomised controlled trials (RCTs) on the effects of bed rest versus early mobilisation (Allen et al. 1999) revealed that no outcomes improved by bed rest and some conditions (including acute low back pain and myocardial infarction) actually worsened significantly in almost half of the studies. Interestingly, from the 1960s, bed rest had been used as an experimental analogue for space flight, and numerous studies had documented the deleterious physiological effects of bed rest in young men.

10.2 Physiological Changes Due to Age, Bed Rest, and Physical Inactivity

Bed rest adversely affects most organ systems. This is of importance for older people because exercise capacity declines with age. The maximum oxygen uptake drops by 5–10% every decade from age 30. The decline is partly because of a decrease in cardiac output as a result of a reduction in cardiac contractility and maximum heart rate. In addition, resistance of the blood vessels increases, and oxygen uptake in skeletal muscle drops as a result of reduced muscle mass and capillarisation. The age-related loss of muscle mass is approximately 1% annually from age 50, and the decline accelerates to 1–2% annually after age 60 (Vandervoort 2002). Maximal muscle strength decreases in parallel to the loss of muscle mass. Thus, an 80-year-old person has about half the muscle strength you find with young people. However, the demand on fitness and muscle strength for specific activities stays more or less the same throughout life. Consequently, deficits appear to be most dominant in tasks where a certain amount of physical capacity is necessary to succeed, for example, climbing stairs, crossing roads, and avoiding an impending fall. This contributes to the fact that especially older patients with little reserve capacity (i.e. the difference between the maximum physical capacity and demand in performing activities of daily living) have an increased risk of developing disability following hospitalisation, where illness and physical inactivity contribute to a further decline in physical capacity.

The physiological changes during bed rest are to some extent similar to the age-related changes. Thus, maximal oxygen uptake declines approximately 1% per day the first month due to changes in the central and peripheral circuits (Convertino 1997). A follow-up of the Dallas Bed Rest and Training Study documented that the 26% decrease in maximal oxygen uptake following 3 weeks of bed rest in 20-year-old men corresponded to the age-related change for the same men 40 years later (McGavock et al. 2009).

Studies on the consequences of bed rest and physical inactivity in healthy older persons have only been published during the last decade, and they have also shown substantial reductions in muscle mass and muscle strength (Kortebein et al. 2008; Suetta et al. 2009). The loss of muscle mass is most dramatic during the first week of immobilisation (Hvid et al. 2014). Notably, one study showed that bed rest also had a negative effect on lower extremity muscle power, that is, the ability to quickly generate high force, which resulted in decreased performance in stair climbing (Kortebein et al. 2008). In addition, it has been demonstrated that it takes longer for older persons to recover from brief periods of muscle disuse compared to young persons (Suetta et al. 2009, 2013; Hvid et al. 2014). It could be argued that hospitalised patients are not confined to complete inactivity, but in healthy older persons, even a reduction in the number of steps from about 6000 to 1400 per day may lead to a 4% reduction of the lower extremity muscle after only 2 weeks (Breen et al. 2013).

Skeletal muscle represents a key element in maintaining metabolic function and as an energy reservoir in catabolic conditions. Skeletal muscle is the largest donor of amino acids in the catabolic state, and this contributes to the loss of muscle mass (Kehlet 1997). Consistent with this, results from a large cohort study documented a significant reduction of muscle mass and muscle strength in community-dwelling older persons who had been hospitalised for more than eight non-consecutive days within a year (Alley et al. 2010).

Alongside changes in the muscles, tendon tensile strength and stiffness decreases, whereby force transmission from the muscle to the bone becomes slower and less precise. The practical implication of this is that the coordination of movements and thereby postural control deteriorates during everyday activities, and it becomes harder to get up from a chair, climb stairs, and prevent a fall.

Other adverse effects of bed rest include an increased risk of constipation (Iovino et al. 2013), pressure ulcers (Lindgren et al. 2004), venous thromboembolism (Emed et al. 2010), and orthostatic hypotension (Feldstein and Weder 2012), of which the latter is fairly prevalent in older patients and related to an increased risk of falling.

10.3 Consequences of Hospitalisation for the Older Patient

Hospital-associated decline in function is common and costly both for the individual and for society. The aetiology of functional decline is unclear; however, the lack of physical activity and exercise during hospital admission clearly contribute through the direct physiological effects of deconditioning. Objectively measured physical activity using accelerometers have shown that daily ambulatory activity in healthy older adults (age >50 years) ranges between 2000 and 9000 steps/day, while the numbers are 1214 steps/day in older adults with disabilities (Tudor-Locke et al. 2011). In contrast, Fisher et al. (2011) showed that patients admitted to the acute care for the elderly took an average of 740 (interquartile range 89–1014) steps/day, and those patients with shorter lengths of stay tended to have higher total steps compared to patients with longer lengths of stay. Results from different studies show that older acutely hospitalised medical patients spend on average 70–83% of their in-hospital time in bed and only 3–5% standing or walking (Brown et al. 2009; Fisher et al. 2011; Pedersen et al. 2013) despite that in most cases physical inactivity is not a result of severe disease (Brown et al. 2004; Fisher et al. 2011). Furthermore, it appears that the frequency of ambulation may be as low for patients independent in walking as for those dependent (Callen et al. 2004). Similar to the findings in acutely admitted medical patients, physical activity level after surgery for hip fracture is very low with an average of 99% of the day either lying or sitting and 1% either standing or walking (Davenport et al. 2015).

It is evident that physical inactivity during hospitalisation is an independent predictor of self-reported functional decline in basic activities (eating, toileting, bath, dressing, toilette) (Fig. 10.1, Panel 1) and nursing home care and death (Boyd et al. 2008; Brown et al. 2004, 2009; Covinsky et al. 2003; Gill et al. 2010). Data from both medical and surgical hospital units suggest that the incidence of iatrogenic disability (i.e. an unintended adverse condition resulting from the activity/treatment of health care providers or institutions) between the time of hospital admission and discharge may be as high as 12% and that the vast majority of the cases could be attributed to low mobilisation including excessive bed rest and lack of exercise (Sourdet et al. 2015).

Hospitalisation-associated disability typically occurs in older patients who have several impairments including comorbidity, cognitive impairment, depression, and limited social support prior to an acute illness (Covinsky et al. 2011). Thus, the risk of loss of function in relation to hospitalisation is highest among

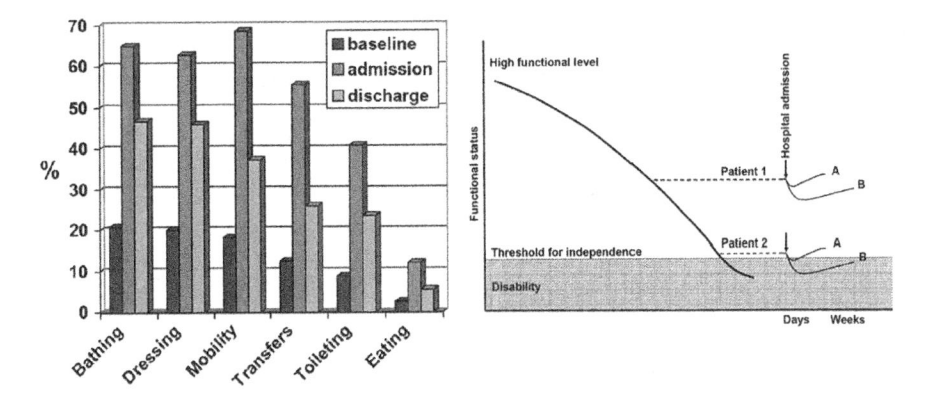

Fig. 10.1 Hospital-associated disability. Panel 1 (left) shows the proportion of older medical patients who required personal assistance in daily activities two weeks prior to admission, at admission, and at discharge (Mudge et al. 2010). Panel 2 (right) shows a model for suggested outcomes of 'fast-track treatment' including mobilisation during hospitalisation (A) and 'usual care' (B) for two patients with different functional status at hospital admission

the oldest, and many do not regain their pre-morbid level of functioning after discharge (Boyd et al. 2008; Brown et al. 2009). Approximately one-third of older medical patients experience decline in activities of daily living (ADL, i.e. typically problems with bathing, dressing, eating, transferring, and toileting) from 2 weeks prior to hospital admission to the time of discharge from hospital, and more than 50% of medical patients older than 85 years leave the hospital with a major new ADL disability (Covinsky et al. 2003). Moreover, the prognosis for functional recovery is poor in older adults discharged after hospitalisation for medical illness, when a new or additional disability in ADL has occurred (Boyd et al. 2008). Even after 1 year, less than 50% of older medical patients have recovered to their pre-illness level, and rates of nursing home placement and death are high (Boyd et al. 2008; Brown et al. 2009). In addition, the risk of readmission increases with the degree of functional impairment at admission, and functioning at discharge is a stronger predictor of readmission than comorbidity and demography (Shih et al. 2016). There is a similar pattern in the loss of independence amongst older adults who are exposed to bed rest following surgery. A large retrospect cohort study investigated loss of independence after surgical procedures in patients 65 years and older and found that 60% of the patients experienced a greater or lesser loss of independence (Berian et al. 2016). Loss of independence increased significantly with age, and occurred in 50% of those aged 65–74 years, 67% of those aged 75–84 years, and 84% of those 85 years and older (Berian et al. 2016). Finally, loss of independence increased the risk of readmission by 70%.

10.4 Physical Activity and Exercise During Hospitalisation

While patients experience a decline in physical functioning in comparison to their habitual level, hospital staff typically experience that older patients get better and gradually need less help during the hospital admission (Mudge et al. 2010). This is in agreement with studies showing that muscle strength and functional capacity remains unchanged or improves during hospitalisation (Bodilsen et al. 2013; Karlsen et al. 2016). The mismatch in the experiences may be because the patients get worse results in physical tests due to illness at the time of admittance. When test results have improved at discharge, this is not necessarily because the patients' functional capacity has improved but may be because they have recovered.

The question is how much physical activity is needed to prevent or reduce the loss of muscle mass and function. A Danish descriptive study showed that functional performance of the lower extremities improved more during hospital admission in geriatric patients with higher activity levels (Karlsen et al. 2016). Preliminary results from the American STRIDE study indicate that an interdisciplinary approach consisting of targeted gait and balance assessment by a physical therapist, followed by daily walks supervised by a recreation therapy assistant, may result in shorter in-hospital stay and a higher proportion of patients discharged directly home (Hastings et al. 2014). Further, loss of community mobility one month post-discharge was prevented by a simple mobility programme consisting of ambulation 1–2 times a day combined with a behavioural intervention that focused on goal setting and addressing mobility barriers (Brown et al. 2016). Importantly, mobilisation was safe, with no falls reported in the intervention group and three falls in the control group (Brown et al. 2016). Finally, data suggest that walking activity during hospitalisation is a predictor of 30-day readmission in older acutely ill people (Fisher et al. 2016).

Relatively few RCTs have been published regarding exercise in older hospitalised patients. A Cochrane review (de Morton et al. 2007) investigated the effect of exercise versus usual care on functional outcomes at discharge among older acutely hospitalised medical patients. Exercise was defined as any physical intervention by therapists alone or as a multidisciplinary intervention designed to maintain or improve the patients' strength or function performed. Seven RCTs and two cluster-randomised trials were identified, and all trials reported exercise intervention to commence within the first days of admission. The content and dosage (frequency, repetition, duration, or intensity) were generally not well described. The results showed that multidisciplinary interventions, which include exercise, may increase the proportion of patients discharged directly home and reduce length and cost of hospital stay for acutely hospitalised older medical patients. A more recent systematic review (Kosse et al. 2013) included 13 studies that investigated the effects of early in-hospital physical rehabilitation compared to usual care among acutely hospitalised geriatric patients. Both exercise-only programmes (physiotherapy or occupational therapy) and multidisciplinary programmes with an exercise component were included. The methodological quality was mostly moderate, and the description of the exercise programmes was poor. Exercise was safe, adherence rates were high for most studies, and patient satisfaction was higher compared to those who received usual care. At discharge, physical performance had improved more in patients who received exercise, and they were less likely to be discharged to a nursing home compared to patients who received usual care (Fig. 10.1, panel 2). Furthermore, physical functioning after discharge improved more if the interventions continued after hospital discharge.

There is increasing evidence that rehabilitation regimes comprising resistance exercise are particularly effective at targeting the functional deteriorations observed with bed rest and hospitalisation (Suetta et al. 2007). But although resistance exercise has been proved to be safe and effective in geriatric outpatients and frail nursing home residents (Fiatarone et al. 1994; Harridge et al. 1999), the effects of resistance exercise during hospitalisation of acutely ill geriatric patients have not yet been investigated. However, a non-randomised study (Sullivan et al. 2001) indicated that the progressive resistance exercise may result in an increase in both muscle strength, sit-to-stand performance, and maximal gait speed among frail elderly patients recuperating from acute illnesses. Importantly, in contrast to the vast majority of other exercise studies, the intervention in this study was initiated while the patients were in a geriatric rehabilitation and recuperative care unit, and none of the patients experienced any complications as a result of the training.

The evidence-based enhanced recovery protocols, also called fast-track surgery, were introduced in the 1990s and has since been used in a variety of elective surgical procedures, including total joint replacement and cardiopulmonary bypass surgery, but also in emergency surgery, for example, after hip fracture. The fast-track protocols aim to reduce organ dysfunctions due to surgical stress and to improve postoperative recovery, and the protocol includes spinal anaesthesia, multimodal opioid-sparing analgesia (i.e. a combination of different types of analgesics other than opioids to achieve the best pain relief), appropriate fluid management, early mobilisation, and functional discharge criteria. In addition to a positive effect on post-surgical complications, there may be an added benefit of reduced length of hospital stay (LOS), which may reduce the risk of hospital-acquired infections, thromboembolic events, and delirium to which older people may be especially vulnerable. A recent systematic review underlines that early commencement of physiotherapy and a weekend service may improve function, reduce length of hospital stay, and lead to higher probability of discharge directly home in the acute phase following total knee arthroplasty (Haas et al. 2016). Following total hip arthroplasty, where patients usually are somewhat older, it appears that early physiotherapy commencement needs to be combined with interventions from other allied health professions in order to obtain a higher probability of discharge directly home. In agreement with these results, it has been shown that early commencement of daily resistance exercise (knee extension) as a supplement to physiotherapy resulted in shorter length of hospital stay compared to physiotherapy alone (Suetta et al. 2004). Importantly, enhanced post-surgical recovery programmes among older patients are safe (Haas et al. 2016; Paton et al. 2014; Suetta et al. 2004).

In cardiac surgery, fast-track treatment has become the global standard of care, and patients who have gone through elective coronary stenting may exercise up to submaximal level starting the day after surgery since this does not increase the incidence of stent thrombosis or postoperative complications (Soga et al. 2010). After coronary bypass surgery, a specialised and supervised cardiac rehabilitation programme as part of a multidisciplinary cardiac rehabilitation programme should start as early as possible (Vanhees et al. 2012). Exercise intensity should be submaximal aerobic exercise at 40–80% of peak oxygen uptake in combination with resistance exercise at 40–80% of maximum muscle strength. The restriction is that training of upper extremities and exercises that causes severe increase in blood pressure is contraindicated in the first eight postoperative weeks to avoid thoracic shear and pressure stress (Vanhees et al. 2012).

Patients with hip fracture are often characterised by being old, having chronic illnesses, low muscle strength, and functional limitations. A recent meta-analysis with meta-regression showed that for these patients, inclusion of supervised progressive resistance exercise in structured exercise programmes that continues after discharge appears to be important for mobility (Diong et al. 2016). Progressive resistance exercise during hospital admission is feasible (Kronborg et al. 2014) and part of an interdisciplinary fast-track treatment with particular focus on comorbidity, pain relief, hydration, oxygenation, nutrition, elimination of delirium, and mobilisation (Taraldsen et al. 2014). Comprehensive geriatric care appears to be beneficial and includes rehabilitation focused on mobilisation progressive exercises based on the patients' ability, surgical procedure and pre-fracture function, ward routines focused on enhancing physical activity including splitting up long periods of sitting/lying, eating in the dining room and using communal areas, and participation in activities of daily living. Compared to the results among patients who were managed with standard orthopaedic care, the comprehensive geriatric care resulted in more time standing/walking and better basic mobility during the first four postoperative days (Taraldsen et al. 2014). Furthermore, the benefit from the comprehensive geriatric care was still present 4 and 12 months post-fracture, where more patients were able to walk, had better self-reported mobility, and gait performance (Thingstad et al. 2016).

The treatment of patients after hip fracture can be somewhat challenging, because some of the patients are characterised by physical and cognitive disability. However, data suggest that the relative improvement in physical function as a result of intensive training during hospitalisation is comparable in patients with normal cognition and patients with cognitive dysfunction (Mitchell et al. 2016). Nevertheless, persons with dementia have substantially lower odds of receiving hospital-based rehabilitation, and thus it is important to ensure that rehabilitation is offered to patients with dementia (Mitchell et al. 2016).

10.5 Effects of Protein Supplementation

Besides the negative effects of physical inactivity, inadequate dietary intake is one of the major factors contributing to the hospital-associated decline in function observed in many older patients (Ferrando et al. 2010). The catabolic stress response coupled with inactivity and inadequate protein intake result in a further loss of muscle mass and delayed functional recovery (Ferrando et al. 2010). Moreover, malnutrition is an independent predictor of subsequent hospital readmission and is associated with higher mortality after hospital discharge. Yet, in older hospitalised patients, as many as 21% of older hospitalised patients may receive less than 50% of their daily dietary requirement including protein (Sullivan et al. 1999). Consequently, protein supplementation is one of cornerstones of fast-track rehabilitation, and the use of protein supplementation has shown to reduce complications, mortality, and hospital readmissions in patients over the age of 65 (Wells and Dumbrell 2006). Whether dietary supplementation increases the effect of resistance type of exercise in the elderly has been to some debate, but in a recent meta-analysis from Cermak and co-workers, they concluded that protein supplementation augments the adaptive response of skeletal muscles to resistance exercise training in healthy older populations (Cermak et al. 2012). More importantly, it has been shown that supplementation with essential amino acids can preserve muscle mass in older adults during extended bed rest (Ferrando et al. 2010). Collectively, it seems important to ensure adequate protein intake in older hospitalised individuals, both to prevent muscle atrophy during bed rest and to augment the beneficial effect of resistance exercise on muscle mass and muscle strength.

10.6 Contraindications to Exercise in Older Patients

In general, the contraindications for exercise are the same for old and young persons and overall, avoiding physical activity carries greater risks than engaging in physical activity. However, special precautions are necessary in acutely ill patients, where it is important to refrain from intensive workouts until the patients are in a stable condition (Pedersen and Saltin 2015; Volaklis and Tokmakidis 2005). In addition, competing diseases must be taken into account before commencing an exercise regimen. That said, the number of absolute contraindications to exercise, even in frail older individuals, are limited and in most cases, despite the underlying disease; the most important point is that the patient is in a stable condition (Pedersen and Saltin 2015; Volaklis and Tokmakidis 2005). This is underlined by the fact that even in frail patients with chronic heart failure, the application of specific resistance exercise programmes as a supplement to conventional aerobic exercise is safe and recommended as long as the intensity is reduced to about 40–60% of VO_{2max} and/or maximal voluntary contraction (MVC) (Volaklis and Tokmakidis 2005). Detailed information about absolute contraindications to specific diseases can be found in an extended review (Pedersen and Saltin 2015). Increased focus on the benefits and risks of physical activity, and consequently research in the field, may lead to revision of some contraindications.

10.7 Summary of What Is Currently Known

- Hospitalisation is associated with an increased risk of hospital-associated disability and decline in functional performance (ADL) among older patients

- Physical inactivity during hospitalisation is an independent predictor of self-reported functional decline in basic activities
- Bed rest and physical inactivity rapidly (within 4–5 days) leads to a loss of muscle mass and muscle strength in both young and older adults
- Older individuals need longer time to recover from a period of muscle disuse
- The functional decline is costly in both economic and human terms
- Focus on mobilisation and training during hospitalisation has only been present in recent decades
- Mobilisation and exercise during hospitalisation is safe and results in improved physical performance and an increased chance of being discharged back to one's own home

10.8 Summary of What Is Currently Unknown

What can and should be done to best counteract loss of muscle mass, muscle strength, and hospitalisation-associated disability is still unclear. There is a need for:

- Research regarding which type, intensity, and dose of physical activity/exercise that should be recommended for different patient groups in order to improve functional outcomes
- Research regarding outcome measures that are valid, with a minimum of floor and ceiling effects and sensitivity to change
- Practice-based evidence research in rehabilitation (Horn et al. 2012), since RCT studies most often are performed in very selected patients (typically 10–15% of the total group). Patients with multiple co-morbidities are often excluded, and this limits the generalisability of the results
- Interventions investigating the effects of changes of work culture and work procedures
- More information about how the hospital environment encourages/motivates patients to get out of bed and be more active
- Qualitative research regarding motivation and barriers for physical activity and exercise in hospitalised patients and motivation and barriers for encouraging this behaviour among staff

10.9 The Key Practical Implications of What Is Currently Known

Given the rapid onset of decline in muscle function early, targeted physical activity and training would have the potential to delay or counteract the loss of muscle mass during hospitalisation. Based on evidence, the recommendation for exercise in older persons with different co-morbidities typically is supervised exercise comprising endurance training, resistance exercise, and balance training (Pedersen et al. 2015). However, in some acutely ill patient populations, high-intensity exercise interventions are medically contraindicated or simply not feasible, and recent data suggest that even relatively low-intensity, short-duration bouts of physical activity such as weight bearing or walking confer some benefit.

The most basic intervention during hospitalisation should therefore be to ensure that the patients get out of bed and ambulated several times a day if at all possible, and this is a multidisciplinary task (de Morton et al. 2007). Function-focused care (Resnick et al. 2016), which includes that patients are supported to perform daily activities, could be a means to reduce the risk of functional decline during hospitalisation. And if at all possible, a few simple exercises such as getting up from a chair and calf raises (Pedersen et al. 2015) should be performed preferably several times daily. Following instruction, these exercises can be performed unsupervised in patients who are not at risk of falling.

Needless to say, individually targeted physiotherapy should be offered to frail patients. Since lower body strength is needed for mobility and a variety of daily activities such as getting out of chair/bed, walking, and climbing stairs (Ploutz-Snyder et al. 2002; Stenroth et al. 2015), resistance exercise especially for the thigh and calf muscles should be included. Performing progressive resistance exercise during hospital admission can be done on an exercise machine but does not require expensive equipment. Using ankle weights and elastic bands for external loading is sufficient and progressive task-specific exercises such as rising from a chair and calf raises using weight vests have been shown to improve function (Bean et al. 2009) and reduce the need to modify tasks of everyday life (Manini et al. 2007) among low-functioning older adults.

For bed-bound patients and patients who are unable to perform resistance exercises, neuromuscular electrical stimulation (NMES), a technique that consists of generating muscle contractions with portable devices connected to surface electrodes (Maffiuletti 2010), could be an option. This modality has been shown to be effective in treating impaired muscles as it has the potential to preserve muscle-protein synthesis and prevent muscle atrophy during immobilisation Gibson et al. 1988). Thus, NMES added to usual care proved to be more effective than usual care alone for preventing muscle weakness in critically ill patients (Maffiuletti et al. 2013).

10.10 Vital Signs and Functional Status

Traditionally, vital signs of multiple physiological body functions are monitored to determine the degree of illness of a patient. Most medical settings use an early warning score (EWS), which is based on the six cardinal vital signs (respiratory rate, oxygen saturation, body temperature, blood pressure, heart rate, and level of consciousness). Since functional status during hospital admission predicts health outcomes after hospitalisation, it has been suggested that functional status over the course of hospitalisation be included as a vital sign that can help guide care, and serve as a guidepost of clinical wellbeing (Covinsky et al. 2011). A large proportion of patients report that they had a decline in function between when the disease started and until they were hospitalised, and consequently it is very important to assess the level of function before the illness, both physically and cognitively, and whether this has changed before admission. Covinsky et al. (2011) suggest asking the following question regarding difficulty with each of the ADLs (taking a bath or shower, getting dressed, transferring (getting out of bed and out of a chair), using the toilet, eating, and walking across a room): 'On the day of admission did you have any difficulty "doing the task"? Did you have any difficulty "doing the task" before the onset of the problem that led to your being hospitalized?' If the patient reports difficulty, assess need for help: 'What help do you need? Who helps you? Do you get enough help?' Assessment tools such as the Katz Index of Independence in Activities of Daily Living and the Barthel Index can be used. Assessment of function through interviews should be followed by measures and assessment of performance, that is, lower extremity function and mobility, which should be repeated in relation to daily rounds.

Monitoring mobility on a daily basis will put focus on the importance of mobility and help identify patients who need help and support to become more mobile. In acutely admitted older medical patients, the ability to get up from a chair without using the arms has been shown to identify mobility limitation 30 days after hospital discharge (Bodilsen et al. 2016). In patients with hip fracture, basic mobility (i.e. ability to independently get out of bed, out of a chair, and walk) during the first three days postoperatively has shown to be predictive of postoperative medical complications, hospital length of stay, discharge, and one-month mortality in patients who were admitted from their own home (Foss et al. 2006).

Knowledge of the patient's functional level in addition to the medical condition helps when planning an individualised intervention targeted at getting the patient back to his/her habitual functional level. In some patients, treatment will require supervised exercise and help with mobilisation, in others it may be sufficient with information and encouragement to maintain daily activities and carry out a few simple unsupervised exercises.

10.11 Conclusion

Physical activity during hospital admission has only been on the agenda during the last few decades. Thus, there is a great need for research regarding what can and should be done to best counteract loss of muscle mass, muscle strength, and hospitalisation-associated disability. Nevertheless, existing evidence support that in-hospital exercise mainly of the lower extremities is both feasible and beneficial in older medical and surgical patients to counteract the detrimental effects of illness combined with bed rest and physical inactivity. However, exercise cannot stand alone but has to be accompanied with interdisciplinary function-focused care, which includes that patients are supported to ambulate and perform daily activities if the goal is to reduce the risk of hospital-associated disability. In addition, protein supplementation should be offered in order to help preserve muscle mass during the catabolic crises and increase the effect of exercise.

Functioning at discharge is a strong predictor of readmission, and consequently it is important to assess the patients' pre-morbid functional status and monitor functional status as a vital sign during hospital admission. This information is also important when care is provided with the patient, which involves goal setting and addressing mobility barriers. Finally, it is important to focus on how the environmental surroundings can promote mobility.

Suggested Further Reading

- Boyd, C. M., Landefeld, C. S., Counsell, S. R., Palmer, R. M., Fortinsky, R. H., Kresevic, D., Burant, C., Covinsky, K. E. (2008). Recovery of activities of daily living in older adults after hospitalization for acute medical illness. *Journal of the American Geriatrics Society, 56* (12), 2171–2179.

- Pedersen, B. K., & Saltin, B. (2015). Exercise as medicine – Evidence for prescribing exercise as therapy in 26 different chronic diseases. *Scandinavian Journal of Medicine and Science in Sports*, 25(Suppl 3), 1–72.
- Swedish National Institute of Public Health. (2010). Physical Activity in the prevention and treatment of disease. Available at http://www.fyss.se/fyss-in-english/chapters-in-fyss/

References

Allen, C., Glasziou, P., & Del Mar, C. (1999). Bed rest: A potentially harmful treatment needing more careful evaluation. *Lancet*, 354(9186), 1229–1233.

Alley, D. E., Koster, A., Mackey, D., Cawthon, P., Ferrucci, L., Simonsick, E. M., et al. (2010). Hospitalization and change in body composition and strength in a population-based cohort of older persons. *Journal of the American Geriatrics Society*, 58(11), 2085–2091.

Bean, J. F., Kiely, D. K., LaRose, S., O'Neill, E., Goldstein, R., & Frontera, W. R. (2009). Increased velocity exercise specific to task training versus the National Institute on Aging's strength training program: Changes in limb power and mobility. *Journals of Gerontology. Series A, Biological Sciences and Medical Sciences*, 64((9), 983–991.

Berian, J. R., Mohanty, S., Ko, C. Y., Rosenthal, R. A., & Robinson, T. N. (2016). Association of loss of independence with readmission and death after discharge in older patients after surgical procedures. *Journal of the American Medical Association Surgery*, 151(9), e161689.

Bodilsen, A. C., Pedersen, M. M., Petersen, J., Beyer, N., Andersen, O., Smith, L. L., Kehlet, H., & Bandholm, T. (2013). Acute hospitalization of the older patient: Changes in muscle strength and functional performance during hospitalization and 30 days after discharge. *American Journal of Physical Medicine and Rehabilitation*, 92(9), 789–796.

Bodilsen, A. C., Klausen, H. H., Petersen, J., Beyer, N., Andersen, O., Jørgensen, L. M., Juul-Larsen, H. G., & Bandholm, T. (2016). Prediction of mobility limitations after hospitalization in older medical patients by simple measures of physical performance obtained at admission to the emergency department. *PLoS One*, 11(5), e0154350.

Boyd, C. M., Landefeld, C. S., Counsell, S. R., Palmer, R. M., Fortinsky, R. H., Kresevic, D., Burant, C., & Covinsky, K. E. (2008). Recovery of activities of daily living in older adults after hospitalization for acute medical illness. *Journal of the American Geriatrics Society*, 56(12), 2171–2179.

Breen, L., Stokes, K. A., Churchward-Venne, T. A., Moore, D. R., Baker, S. K., Smith, K., et al. (2013). Two weeks of reduced activity decreases leg lean mass and induces "anabolic resistance" of myofibrillar protein synthesis in healthy elderly. *Journal of Clinical Endocrinology and Metabolism, 98*(6), 2604–2612.

Brown, C. J., Friedkin, R. J., & Inouye, S. K. (2004). Prevalence and outcomes of low mobility in hospitalized older patients. *Journal of the American Geriatrics Society, 52*(8), 1263–1270.

Brown, C. J., Roth, D. L., Allman, R. M., Sawyer, P., Ritchie, C. S., & Roseman, J. M. (2009). Trajectories of life-space mobility after hospitalization. *Annals of Internal Medicine, 150*(6), 372–378.

Brown, C. J., Foley, K. T., Lowman, J. D., Jr., MacLennan, P. A., Razjouyan, J., Najafi, B., Locher, J., & Allman, R. M. (2016). Comparison of posthospitalization function and community mobility in hospital mobility program and usual care patients: A randomized clinical trial. *Journal of the American Medical Association Internal Medicine, 176*(7), 921–927.

Callen, B. L., Mahoney, J. E., Grieves, C. B., Wells, T. J., & Enloe, M. (2004). Frequency of hallway ambulation by hospitalized older adults on medical units of an academic hospital. *Geriatric Nursing, 25*(4), 212–217.

Cermak, N. M., Res, P. T., de Groot, L. C., Saris, W. H., & van Loon, L. J. (2012). Protein supplementation augments the adaptive response of skeletal muscle to resistance-type exercise training: A meta-analysis. *American Journal of Clinical Nutrition, 96*(6), 1454–1464.

Convertino, V. A. (1997). Cardiovascular consequences of bed rest: Effect on maximal oxygen uptake. *Medicine and Science in Sports and Exercise, 29*(2), 191–196.

Covinsky, K. E., Palmer, R. M., Fortinsky, R. H., Counsell, S. R., Stewart, A. L., Kresevic, D., Burant, C. J., & Landefeld, C. S. (2003). Loss of independence in activities of daily living in older adults hospitalized with medical illnesses: Increased vulnerability with age. *Journal of the American Geriatrics Society, 51*(4), 451–458.

Covinsky, K. E., Pierluissi, E., & Johnston, C. B. (2011). Hospitalization-associated disability: "She was probably able to ambulate, but I'm not sure". *Journal of the American Medical Association, 306*(16), 1782–1793.

Davenport, S. J., Arnold, M., Hua, C., Schenck, A., Batten, S., & Taylor, N. F. (2015). Physical activity levels during acute inpatient admission after hip fracture are very low. *Physiotherapy Research International, 20*(3), 174–181.

de Morton, N. A., Keating, J. L., & Jeffs, K. (2007). Exercise for acutely hospitalised older medical patients. *Cochrane Database of Systematic Reviews, 1*, CD005955.

Diong, J., Allen, N., & Sherrington, C. (2016). Structured exercise improves mobility after hip fracture: A meta-analysis with meta-regression. *British Journal of Sports Medicine, 50*(6), 346–355.

Emed, J. D., Morrison, D. R., Des Rosiers, L., & Kahn, S. R. (2010). Definition of immobility in studies of thromboprophylaxis in hospitalized medical patients: A systematic review. *Journal of Vascular Nursing, 28*(2), 54–66.

Feldstein, C., & Weder, A. B. (2012). Orthostatic hypotension: A common, serious and underrecognized problem in hospitalized patients. *Journal of the American Society of Hypertension, 6*(1), 27–39.

Ferrando, A. A., Paddon-Jones, D., Hays, N. P., Kortebein, P., Ronsen, O., Williams, R. H., McComb, A., Symons, T. B., Wolfe, R. R., & Evans, W. (2010). EAA supplementation to increase nitrogen intake improves muscle function during bed rest in the elderly. *Clinical Nutrition, 29*(1), 18–23.

Fiatarone, M. A., O'Neill, E. F., Ryan, N. D., Clements, K. M., Solares, G. R., Nelson, M. E., Roberts, S. B., Kehayias, J. J., Lipsitz, L. A., & Evans, W. J. (1994). Exercise training and nutritional supplementation for physical frailty in very elderly people. *New England Journal of Medicine, 330*(25), 1769–1775.

Fisher, S. R., Goodwin, J. S., Protas, E. J., Kuo, Y. F., Graham, J. E., Ottenbacher, K. J., & Ostir, G. V. (2011). Ambulatory activity of older adults hospitalized with acute medical illness. *Journal of the American Geriatrics Society, 59*(1), 91–95.

Fisher, S. R., Graham, J. E., Ottenbacher, K. J., Deer, R., & Ostir, G. V. (2016). Inpatient walking activity to predict readmission in older adults. *Archives of Physical Medicine and Rehabilitation, 97*(9 Suppl), S226–S231.

Foss, N. B., Kristensen, M. T., & Kehlet, H. (2006). Prediction of postoperative morbidity, mortality and rehabilitation in hip fracture patients: The cumulated ambulation score. *Clinical Rehabilitation, 20*(8), 701–708.

Gibson, J. N., Smith, K., & Rennie, M. J. (1988). Prevention of disuse muscle atrophy by means of electrical stimulation: Maintenance of protein synthesis. *Lancet, 2*(8614), 767–770.

Gill, T. M., Allore, H. G., Gahbauer, E. A., & Murphy, T. E. (2010). Change in disability after hospitalization or restricted activity in older persons. *Journal of the American Medical Association, 304*(17), 1919–1928.

Haas, R., Sarkies, M., Bowles, K. A., O'Brien, L., & Haines, T. (2016). Early commencement of physical therapy in the acute phase following elective lower limb arthroplasty produces favorable outcomes: A systematic review and meta-analysis examining allied health service models. *Osteoarthritis and Cartilage, 24*(10), 1667–1681.

Harridge, S. D., Kryger, A., & Stensgaard, A. (1999). Knee extensor strength, activation, and size in very elderly people following strength training. *Muscle and Nerve, 22*(7), 831–839.

Hastings, S. N., Sloane, R., Morey, M. C., Pavon, J. M., & Hoenig, H. (2014). Assisted early mobility for hospitalized older veterans: Preliminary data from the STRIDE program. *Journal of the American Geriatrics Society, 62*(11), 2180–2184.

Horn, S. D., DeJong, G., & Deutscher, D. (2012). Practice-based evidence research in rehabilitation: An alternative to randomized controlled trials and traditional observational studies. *Archives of Physical Medicine and Rehabilitation, 93*(8 Suppl), S127–S137.

Hvid, L. G., Suetta, C., Nielsen, J. H., Jensen, M. M., Frandsen, U., Ørtenblad, N., Kjaer, M., & Aagaard, P. (2014). Aging impairs the recovery in mechanical muscle function following 4 days of disuse. *Experimental Gerontology, 52*, 1–8.

Iovino, P., Chiarioni, G., Bilancio, G., Cirillo, M., Mekjavic, I. B., Pisot, R., & Ciacci, C. (2013). New onset of constipation during long-term physical inactivity: A proof-of-concept study on the immobility-induced bowel changes. *PLoS One, 8*(8), e72608.

Karlsen, A., Loeb, M. R., Andersen, K. B., Joergensen, K. J., Scheel, F. U., Turtumoeygard, I. F., Perez, A. L., Kjaer, M., & Beyer, N. (2016). Improved functional performance in geriatric patients during hospital stay. *American Journal of Physical Medicine & Rehabilitation, 96*(5), e78–e84.

Kehlet, H. (1997). Multimodal approach to control postoperative pathophysiology and rehabilitation. *British Journal of Anaesthesia, 78*(5), 606–617.

Kortebein, P., Symons, T. B., Ferrando, A., Paddon-Jones, D., Ronsen, O., Protas, E., Conger, S., Lombeida, J., Wolfe, R., & Evans, W. J. (2008). Functional impact of 10 days of bed rest in healthy older adults. *Journals of Gerontology. Series A, Biological Sciences and Medical Sciences, 63*(10), 1076–1081.

Kosse, N. M., Dutmer, A. L., Dasenbrock, L., Bauer, J. M., & Lamoth, C. J. (2013). Effectiveness and feasibility of early physical rehabilitation programs for geriatric hospitalized patients: A systematic review. *BMC Geriatrics, 13*, 107. https://doi.org/10.1186/1471-2318-13-107.

Kronborg, L., Bandholm, T., Palm, H., Kehlet, H., & Kristensen, M. T. (2014). Feasibility of progressive strength training implemented in the acute ward after hip fracture surgery. *PLoS One, 9*(4), e93332.

Lindgren, M., Unosson, M., Fredrikson, M., & Ek, A. C. (2004). Immobility – A major risk factor for development of pressure ulcers among adult hospitalized patients: A prospective study. *Scandinavian Journal of Caring Sciences, 18*(1), 57–64.

Maffiuletti, N. A. (2010). Physiological and methodological considerations for the use of neuromuscular electrical stimulation. *European Journal of Applied Physiology, 110*(2), 223–234.

Maffiuletti, N. A., Roig, M., Karatzanos, E., & Nanas, S. (2013). Neuromuscular electrical stimulation for preventing skeletal-muscle weakness and wasting in critically ill patients: A systematic review. *BMC Medicine, 11*, 137.

Manini, T., Marko, M., VanArnam, T., Cook, S., Fernhall, B., Burke, J., & Ploutz-Snyder, L. (2007). Efficacy of resistance and task-specific exercise in older adults who modify tasks of everyday life. *Journals of Gerontology. Series A, Biological Sciences and Medical Sciences, 62*(6), 616–623.

Manton, K. G., Corder, L. S., & Stallard, E. (1993). Estimates of change in chronic disability and institutional incidence and prevalence rates in the U.S. elderly population from the 1982, 1984, and 1989 National Long Term Care Survey. *Journal of Gerontology, 48*(4), S153–S166.

McGavock, J. M., Hastings, J. L., Snell, P. G., McGuire, D. K., Pacini, E. L., Levine, B. D., & Mitchell, J. H. (2009). A forty-year follow-up of the Dallas bed rest and training study: The effect of age on the cardiovascular response to exercise in men. *Journals of Gerontology. Series A, Biological Sciences and Medical Sciences, 64*((2), 293–299.

Mitchell, R., Harvey, L., Brodaty, H., Draper, B., & Close, J. (2016). Hip fracture and the influence of dementia on health outcomes and access to hospital-based rehabilitation for older individuals. *Disability and Rehabilitation, 14*, 1–10.

Mudge, A. M., O'Rourke, P., & Denaro, C. P. (2010). Timing and risk factors for functional changes associated with medical hospitalization in older patients. *Journals of Gerontology. Series A, Biological Sciences and Medical Sciences, 65*(8), 866–872.

Paton, F., Chambers, D., Wilson, P., Eastwood, A., Craig, D., Fox, D., Jayne, D., & McGinnes, E. (2014). Effectiveness and implementation of enhanced recovery after surgery programmes: A rapid evidence synthesis. *BMJ Open, 4*(7), e005015.

Pedersen, B. K., & Saltin, B. (2015). Exercise as medicine – Evidence for prescribing exercise as therapy in 26 different chronic diseases. *Scandinavian Journal of Medicine and Science in Sports, 25*(Suppl 3), 1–72.

Pedersen, M. M., Bodilsen, A. C., Petersen, J., Beyer, N., Andersen, O., Lawson-Smith, L., Kehlet, H., & Bandholm, T. (2013). Twenty-four-hour mobility during acute hospitalization in older medical patients. *The Journals of Gerontology. Series A, Biological Sciences and Medical Sciences, 68*(3), 331–337.

Pedersen, M. M., Petersen, J., Bean, J. F., Damkjaer, L., Juul-Larsen, H. G., Andersen, O., Beyer, N., & Bandholm, T. (2015). Feasibility of progressive sit-to-stand training among older hospitalized patients. *PeerJ, 3*, e1500.

Ploutz-Snyder, L. L., Manini, T., Ploutz-Snyder, R. J., & Wolf, D. A. (2002). Functionally relevant thresholds of quadriceps femoris strength. *The Journals of Gerontology. Series A, Biological Sciences and Medical Sciences, 57*(4), B144–B152.

Resnick, B., Wells, C., Galik, E., Holtzman, L., Zhu, S., Gamertsfelder, E., Laidlow, T., & Boltz, M. (2016). Feasibility and efficacy of function-focused Care for Orthopedic Trauma Patients. *Journal of Trauma Nursing, 23*(3), 144–155.

Roubenoff, R. (2000). Sarcopenia: A major modifiable cause of frailty in the elderly. *Journal of Nutrition Health and Aging, 4*(3), 140–142.

Shih, S. L., Zafonte, R., Bates, D. W., Gerrard, P., Goldstein, R., Mix, J., Niewczyk, P., Greysen, S. R., Kazis, L., Ryan, C. M., & Schneider, J. C. (2016). Functional status outperforms comorbidities as a predictor of 30-day acute care readmissions in the inpatient rehabilitation population. *Journal of the American Medical Directors Association, 17*(10), 921–926.

Soga, Y., Yokoi, H., Ando, K., Shirai, S., Sakai, K., Kondo, K., Goya, M., Iwabuchi, M., & Nobuyoshi, M. (2010). Safety of early exercise training after elective coronary stenting in patients with stable coronary artery disease. *European Journal of Cardiovascular Prevention and Rehabilitation, 17*(2), 230–234.

Sourdet, S., Lafont, C., Rolland, Y., Nourhashemi, F., Andrieu, S., & Vellas, B. (2015). Preventable iatrogenic disability in elderly patients during hospitalization. *Journal of the American Medical Directors Association, 16*(8), 674–681.

Stenroth, L., Sillanpää, E., McPhee, J. S., Narici, M. V., Gapeyeva, H., Pääsuke, M., Barnouin, Y., Hogrel, J. Y., Butler-Browne, G., Bijlsma, A., Meskers, C. G., Maier, A. B., Finni, T., & Sipilä, S. (2015). Plantarflexor muscle-tendon properties are associated with mobility in healthy older adults. *The Journals of Gerontology. Series A, Biological Sciences and Medical Sciences, 70*(8), 996–1002.

Suetta, C., Magnusson, S. P., Rosted, A., Aagaard, P., Jakobsen, A. K., Larsen, L. H., Duus, B., & Kjaer, M. (2004). Resistance training in the early postoperative phase reduces hospitalization and leads to muscle hypertrophy in elderly hip surgery patients–a controlled, randomized study. *Journal of the American Geriatrics Society, 52*(12), 2016–2022.

Suetta, C., Magnusson, S. P., Beyer, N., & Kjaer, M. (2007). Effect of strength training on muscle function in elderly hospitalized patients. *Scandinavian Journal of Medicine and Science in Sports, 17*(5), 464–472.

Suetta, C., Hvid, L. G., Justesen, L., Christensen, U., Neergaard, K., Simonsen, L., Ortenblad, N., Magnusson, S. P., Kjaer, M., & Aagaard, P. (2009). Effects of aging on human skeletal muscle after immobilization and retraining. *Journal of Applied Physiology (1985), 107*(4), 1172–1180.

Suetta, C., Frandsen, U., Mackey, A. L., Jensen, L., Hvid, L. G., Bayer, M. L., Petersson, S. J., Schrøder, H. D., Andersen, J. L., Aagaard, P., Schjerling, P., & Kjaer, M. (2013). Ageing is associated with diminished muscle re-growth and myogenic precursor cell expansion early after immobility-induced atrophy in human skeletal muscle. *Journal of Physiology, 591*(15), 3789–3804.

Sullivan, D. H., Sun, S., & Walls, R. C. (1999). Protein-energy undernutrition among elderly hospitalized patients: A prospective study. *Journal of the American Medical Association, 281*(21), 2013–2019.

Sullivan, D. H., Wall, P. T., Bariola, J. R., Bopp, M. M., & Frost, Y. M. (2001). Progressive resistance muscle strength training of hospitalized frail elderly. *American Journal of Physical Medicine and Rehabilitation, 80*(7), 503–509.

Taraldsen, K., Sletvold, O., Thingstad, P., Saltvedt, I., Granat, M. H., Lydersen, S., & Helbostad, J. L. (2014). Physical behavior and function early after hip fracture surgery in patients receiving comprehensive geriatric care or orthopedic care – A randomized controlled trial. *The Journals of Gerontology. Series A, Biological Sciences and Medical Sciences, 69*(3), 338–345.

Thingstad, P., Taraldsen, K., Saltvedt, I., Sletvold, O., Vereijken, B., Lamb, S. E., & Helbostad, J. L. (2016). The long-term effect of comprehensive geriatric care on gait after hip fracture: The Trondheim hip fracture trial–a randomised controlled trial. *Osteoporosis International, 27*(3), 933–942.

Tudor-Locke, C., Craig, C. L., Aoyagi, Y., Bell, R. C., Croteau, K. A., De Bourdeaudhuij, I., Ewald, B., Gardner, A. W., Hatano, Y., Lutes, L. D., Matsudo, S. M., Ramirez-Marrero, F. A., Rogers, L. Q., Rowe, D. A., Schmidt, M. D., Tully, M. A., & Blair, S. N. (2011). How many steps/day are enough? For older adults and special populations. *International Journal of Behavioral Nutrition and Physical Activity, 8*, 80.

Vandervoort, A. A. (2002). Aging of the human neuromuscular system. *Muscle & Nerve, 25*(1), 17–25.

Vanhees, L., Rauch, B., Piepoli, M., van Buuren, F., Takken, T., Börjesson, M., Bjarnason-Wehrens, B., Doherty, P., Dugmore, D., & Halle, M. (2012). Writing group, EACPR. Importance of characteristics and modalities of physical activity and exercise in the management of cardiovascular health in individuals with cardiovascular disease (part III). *European Journal of Preventive Cardiology, 19*(6), 1333–1356.

Volaklis, K. A., & Tokmakidis, S. P. (2005). Resistance exercise training in patients with heart failure. *Sports Medicine, 35*(12), 1085–1103.

Wells, J. L., & Dumbrell, A. C. (2006). Nutrition and aging: Assessment and treatment of compromised nutritional status in frail elderly patients. *Clinical Interventions in Aging, 1*(1), 67–79.

Section 3

How to Maximise Participation in Physical Activity Among Older People

Julia K. Wolff

This section will approach physical activity promotion in old age from a psychological perspective. Referring to the ecological model by Dahlgren and Whitehead (1991) that serves as the overall theoretical framework for this handbook (see Chap. 1 for details), the psychological perspective concentrates on the central component of the model: the individual. That is, psychological approaches to promote physical activity in old age target individual factors, such as motivation, attitudes, and strategies.

The following chapters integrate theories and practices from health psychology and developmental psychology. These two disciplines both have a long-standing tradition in investigating the promotion of physical activity in the context of opportunities and challenges over the course of development throughout adulthood and old age. Organised by central gateways to physical activity promotion, the chapters summarise pertinent psychological theories, concepts, and techniques. All of these are critically evaluated with regard to empirical findings and in their applicability to the life circumstances of older adults.

Chapter 11 introduces the relevant psychological theories and summarises important behaviour change techniques for promoting physical activity. It also highlights empirical evidence for validation of theories and effectiveness of techniques among older adults. This information provides the theoretical

---

J. K. Wolff (✉)
Institute of Psychogerontology, Friedrich-Alexander-University, Erlangen-Nuremberg

basis for the following chapters that go into detail on the most important techniques and concepts in physical activity promotion among older adults.

Self-efficacy, meaning the belief of being able to accomplish a task despite difficulties, is an important psychological resource for the initiation and maintenance of physical activity in old age. Chapter 12 provides details on this psychological construct and its theoretical foundation. Empirical evidence on the effects of self-efficacy on physical activity as well as opportunities to promote self-efficacy beliefs in older adults is summarised before concluding with implications for practice.

Each behaviour is enacted in accordance with personal motives of an individual. This is also true for physical activity, and, thus, Chap. 13 focuses on motivational barriers and resources for physical activity in old age. Empirical evidence regarding the relevance of classical motivational factors from health psychological theories, for example, to what extent one identifies with being physically active (e.g., cycling instead of driving as a routine way of moving when people perceive themselves as 'an active person'), subjective norms related to physical activity (e.g., sedentary behaviour viewed as 'normal' in old age), perceptions of risks resulting from not being physically active (e.g., developing functional limitations), and expectancies regarding positive outcomes of physical activity (e.g., staying fit and mobile) and their relevance in old age are discussed. This knowledge is complemented by a summary of research from developmental psychology where the perception of one's own ageing process as positive or negative has been described as an important predictor for physical activity.

Chapter 14 focuses on the role of self-regulation (e.g., monitoring and regulating one's own behaviour) and planning strategies (e.g., plans of when, where, and how to be active) in the promotion of physical activity among older adults. This chapter brings together self-regulatory techniques for changing behaviour from health psychology with self-regulatory theories from developmental psychology. The interplay of age-related changes in cognition, motivation, as well as physical functioning and self-regulatory behaviour are discussed. Contradictory empirical findings on effects of self-regulation on physical activity are summarised with important conclusions for practice.

This section ends with Chap. 15 that deals with tailoring physical activity interventions to the needs of older adults. Acceptability of physical activity as a normal part of life in old age and effectiveness of behaviour change techniques with older people are discussed. This includes empirical evidence on factors associated with physical activity in older people and adaptations to interventions to address common misperceptions around physical activity and the older adult population. The chapter concludes with practical implications for promoting initiation and maintenance of physical activity among older people.

In sum, this section will give an overview on theories and constructs from health psychology and developmental psychology that are investigated in the context of physical activity promotion among older people. In doing so, this section focuses on individual factors that are relevant for promoting physical activity according to the model by Dahlgren and Whitehead (1991; see Chap. 1 for details). It gives important suggestions on how to achieve higher engagement in physical activity in old age that is accompanied with many benefits as outlined in Section 1. Psychological resources such as motivation to be active, self-efficacy, self-views, and planning strategies and their importance for initiation and maintenance of physical activity up into old age are explained. Behaviour change techniques to promote these individual resources and how they may apply to everyday life of older people are discussed. The described individual circumstances and resources as well as intervention techniques interact with the environment (Section 5), healthcare, and social embeddedness (Sections 4 and 6) as well as health status (Section 2) of the person. Many of the findings reported are relevant for current debates in promotion of physical activity as described in Section 7. Thus, individual psychological resources and strategies that can be promoted in physical activity interventions interact with the individual, social, and societal context a person lives in and should be interpreted and applied integrating the knowledge of the other sections and chapters of this handbook.

11

Behaviour Change Theories and Techniques for Promoting Physical Activity Among Older People

Karen Morgan and Maw Pin Tan

11.1 Introduction

Despite the well-established benefits of physical activity for older adults, levels of activity remain low in this population (see Chap. 2). This has led to an increasing focus on interventions to increase physical activity specifically among older adults. This chapter will summarise the most common health psychology models of behaviour change that have been used to guide such interventions. A key component of designing effective interventions is the identification of the behaviour change techniques (BCTs) that work best for older adults in different contexts or settings. Hence, we will highlight important recent advances in developing a taxonomy of behaviour change techniques (Michie et al. 2013).

K. Morgan (✉)
Perdana University-Royal College of Surgeons in Ireland School of Medicine, Perdana University, Serdang, Selangor, Malaysia

Division of Population Health Sciences, Royal College of Surgeons in Ireland, Dublin, Ireland

M. P. Tan
Department of Medicine, Faculty of Medicine, University of Malaya, Kuala Lumpur, Malaysia

11.2 Behaviour Change Theories

In their book, *ABC of Behaviour Change Theories*, Michie and colleagues outlined 83 theories of behaviour and behaviour change that they identified based on a literature review carried out under the direction of an expert group from a range of disciplines (Michie et al. 2014). Seven theories were used in almost three-quarters (73%) of the studies found in their review. These were (in order of frequency of occurrence): the Transtheoretical Model of Change (TTM, also known as the Stages of Change Model), the Theory of Planned Behaviour (TPB), Social Cognitive Theory (SCT), the Information-Motivation-Behavioural-Skills Model (IMB), the Health Belief Model (HBM), Self-Determination Theory (SDT) and the Health Action Process Approach (HAPA). Each of these theories will be summarised here. Each summary will be followed by a brief discussion of studies that have used the theory to explore physical activity, particularly with older adults.

Some studies have assessed more than one of the theories mentioned above. One worth noting is a review of RCTs which included 19,357 participants from 82 studies involving TTM, SCT, TPB among others (Gourlan et al. 2016). A meta-analysis showed a small- to medium-effect size (Cohen's d) on physical activity. Comparing theories, the authors found no one theory to be superior in terms of effect size. They did find that interventions based on a single theory were more effective than those based on multiple theories. The authors note however, that many of the trials they reviewed in which interventions were based on multiple theories did not outline the rationale for their approach. This has been noted in a number of other reviews (e.g. Chase 2013).

11.2.1 The Transtheoretical Model

The TTM or Stages of Change Model (Prochaska and DiClemente 1984) assumes that people move through stages of change and that different psychological processes are involved at each stage. The model encompasses 5 stages of change, 10 change processes, decisional balance, self-efficacy and temptation. The stages as described by Prochaska and DiClemente are:

- Precontemplation: a person in this stage may not be aware of the need to change and is generally not considering changing within the next six months. Individuals may be in denial, be resistant to change, may report more barriers to change and low self-efficacy for change. Self-efficacy was defined by Bandura (1995, p. 2) as 'the belief in one's capabilities to

organize and execute the courses of action required to manage prospective situations.'
- Contemplation: the need for change is acknowledged and consideration is being given to changing within the next six months. ('I will increase my physical activity.') Individuals at this stage may seek and be responsive to information, for example, information about physical activity classes or the benefits of being physically active.
- Preparation: an individual in this stage is ready to change and sets specific goals (e.g. sets a date to start a schedule of physical activity). Making concrete plans is important at this stage.
- Action: in this stage efforts to change behaviour can be observed (e.g. starting a physical activity regime). Realistic goals and social support are important. Moving into this stage can be a challenge for some vulnerable groups (e.g. frail older adults due to fear of injury or falling).
- Maintenance: in this stage an individual has maintained behaviour for more than six months (e.g. adheres to physical activity regime). Self-monitoring can assist with maintenance.

According to this theory, individuals can move back and forward between stages, for example, from preparation back to contemplation and from action back to preparation (e.g. in the case of relapse) and some individuals may stay at a certain stage for long periods. Precontemplation and contemplation are generally considered to be concerned with motivation and intention while preparation involves intention and volition. In some versions of the model, termination (where an individual is confident of not relapsing) (Prochaska and Prochaska 2011) or relapse are added as a sixth stage.

Two sets of processes facilitate movement between stages. These are experiential processes (which aid movement between the first three stages) and behavioural processes (predominately used in the action and maintenance phases). These are outlined in Table 11.1.

As individuals move through stages, decisional balance (the process of comparing potential losses and benefits or the pros and cons associated with behaviour change) shifts. For example, in precontemplation the potential losses/cons associated with change outweigh the benefits or pros of the status quo. In contemplation, the two sides become more balanced (ambivalence). Once the perceived pros outweigh the cons, the individual moves into preparation. Self-efficacy is also dynamic. Initially, self-efficacy for change is likely to be low and the temptation is to maintain the status quo (unhealthy behaviour). However, as self-efficacy increases and temptation is reduced, behaviour

Table 11.1 Experiential and behavioural processes which facilitate movement between stages of change

---

Experiential

Consciousness raising: increasing awareness of the need to change or the reasons to change, for example, finding or seeking information on the benefits of physical activity. The focus may be on cause (e.g. reasons for inactivity), consequences (e.g. negative outcomes associated with inactivity) or cures (how to become more active)

Dramatic relief: paying attention to and expressing feelings about a problem, for example, concern about having a sedentary lifestyle. Testimonies from others can trigger emotions

Environmental reevaluation: this is about noticing the negative effect of unhealthy behaviour and the positive effect of healthy behaviour on others; assessing the impact that change might have more broadly, and how it would change one's social environment, for example, being a role model

Self-reevaluation: assessing how a change (e.g. becoming physically active) might impact on one's own self-image (e.g. wanting to see oneself as a healthy person)

Social liberation: noticing increased social opportunity for change, for example, publically available and accessible facilities for physical activity

Behavioural

Helping relationships: having relationships that are supportive of change, seeking and using social support

Counter conditioning: learning new behaviours that are healthy and substituting them for unhealthy ones, for example, going for a walk instead of watching TV

Stimulus control: managing the environment by reducing cues for unhealthy behaviours, for example, moving the TV and increasing those for healthy behaviour and having walking shoes visible/easily accessible at all times

Reinforcement management: having rewards for healthy behaviour

Self-liberation: believing in one's ability to change and committing to change

---

change can occur and be maintained. Relapse can occur where temptation exceeds maintenance self-efficacy.

The TTM has proved to be popular as a theory used to guide interventions. However, the evidence for its efficacy is mixed. Bully et al. (2015) reviewed theory-based interventions for lifestyle modifications (including physical activity) in primary care settings. Of 17 studies identified, 13 used the TTM. Six addressed physical activity alone or in combination with other behaviour(s). Half of the studies showed the effect of an intervention on activity. Only two studies included older adults specifically. One of these demonstrated an intervention effect, the other did not. The study which showed a positive effect of an intervention used a counselling intervention (delivered by nurses) for older women (average age 74 years) and was effective over a 12-month period (Mairki et al. 2006). This and other reviews (Bridle et al. 2005; Hutchison et al. 2009) noted that lack of model specification and poor application of the model are a concern.

As part of a project which examined theory-based psychosocial determinants of physical activity and fall risks in community-dwelling older adults, Kosma and Cardinal (2016) assessed stage of change of participants. They found that those in the 'action' stage reported less cons of being physically active than those in the precontemplation, contemplation or preparation stages. Physical activity increased and falls risks decreased across the stages. Processes of change and decisional balance were also assessed; however, the only predictor of physical activity was self-efficacy. The implication for intervention design being that older adults should be given opportunities to build self-efficacy through guided experience as this may be more important than cognitive evaluations of the pros and cons of being physically active (see Chap. 12 for details on self-efficacy).

Although the TTM has been heavily criticised (West 2005), it remains a very popular theory in health promotion. Bridle et al. noted that TTM interventions tend to be more intense (perhaps due to personalisation) which may contribute to the effects observed in some studies (Bridle et al. 2005). Studies with older adults lend some support to the idea that personalisation is important (Gellert et al. 2014b; van Stralen et al. 2011).

11.2.2 The Theory of Planned Behaviour

The TPB (Ajzen 1985) evolved from the Theory of Reasoned Action (Fishbein and Ajzen 1975) and proposes that behaviour is determined by behavioural intention. The key determinants of this behavioural intention are: (a) attitudes (outcome expectancies or beliefs about the outcomes of a behaviour and the value of these outcomes), (b) subjective norms or the influence of the social environment (social pressure to maintain the status quo or to change or beliefs about what other people think you should do) and (c) perceived behavioural control (personal beliefs about control over the resources and skills required to perform a behaviour, including in difficult situations), see Chap. 13 for details on these concepts.

Interventions designed based on the TPB initially focused on increasing behavioural intention; however there is a now well-documented intention-behaviour gap, that is, the gap between what individuals intend to do and what they actually do. A 2012 systematic review and meta-analysis, which focused specifically on the intention-behaviour gap in the context of physical activity, included 10 studies and 3,899 participants (albeit all aged less than 64 years). Only 54% of those who intended to be physically active at public guideline levels actually were (Rhodes and de Bruijn 2013). The authors suggested that while there was strong evidence that intention is necessary for physical activity to occur (only 2% of non-intenders were subsequently physically active), this alone is not sufficient for behaviour.

Hardeman et al. (2010) conducted a systematic review of studies which applied the TPB to a behaviour change intervention and/or the evaluation of a behaviour change intervention. The review identified 30 papers and 24 studies (3 included physical activity as an outcome variable). Interventions included strategies such as the provision of information, persuasion, planning, social support, goal setting and skills building. What Hardeman et al. highlighted was that while all studies used the TPB to guide measurement, only half used it in the actual development of the intervention. The authors also commented on the poor quality of many studies and the lack of reporting in terms of the targeted component of the TPB in the interventions.

There has been much criticism of TPB and considerable debate about whether it should be retired or extended (Sniehotta et al. 2014, 2015). It has been proposed that the TPB needs to be revised to include planning activities (Conner et al. 2002) and implementation intentions ('if-then' plans that specify when, where and how a behaviour will be enacted) (Webb and Sheeran 2007). A 2011 meta-analysis of the effect of implementation intentions on physical activity found an overall small to medium effect of interventions (Bélanger-Gravel et al. 2013). It has been suggested that planning and implementation intentions maybe particularly helpful for those who experience difficulties enacting certain behaviours, for example (Allan et al. 2013; Hall et al. 2012). Planning is further discussed in Chap. 14.

A 2014 study which specifically looked at implementation intentions related to physical activity in a sample of older women ($N = 75$) with an average age of 74 years found that implementation intentions significantly enhanced physical activity over the study period of 4 weeks with a moderate effect size (Hall et al. 2014). In this study, women with stronger executive control saw the most benefit from using implementation intentions. On the other hand, a TPB-based RCT designed to promote physical activity and healthy eating among older adults with type 2 diabetes and cardiovascular disease was less successful (183 participants; average age 61 years). The intervention focused on attitudes, perceived barriers, social support, planning for change and fostering control (White et al. 2012). The study showed some change in physical activity but this was not sustained at the six-week follow-up.

Overall few studies have used the TPB to design and/or evaluate interventions to increase physical activity in older adults. Extending the theory to incorporate other important determinants of behaviour may be useful.

11.2.3 Social Cognitive Theory

SCT (Bandura 1995) proposes that how an individual functions is the result of dynamic interactions between behaviour, personal and environmental factors. This is often referred to as reciprocal determinism. For example, the likelihood of engaging in a particular behaviour (e.g. being physically active) may be increased by individual or personal factors, for example, outcome expectancies or self-efficacy. This may impact norms in a social group, which in turn may impact individual outcome expectancies/motivation and thus increase the likelihood of the behaviour occurring again.

SCT theory describes five basic capabilities that explain human cognition and behaviour. *Symbolising capability* refers to the ability to form, use and store symbols. This allows individuals to ascribe meaning to experiences and create cognitive models which guide future behaviour. Individuals plan future actions (e.g. being physically active), anticipate outcomes (e.g. risk of falling/injury) and set goals using *forethought capability.* Learning can occur through observing the actions of others and the consequences of these actions, allowing individuals to avoid trial and error processes that might be risky. This is referred to as *vicarious capability.* In the context of physical activity in older adults, observing others engaging in activities is an opportunity for learning. The *self-regulatory capability* allows individuals to monitor and change behaviour in response to feedback. Where there is incongruity between behaviour and the standard against which it is being measured, change may be prompted. Finally, the *self-reflective capability* refers to the ability to evaluate experience. Individuals beliefs about their ability to cope with certain situations or behave in certain ways are derived from reflection. These beliefs or perceptions are also known as self-efficacy.

In a systematic review and meta-analysis of 44 studies of physical activity and SCT, Young et al. (2014) identified 55 different SCT models of physical activity. Each of these included at least one measure of self-efficacy and outcome expectations. Less than half (22 of 55) models included all of the major SCT constructs. In all, 10 of the 55 models were applied in older populations. Overall, the majority of studies were of poor quality. Self-efficacy and goals were associated with physical activity. No association between outcome expectancies and physical activity was recorded. The effect was moderated by methodological quality and also by age (the effect was larger as quality and age increased). The authors concluded that SCT theory is a useful theory for explaining physical activity behaviour (with particular potential in older populations) but that there is a need for more high-quality studies that test-specific techniques which operationalise the behaviour change constructs in SCT (Young et al. 2014). A more detailed discussion of self-efficacy is included in Chap. 12.

11.2.4 The Information-Motivation-Behavioural-Skills Model

The IMB model (Fisher and Fisher 1992; Fisher et al. 1996) is concerned with adherence. In this model, information is knowledge about a medical condition and its management. Motivation includes personal motivation (attitude to adherence), social support and subjective norms. Behavioural skills are the skills, tools or strategies necessary to perform the behaviour.

The IMB was initially developed to explain HIV-related health behaviours and although predominantly used as a model to consider risky sexual behaviour, it is increasingly being considered as a theory for understanding health behaviours in patients who have chronic illnesses. Chang et al. (2014) systematically reviewed RCTs which included intervention strategies based on the IMB. Of the 12 identified, only 1 study examined physical activity (alongside other lifestyle factors) in patients with type 2 diabetes (average age 58 years). In this study (carried out in Puerto Rico), attitudes to exercise were associated with behavioural skills that were independently associated with exercise behaviour. No association was found for social norms for physical activity or information about physical activity (Osborn et al. 2010). This study also called for the detailed and transparent reporting of how the IMB is operationalised in studies.

The IMB may be a useful model to consider when working with older patients to increase physical activity as part of a self-care or self-management regimes.

11.2.5 The Health Belief Model

The HBM (Becker 1974; Rosenstock 1974; Stretcher et al. 1997) proposes that the likelihood an individual will engage in a particular health behaviour, for example, being physically active, depends on their perception of (a) the severity of potential illness (b) their susceptibility to that illness (c) the benefits of taking preventative action (see Chap. 13) and (d) the cost of or barriers to taking action. The HBM views demographic factors (e.g. age, gender, ethnicity, socioeconomic status) and socio-psychological factors (e.g. personality, social norms) as important influencers of these perceptions.

Assessing the severity of illness (e.g. 'I believe cardiovascular disease is very serious.') and perceived susceptibility (e.g. 'I am not physically active and so vulnerable to cardiovascular disease.') forms a threat evaluation. This is followed by a behavioural evaluation, in which an individual assesses the benefits of taking action (e.g. 'being physically active would improve my health') versus the cost of doing so (e.g. 'joining the gym is expensive'). This is somewhat similar to decisional balance in the TTM. Cues-to-action prompt behaviour change. These can be internal (e.g. being out of breath) or external (e.g. a media campaign to promote activity or interaction with friends who are active). Where threat evaluation is low, stronger cues are required to trigger action. The concept of self-efficacy has also been incorporated into the model in order that it might better explain habitual behaviour (Rosenstock 1990). Promoting health behaviour, therefore, may concentrate on increasing the threat evaluation, increasing cues to action or focus on barriers and benefits to tip the balance in favour of action.

A meta-analysis by Carpenter (2010) included 18 studies (n = 2,702) and concluded that the different HBM constructs were of varied and weak predictive power in relation to health behaviour. In relation to physical activity, a community-based HBM theory-based intervention that took place over four months in senior centres in the United States was found to increase minutes of physical activity and step count (Fitzpatrick et al. 2008). Few other studies have examined HBM and physical activity or considered older adults, although some recent studies have suggested the model could be applied to the area of falls prevention which is closely linked with physical activity.

11.2.6 Self-Determination Theory

The SDT is a framework or meta-theory for the study of motivation, personality and well-being (Deci and Ryan 2008). The SDT assumes individuals actively seek opportunities to grow and that new experiences are essential to development. According to this theory, individuals have three innate needs and when these needs are met, optimal growth and function is facilitated. These needs are the need for competence (the need to learn new skills, gain mastery), relatedness (the need to experience connection with others or belonging) and autonomy (the need to feel in control or to have choice).

Where an environment is supportive of these needs, intrinsic motivation is fostered, that is, motivation due to inherent interest. There are different types of motivation that drive behaviour. These are amotivation (unregulated motivation with no intention to engage in a behaviour), intrinsic motivation and extrinsic motivation (doing something as a means to achieve an outcome external to the behaviour itself, e.g. reward). The SDT framework comprises a number of theories, each concerned with an aspect of motivation (see Deci and Ryan 2007, for detailed discussion). Intrinsic or internalised motivation is seen as an important driver of behaviour and sustained change. SDT also highlights the importance of considering the nature of goals and that individuals are more motivated to achieve goals framed as being important to meeting their basic needs of being competent, connected and having choice.

A systematic review of 66 studies which assessed the relationship between the SDT and physical activity reported a positive association between more autonomous forms of motivation and exercise behaviour (Teixeira et al. 2012). A detailed discussion of motivation is included in Chap. 13. A small feasibility study based in Korea using a mixed-methods approach to evaluate a 13-month SDT-based exercise programme for older adults suggests SDT-based interventions may be worth exploring with this population (Lee et al. 2016).

11.2.7 The Health Action Process Approach

The HAPA model (Schwarzer 1992, 2008) proposes that behaviour change is achieved as the result of a two-phase/stage process. The first stage centres on motivation and the development of an intention. This process includes risk perception (e.g. 'I am at risk of getting ill'), outcome expectancies (e.g. 'if I exercise I am less likely to get ill') and perceived action self-efficacy or belief in one's ability to perform an action. (e.g. 'I can follow a weekly exercise schedule.') Positive outcome expectancies and perceived action self-efficacy are necessary in order for an intention to change behaviour to be formed (see Chap. 13). The second phase, called the volitional phase, concerns the initiation and maintenance of behaviour. This is achieved through forming action planning and coping planning (see Chap. 14). Coping self-efficacy (belief in the ability to maintain one's actions) and recovery self-efficacy (belief in the ability to resume action after failure) are important in this phase (see Chap. 12).

It has been suggested that among older adults the motivation for maintenance and loss prevention is higher than that of younger adults (Freund 2006), and they may perceive more risks associated with engaging rather than not engaging in health behaviours. Caudroit and colleagues (2011) targeted retirees in a study which aimed to examine the HAPA in a sample of 120 individuals over a 6-month period. Specifically, they examined the roles of self-efficacy, risk perception and outcome expectancies in predicting physical activity. Results indicated that self-efficacy and risk perception were important in intention formation, however the effect for outcome expectancies was not significant. Planning was not associated with activity, a finding it is suggested may indicate that when older individuals are motivated to engage in physical activity, their intentions are translated directly into action. Perhaps, for retirees, less planning (see Chap. 14) is required when their motivation is high as they have more autonomy over their time than those in paid employment.

A theory-based qualitative study carried out in the United Kingdom suggests that an individualised approach to increasing physical activity is required in the period of transition to retirement (McDonald et al. 2015). While certain barriers to being physically active (e.g. time) may be removed, other barriers may become more salient (e.g. financial cost). The findings suggest that transition to retirement may be a favourable time to promote physical activity and that the patterns of physical activity may develop over the different phases of retirement. A discussion in relation to making physical activity personally relevant to older adults is included in Chap. 15.

11.3 From Theory to Techniques

As previously noted, several reviews of theory-driven or theory-based interventions have highlighted a need for authors to include more detailed descriptions of how theoretical concepts are operationalised. A theoretical understanding of behaviour and behaviour change is essential to ensure the development of effective interventions (Davis et al. 2015). Focusing on specific BCTs rather than broader theoretical concepts is seen an important step forward in developing and evaluating interventions. A BCT can be defined as:

> an active component of an intervention designed to change behaviour. The defining characteristics of a BCT are that it is 'observable, replicable, irreducible' a component of an intervention designed to change behaviour and a postulated active ingredient within the intervention. It is thus the smallest component compatible with retaining the postulated active ingredients, i.e. the proposed mechanisms of change, and can be used alone or in combination with other BCTs. (Michie and Johnston 2013, p. 182)

The BCT Taxonomy version 1 (BCTTv1) is a comprehensive and structured classification of BCTs (Michie et al. 2013). This taxonomy was developed using a Delphi-type approach, includes 93 BCTs grouped in 16 clusters and represents a significant advance in the development of new interventions, as well as facilitating the accurate and faithful replication of existing interventions. It also provides a schema for systematic reviews endeavouring to synthesise information about BCTs from many studies. Online training in the use of the BCTTv1 has been developed, and includes access to a range of resources and support (see www.bct-taxonomy.com). The BCTTv1 was developed in the context of the COM-B (capability, opportunity, motivation and behaviour) change framework (Michie et al. 2011), a new behaviour change framework—the 'COM-B system' which the authors hope will overcome limitations in existing frameworks. This framework is described in detail in the introduction of this handbook. An overview and discussion of the effects of specific BCTs on physical activity in older adults is included in the following chapters in this handbook (12, 13, 14 and 15).

11.4 Practical Implications

Understanding older adult's perspectives on physical activity in context and assessing the acceptability of different interventions to them is essential if behaviour change is to be achieved at population level (see Chap. 15). Much of what we know about promoting physical activity has been learned from studies that do not include older adults. Indeed studies with older adults suggest that merely transferring models that work with other populations will not be sufficient and in fact could have negative impacts (e.g. French et al. 2014).

Research on the HAPA model suggests that perhaps planning is not viewed as a useful strategy by older adults (Caudroit et al. 2011; Warner et al. 2016). It has also been suggested that framing messages in terms of health or focusing on health benefits might not be the best strategy for increasing physical activity in community-dwelling older adults. Looking at the literature on quality of life (QoL) and QoL assessment, we know that over emphasising physical health prevents an accurate and full understanding of QoL. For many older adults, health is no longer the most important component of QoL (Morgan and McGee 2016). So perhaps health benefits are similarly regulated to secondary benefit status when it comes to physical activity. Focusing on the social aspects of physical activity might be a more useful strategy with older adults.

Focusing on self-efficacy is a recommendation from a number of studies (e.g. Kosma and Cardinal 2016); Young et al.'s (2014) meta-analysis of SCT found that self-efficacy and goal setting were associated with physical activity while studies using SDT have been positive about its potential for use with older populations (Lee et al. 2016; Teixeira et al. 2012). Future interventions could focus on specific strategies to build physical activity self-efficacy.

Older adults may also benefit more from personalised or age-tailored interventions (Gellert et al. 2014a). The older population is a very large and growing one (see Chap. 2), and it is not homogenous. Future studies must not just acknowledge this but allow for it in their design. It has been suggested, for example, that *N*-of-1 trials are an important additional method of testing BCTs. Nyman et al. (2016) highlight the potential of *N*-of-1 studies to test multiple BCTs in the same individual to see which are most effective. This could potentially allow a high degree of intervention tailoring.

Another important consideration is extending study designs to include populations of older adults in developing countries and cultures different to those that predominate the current studies. One study carried out with Arab women (mostly aged over 50 years) in Qatar found that social/cultural barriers to being physically active included traditional values and taboos about women going out in public without a male relative (Donnelly et al. 2012). The built environment in many developing countries does not encourage physical activity (e.g. no walkways, lack of public transport) and harsh climates also need to be considered. On the other hand, collectivist cultures such as those seen in the Middle East and Asia, could provide a powerful basis for exploring motivation, social norms and social support in relation to changing physical activity levels. Individualistic cultures emphasise the self, and this is reflected in the models discussed which highlight the importance of components like self-efficacy, self-regulation and self-determination. Collectivist cultures (70% of the world, Triandis 1989) are group oriented, and roles may be determined by the group. This leads to differences in decision-making (prioritising the individual or the collective) and in how responsibility is viewed. Collectivist cultures are more likely to allow external explanations of outcomes (successful or otherwise) (Leake and Black 2005).

11.5 Conclusion

Health psychology theories provide important frameworks within which we can consider health behaviours, including physical activity. The theories outlined in the chapter have contributed enormously to our understanding of human needs, motivations, cognition and behaviours. Theoretical limitations and poor and unspecified operationalisation of theoretical constructs however has hampered progress in designing and implementing interventions to change behaviour. The COM-B framework and BCTTv1, therefore, represent exciting and important developments in the field and their use should facilitate significant progress in implementing behaviour change interventions. There are limited theory-based intervention studies carried out with older populations which makes it difficult to make specific recommendations about which theories to use. However, there are some practical implications of the research which has been conducted that can be used as a starting point.

Older adults have been underrepresented in studies conducted to date despite the potential for health and well-being benefits from increasing physical activity in this population. Globalisation also requires the consideration of groups of older adults across the world and the specific challenges and opportunities their circumstances may present.

Suggested Further Reading

- Michie, S., Richardson, M., Johnston, M., Abraham, C., Francis, J., Hardeman, W., Eccles, M. P., Cane, J., & Wood, C. E. (2013). The behavior change technique taxonomy (v1) of 93 hierarchically clustered techniques: Building an international consensus for the reporting of behavior change interventions. *Annals of Behaviour Medicine, 46,* 81–95. https://doi.org/10.1007/s12160-013-9486-6.
- Michie, S., West, R., Campbell, R., Brown, J., & Gainforth, H. (2014). *ABC of behaviour change theories.* Great Britain: Silverback Publishing.

References

Ajzen, I. (1985). From intentions to actions: A theory of planned behavior. In J. Kuhl & J. Beckman (Eds.), *Action-control: From cognition to behavior* (pp. 11–39). Heidelberg: Springer.

Allan, J. L., Sniehotta, F. F., & Johnston, M. (2013). The best laid plans: Planning skill determines the effectiveness of action plans and implementation intentions. *Annals of Behavioral Medicine, 46*(1), 114–120. https://doi.org/10.1007/s12160-013-9483-9.

Bandura, A. (1995). *Self efficacy in changing societies.* New York: Cambridge University Press.

Becker, M. H. (1974). The health belief model and personal health behavior. *Health Education Monographs., 2*(4), 324–508.

Bélanger-Gravel, A., Godin, G., & Amireault, S. (2013). A meta-analytic review of the effect of implementation intentions on physical activity. *Health Psychology Review, 7*(1), 23–54. https://doi.org/10.1080/17437199.2011.560095.

Bridle, C., Riemsma, R. P., Pattenden, J., Sowden, A. J., Mather, L., Watt, I. S., & Walker, A. (2005). Systematic review of the effectiveness of health behavior interventions based on the transtheoretical model. *Psychology & Health, 20*(3), 283–301. https://doi.org/10.1080/08870440512331333997.

Bully, P., Sánchez, Á., Zabaleta-del-Olmo, E., Pombo, H., & Grandes, G. (2015). Evidence from interventions based on theoretical models for lifestyle modification (physical activity, diet, alcohol and tobacco use) in primary care settings: A systematic review. *Preventive Medicine, 76*(Supplement), S76–S93. https://doi.org/10.1016/j.ypmed.2014.12.020.

Carpenter, C. J. (2010). A meta-analysis of the effectiveness of health belief model variables in predicting behavior. *Health Communication, 25*(8), 661–669. https://doi.org/10.1080/10410236.2010.521906.

Caudroit, J., Stephan, Y., & Le Scanff, C. (2011). Social cognitive determinants of physical activity among retired older individuals: An application of the health action process approach. *British Journal of Health Psychology, 16*(Pt 2), 404–417. https://doi.org/10.1348/135910710x518324.

Chang, S. J., Choi, S., Kim, S.-A., & Song, M. (2014). Intervention strategies based on information-motivation-behavioral skills model for health behavior change: A systematic review. *Asian Nursing Research, 8*(3), 172–181. https://doi.org/10.1016/j.anr.2014.08.002.

Chase, J. A. (2013). Physical activity interventions among older adults: A literature review. *Research & Theory for Nursing Practice, 27*(1), 53–80.

Conner, M., Norman, P., & Bell, R. (2002). The theory of planned behavior and healthy eating. *Health Psychology, 21*(2), 194–201.

Davis, R., Campbell, R., Hildon, Z., Hobbs, L., & Michie, S. (2015). Theories of behaviour and behaviour change across the social and behavioural sciences: A scoping review. *Health Psychology Review, 9*(3), 323–344. https://doi.org/10.1080/17437199.17432014.17941722. Epub 17432014 Aug 17437198.

Deci, E., & Ryan, R. (2007). *Self-determination theory: Basic psychological needs in motivation, development, and wellness*. New York: The Guilford Press.

Deci, E., & Ryan, R. (2008). Self-determination theory: A macrotheory of human motivation, development and health. *Canadian Psychology/Psychologie Canadienne, 49*(3), 182–185.

Donnelly, T. T., Al Suwaidi, J., Al Enazi, N. R., Idris, Z., Albulushi, A. M., Yassin, K., et al. (2012). Qatari women living with cardiovascular diseases-challenges and opportunities to engage in healthy lifestyles. *Health Care for Women International, 33*(12), 1114–1134. https://doi.org/10.1080/07399332.07392012.07712172.

Fishbein, M., & Ajzen, I. (1975). *Belief, attitude, intention and behavior: An introduction to theory and research*. Reading: Addison-Wesley.

Fisher, J. D., & Fisher, W. A. (1992). Changing AIDS-risk behavior. *Psychological Bulletin, 111*, 455–474.

Fisher, J. D., Fisher, W. A., Misovich, S. J., Kimble, D. L., & Malloy, T. E. (1996). Changing AIDS risk behavior: Effects of an intervention emphasizing AIDS risk reduction information, motivation, and behavioral skills in a college student population. *Health Psychology, 15,* 114–123.

Fitzpatrick, S. E., Reddy, S., Lommel, T. S., Fischer, J. G., Speer, E. M., Stephens, H., et al. (2008). Physical activity and physical function improved following a community-based intervention in older adults in Georgia senior centers. *Journal of Nutrition for the Elderly, 27*(1–2), 135–154. https://doi.org/10.1080/01639360802060223.

French, D. P., Olander, E. K., Chisholm, A., & Mc Sharry, J. (2014). Which behaviour change techniques are most effective at increasing older adults' self-efficacy and physical activity behaviour? A systematic review. *Annals of Behavioral Medicine, 48*(2), 225–234. https://doi.org/10.1007/s12160-014-9593-z.

Freund, A. M. (2006). Age-differential motivational consequences of optimization versus compensation focus in younger and older adults. *Psychology & Aging, 21*(2), 240–252. https://doi.org/10.1037/0882-7974.21.2.240.

Gellert, P., Ziegelmann, J. P., Krupka, S., Knoll, N., & Schwarzer, R. (2014a). An age-tailored intervention sustains physical activity changes in older adults: A randomized controlled trial. *International Journal of Behavioral Medicine, 21*(3), 519–528. https://doi.org/10.1007/s12529-013-9330-1.

Gellert, P., Ziegelmann, J. P., Krupka, S., Knoll, N., & Schwarzer, R. (2014b). An age-tailored intervention sustains physical activity changes in older adults: A randomized controlled trial. *International Journal of Behavioral Medicine, 21*(3), 519–528. https://doi.org/10.1007/s12529-013-9330-1.

Gourlan, M., Bernard, P., Bortolon, C., Romain, A. J., Lareyre, O., Carayol, M., et al. (2016). Efficacy of theory-based interventions to promote physical activity. A meta-analysis of randomised controlled trials. *Health Psychology Review, 10*(1), 50–66. https://doi.org/10.1080/17437199.2014.981777.

Hall, P. A., Zehr, C. E., Ng, M., & Zanna, M. P. (2012). Implementation intentions for physical activity in supportive and unsupportive environmental conditions: An experimental examination of intention–behavior consistency. *Journal of Experimental Social Psychology, 48*(1), 432–436. https://doi.org/10.1016/j.jesp.2011.09.004.

Hall, P. A., Zehr, C., Paulitzki, J., & Rhodes, R. (2014). Implementation intentions for physical activity behavior in older adult women: An examination of executive function as a moderator of treatment effects. *Annals of Behavioral Medicine, 48*(1), 130–136. https://doi.org/10.1007/s12160-013-9582-7.

Hardeman, W., Johnston, M., Johnston, D., Bonetti, D., Wareham, N., & Kinmonth, A. L. (2010). Application of the theory of planned behaviour in behaviour change interventions: A systematic review. *Psychology & Health, 17*(2), 123–158. https://doi.org/10.1080/08870440290013644a.

Hutchison, A. J., Breckon, J. D., & Johnston, L. H. (2009). Physical activity behavior change interventions based on the transtheoretical model: A systematic review. *Health Education Behaviour, 36*(5), 829–845.

Kosma, M., & Cardinal, B. J. (2016). The Transtheoretical model, physical activity, and falls risks among diverse older adults. *Activities, Adaptation & Aging, 40*(1), 35–52. https://doi.org/10.1080/01924788.2016.1127051.

Leake, D., & Black, R. (2005). *Essential tools: Improving secondary education and transition for youth with disabilities. Cultural and linguistic diversity: Implications for transition personnel.* Minneapolis: ICI Publications Office.

Lee, M., Kim, M. J., Suh, D., Kim, J., Jo, E., & Yoon, B. (2016). Feasibility of a self-determination theory-based exercise program in community-dwelling south Korean older adults: Experiences from a 13-month trial. *Journal of Aging and Physical Activity, 24*(1), 8–21. https://doi.org/10.1123/japa.2014-0056.

Mairki, A., Bauer, G. F., Nigg, C. R., Conca-Zeller, A., & Gehring, T. M. (2006). Transtheoretical model-based exercise counselling for older adults in Switzerland: Quantitative results over a 1-year period. *Sozial- und Präventivmedizin, 51*(5), 273–280.

McDonald, S., O'Brien, N., White, M., & Sniehotta, F. F. (2015). Changes in physical activity during the retirement transition: A theory-based, qualitative interview study. *International Journal of Behavioral Nutrition and Physical Activity, 12*, 25. https://doi.org/10.1186/s12966-015-0186-4.

Michie, S., & Johnston, M. (2013). Behavior change techniques. In M. D. Gellman & J. R. Turner (Eds.), *Encyclopaedia of behavioral medicine* (pp. 182–187). New York: Springer.

Michie, S., van Stralen, M. M., & West, R. (2011). The behaviour change wheel: A new method for characterising and designing behaviour change interventions. *Implementation Science, 6*, 42. https://doi.org/10.1186/1748-5908-6-42.

Michie, S., Richardson, M., Johnston, M., Abraham, C., Francis, J., Hardeman, W., et al. (2013). The behavior change technique taxonomy (v1) of 93 hierarchically clustered techniques: Building an international consensus for the reporting of behavior change interventions. *Annals of Behavioral Medicine, 46*(1), 81–95. https://doi.org/10.1007/s12160-013-9486-6.

Michie, S., West, R., Campbell, R., Brown, J., & Gainforth, H. (2014). *ABC of behaviour change theories.* London: Silverback Publishing.

Morgan, K., & McGee, H. (2016). Quality of life. In Y. Benyamini, M. Johnston, & E. Karademas (Eds.), *Health assessment.* Boston: Hogrefe Publishing. http://hogrefe.ciando.com/img/books/extract/161676452X_lp.pdf.

Nyman, S. R., Goodwin, K., Kwasnicka, D., & Callaway, A. (2016). Increasing walking among older people: A test of behaviour change techniques using factorial randomised N-of-1 trials. *Psychology & Health, 31*(3), 313–330. https://doi.org/10.1080/08870446.2015.1088014.

Osborn, C. Y., Amico, R., Fisher, W. A., Egede, L. E., & Fisher, J. D. (2010). An information—motivation—behavioral skills analysis of diet and exercise behavior in Puerto Ricans with diabetes. *Journal of Health Psychology, 15*(8), 1201–1213.

Prochaska, J. O., & DiClemente, C. C. (1984). *The Transtheoretical approach: Crossing traditional boundaries of therapy.* Homewood: Dow Jones Irwin.

Prochaska, J. O., & Prochaska, J. M. (2011). Behavior change. In C. Heverling & T. Reilly (Eds.), *Population health creating a culture of wellness*. Burlington: Jones & Bartlett Learning, LLC.

Rhodes, R. E., & de Bruijn, G.-J. (2013). How big is the physical activity intention–behaviour gap? A meta-analysis using the action control framework. *British Journal of Health Psychology, 18*, 296–309. https://doi.org/10.1111/bjhp.12032.

Rosenstock, I. (1974). Historical origins of the health belief model. *Health Education Monographs., 2*(4), 354–386.

Rosenstock, I. (1990). The health belief model: Explaining health behavior through expectancies. In K. Glanz, F. M. Lewis, & B. Rimer (Eds.), *Health behavior and health education: Theory, research, and practice*. San Francisco: Jossey-Bass.

Schwarzer, R. (1992). Self-efficacy in the adoption and maintenance of health behaviors: Theoretical approaches and a new model. In R. Schwarzer (Ed.), *Self-efficacy: Thought control of action* (pp. 217–243). Washington, DC: Hemisphere Publishing Corp.

Schwarzer, R. (2008). Modeling health behavior change: How to predict and modify the adoption and maintenance of health behaviors. *Applied Psychology: An International Review, 57*, 1–29. https://doi.org/10.1111/j.1464-0597.2007.00325.x

Sniehotta, F. F., Presseau, J., & Araújo-Soares, V. (2014). Time to retire the theory of planned behaviour. *Health Psychology Review, 8*(1), 1–7.

Sniehotta, F. F., Presseau, J., & Araújo-Soares, V. (2015). On the development, evaluation and evolution of health behaviour theory. *Health Psychology Review, 9*(2), 176–189. https://doi.org/10.1080/17437199.2015.1022902.

Stretcher, V. J., Champion, V. L., & Rosenstock, L. M. (1997). The health belief model and health behavior. In D. S. Goshman (Ed.), *Handbook of health behavior research* (Vol. 1, pp. 71–91). New York: Plenum Press.

Teixeira, P. J., Carraça, E. V., Markland, D., Silva, M. N., & Ryan, R. M. (2012). Exercise, physical activity, and self-determination theory: A systematic review. *The International Journal of Behavioral Nutrition and Physical Activity, 9*, 78–78. https://doi.org/10.1186/1479-5868-9-78.

Triandis, H. C. (1989). Cross-cultural studies of individualism and collectivism. *Nebraska Symposium on Motivation, 37*, 43–133.

van Stralen, M. M., de Vries, H., Mudde, A. N., Bolman, C., & Lechner, L. (2011). The long-term efficacy of two computer-tailored physical activity interventions for older adults: Main effects and mediators. *Health Psychology, 30*(4), 442–452. https://doi.org/10.1037/a0023579.

Warner, L. M., Wolff, J. K., Ziegelmann, J. P., Schwarzer, R., & Wurm, S. (2016). Revisiting self-regulatory techniques to promote physical activity in older adults: Null-findings from a randomised controlled trial. *Psychology & Health*, 1–21. https://doi.org/10.1080/08870446.2016.1185523.

Webb, T. L., & Sheeran, P. (2007). How do implementation intentions promote goal attainment? A test of component processes. *Journal of Experimental Social Psychology, 43*, 295–302.

West, R. (2005). Time for a change: Putting the transtheoretical (stages of change) model to rest. *Addiction, 100*(58), 1036–1039.

White, K. M., Terry, D. J., Troup, C., Rempel, L. A., Norman, P., Mummery, K., et al. (2012). An extended theory of planned behavior intervention for older adults with type 2 diabetes and cardiovascular disease. *Journal of Aging & Physical Activity, 20*(3), 281–299.

Young, M. D., Plotnikoff, R. C., Collins, C. E., Callister, R., & Morgan, P. J. (2014). Social cognitive theory and physical activity: A systematic review and meta-analysis. *Obesity Reviews, 15*(12), 983–995. https://doi.org/10.1111/obr.12225.

12

Self-Efficacy and Its Sources as Determinants of Physical Activity among Older People

Lisa M. Warner and David P. French

12.1 Introduction

Throughout life, there are a variety of barriers for being physically active and the ageing process can add to these barriers. Therefore, regularly engaging in an active lifestyle is a challenging task for most people. It is also the case that people differ greatly in how limiting they *perceive* the same barriers. For example, one person may not enjoy the prospect of walking by themselves, whereas another person may relish the opportunity to enjoy some time by themselves. As a consequence there are older adults with various functional limitations who still exercise regularly whereas others remain sedentary even though they do not experience functional limitations. Many of these discrepancies can be explained by different levels of perceived *self-efficacy* for physical activity.

Bandura, the founder of the concept, describes self-efficacy as "the conviction that one can successfully execute the behaviour required to produce the outcomes" (Bandura 1977, p. 193). Self-efficacy can be understood as the belief in being able to accomplish a task despite setbacks and barriers. Persons

---

L. M. Warner (✉)
Department of Health Psychology and Social, Organization and Economic Psychology, Freie Universität Berlin, Berlin, Germany

Department of Psychology, MSB Medical School Berlin, Berlin, Germany

D. P. French
Manchester Centre for Health Psychology, School of Health Sciences, University of Manchester, Manchester, UK

with high levels of self-efficacy tend to feel more capable, choose more ambitious goals, and invest more effort into attaining their goals. With respect to physical activity, being self-efficacious, for example, means that one feels capable of regularly walking for 30 minutes a day, even when there are suboptimal weather conditions. While repeatedly overcoming the initial hesitation to go for a walk in cold and rainy weather, someone might soon not hesitate to engage in physical activity under these circumstances and perceive increased abilities for future activity—precisely because they overcame earlier barriers. Initial levels of self-efficacy hence increase the likelihood of successful performance, which then proves people's capabilities—and establish the self-fulfilling prophecy effect that self-efficacy beliefs can have (Lackner et al. 1996).

Empirical research shows a close relationship between self-efficacy beliefs and being physically active in younger and older adults (Bauman et al. 2012; van Stralen et al. 2009). Further, interventions are more successful to increase physical activity if they include behaviour change techniques to prompt self-efficacy (Williams and French 2011). This link between physical activity and self-efficacy could be even more pronounced in older than younger adults (Schwarzer and Renner 2000; Young et al. 2014). In sum, there are a number of theoretical and empirical grounds for considering self-efficacy for physical activity when designing programmes to promote physical activity to suit the particular needs of older people.

12.2 What Is Self-Efficacy and What Is It Not?

There are literally dozens of different constructs that have been proposed to relate to the idea of "control" as an important aspect of human behaviour and functioning (Skinner 1996). To ensure clarity, it is helpful to distinguish the concept of self-efficacy from similar concepts. Self-efficacy should not be mistaken for objective *capabilities*. Self-efficacy is the *subjective belief* individuals hold about their capabilities. Therefore, self-efficacy does not necessarily have to be related to an individual's actual abilities (Bandura 1997). Self-efficacy beliefs are related to *optimism*, but they can be distinguished by detecting the causes for the positive outlook into the future: Whereas optimists predict that the future will be bright no matter what they do (e.g., fortunate circumstances, help, chance), self-efficacious individuals believe that they can be successful by means of their own abilities and actions (Alarcon et al. 2013). A similar principle applies to distinguishing self-efficacy from the concept of *locus of control*.

This concept distinguishes external causes for an outcome, such as luck or the difficulty of a task, from internal causes, such as ability or effort. Individuals with an internal locus of control hence believe that the reason for an outcome lies within themselves but they do not necessarily believe that they can positively influence this internal factor (Warner and Schwarzer, in press). Despite the empirical association of having an internal locus of control and perceiving self-efficacy (Judge et al. 2002), the two constructs can hence be considered as being theoretically distinct.

Another construct similar to self-efficacy is *perceived behavioural control* (PBC). Some authors use self-efficacy and PBC interchangeably (e.g., Fishbein and Cappella 2006) and some prefer to distinguish them (e.g., Ajzen 2002). If one takes a look at the measures that should be used to assess both constructs, it becomes apparent in which way they should differ: items to measure PBC usually include a statement about the ease or difficulty of an undertaking, such as "It is easy/difficult for me to….". In comparison, self-efficacy items usually incorporate the "can-do" component, such as "I am sure that I can do…". Therefore, some authors refer to self-efficacy as the "can-do cognition" (Schwarzer and Warner 2013, p. 113). It is notable that there is often considerable overlap in measures designed to measure self-efficacy or PBC (Johnston et al. 2014). It has been argued that the distinction between self-efficacy and PBC is less important for physical activity (French 2015) where easy/difficult and confident/unconfident are highly associated but is more important for behaviours such as alcohol consumption (Cooke et al. 2016), where the association is much lower.

In contrast to related constructs, the most important distinction criterion to distinguish self-efficacy from other concepts is, hence, that it infers *internal attribution*: it is a subjective perception of one's own capabilities. It pertains to competence and future behaviour. One commonly used scale for general physical activity in older adults is the Self-Efficacy for Exercise Scale (Resnick and Jenkins 2000). More detailed guidelines on the construction of self-efficacy measures can be found in a comprehensive book chapter by Bandura (2006).

Some authors also distinguish initiation, maintenance, and recovery self-efficacy (Higgins et al. 2014; McAuley et al. 2003). For example, Kassavou et al. (2014) found that continued attendance at walking groups in a sample of (mainly) older adults (90% were between 40 and 79 years old) was predicted by recovery self-efficacy, that is, confidence in the capacity to resume attendance having stopped, but not maintenance self-efficacy, that is, confidence in the capacity to continually attend.

12.3 How Does Self-Efficacy Fit into Health Behaviour Change Theories?

The concept of self-efficacy was originally developed by Bandura as the key construct within the social cognitive theory (SCT; for details, see Chap. 11; Bandura 1977, 1997). He states that unless people *believe that they can* engage in a behaviour and that engaging in this behaviour would *produce the desired outcome*, they would not perceive any incentive to initiate the behaviour or to persevere in the face of difficulties (Bandura 1977). The theory hence predicts that humans act if they think the action will produce a desired outcome, if they have favourable *outcome expectancies* (for details, see Chap. 13), if they think they are able to produce these outcomes by means of their own behaviour, and if they perceive *self-efficacy*. For example, someone may believe they are able to achieve the recommended level of 150 minutes of moderate or vigorous physical activity per week (self-efficacy). Unless this person believes that this behaviour would contribute achieving an outcome such as increased fitness, maintained physical functioning, or weight loss (outcome expectancies) which relates to a personally valued goal, they will not deliberately attempt to engage in the behaviour. Besides these core elements of social cognitive theory—self-efficacy, goals, and outcome expectancies—Bandura further acknowledges the role of hindering and facilitating sociostructural factors (see Fig. 12.1 for an overview of SCT).

According to Benight and Bandura (2004), one of the most prominent sociostructural facilitators within SCT is *social support*. Several mediating pathways and interactions (moderating effects) between social support and self-efficacy have been discussed in the coping context (Schwarzer and Knoll 2007). Because of its predictive power for various health behaviours,

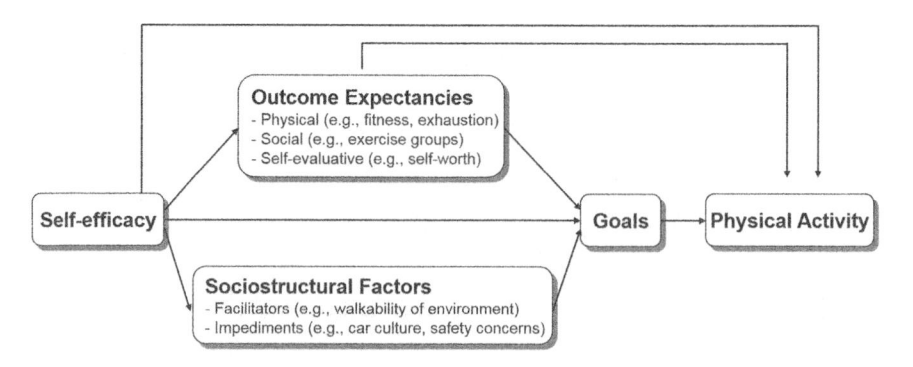

Fig. 12.1 Illustration of the social cognitive theory for physical activity in older adults

self-efficacy has become an indispensable part of many theories of health behaviour change. In most of these theories, self-efficacy does not only affect health behaviour directly but is often proposed to have an indirect effect as well, by prompting other determinants in the behaviour change process. Health behaviour change theories such as the health action process approach (Schwarzer 2008), protection motivation theory (Maddux and Rogers 1983), the revised health belief model (Rosenstock et al. 1988), and the transtheoretical model (Prochaska and DiClemente 1982) have therefore incorporated control beliefs into their frameworks as well (for details on health behaviour change theories, see Chap. 11).

12.4 Self-Efficacy for Physical Activity in Older Adults

Self-efficacy is a reliable predictor of many health-related behaviours, such as healthy eating, screening, and alcohol consumption, and has been shown to reliably predict changes in many health-related behaviours too (Luszczynska and Schwarzer 2015). In line with this, self-efficacy is the social cognition construct that is most consistently found to be associated with physical activity in adults (Bauman et al. 2012). It is also one of the most consistent predictors of physical activity initiation and uptake in adults aged 50 years and older (Koeneman et al. 2011; van Stralen et al. 2009). Further, although self-efficacy has mediated the effects of few interventions to increase physical activity (Rhodes and Pfaeffli 2010), at least partly as many interventions fail to change self-efficacy. Overall, there is good reason to believe that self-efficacy has a causal role in changing physical activity behaviour (French 2013), especially in adults aged 60 years and older (French et al. 2014).

Despite the large number of studies underpinning the effect of self-efficacy on physical activity, there is surprisingly little research on the origins of self-efficacy beliefs in the health behaviour domain. This lack of firm evidence may explain why many interventions fail to promote behaviour change. Given this, Bandura's theoretical assumptions on the sources upon which humans build their self-efficacy beliefs are therefore still a solid theoretical basis and often cited. Only recently, empirically driven methods to detect the most effective sources of self-efficacy for physical activity have been established, which rely on the use of taxonomies of behaviour change techniques that can be considered the "active ingredients" in behaviour change interventions (for details on the BCT taxonomy, see Chap. 11; Abraham and Michie 2008; Michie et al. 2011, 2013).

The development of such taxonomies has allowed the use of moderator analyses in meta-analyses, to investigate which behaviour change techniques are associated with larger changes in self-efficacy for physical activity in previous intervention studies (Olander et al. 2013; Williams and French 2011), including studies among older adults (French et al. 2014).

12.5 The Sources of Self-Efficacy

According to Bandura, *mastery experience* is "the most effective source of efficacy information because they provide the most authentic evidence of whether one can master whatever it takes to succeed" (1997, p. 80). Wood and Bandura (1989) state that individuals' beliefs and individuals' actions can be mutually reinforcing, suggesting an upward spiral between mastery experiences and self-efficacy. Most older people will have personal experiences with being physically active at least at some point in their life. Therefore, disentangling mastery experience and self-efficacy can be challenging for empirical research (for further discussion of reciprocal causality between mastery experience and self-efficacy, see French 2013).

In order to prompt mastery experience in interventions to promote physical activity in older adults, different behaviour change techniques have been applied. The technique most often used is to incorporate exercise sessions into an intervention programme to offer the opportunity for authentic mastery experience with the behaviour (Ashford et al. 2010). A trial by McAuley et al. (2005), for example, found that those adults aged 60–75 who attended the exercise groups within an intervention programme more frequently finished the programme with higher self-efficacy beliefs. Another way to activate mastery experience can be to let people *remember or retell positive activity experiences* they made (Bandura 1997). This technique is, for example, used in the well-established Motivational Interviewing approach (Miller and Rollnick 2002). In line with this, the more often older adults are active and the more salient their mastery experience is, the more likely they will increase their self-efficacy to be active.

For many older adults, however, mastery experiences may have last occurred some considerable time ago. A technique suggested by Bandura to build mastery experiences is to split up goals into smaller steps that can be more easily achieved (1997). For an improvement of self-efficacy beliefs towards more physical activity among adults over 60 years of age, the technique of *setting graded tasks* indeed seems to be a promising approach, as a meta-analysis found interventions to be more effective if they included this behaviour change technique (French et al. 2014).

A technique often used to display efforts and progress along the way to successful behaviour change, which is constantly found to be one of the strongest behaviour change techniques to increase physical activity in young and middle-aged groups is *self-monitoring* (Michie et al. 2009). Caution is, however, warranted when using self-monitoring as a behaviour change technique in interventions to promote physical activity in older adults: self-monitoring *of the behaviour* was found to decrease the likelihood of an intervention to be effective in a meta-analysis among people aged 60 years and over (French et al. 2014). This may be as many older adults are not very active (Scholes and Mindell 2013), and receiving feedback on this lack of physical activity may indicate a lack of mastery. Prompting to self-monitor the *behavioural outcomes* instead of the behaviour per se was, however, associated with increased self-efficacy in this meta-analysis. This suggests that older adults should rather be advised to focus on the positive changes they perceive as a result of being active, than the mere activity (French et al. 2014). In the words of an older person in an orthopaedic rehabilitation programme, *When I saw the improvements I was making, that helped me keep going and helped me do a little bit more* (Resnick 2002).

To make the most of newly gained mastery experiences, interventions can prepare older adults for temporal setbacks and lapses to help avoid what Marlatt and Gordon (1985) call the *abstinence violation effect*. As most people have a tendency to interpret lapses as a sign of incapability, they run the risk of dropping all effort and experiencing a full relapse. When they learn to attribute lapses to external causes, such as to the end of a stressful day or to a highly tempting situation, self-efficacy can be maintained and trained for future risk situations.

Although not always named among the sources of self-efficacy, Bandura also identifies *mental imagery* as another possible origin of self-efficacy beliefs (Bandura 1977) and demonstrates its use to treat phobias. Among sedentary adults, imagining the outcomes of physical activity (*approach imagery*) as well as the steps that need to be fulfilled to attain their goals related to physical activity (*process imagery*) might also be a way to establish a sense of mastery and enhance self-efficacy beliefs (Chan and Cameron 2012).

Vicarious experience, such as seeing others succeed at a task or enjoy a behaviour can activate beliefs of being able to achieve similar outcomes with similar behaviours—especially among those who have low beliefs in their own capabilities. This is why this technique is often applied in self-help groups, in which people, who have already mastered a certain problem, teach others how to manage this problem as well, thereby modelling successful goal pursuit. Seeing others succeed at a behaviour increases self-efficacy also because it provides observers with strategies and techniques needed to attain desired goals or to overcome certain barriers (Bandura 1997). Qualitative research points to the fact that older adults consider the absence of role models to be a barrier to regular physical activity (Allender et al. 2006). Also role models are often named when participants are interviewed about the foundations of their self-efficacy beliefs (Resnick 2002). An older person interviewed during rehabilitation at a geriatric hospital, for example, said *I saw a couple of women from my church. They were at the end of the therapy and I watched a few of them go up the stairs. I was surprised to see them. They had done gone where I am going, and I found that encouraging* (Resnick 2002). Self-disclosing coping models—role models that had to face the same difficulties—with similar characteristics as the observer, like age, gender, or level of expertise are assumed to be particularly effective (Bandura 1997). Systematic research on the effectiveness of different models is, however, scarce in the area of physical activity among older adults and so it is unclear what the salient dimensions by which older people use to judge similarity are. Modelling should not be mistaken for mere normative feedback: providing normative information on others' behaviour was found to decrease the effectiveness of interventions to promote self-efficacy for physical activity among adults older than 60 years (French et al. 2014).

A related strategy to providing vicarious experience is *self-modelling*. This technique was, for example, applied in an intervention to increase physical activity among stroke survivors (average sample age of 63 years, age range 33–93). They were provided with written material that did not only describe the exercises prescribed by the physiotherapists at the end of their rehabilitation programme but also included photos of the respective patient performing these exercises in the clinic. These leaflets were posted on easily observable spots at patients' homes to prompt self-modelling (Shaughnessy and Resnick 2009). Even though theoretically promising, the effectiveness of this strategy cannot be quantified or evaluated yet, as there are too few interventions that have applied it and most are embedded into larger programmes.

Verbal or social persuasion is the assurance of other people that they believe in a person's capabilities (Bandura 1997). Verbal persuasion has been shown to be most effective when it derives from credible sources such as health professionals (Perloff 1993). If, however, someone already possesses a strong belief in *not* being able to succeed, maybe even underlined by negative experiences with physical activity in the past, verbal persuasion is more likely to result in lower than in higher self-efficacy (Bandura 1997). Therefore, this source of self-efficacy needs to be addressed with care and experience to avoid reactance (Miller et al. 2007).

One longitudinal study on older adults found *self-persuasion* to be positively related to later self-efficacy for physical activity in adults aged 65 and older (Warner et al. 2014) and other researchers found "just do it"-self-talk to be a good predictor of exercise in later adulthood (aged 56 and older; O'Brien Cousins and Gillis 2005). Manipulations of *motivational self-talk* were also shown to have a positive association with physical activity levels in obese populations of broad age (aged 28–77 years; but note that there was no effect of self-talk on self-efficacy in this meta-analysis; Olander et al. 2013) and in athletes (Hardy 2006). This promising technique needs more research on whether it could also be effective to enhance regular physical activity among older adults.

Immediately prior to performing challenging tasks, most people perceive *somatic and affective states* such as a feeling of apprehension, a fast-beating heart, sweaty hands, or more general fatigue, aches, or pains. If such somatic and affective states are *subjectively interpreted* as unpreparedness, anticipation of poor performance or inability to perform physical activity they can decrease individuals' self-efficacy and subsequent physical activity (Bandura 1997). Along this line, research shows that feeling fit is an important precondition for self-efficacy for physical activity among older adults (O'Brien Cousins and Tan 2002) and that measures of perceived health (e.g., ratings of vitality) are more strongly associated with self-efficacy for physical activity than more objective measures of health (e.g., presence of illnesses) among older adults (O'Brien Cousins 2000; Perkins et al. 2009; Warner et al. in press).

Older adults are often uncertain of whether exercising would be without risk for their health (O'Brien Cousins 2000), so encouragement of a health professional to perform light to moderate physical activity despite certain health problems might help to avoid misinterpretations of bodily symptoms. Relatedly, it is a key concern of many older people when attending exercise classes that the person running such classes is competent and trustworthy and will prevent older adults from overexerting, injuring or otherwise harming themselves (Devereux-Fitzgerald et al. 2016). Another possibility to encounter concerns towards the risks of physical activity in older adults would be to create safe opportunities for exercise that lessen the fear of injuries or social evaluation by younger or fitter individuals by providing professional guidance and age-matched exercise groups.

Bandura (1997) suggested that mastery experience is the most effective source, followed by vicarious experience (role modelling), verbal persuasion, and physiological feedback. To assess the *sources of self-efficacy for physical activity*, Warner et al. (2014) validated six scales. Some prospective studies confirm mastery experience to be the strongest source of self-efficacy for physical activity for older adults and further suggest that feeling healthy and perceiving low negative affect before being active as well as the use of motivational self-talk predict self-efficacy for physical activity in adults aged 65 years and older (Warner et al. 2011, 2014). Also few studies have looked at the *conjoint effects* of targeting several sources of self-efficacy in physical activity interventions. These studies assume that prompting some of the sources might only be effective if combined with prompts from a different source. Only one intervention study in the exercise domain (Wise and Trunnell 2001) experimentally tested three of the self-efficacy sources against each other and in combination (mastery experience, vicarious experience, verbal persuasion). It found that mastery experience was effective no matter in which combination of sources but that verbal persuasion was only effective if preceded by performance accomplishment (mastery experience) of the tested physical task (bench pressing) among women aged 18–40 years.

12.6 Further Possible Sources of Self-Efficacy

Based on several qualitative studies on the barriers and benefits perceived by older adults, O'Brien Cousins (2000, p. 290) came to the conclusion that "Older adults tend to limit their activity choices to walking, gardening, and some forms of dancing, perhaps because they are seeking the most enjoyable, age-appropriate activities and perhaps because they do not feel skilled at other things." This focus on specific forms of physical activity is important when considering interventions to promote self-efficacy for physical activity, for at least two reasons.

First, many older adults are inactive and physically deconditioned. For this reason, many older adults do not feel that performing physical activity for its own sake is sensible or appropriate (McGowan et al. in press). Their outcome expectancies and self-efficacy in relation to physical activity are therefore both likely to be low. Given this, those seeking to encourage older people to be more active would not prime these negative beliefs if they talk about activities that older people see as being more appropriate such as dancing. The key point here is not to label activities that involve physical activity as physical activity, as they are likely to be more acceptable and stimulate more confidence when described in different terms (e.g., neighbourhood sightseeing tours, ballroom dancing; see Chap. 15 for details on acceptability of physical activity).

Relatedly, putting more emphasis on encouraging those forms of physical activity that older adults find *enjoyable* could be an important way to foster self-efficacy. It is often the case that activities that are seen as enjoyable are also seen as being easier to perform (Kraft et al. 2005), presumably as this removes barriers to doing them such as lack of interest or competing goals. The suggestion to increase the fun in physical activity is backed up by socio-emotional selectivity theory (Carstensen 1992). Carstensen suggests that the process of ageing is accompanied by an inclination towards activities and social contacts that initiate short-term positive affect (Carstensen and Mikels 2005). This *positivity effect* is also supported by the finding that adults aged 61 years and older remember positively framed messages better than loss-framed messages in intervention material to increase physical activity (Notthoff and Carstensen 2014). Enjoyable physical activities that yield possibilities to experience positive social interactions hence seem to be promising to enhance the likelihood of regular exercise among older adults.

Second, another possible way to increase self-efficacy for physical activity especially among older adults, might be to tackle their views on ageing. Levy et al. (2002) propose that *ageing stereotypes* and *views on ageing* affect health and health behaviours also via self-efficacy beliefs. Even though first attempts have been made to increase views on ageing to promote older adults' physical activity, the effects on self-efficacy beliefs are still to be investigated (for details on effects of self-perceptions of ageing on physical activity, see Chap. 12; Wolff et al. 2014).

12.7 Food for Thought for Future Research

The construct of self-efficacy has been studied for several decades but there are still exciting open research questions and debates. Some of these open questions concern the measurement and conceptualisation of the construct in general and others more directly relate to older adults' physical activity. A debate reactivated by Williams and Rhodes (2016) relates to the confoundedness of self-efficacy measures with other constructs from behaviour changes theories. A way to find out how participants interpret self-efficacy items and whether they confound them with similar theoretical constructs in order to render future self-efficacy scales less confounded would be to conduct think-aloud studies (French et al. 2007).

Another problem known from other behavioural domains that may arise when study participants rate their self-efficacy beliefs at the beginning of an intervention is that self-efficacy beliefs can be too high. When people overestimate their abilities, this can decrease the chance for successful behaviour change (Staring and Breteler 2004; Vancouver et al. 2002). McAuley and colleagues, for example, observed that self-efficacy levels among adults 65 years of age on average may decrease towards the end of a physical activity programme due to participants' realisation that keeping up activities after the structured intervention ends is more challenging than they originally anticipated (McAuley et al. 2003). Some authors, therefore, suggest to offer home-based exercise programmes instead of structured group exercises to increase self-efficacy beliefs that persist after the structured programme has ended (Higgins et al. 2014).

A key issue that warrants further consideration is how the role of self-efficacy changes over time. As previously discussed, there is now good evidence that self-efficacy is important in the success of attempts to initiate increases in physical activity. However, our understanding of the role of self-efficacy in the *maintenance* of increases in physical activity is comparatively rudimentary. In particular, what behaviour change techniques are most successful at helping people maintain levels of self-efficacy for physical activity, and how these are different from those that bring about initial changes in self-efficacy.

Another neglected avenue for research concerns the specification in social cognitive theory that the environment interacts in a dynamic way with self-efficacy and behaviour (Bandura 1977). Despite this theorising, there is still a dearth of evidence on what features of the environment are likely to facilitate high levels of self-efficacy. One possibility would be that social environments that have more positive stereotypes of ageing that emphasise capability rather than passivity may promote increased self-efficacy at a population level. Alternatively, physical environments that promote increased walking may do so by increasing the self-efficacy of people within those environments, by removing barriers such as fear of falling or violence (Booth et al. 2000; Fleig et al. 2016).

12.8 Practical Implications

Even though it is too early to develop definitive guidelines on how to best enhance self-efficacy in older adults, we tried to summarise behaviour change strategies that could be used to induce the sources of self-efficacy for physical activity in older adults in Fig. 12.2.

Policymakers and interventionists should bear in mind that mastery experiences are the key source of self-efficacy in any age group. Therefore, we

Source	Mode of Induction
Mastery experience	Opportunities for performance (e.g., safe opportunities to exercise) Reactive positive activity experiences (e.g., exercise biographies) Graded mastery experiences (e.g., set smaller goals) Self-monitoring of behavioural outcome (e.g., diary on numbers of stairs without break) Mental imagery (e.g., imagery of success or progress)
Vicarious experience	Life Modelling (e.g., exercise groups) Symbolic Modelling (e.g., Videos, Testimonials) Self Modelling (e.g., pictures of self exercising)
Verbal persuasion	Encouragement from health professional (e.g., from GP) Motivational self-talk (e.g., "just do it" attitude)
Somatic and affective states	Attribution (e.g., clarification of bodily symptoms) Opportunities for performance (e.g., under supervision of trainer, but not the public)

Fig. 12.2 Summary of the modes of induction for the four sources of self-efficacy for physical activity among older adults

recommend to elicit the particular barriers for mastery experiences with physical activity in old age (physical, environmental, social but also subjective barriers including views on ageing and perceived physiological and affective states) and bear them in mind during intervention development. To build mastery experiences step by step, indirect modes of induction such as writing a biography about one's previous positive physical activity experiences or imagining success and the necessary steps towards it before starting to exercise might be successful among older adults. Also some bodily symptoms such as heart rate increases or shortness of breath should be explained, before inexperienced older adults are asked to exercise. Once exercise sessions are initiated, close supervision and a group context can be recommended. A promising avenue to promote self-efficacy for physical activity in older adults might also be to highlight the fun and social benefits physical activity has to offer.

12.9 Conclusions

Self-efficacy is clearly an important cognition for the initiation and maintenance of regular physical activity in every age group but particularly in older adults as they face more (objective and subjective) barriers than younger age groups. Knowing more about the foundations of self-efficacy beliefs can help to eliminate some of these barriers (e.g., safe opportunities such as exercise groups for cardiac patients) and assist older adults in finding ways to overcome other barriers (e.g., subjective barriers, misinterpretations of bodily symptoms). This chapter clarifies the important role of self-efficacy beliefs for physical activity among older adults and summarises many ways in how to improve self-efficacy. With that, we hope that this chapter encourages interventionists and researchers to keep on prompting and investigating self-efficacy to find ways how to address it even more effectively in future physical activity programmes for older adults. With that said, we would like to conclude in Bandura's (2004, p. 162) words, "As you venture forth to promote your own health and that of others, may the efficacy force be with you."

Suggested Further Readings

- Bandura, A. (1997). *Self-efficacy: The exercise of control.* New York: Freeman.
- French, D. P., Olander, E., Chisholm, A., & Mc Sharry, J. (2014). Which behaviour change techniques are most effective at increasing older adults' self-efficacy and physical activity behaviour? A systematic review. *Annals of Behavioral Medicine, 48*(2), 225–234. https://doi.org/10.1007/s12160-014-9593-z.
- Warner, L. M., Schüz, B., Wolff, J. K., Parschau, L., Wurm, S., & Schwarzer, R. (2014). Sources of self-efficacy for physical activity. *Health Psychology, 33*(11), 1298–1308. https://doi.org/10.1037/hea0000085.

References

Abraham, C., & Michie, S. (2008). A taxonomy of behavior change techniques used in interventions. *Health Psychology, 27*(3), 379–387.

Ajzen, I. (2002). Perceived behavioral control, self-efficacy, locus of control, and the theory of planned behavior. *Journal of Applied Social Psychology, 32*(4), 665–683. https://doi.org/10.1111/j.1559-1816.2002.tb00236.x.

Alarcon, G. M., Bowling, N. A., & Khazon, S. (2013). Great expectations: A meta-analytic examination of optimism and hope. *Personality and Individual Differences, 54*(7), 821–827. https://doi.org/10.1016/j.paid.2012.12.004.

Allender, S., Cowburn, G., & Foster, C. (2006). Understanding participation in sport and physical activity among children and adults: A review of qualitative studies. *Health Education Research, 21*(6), 826–835.

Ashford, S., Edmunds, J., & French, D. P. (2010). What is the best way to change self-efficacy to promote lifestyle and recreational physical activity? A systematic review with meta-analysis. *British Journal of Health Psychology, 15*(2), 265–288. https://doi.org/10.1348/135910709X461752.

Bandura, A. (1977). Self-efficacy: Toward a unifying theory of behavioral change. *Psychological Review, 84*(2), 191–215. https://doi.org/10.1037/0033-295x.84.2.191.

Bandura, A. (1997). *Self-efficacy: The exercise of control.* New York: Freeman.

Bandura, A. (2004). Health promotion by social cognitive means. *Health Education & Behavior, 31*(2), 143–164. https://doi.org/10.1177/1090198104263660.

Bandura, A. (2006). Guide for constructing self-efficacy scales. In F. Pajares & T. Urdan (Eds.), *Self-efficacy beliefs of adolescents* (Vol. 5, pp. 307–337). Greenwich: Information Age Publishing.

Bauman, A. E., Reis, R. S., Sallis, J. F., Wells, J. C., Loos, R. J. F., & Martin, B. W. (2012). Correlates of physical activity: Why are some people physically active and others not? *The Lancet, 380*(9838), 258–271. https://doi.org/10.1016/S0140-6736(12)60735-1.

Benight, C. C., & Bandura, A. (2004). Social cognitive theory of posttraumatic recovery: The role of perceived self-efficacy. *Behaviour Research & Therapy, 42*(10), 1129–1148. https://doi.org/10.1016/j.brat.2003.08.008.

Booth, M. L., Owen, N., Bauman, A., Clavisi, O., & Leslie, E. (2000). Social-cognitive and perceived environment influences associated with physical activity in older Australians. *Preventive Medicine: An International Journal Devoted to Practice and Theory, 31*(1), 15–22. https://doi.org/10.1006/pmed.2000.0661.

Carstensen, L. L. (1992). Social and emotional patterns in adulthood: Support for socioemotional selectivity theory. *Psychology and Aging, 7*(3), 331–338. https://doi.org/10.1037//0882-7974.7.3.331.

Carstensen, L. L., & Mikels, J. A. (2005). At the intersection of emotion and cognition: Aging and the positivity effect. *Current Directions in Psychological Science, 14*(3), 117–121. https://doi.org/10.1111/j.0963-7214.2005.00348.x.

Chan, C., & Cameron, L. (2012). Promoting physical activity with goal-oriented mental imagery: A randomized controlled trial. *Journal of Behavioral Medicine, 35*(3), 347–363. https://doi.org/10.1007/s10865-011-9360-6.

Cooke, R., Dahdah, M., Norman, P., & French, D. P. (2016). How well does the theory of planned behaviour predict alcohol consumption? A systematic review and meta-analysis. *Health Psychology Review, 10*(2), 148–167. https://doi.org/10.1080/17437199.2014.947547.

Devereux-Fitzgerald, A., Powell, R., Dewhurst, A., & French, D. P. (2016). The acceptability of physical activity interventions to older adults: A systematic review and meta-synthesis. *Social Science & Medicine, 158*, 14–23. https://doi.org/10.1016/j.socscimed.2016.04.006.

Fishbein, M., & Cappella, J. N. (2006). The role of theory in developing effective health communications. *Journal of Communication, 56*(Suppl 1), S1–S17. https://doi.org/10.1111/j.1460-2466.2006.00280.x.

Fleig, L., Ashe, M. C., Voss, C., Therrien, S., Sims-Gould, J., McKay, H. A., & Winters, M. (2016). Environmental and psychosocial correlates of objectively measured physical activity among older adults. *Health Psychology, 35*(12), 1364–1372. https://doi.org/10.1037/hea0000403.

French, D. P. (2013). The role of self-efficacy in changing health-related behaviour: Cause, effect or spurious association? *British Journal of Health Psychology, 18*(2), 237–243. https://doi.org/10.1111/bjhp.12038.

French, D. P. (2015). Self-efficacy and health. In J. D. Wright (Ed.), *International encyclopedia of the social and behavioral sciences* (Vol. 21, 2nd ed., pp. 509–514). Oxford: Elsevier.

French, D. P., Cooke, R., McLean, N., Williams, M., & Sutton, S. (2007). What do people think about when they answer theory of planned behaviour questionnaires?: A 'think aloud' study. *Journal of Health Psychology, 12*(4), 672–687.

French, D. P., Olander, E., Chisholm, A., & Mc Sharry, J. (2014). Which behaviour change techniques are most effective at increasing older adults' self-efficacy and physical activity behaviour? A systematic review. *Annals of Behavioral Medicine, 48*(2), 225–234. https://doi.org/10.1007/s12160-014-9593-z.

Hardy, J. (2006). Speaking clearly: A critical review of the self-talk literature. *Psychology of Sport and Exercise, 7*(1), 81–97. https://doi.org/10.1016/j.psychsport.2005.04.002.

Higgins, T. J., Middleton, K. R., Winner, L., & Janelle, C. M. (2014). Physical activity interventions differentially affect exercise task and barrier self-efficacy: A meta-analysis. *Health Psychology, 33*(8), 891–903. https://doi.org/10.1037/a0033864.

Johnston, M., Dixon, D., Hart, J., Glidewell, L., Schröder, C., & Pollard, B. (2014). Discriminant content validity: A quantitative methodology for assessing content of theory-based measures, with illustrative applications. *British Journal of Health Psychology, 19*(2), 240–257. https://doi.org/10.1111/bjhp.12095.

Judge, T. A., Erez, A., Bono, J. E., & Thoresen, C. J. (2002). Are measures of self-esteem, neuroticism, locus of control, and generalized self-efficacy indicators of a common core construct? *Journal of Personality and Social Psychology, 83*(3), 693–710. https://doi.org/10.1037/0022-3514.83.3.693.

Kassavou, A., Turner, A., Hamborg, T., & French, D. P. (2014). Predicting maintenance of attendance at walking groups: Testing constructs from three leading maintenance theories. *Health Psychology, 33*(7), 752–756. https://doi.org/10.1037/hea0000015.

Koeneman, M. A., Verheijden, M. W., Chinapaw, M. J. M., & Hopman-Rock, M. (2011). Determinants of physical activity and exercise in healthy older adults: A systematic review. *International Journal of Behavioral Nutrition and Physical Activity, 8*, 142–142.

Kraft, P., Rise, J., Sutton, S., & Røysamb, E. (2005). Perceived difficulty in the theory of planned behaviour: Perceived behavioural control or affective attitude? *British Journal of Social Psychology, 44*(3), 479–496. https://doi.org/10.1348/014466604x17533.

Lackner, J. M., Carosella, A. M., & Feuerstein, M. (1996). Pain expectancies, pain, and functional self-efficacy expectancies as determinants of disability in patients with chronic low back disorders. *Journal of Consulting and Clinical Psychology, 64*(1), 212–220. https://doi.org/10.1037/0022-006X.64.1.212.

Levy, B. R., Slade, M. D., & Kasl, S. V. (2002). Longitudinal benefit of positive self-perceptions of aging on functional health. *The Journals of Gerontology Series B:*

Psychological Sciences and Social Sciences, 57(5), P409–P417. https://doi.org/10.1093/geronb/57.5.P409.

Luszczynska, A., & Schwarzer, R. (2015). Social-cognitive theory. In M. Conner & P. Norman (Eds.), *Predicting and changing health behaviour* (pp. 225–251). Maidenhead: McGraw Hill Open University Press.

Maddux, J. E., & Rogers, R. W. (1983). Protection motivation and self-efficacy: A revised theory of fear appeals and attitude change. *Journal of Experimental Social Psychology, 19*(5), 469–479. https://doi.org/10.1016/0022-1031(83)90023-9.

Marlatt, G. A., & Gordon, J. R. (1985). *Relapse prevention: Maintenance strategies in the treatment of addictive behaviors.* New York: Guilford Press.

McAuley, E., Jerome, G. J., Marquez, D. X., Elavsky, S., & Blissmer, B. (2003). Exercise self-efficacy in older adults: Social, affective, and behavioral influences. *Annals of Behavioral Medicine, 25*(1), 1–7. https://doi.org/10.1207/S15324796ABM2501_01.

McAuley, E., Elavsky, S., Jerome, G. J., Konopack, J. F., & Marquez, D. X. (2005). Physical activity-related well-being in older adults: Social cognitive influences. *Psychology and Aging, 20*(2), 295–302.

McGowan, L. J., Devereux-Fitzgerald, A., Powell, R., & French, D. P. (in press). How acceptable do older adults find the concept of being physically active? A systematic review and meta-synthesis. *International Review of Sport and Exercise Psychology*, 1–24.

Michie, S., Abraham, C., Whittington, C., McAteer, J., & Gupta, S. (2009). Effective techniques in healthy eating and physical activity interventions: A meta-regression. *Health Psychology, 28*(6), 690–701. https://doi.org/10.1037/a0016136.

Michie, S., Ashford, S., Sniehotta, F. F., Dombrowski, S. U., Bishop, A., & French, D. P. (2011). A refined taxonomy of behaviour change techniques to help people change their physical activity and healthy eating behaviours: The CALO-re taxonomy. *Psychology & Health, 26*(11), 1479–1498. https://doi.org/10.1080/08870446.2010.540664.

Michie, S., Richardson, M., Johnston, M., Abraham, C., Francis, J., Hardeman, W., et al. (2013). The behavior change technique taxonomy (v1) of 93 hierarchically clustered techniques: Building an international consensus for the reporting of behavior change interventions. *Annals of Behavioral Medicine, 46*(1), 81–95. https://doi.org/10.1007/s12160-013-9486-6.

Miller, W. R., & Rollnick, S. (2002). *Motivational interviewing: Preparing people for change.* New York: Guilford.

Miller, C. H., Lane, L. T., Deatrick, L. M., Young, A. M., & Potts, K. A. (2007). Psychological reactance and promotional health messages: The effects of controlling language, lexical concreteness, and the restoration of freedom. *Human Communication Research, 33*(2), 219–240. https://doi.org/10.1111/j.1468-2958.2007.00297.x.

Notthoff, N., & Carstensen, L. L. (2014). Positive messaging promotes walking in older adults. *Psychology and Aging, 29*(2), 329–341. https://doi.org/10.1037/a0036748.

O'Brien Cousins, S. (2000). "My heart couldn't take it": Older women's beliefs about exercise benefits and risks. *The Journals of Gerontology. Series B, Psychological Sciences and Social Sciences, 55*(5), 283–294. https://doi.org/10.1093/geronb/55.5.P283.

O'Brien Cousins, S., & Gillis, M. M. (2005). "Just do it… before you talk yourself out of it": The self-talk of adults thinking about physical activity. *Psychology of Sport and Exercise, 6*(3), 313–334. https://doi.org/10.1016/j.psychsport.2004.03.001.

O'Brien Cousins, S., & Tan, M. (2002). Sources of efficacy for walking and climbing stairs among older adults. *Physical & Occupational Therapy in Geriatrics, 20*(3), 51–68. https://doi.org/10.1300/J148v20n03_04.

Olander, E. K., Fletcher, H., Williams, S., Atkinson, L., Turner, A., & French, D. P. (2013). What are the most effective techniques in changing obese individuals' physical activity self-efficacy and behaviour: A systematic review and meta-analysis. *International Journal of Behavioral Nutrition and Physical Activity, 10*(1), 29–29. https://doi.org/10.1186/1479-5868-10-29.

Perkins, H. Y., Baum, G. P., Taylor, C. L. C., & Basen-Engquist, K. M. (2009). Effects of treatment factors, comorbidities and health-related quality of life on self-efficacy for physical activity in cancer survivors. *Psycho-Oncology, 18*(4), 405–411. https://doi.org/10.1002/pon.1535.

Perloff, R. M. (1993). *The dynamics of persuasion*. Hillsdale/England: Lawrence Erlbaum Associates.

Prochaska, J. O., & DiClemente, C. C. (1982). Transtheoretical therapy: Toward a more integrative model of change. *Psychotherapy: Theory, Research & Practice, 19*(3), 276–288. https://doi.org/10.1037/h0088437.

Resnick, B. (2002). Geriatric rehabilitation: The influence of efficacy beliefs and motivation. *Rehabilitation Nursing: The Official Journal of The Association of Rehabilitation Nurses, 27*(4), 152–159.

Resnick, B., & Jenkins, L. S. (2000). Testing the reliability and validity of the self-efficacy for exercise scale. *Nursing Research, 49*(3), 154–159. https://doi.org/10.1097/00006199-200005000-00007.

Rhodes, R. E., & Pfaeffli, L. A. (2010). Mediators of physical activity behaviour change among adult non-clinical populations: A review update. *International Journal of Behavioral Nutrition and Physical Activity, 7*, 37. https://doi.org/10.1186/1479-5868-7-37.

Rosenstock, I. M., Strecher, V. J., & Becker, M. H. (1988). Social learning theory and the health belief model. *Health Education & Behavior, 15*(2), 175–183. https://doi.org/10.1177/109019818801500203.

Scholes, S., & Mindell, J. (2013). Physical activity in adults. In R. Craig & J. Mindell (Eds.), *Health survey for England 2012* (Vol. 1, pp. 1–49). London: Health and Social Care Information Centre.

Schwarzer, R. (2008). Modeling health behavior change: How to predict and modify the adoption and maintenance of health behaviors. *Applied Psychology, 57*(1), 1–29. https://doi.org/10.1111/j.1464-0597.2007.00325.x.

Schwarzer, R., & Knoll, N. (2007). Functional roles of social support within the stress and coping process: A theoretical and empirical overview. *International Journal of Psychology, 42*(4), 243–252. https://doi.org/10.1080/00207590701396641.

Schwarzer, R., & Renner, B. (2000). Social-cognitive predictors of health behavior: Action self-efficacy and coping self-efficacy. *Health Psychology, 19*(5), 487–495.

Schwarzer, R., & Warner, L. M. (2013). Perceived self-efficacy and its relationship to resilience. In S. Prince-Embury & D. H. Saklofske (Eds.), *Resilience in children, adolescents, and adults: Translating research into practice* (pp. 139–150). New York: Springer.

Shaughnessy, M., & Resnick, B. M. (2009). Using theory to develop an exercise intervention for patients post stroke. *Topics in Stroke Rehabilitation, 16*(2), 140–146. https://doi.org/10.1310/tsr1602-140.

Skinner, E. A. (1996). A guide to constructs of control. *Journal of Personality and Social Psychology, 71*(3), 549–570. https://doi.org/10.1037/0022-3514.71.3.549.

Staring, A. B. P., & Breteler, M. H. M. (2004). Decline in smoking cessation rate associated with high self-efficacy scores. *Preventive Medicine, 39*(5), 863–868. https://doi.org/10.1016/j.ypmed.2004.03.025.

van Stralen, M. M., De Vries, H., Mudde, A. N., Bolman, C., & Lechner, L. (2009). Determinants of initiation and maintenance of physical activity among older adults: A literature review. *Health Psychology Review, 3*(2), 147–207. https://doi.org/10.1080/17437190903229462.

Vancouver, J. B., Thompson, C. M., Tischner, E. C., & Putka, D. J. (2002). Two studies examining the negative effect of self-efficacy on performance. *Journal of Applied Psychology, 87*(3), 506–516. https://doi.org/10.1037//0021-9010.87.3.506.

Warner, L. M., & Schwarzer, R. (in press). Self-efficacy. In K. S. M. L. Robbins (Ed.), *The Wiley encyclopedia of health psychology: Volume II, the social bases of health behavior*. New York: Wiley-Blackwell.

Warner, L. M., Schüz, B., Knittle, K., Ziegelmann, J. P., & Wurm, S. (2011). Sources of perceived self-efficacy as predictors of physical activity in older adults. *Applied Psychology: Health and Well-Being, 3*(2), 172–192. https://doi.org/10.1111/j.1758-0854.2011.01050.x.

Warner, L. M., Schüz, B., Wolff, J. K., Parschau, L., Wurm, S., & Schwarzer, R. (2014). Sources of self-efficacy for physical activity. *Health Psychology, 33*(11), 1298–1308. https://doi.org/10.1037/hea0000085.

Warner, L. M., Wolff, J. K., Spuling, S. M., & Wurm, S. (in press). Perceived somatic and affective barriers for self-efficacy and physical activity. *Journal of Health Psychology*. https://doi.org/10.1177/1359105317705979.

Williams, S. L., & French, D. P. (2011). What are the most effective intervention techniques for changing physical activity self-efficacy and physical activity behaviour-and are they the same? *Health Education Research, 26*(2), 308–322. https://doi.org/10.1093/her/cyr005.

Williams, D. M., & Rhodes, R. E. (2016). The confounded self-efficacy construct: Conceptual analysis and recommendations for future research. *Health Psychology Review, 10*(2), 113–128. https://doi.org/10.1080/17437199.2014.941998.

Wise, J. B., & Trunnell, E. P. (2001). The influence of sources of self-efficacy upon efficacy strength. *Journal of Sport & Exercise Psychology, 23*(4), 268–280.

Wolff, J. K., Warner, L. M., Ziegelmann, J. P., & Wurm, S. (2014). What do targeting positive views on ageing add to a physical activity intervention in older adults? Results from a randomised controlled trial. *Psychology & Health, 29*(8), 915–932. https://doi.org/10.1080/08870446.2014.896464.

Wood, R., & Bandura, A. (1989). Social cognitive theory of organizational management. *Academy of Management Review, 14*(3), 361–384.

Young, M. D., Plotnikoff, R. C., Collins, C. E., Callister, R., & Morgan, P. J. (2014). Social cognitive theory and physical activity: A systematic review and meta-analysis. *Obesity Reviews, 15*, 983–995. https://doi.org/10.1111/obr.12225.

13

Motivational Barriers and Resources for Physical Activity Among Older People

Verena Klusmann and Nanna Notthoff

13.1 Introduction

Imagine wanting to assist an older person in becoming physically active or in increasing their activity to a health-enhancing level. As you begin, you realise that physical activity is neither part of his or her self-concept (i.e., he or she does not self-identify as an "active person") nor are there significant exercising role models in his or her past or present social environment (e.g., no friends or relatives of the same age exercise regularly). Further, you worry that the person may feel invulnerable to the risk of developing a health problem and may not be convinced that exercise entails any benefits at all. Above all, your target person may think that ageing comes with inevitable physical and social losses. All of this seems a bit exaggerated? On second thought, it might not be too unrealistic. The large number of inactive people is evidence for these motivational barriers. For our fictitious individual, hardly any other idea would seem more far-fetched than beginning to be more physically active. Any personal competencies like exercise skills or the necessary physical

V. Klusmann (✉)
Department of Psychology, Psychological Assessment & Health Psychology, University of Konstanz, Konstanz, Germany

Department of Human and Health Sciences, Institute for Public Health and Nursing Research, Division for Health Promotion & Prevention, University of Bremen, Bremen, Germany

N. Notthoff
Department of Psychology, Humboldt University Berlin, Berlin, Germany

conditions would be irrelevant, and considerations of fostering self-efficacy (see Chap. 12) or implementation strategies (see Chap. 14) would be premature and futile. Thus, this chapter deals with central concepts of motivational barriers and resources for physical activity with special attention to older adults. After introducing and defining each of the constructs, corresponding empirical evidence will be discussed, and finally, practical implications will be presented as appropriate.

13.2 Self-Identity

Self-identity refers to being situated in a specific role (Stets and Burke 2003). According to Identity Theory, people's goals are based on their identities, and people strive to maintain consistency between identity and behaviour in pursuing their goals (Gecas and Burke 1995). The mechanisms for how this happens can be drawn from Social Cognitive Theory (see Chap. 11). For example, a person who identifies as an exerciser could have high levels of exercise-related self-efficacy (belief to be able to exercise, even in the face of obstacles), a reliable predictor of behaviour (see Chap. 12).

People who seriously pursue athletic endeavours tend to identify with these activities. This was demonstrated in a study of master cyclists (35–69 years) who described cycling as part of their identity that distinguished them from other people (Appleby and Dieffenbach 2016). One does not have to be an athlete to identify as an "exerciser" or physically active person. Among participants (58–95 years) in exercise classes in an assisted living facility, many people agreed that physical activity was part of their identity. The more they agreed, the more active they were and the more they intended to continue their activities in the future (Strachan et al. 2010).

The relationship between exercise identity and physical activity engagement seems to be bi-directional. In a sample of members of a 24-hour fitness facility (18–94 years), the more people exercised, the more they perceived physical changes in their bodies, which in turn led them to identify more as exercisers (Mullen 2011). This was true for the entire age range. An external prompt may be effective to jumpstart this process. Hardcastle and Taylor (2005) showed that middle-aged and older adults (43–77 years) who had received a prescription from their general practitioner to participate in a ten-week exercise program to improve their general fitness or health began to form an exercise identity. Contributing factors were physical activities' becoming part of people's routine, experiencing physical activity as meaningful and as a way to feel accomplished, and making social connections. Thus far, intervention studies aimed at modifying physical activity identity in older adults and affecting their behaviour have not been conducted. In younger adults, findings on whether changes in identity also result in changes in behaviour seem to be mixed according to a recent review (Rhodes et al. 2016).

From a provider's perspective, the idea of how well exercise aligns with older adults' identity also seems to be important. The degree to which exercise fits with older adults' identity was one of the main factors determining whether or not older adults took up exercise according to interviews with instructors (Hawley-Hague et al. 2016). The instructors stated that family members and health professionals sometimes undermined the process of physical activities' becoming integrated into older adults' identity when they communicated their belief that exercise was not suitable beyond a certain age. Thus, in considering whether and how physical activity becomes part of older adults' identity, one also has to take into consideration views of ageing (cf. Whaley and Ebbeck 2002). Ageing is often viewed as associated with physical limitations, which may prevent physical activity from becoming part of an older adult's identity (see also paragraphs 13.4 on subjective norms and 13.5 on self-perceptions of ageing).

13.3 Autonomous Versus Controlled Motivation

Unlike other concepts of motivation, Self-Determination Theory (SDT) focuses on type, rather than amount of motivation (Deci and Ryan 2008). In its original form (see also Chap. 11), SDT differentiated between intrinsic and extrinsic motivation with intrinsic motivation coming from within a person (e.g., an activity is performed for enjoyment) and extrinsic motivation being a result of external pressures (e.g., an activity is performed for a reward). People's motivation for behaviour can shift on a continuum from autonomous to controlled motivation, comprising external and so-called introjected regulation, the latter referring to internalised rewards and punishments (Deci and Ryan 2008).

Only recently, has SDT been applied to studying physical activity of older adults. The idea that higher levels of autonomous motivation for physical activity are associated with greater activity participation was confirmed in several quantitative and qualitative studies. Ferrand et al. (2012, 2014) showed that the amount of physical activity older enrolees (63–89 years) in a French activity program engaged in depended on their motivational profile. Participants in the cluster characterised by a higher degree of autonomous motivation were more active than those in the cluster characterised by a somewhat higher degree of controlled motivation. SDT motivational profiles also seem to predict whether or not people maintain or take up physical activity in retirement (Beck et al. 2010).

SDT has successfully been used as a basis for the design of interventions aimed at promoting physical activity in older adults. Thus far, it is unclear whether it is superior to other theoretical models. Friederichs et al. (2015) showed that both an SDT-based intervention and a traditional condition based on several other theories (Theory of Planned Behaviour, Social Cognitive Theory, Self-regulation Theory, and Transtheoretical Model; see Chap. 11) and involving tailored advice increased physical activity more than the waitlist control condition (18–70 years). The SDT-based intervention was more effective for promoting total minutes of activity, whereas the traditional approach was more effective for increasing the number of days on which participants engaged in at least 30 minutes of activity (Friederichs et al. 2015). In encouraging sedentary older adults to walk more, an SDT-based approach was superior to simply referring people to an exercise class or providing them with a structured walking program (Van Hoecke et al. 2014).

Interventions to date have sought to increase autonomous motivation by targeting the three psychological needs—autonomy, competence, and relatedness—that are proposed to be the underlying mechanisms. Van Hoecke et al. (2014) confirmed that individual counselling sessions were successful in promoting the satisfaction of the three needs and that participants experienced gains in autonomous motivation as a result. The relevance of the three needs for autonomous motivation was also recognised by participants themselves in another study (Lee et al. 2016). Interviews with participants of a French activity program showed that having an opportunity to assist with leading a program (autonomy) and feeling socially connected with other group members (relatedness) increased autonomous motivation. Concerns about age-related physical limitations, in contrast, led to higher controlled motivation (Ferrand et al. 2014).

However, the satisfaction of psychological needs can also be cited as a reason for being sedentary. Although one of the main motivations for remaining physically active in retirement was being part of a social group, inactive retirees found other ways to satisfy their need for relatedness. Furthermore, not fitting in with an exercise group was also one of the reasons why people discontinued physical activity. The importance of these psychological needs may differ between men and women. Relatedness seems to be more significant for women than for men. It should also be recognised that the association between psychological needs, motivational profiles, and physical activity is multi-directional. For example, increases in physical activity participation can lead to feelings of achievement and competence (Beck et al. 2010; Solberg et al. 2012).

13.4 Subjective Norms

The idea that subjective norms influence behaviour has been incorporated in several theories of health behaviour change (see Chap. 11). The term subjective norm refers to the likely or anticipated pressure from social partners such as family members and friends, but also health professionals to perform a behaviour and the motivation to give into this pressure. In other words, a person's subjective norm is his or her impression of what important social partners believe the person ought to do. Importantly, subjective norms should be distinguished from social norms, which are normative beliefs that are present in society as a whole.

Although subjective norms as a construct within the Theory of Planned Behaviour (see Chap. 11) have been broadly applied to understanding the uptake and maintenance of physical activity and designing intervention studies aimed at promoting it, few studies have included older adults, as documented in a recent review (Koeneman et al. 2011). Only 1 of the 30 included studies examined the influence of subjective norms on older adults' attendance in a physical activity program.

From the limited available evidence, it appears that subjective norms can be useful for predicting older adults' intentions to be physically active; however, they do not tend to reliably predict behaviour. For example, subjective norms predicted the intention of older adults aged 65–90 years enrolled in an exercise program to attend classes regularly (Lucidi et al. 2006). Actual class attendance was unrelated to participants' subjective norms. Likewise, subjective norms predicted older women's intention to meet the World Health Organization's (WHO) recommendations for aerobic physical activity (150 minutes of moderate activity per week or 75 minutes of vigorous activity per week), but not whether they actually met these recommendations (Vallance et al. 2011). The construct of subjective norms is not the only one of the Theory of Planned Behaviour components that only tends to predict older adults' intention to be physically active, but not their behaviour (Dean et al. 2007).

Findings regarding which factor in the Theory of Planned Behaviour—subjective norms, perceived behavioural control, or attitudes (see paragraph 13.7 on outcome expectancies)—best predicts intention to be active or actual activity are mixed. Two studies showed that although the Theory of Planned Behaviour as a whole predicted older adults' intention to be physically active, when the three factors were considered separately, only perceived behavioural control was relevant (Brenes et al. 1998; Galea and Bray 2006).

In sum, the available evidence suggests that subjective norms could be useful for predicting the intention of older adults who are already affiliated with a physical activity program to attend program sessions regularly. It remains unclear whether subjective norms can explain shortfalls of activity in sedentary older adults. Interventions aimed at changing subjective norms and the effects of such changes on physical activity intention and behaviour seem to be lacking, possibly because existing observational studies have documented that subjective norms do not reliably predict actual behaviour. If subjective norms were the target in a behavioural intervention, measures should be taken to reduce the intention-behaviour gap (see Chap. 14).

13.5 Self-Perceptions of Ageing

Recent research has demonstrated that how people view their own and others' ageing has the potential to determine whether they engage in health-promoting behaviours (for an overview see Miche et al. 2015). People, who in midlife associated their own ageing with fewer negative changes, lived a full 7.6 years (median) longer than their peers (Levy et al. 2002). When compared with recent data (Nusselder et al. 2009) on increased life expectancy through not smoking (4.3 years for men, 4.1 years for women) or high levels of physical activity (3.5 years for men, 3.4 years for women), these "added years" that seem to depend on ageing self-perceptions are especially impressive.

Levy (2009) postulates that age stereotypes exert their influence on health, well-being, and longevity through having pertinent behavioural consequences like healthy practices such as participating in exercise (see Levy and Myers 2004). That age expectations of decline seem to act as a barrier to physical activity has been shown by large-scale surveys (Meisner et al. 2013; Sarkisian et al. 2005). The study by Meisner et al. (2013) indicated a "matching effect," that is, more positive ageing-related expectations regarding physical health (but not expectations about mental health or cognitive function) were associated with strenuous sport and recreational physical activities in those adults (41–97 years) without functional limitations. Consequentially, negative expectations may make people think that they are unable to engage in strenuous activities due to their advanced age and, subsequently, they may dis-identify (see paragraph 13.2 on self-identity) and disengage from these activities.

Studies using data from the German Aging Survey showed that positive images of ageing increased sports participation in middle-aged adults (40–64 years) and leisure-time walking in older adults (65–85 years; Wurm et al. 2010). Given a positive view on ageing, even older people in poor health walked as regularly as their healthy peers. Shedding some light on underlying mechanisms, Wurm et al. (2013) found that after a serious health event, older people were inclined to utilise productive strategies like selective optimisation and compensation (see Chaps. 14 and 15) if they did not equate ageing with physical losses. Those with negative images of ageing, in contrast, did less for their health, which eventually resulted in lower life satisfaction and worse subjective health.

Interventions fostering a positive view on ageing in older adults may be successful in not only improving self-perceptions of ageing, but also increasing physical activity. In one intervention, images of older adults were changed by correcting false beliefs about ageing and teaching participants to identify and modify automatic counterproductive thoughts (Wolff et al. 2014). Positive age stereotypes may even be strengthened via subliminal priming (Levy et al. 2014). Evoked mastery experiences through becoming physically active, in turn, may help to buffer otherwise worsened ageing evaluations (Klusmann et al. 2012). This is in line with Meisner and colleagues' (2013) assumption that interventions to promote realistic ageing expectations regarding physical health should be particularly effective for increasing physical activity in older adults; they combat fatalistic thinking and stereotype-congruent disengagement. On a societal level, fostering positive intergenerational interactions, education about age and ageing, and changing media portrayals of older people have been suggested (Kotter-Grühn 2015). Interventions could also make use of the matching effect and use role models to combat stereotypes of ageing (Horton 2010).

13.6 Risk Perceptions

Perceptions of risk are crucial for motivating people to adopt protective behaviours like physical activity, especially in old age (Renner et al. 2007; Schwarzer and Renner 2000). Commonly, it is assumed that threat appraisals result from perceived susceptibility or vulnerability and severity of disease (Stretcher et al. 1997; van der Pligt 1998).

Experts commonly judge and compare risk factors by combining the likelihood of occurrence and the severity of adverse outcomes (Fischhoff et al. 2000; Slovic 2000). Communicating a health threat in a way common in public health campaigns aimed at disease prevention can only solve part of the problem, however (Hamilton and Lobel 2015). In order to take protective action, people need to not only be aware of a risk *in general*, but they need to feel *personally* at risk (Schwarzer 2008). Lay people's assessments are a function of the triggered affective responses (e.g., worry and perceived dread) and the familiarity and estimated controllability of a health threat (Slovic 1987; Slovic et al. 2005). Motivating people for proper action might work best if one tackles anticipatory emotions, possibly by using affect-rich images and narratives (Sheeran et al. 2014; Slovic and Peters 2006).

Both the adequacy and the adaptiveness of lay people's judgements have been subject to controversial debates (for an overview see Renner and Schupp 2011). It is an often replicated finding that people accept high-risk health information to a lesser degree than low-risk information, often referred to as self-defensive bias (Ditto 2009; Helzer and Dunning 2012; Van 't Riet and Ruiter 2013). However, a lack of reassurance after receiving low-risk feedback has also been observed (e.g., Gamp and Renner 2015). The Cue-Adaptive Reasoning Account (Renner 2004) explained how people reasonably invest resources to scrutinise negative and unexpected risk information, what prevents them from both an unnecessary investment and a rash termination of already-taken protective actions (Renner and Schupp 2011).

Comparing participants under the age of 31 years with older adults (31–84 years) from a German sample revealed that the perception of risk significantly predicted the intention for protective behaviour in older adults, but had no substantial effect for younger adults (Schwarzer and Renner 2000). Other studies confirmed that risk perceptions had a particular influence on motivation for physical activity in older adults (Renner et al. 2007).

It seems obvious that older people also perceive greater risks in absolute terms, given declining major biological systems and increasing objective prevalence for chronic diseases, accompanied by a rising priority for health (e.g., Ebner et al. 2006; Schindler and Staudinger 2008). Older people indeed perceive a heightened absolute risk for the development of cardiovascular diseases (Hamilton and Lobel 2012; Meischke et al. 2000; Renner et al. 2000, 2007), but show lower risk perceptions for stroke, diabetes, as well as breast and lung cancer compared to younger age groups (Adriaanse et al. 2008; Hamilton and Lobel 2012; Harwell et al. 2005). Albeit older people with a high body mass index perceive a higher risk of heart disease (e.g., Renner et al. 2000), a substantial proportion of—especially male—participants still disagreed that their heightened body weight was a health risk (Gregory et al. 2008). Since physical exercise is especially beneficial for cardiovascular health, the heightened risk perception in old age might help to boost motivation in this regard. Despite this, the mixed evidence leads over to the issue of biases that have been observed to influence people's subjective risk estimates.

Acknowledging that one's risk increases in old age does not necessarily imply that people become less optimistic about their risk in comparison with their peers. Unrealistic optimism was observed in middle-aged and older adults as well (Hamilton and Lobel 2012; Renner et al. 2000) and might be explained by increasing compensatory social downward comparisons in the face of experienced age-related declines (Bauer et al. 2008).

13.7 Outcome Expectancies

The value of the expected outcomes is essential in determining someone's readiness to act (e.g., Atkinson 1957). Having been established as a core concept in enabling behaviour change by Social Cognitive Theory, different labels like perceived benefit (Health Belief Model) or behavioural beliefs (Theory of Planned Behaviour) have been used (see Chap. 11).

The basic idea is that without the expectation of a resultant benefit, health behaviour lacks its justification, and consequently, the likelihood of disengagement increases. For example, people might agree that they could wear a helmet when riding a bicycle, but whether they decide to do so crucially depends on being convinced that wearing a helmet actually increases safety. Outcome expectancies have the form of if-then assumptions (like "If I engage in physical activity, then I will…") that refer to expected consequences of actions or behaviours that differ in the degree of desirability and probability (Bandura 2001; Heckhausen 1977). A thorough contemplation process with balancing of pros and cons of anticipated behavioural outcomes precedes the formation of outcome expectancies. Following a dynamic perspective, outcome expectancies are important for moving people from a pre-intending to an intending, that is, a pre-active stage of behaviour change (Schwarzer 2008). Outcome expectancies have been shown to translate threat appraisals and risk perceptions into action (see paragraph 13.6 on risk perceptions) and are an important mediator between self-efficacy beliefs and physical exercise (see Chap. 12; Gellert et al. 2012).

Classically, outcome expectancies ascribe value to an action due to presumed positive psychological effects (e.g., fun, relaxation, companionship), body image (e.g., appearance, self-image, confidence), or health benefits (Steinhardt and Dishman 1989; Schwarzer 2008). Outcome expectancies focusing on consequences closely tied to the behaviour itself are a better predictor of physical activity than distal ones. Specifically, affective expectations directly related to emotional states during or directly after physical activity affected intentions and behaviour in older adults (60–95 years) the most (Gellert et al. 2012). An age-tailored intervention targeting present orientation and emotional benefits of exercise together with components of goal attainment led to superior maintenance of physical activity in 60+ year-old adults (Gellert et al. 2014). The crucial importance of proximal, emotional outcome expectancies for physical activity enhancement in old age is substantiated by research on the role of affective attitudes (e.g., Conner et al. 2015) and fits with the idea of Socioemotional Selectivity Theory, assuming an increased focus on emotionally gratifying experiences in the here and now in older compared to younger age (e.g., Carstensen and Mikels 2005; see also Chaps. 12 and 14).

Adding to these findings, we recently demonstrated the importance of a positive dynamic through the actual *fulfilment* of outcome expectancies in the time course of exercise adoption and maintenance (Klusmann et al. 2016). Outcome expectancy fulfilment was the predominant predictor for differentiating between successful and unsuccessful behaviour changes and proximal outcome expectancies concerning emotional rewards were most meaningful in this regard. Outcome expectancies gain volitional relevance, especially if our expectations are met. Only then is it worth investing the effort; the behaviour change process is fuelled in terms of an upwards spiral (Loehr et al. 2014; Rothman 2000). An absence of desired outcomes, in contrast, results in a standstill, in which good intentions weaken or fade, and a sustainable change of habits becomes very unlikely.

Interestingly, in the above-mentioned study (Klusmann et al. 2016), older participants aged 60+ years were slightly less successful in their attempts to increase physical activity than younger adults. Higher age was associated with somewhat less endorsement of outcome expectancies and correspondingly fewer fulfilments.

13.8 Practical Implications

Remember our example from the beginning of the chapter: We were to realise that as long as central motivational requirements are unmet, any efforts to foster self-efficacy (see Chap. 12) or initiate volitional processes of behaviour change (see Chap. 14) seem premature and futile. Conversely, if our hypothetical person were to recognise the potentials of age and ageing and thus, were to have favourable self-perceptions of ageing, were to be convinced by the beneficial outcomes of physical activity, were to have an exercise identity, and were to be intrinsically motivated, a reasonable basis for health behaviour change could be established. In the following we will illustrate possible gateways for overcoming barriers and activating motivational resources for physical activity up to old age.

Whether or not older adults identify as exercisers seems to crucially depend on the terminology used to describe physical activity. Older adults seem to use terms other than exercise—for example, "physically active"—to describe themselves (Whaley and Ebbeck 2002). Thus, the name of an exercise class could determine whether it aligns with older adults' identity and is well received within this age group (Hawley-Hague et al. 2016). Using the terms "exercise" or "falls prevention" could be a deterrent whereas "movement" may be more appealing; it may signal that the class is comprised of a variety of activities and that every participant will be able to find something suitable without having to self-identify as frail and at risk of falling (Nyman 2011).

Besides choosing appropriate names for activity programs aimed at older adults, creating an environment that fosters the integration of physical activity into older adults' identity can mean ensuring that social partners including health professionals express the opinion that physical activity is a life-long pursuit. Among regularly active older people, physical activity identity can develop further on its own as long as the older adults observe effects of their activity, for example, physical changes or feelings of achievement (see also paragraph 13.7 on outcome expectancies).

To increase the amount of favourable autonomous motivation, it seems advantageous to let participants take an active role in activity programs (cf. Ferrand et al. 2014) and to facilitate the development of a sense of togetherness or unity, for example, by explicitly supporting processes of group bonding, especially in women (Beck et al. 2010). However, one is well advised to also consider the risk of negative group dynamics, group members agreeing on "age-appropriate" sedentary behaviour, or people not fitting in.

For older people who already participate in an activity program, it seems useful to address subjective norms to increase their commitment (cf. Lucidi et al. 2006). However, subjective norms probably cannot prevent activity shortfalls, and it is more than doubtful whether tackling personal norms can stimulate newly adopted engagement.

The intriguing effects of favourable ageing self-perceptions boosting physical activity up to old age have taught us that taking means to support positive images of ageing will pay off. One can choose to directly combat negative age stereotypes through either correcting false beliefs or practising productive thinking (cf. Wolff et al. 2014). Alternatively, positive ageing perceptions might unobtrusively be strengthened by providing positive experiences with one's ageing body, helping people realise that fitness resources can be activated and that they are still powerful and capable (cf. Klusmann et al. 2012). Also, role models combating age stereotypes could be useful (Horton 2010). However, promoting master athletes entails the risk of older people's dis-identification. Role models should thus show characteristics as similar as possible to a peer of the target audience.

For risk communication, Renner and Schupp (2011) point out the following central principles: People should be informed about absolute risk using natural frequencies (conditional probabilities are hardly understood by both lay people and experts; Gigerenzer et al. 2008) as well as about the relative risk by comparing different hazards (to provide anchors for orientation and help people deal with both small numbers of probabilities and probabilities that exceed a 50–50 chance; Lipkus 2007; Weinstein 2000). To circumvent high-risk stereotypes that facilitate downward comparisons and negotiation of risk, recipients should be informed about their risk relative to similar others or receive personalised risk information (Hahn and Renner 1998; Harris et al. 2008; cf. Perloff and Fetzer 1986). Negative as well as positive feedback should be of high quality, since information conflicting with pre-existing risk perceptions is scrutinised carefully (Renner 2004). Finally, effective risk communication should disclose feasible ways to reduce risk and to increase healthy behaviour (Sheeran et al. 2014).

Maintenance problems of physical activity in old age might be overcome by fostering realistic outcome expectancies (Evers et al. 2012; Renner et al. 2012). Before starting to exercise, people mostly focus on the aversive beginning and thus underestimate enjoyment (Ruby et al. 2011). Expectancy adjustment might help people focus on accomplishable outcomes and make people see the attained outcomes that may reinforce behaviour change. Indeed, teaching exercise trainers strategies to promote positive emotions during exercise sessions increases adherence (Jekauc 2015) and, likewise, affective short-term messages produce higher levels of physical activity (Morris et al. 2015). A final note on a popular strategy: Broaching the issue of age-related physical limitations seems contraindicated in multiple ways. As we have come to know, it equally leads to higher levels of unfavourable controlled motivation and evokes less effective outcome expectancies.

13.9 Conclusion

Overall, the concepts introduced in this chapter have qualified as useful tools for understanding the activity of older adults and designing interventions to promote it. As is state-of-the-art in the health promotion profession, the development of effective interventions and programs is based on a thorough need and capacity assessment that considers the particular features of people and settings. With ageing, diversity of people increases; thus, there will hardly be any fixable one-fits-all approach to motivate older people for physical activity. Integrative approaches in which several concepts are combined to meet the specific needs of a target person or a target group of older people may be best.

Suggested Further Reading

- Gigerenzer, G., Gaissmaier, W., Kurz-Milcke, E., Schwartz, L.M., & Woloshin, S. (2008). Helping doctors and patients make sense of health statistics. *Psychological Science in the Public Interest, 8*, 53–96.
- Meisner, B. A., Weir, P. L., & Baker, J. (2013). The relationship between aging expectations and various modes of physical activity among aging adults. *Psychology of Sport and Exercise, 14*, 569–576.
- Strachan, S. M., Brawley, L. R., Spink, K., & Glazebrook, K. (2010). Older adults' physically-active identity: Relationships between social cognitions, physical activity and satisfaction with life. *Psychology of Sport and Exercise, 11*(2), 114–121.

References

Adriaanse, M. C., Twisk, J. W., Dekker, J. M., Spijkerman, A. M., Nijpels, G., Heine, R. J., & Snoek, F. J. (2008). Perceptions of risk in adults with a low or high risk profile of developing type 2 diabetes; A cross-sectional population-based study. *Patient Education and Counseling, 73*, 307–312.

Appleby, K. M., & Dieffenbach, K. (2016). "Older and faster": Exploring elite masters cyclists' involvement in competitive sport. *Sport Psychologist, 30*, 13–23.

Atkinson, J. W. (1957). Motivational determinants of risk-taking behavior. *Psychological Review, 64*, 359–372.

Bandura, A. (2001). Social cognitive theory: An agentic perspective. *Annual Review of Psychology, 52*, 1–26.

Bauer, I., Wrosch, C., & Jobin, J. (2008). I'm better off than most other people: The role of social comparisons for coping with regret in young adulthood and old age. *Psychology and Aging, 23*, 800–811.

Beck, F., Gillison, F., & Standage, M. (2010). A theoretical investigation of the development of physical activity habits in retirement. *British Journal of Health Psychology, 15*, 663–679.

Brenes, G. A., Strube, M. J., & Storandt, M. (1998). An application of the theory of planned behavior to exercise among older adults. *Journal of Applied Social Psychology, 28*, 2274–2290.

Carstensen, L. L., & Mikels, J. A. (2005). At the intersection of emotion and cognition: Aging and the positivity effect. *Current Directions in Psychological Science, 14*, 117–121.

Conner, M., McEachan, R., Taylor, N., O'Hara, J., & Lawton, R. (2015). Role of affective attitudes and anticipated affective reactions in predicting health behaviors. *Health Psychology, 34*, 642–652.

Dean, R. N., Farrell, J. M., Kelley, M. L., Taylor, M. J., & Rhodes, R. E. (2007). Testing the efficacy of the theory of planned behavior to explain strength training in older adults. *Journal of Aging and Physical Activity, 15*(1), 1–12.

Deci, E. L., & Ryan, R. M. (2008). Self-determination theory: A macrotheory of human motivation, development, and health. *Canadian Psychology, 49*, 182–185.

Ditto, P. H. (2009). Passion, reason, and necessity a quantity-of-processing view of motivated reasoning. In T. Bayne & J. Fernández (Eds.), *Delusion and self-deception: Affective and motivational influences on belief formation* (pp. 23–53). New York: Psychology Press.

Ebner, N. C., Freund, A. M., & Baltes, P. B. (2006). Developmental changes in personal goal orientation from young to late adulthood: From striving for gains to maintenance and prevention of losses. *Psychology and Aging, 21*, 664–678.

Evers, A., Klusmann, V., Ziegelmann, J. P., Schwarzer, R., & Heuser, I. (2012). Long-term adherence to a physical activity intervention: The role of telephone-assisted vs. self-administered coping plans and strategy use. *Psychology & Health, 27*, 784–797.

Ferrand, C., Nasarre, S., Hautier, C., & Bonnefoy, M. (2012). Aging and well-being in French older adults regularly practicing physical activity: A self-determination perspective. *Journal of Aging and Physical Activity, 20*, 215–230.

Ferrand, C., Martinent, G., & Bonnefoy, M. (2014). Exploring motivation for exercise and its relationship with health-related quality of life in adults aged 70 years and older. *Ageing and Society, 34*, 411–427.

Fischhoff, B., Bostrom, A., & Quadrel, M. J. (2000). Risk perception and communication. In T. Connolly, H. R. Arkes, & K. R. Hammond (Eds.), *Judgment and decision making: An interdisciplinary reader* (pp. 479–499). New York: Cambridge University Press.

Friederichs, S. A., Oenema, A., Bolman, C., & Lechner, L. (2015). Long term effects of self-determination theory and motivational interviewing in a web-based physical activity intervention: Randomized controlled trial. *International Journal of Behavioral Nutrition and Physical Activity, 12*(1), 1–12.

Galea, M. N., & Bray, S. R. (2006). Predicting walking intentions and exercise in individuals with intermittent claudication: An application of the theory of planned behavior. *Rehabilitation Psychology, 51*, 299–305.

Gamp, M., & Renner, B. (2015). Experience-based health risk feedback and lack of reassurance. *Health Psychology and Behavioral Medicine, 3*, 410–423.

Gecas, V., & Burke, P. J. (1995). Self and identity. In K. Cook, G. A. Fine, & J. S. House (Eds.), *Sociological perspectives in social psychology* (pp. 41–67). Boston: Allyn & Bacon.

Gellert, P., Ziegelmann, J. P., & Schwarzer, R. (2012). Affective and health-related outcome expectancies for physical activity in older adults. *Psychology & Health, 27*, 816–828.

Gellert, P., Ziegelmann, J. P., Krupka, S., Knoll, N., & Schwarzer, R. (2014). An age-tailored intervention sustains physical activity changes in older adults: A randomized controlled trial. *International Journal of Behavioral Medicine, 21*, 519–528.

Gigerenzer, G., Gaissmaier, W., Kurz-Milcke, E., Schwartz, L. M., & Woloshin, S. (2008). Helping doctors and patients make sense of health statistics. *Psychological Science in the Public Interest, 8*, 53–96.

Gregory, C. O., Blanck, H. M., Gillespie, C., Maynard, L. M., & Serdula, M. K. (2008). Perceived health risk of excess body weight among overweight and obese men and women: Differences by sex. *Preventive Medicine, 47*, 46–52.

Hahn, A., & Renner, B. (1998). Perception of health risks: How smoker status affects defensive optimism. *Anxiety, Stress and Coping, 11*, 93–112.

Hamilton, J. G., & Lobel, M. (2012). Passing years, changing fears? Conceptualizing and measuring risk perceptions for chronic disease in younger and middle-aged women. *Journal of Behavioral Medicine, 35*, 124–138.

Hamilton, J. G., & Lobel, M. (2015). Psychosocial factors associated with risk perceptions for chronic diseases in younger and middle-aged women. *Women Health, 55*, 921–942.

Hardcastle, S., & Taylor, A. H. (2005). Finding an exercise identity in an older body: "It's redefining yourself and working out who you are". *Psychology of Sport and Exercise, 6*, 173–188.

Harris, P. R., Griffin, D. W., & Murray, S. (2008). Testing the limits of optimistic bias: Event and person moderators in a multilevel framework. *Journal of Personality and Social Psychology, 95*, 1225–1237.

Harwell, T. S., Blades, L. L., Oser, C. S., Dietrich, D. W., Okon, N. J., Rodriguez, D. V., et al. (2005). Perceived risk for developing stroke among older adults. *Preventive Medicine, 41*, 791–794.

Hawley-Hague, H., Horne, M., Skelton, D. A., & Todd, C. (2016). Older adults' uptake and adherence to exercise classes. *Journal of Aging and Physical Activity, 24*, 119–128.

Heckhausen, H. (1977). Achievement motivation and its constructs: A cognitive model. *Motivation and Emotion, 1*, 283–329.

Helzer, E., & Dunning, D. (2012). On motivated reasoning and self-belief. In S. Vazire & T. D. Wilson (Eds.), *Handbook of self-knowledge* (pp. 379–396). New York: Guilford Press.

Horton, S. (2010). Masters athletes as role models? Combating stereotypes of aging. In J. Baker (Ed.), *The masters athlete: Understanding the role of sport and exercise in optimizing aging* (pp. 122–136). London: Routledge.

Jekauc, D. (2015). Enjoyment during exercise mediates the effects of an intervention on exercise adherence. *Psychology, 6*, 48–54.

Klusmann, V., Evers, A., Schwarzer, R., & Heuser, I. (2012). Views on aging and emotional benefits of physical activity: Effects of an exercise intervention in older women. *Psychology of Sport and Exercise, 13*, 236–242.

Klusmann, V., Musculus, L., Sproesser, G., & Renner, B. (2016). Fulfilled emotional outcome expectancies enable successful adoption and maintenance of physical activity. *Frontiers in Psychology, 6*, 1990.

Koeneman, M. A., Verheijden, M. W., Chinapaw, M. J., & Hopman-Rock, M. (2011). Determinants of physical activity and exercise in healthy older adults: A systematic review. *International Journal of Behavioral Nutrition and Physical Activity, 8*, 142.

Kotter-Grühn, D. (2015). Changing negative views of aging: Implications for intervention and translational research. *Annual Review of Gerontology and Geriatrics, 35*, 167–186.

Lee, M., Kim, M. J., Suh, D., Kim, J., Jo, E., & Yoon, B. (2016). Feasibility of a self-determination theory-based exercise program in community-dwelling South Korean older adults: Experiences from a 13-month trial. *Journal of Aging and Physical Activity, 24*, 8–21.

Levy, B. R. (2009). Stereotype embodiment: A psychosocial approach to aging. *Current Directions in Psychological Science, 18*, 332–336.

Levy, B. R., & Myers, L. M. (2004). Preventive health behaviors influenced by self-perceptions of aging. *Preventive Medicine, 39*, 625–629.

Levy, B. R., Slade, M. D., Kunkel, S. R., & Kasl, S. V. (2002). Longevity increased by positive self-perceptions of aging. *Journal of Personality and Social Psychology, 83*, 261–270.

Levy, B. R., Pilver, C., Chung, P. H., & Slade, M. D. (2014). Subliminal strengthening: Improving older individuals' physical function over time with an implicit-age-stereotype intervention. *Psychological Science, 25*, 2127–2135.

Lipkus, I. M. (2007). Numeric, verbal, and visual formats of conveying health risks: Suggested best practices and future recommendations. *Medical Decision Making, 27*, 696–713.

Loehr, V. G., Baldwin, A. S., Rosenfield, D., & Smits, J. A. (2014). Weekly variability in outcome expectations: Examining associations with related physical activity experiences during physical activity initiation. *Journal of Health Psychology, 19*, 1309–1319.

Lucidi, F., Grano, C., Barbaranelli, C., & Violani, C. (2006). Social-cognitive determinants of physical activity attendance in older adults. *Journal of Aging and Physical Activity, 14*, 344–359.

Meischke, H., Sellers, D. E., Goff, D. C., Daya, M. R., Meshack, A., Taylor, J., & Hand, M. M. (2000). Factors that influence personal perceptions of the risk of an acute myocardial infarction. *Behavioral Medicine, 26*, 4–13.

Meisner, B. A., Weir, P. L., & Baker, J. (2013). The relationship between aging expectations and various modes of physical activity among aging adults. *Psychology of Sport and Exercise, 14*, 569–576.

Miche, M., Brothers, A., Diehl, M., & Wahl, H. W. (2015). Subjective aging and awareness of aging: Toward a new understanding of the aging self. *Annual Review of Gerontology and Geriatrics, 35*, 1–28.

Morris, B., Lawton, R., McEachan, R., Hurling, R., & Conner, M. (2015). Changing self-reported physical activity using different types of affectively and cognitively framed health messages, in a student population. *Psychology, Health & Medicine, 2015*, 1–10.

Mullen, S. P. (2011). Perceptions of change and certainty regarding the self-as-exerciser: A multistudy report. *Journal of Sport and Exercise Psychology, 33*, 710–733.

Nusselder, W. J., Franco, O. H., Peeters, A., & Mackenbach, J. P. (2009). Living healthier for longer: Comparative effects of three heart-healthy behaviors on life expectancy with and without cardiovascular disease. *BMC Public Health, 9*, 487.

Nyman, S. R. (2011). Psychosocial issues in engaging older people with physical activity interventions for the prevention of falls. *Canadian Journal on Aging, 30*, 45–55.

Perloff, L. S., & Fetzer, B. K. (1986). Self-other judgments and perceived vulnerability to victimization. *Journal of Personality and Social Psychology, 50*, 502–510.

Renner, B. (2004). Biased reasoning: Adaptive responses to health risk feedback. *Personality and Social Psychology Bulletin, 30*, 384–396.

Renner, B., & Schupp, H. (2011). The perception of health risks. In H. Friedman (Ed.), *The Oxford handbook of health psychology* (pp. 637–665). New York: Oxford University Press.

Renner, B., Knoll, N., & Schwarzer, R. (2000). Age and body weight make a difference in optimistic health beliefs and nutrition behaviors. *International Journal of Behavioral Medicine, 7*, 143–159.

Renner, B., Spivak, Y., Kwon, S., & Schwarzer, R. (2007). Does age make a difference? Predicting physical activity of South Koreans. *Psychology and Aging, 22*, 482–493.

Renner, B., Hankonen, N., Ghisletta, P., & Absetz, P. (2012). Dynamic psychological and behavioral changes in the adoption and maintenance of exercise. *Health Psychology, 31*, 306–315.

Rhodes, R. E., Kaushal, N., & Quinlan, A. (2016). Is physical activity a part of who I am? A review and meta-analysis of identity, schema and physical activity. *Health Psychology Review, 10*, 204–225.

Rothman, A. J. (2000). Toward a theory-based analysis of behavioral maintenance. *Health Psychology, 19*, 64–69.

Ruby, M. B., Dunn, E. W., Perrino, A., Gillis, R., & Viel, S. (2011). The invisible benefits of exercise. *Health Psychology, 30*, 67–74.

Sarkisian, C. A., Prohaska, T. R., Wong, M. D., Hirsch, S., & Mangione, C. M. (2005). The relationship between expectations for aging and physical activity among older adults. *Journal of General Internal Medicine, 20*, 911–915.

Schindler, I., & Staudinger, U. M. (2008). Obligatory and optional personal life investments in old and very old age: Validation and functional relations. *Motivation and Emotion, 32*, 23–36.

Schwarzer, R. (2008). Modeling health behavior change: How to predict and modify the adoption and maintenance of health behaviors. *Applied Psychology, 57*, 1–29.

Schwarzer, R., & Renner, B. (2000). Social-cognitive predictors of health behavior: Action self-efficacy and coping self-efficacy. *Health Psychology, 19*, 487–495.

Sheeran, P., Harris, P. R., & Epton, T. (2014). Does heightening risk appraisals change people's intentions and behavior? A meta-analysis of experimental studies. *Psychological Bulletin, 140*, 511–543.

Slovic, P. (1987). Perception of risk. *Science, 236*, 280–285.

Slovic, P. (2000). *The perception of risk*. London: Earthscan Publications.

Slovic, P., & Peters, E. (2006). Risk perception and affect. *Current Directions in Psychological Science, 15*, 322.

Slovic, P., Peters, E., Finucane, M., & MacGregor, D. G. (2005). Affect, risk, and decision making. *Health Psychology, 24*, 35–40.

Solberg, P. A., Hopkins, W. G., Ommundsen, Y., & Halvari, H. (2012). Effects of three training types on vitality among older adults: A self-determination theory perspective. *Psychology of Sport and Exercise, 13*, 407–417.

Steinhardt, M. A., & Dishman, R. K. (1989). Reliability and validity of expected outcomes and barriers for habitual physical activity. *Journal of Occupational Medicine, 31*, 536–546.

Stets, J. E., & Burke, P. J. (2003). A sociological approach to self and identity. In M. R. Leary & J. P. Tangney (Eds.), *Handbook of self and identity* (pp. 128–152). New York: Guilford Press.

Strachan, S. M., Brawley, L. R., Spink, K., & Glazebrook, K. (2010). Older adults' physically-active identity: Relationships between social cognitions, physical activity and satisfaction with life. *Psychology of Sport and Exercise, 11*, 114–121.

Stretcher, V. J., Champion, V. L., & Rosenstock, I. M. (1997). The health belief model and health behavior. In D. S. Goschman (Ed.), *Handbook of health behavior research* (Vol. 1, pp. 71–91). New York: Plenum Press.

Vallance, J. K., Murray, T. C., Johnson, S. T., & Elavsky, S. (2011). Understanding physical activity intentions and behavior in postmenopausal women: An application of the theory of planned behavior. *International Journal of Behavioral Medicine, 18*, 139–149.

Van 't Riet, J., & Ruiter, R. A. C. (2013). Defensive reactions to health-promoting information: An overview and implications for future research. *Health Psychology Review, 7*, 104–136.

van der Pligt, J. (1998). Perceived risk and vulnerability as predictors of precautionary behaviour. *British Journal of Health Psychology, 3*, 1–14.

Van Hoecke, A. S., Delecluse, C., Bogaerts, A., & Boen, F. (2014). The long-term effectiveness of need-supportive physical activity counseling compared with a standard referral in sedentary older adults. *Journal of Aging and Physical Activity, 22*, 186–198.

Weinstein, N. D. (2000). Perceived probability, perceived severity, and health-protective behavior. *Health Psychology, 19*, 65–74.

Whaley, D. E., & Ebbeck, V. (2002). Self-schemata and exercise identity in older adults. *Journal of Aging and Physical Activity, 10*, 245–259.

Wolff, J. K., Warner, L. M., Ziegelmann, J. P., & Wurm, S. (2014). What do targeting positive views on ageing add to a physical activity intervention in older adults? Results from a randomised controlled trial. *Psychology & Health, 29*, 915–932.

Wurm, S., Tomasik, M. J., & Tesch-Römer, C. (2010). On the importance of a positive view on ageing for physical exercise among middle-aged and older adults: Cross-sectional and longitudinal findings. *Psychology & Health, 25*, 25–42.

Wurm, S., Warner, L. M., Ziegelmann, J. P., Wolff, J. K., & Schüz, B. (2013). How do negative self-perceptions of aging become a self-fulfilling prophecy? *Psychology and Aging, 28*, 1088–1097.

14

Self-Regulation and Planning Strategies to Initiate and Maintain Physical Activity Among Older People

Paul Gellert and Andre M. Müller

14.1 Introduction

Behaviour in general is often regulated by non-conscious processes such as habits or automatic responses triggered by environmental cues (Rebar et al. 2016). People just act without much conscious control or planning. In contrast, self-regulation refers to control processes which actively modulate the behaviour in order to bring it in line with set goals and standards (Baumeister and Vohs 2004). Self-regulation usually involves conscious processes as the individual intentionally initiates, regulates, and evaluates behaviour (Baumeister and Vohs 2004). Self-regulation, which is sometimes called volition, is vital throughout various behavioural action phases. It is a key capability when it comes to taking up a new behaviour, which demands high levels of control. Additionally, self-regulation is crucial in the maintenance of a behaviour, which has not yet become a routine. Likewise, shielding the intended behaviour from attractive yet goal-threatening alternatives and recovering from relapses requires successful self-regulation.

P. Gellert (✉)
Institute for Medical Sociology and Rehabilitation Science,
Charité – Universitätsmedizin Berlin, Berlin, Germany

A. M. Müller
Saw Swee Hock School of Public Health, National University of Singapore, Singapore, Singapore

14.2 Theory of Self-Regulation

Although there are a variety of theories and models on human self-regulation such as Self-Regulatory Strength (e.g., Muraven and Baumeister 2000), Delay of Gratification (Mischel et al. 1989), or Automatic Self-Regulation (Bargh 1990; Sheeran et al. 2013), in the following the focus is on the Control Theory of Self-Regulation (Carver and Scheier 1981, 1982), a widely accepted framework to understand and change behaviour.

Carver and Scheier's Control Theory (1981, 1982) outlines the mechanism of self-regulation and its importance for initiating as well as maintaining an intended behaviour. Control here means the mental capacity to implement an intended behaviour while inhibiting other, unintended behaviours. According to this theory, self-regulation is a negative feedback loop (see Fig. 14.1), in which the individual evaluates a present state (input function) to then compare it with a desired status or a set goal (reference value, goal, or standard-comparator).

If there is a difference perceived between the present state and the goal, regulatory processes and behavioural responses (output function) that result in an impact on the behaviour or the environment will be activated by the individual in order to reduce the difference. For example, an older person with limited mobility might set the goal (reference value or goal setting) to engage in a home-based balance training three times a week. The reference value or goal may be embedded in a goal hierarchy where subordinate goals (e.g., balance exercise three times a week) serve superordinate goals (e.g., prevent falls). If this person performed the balance exercise two times per week,

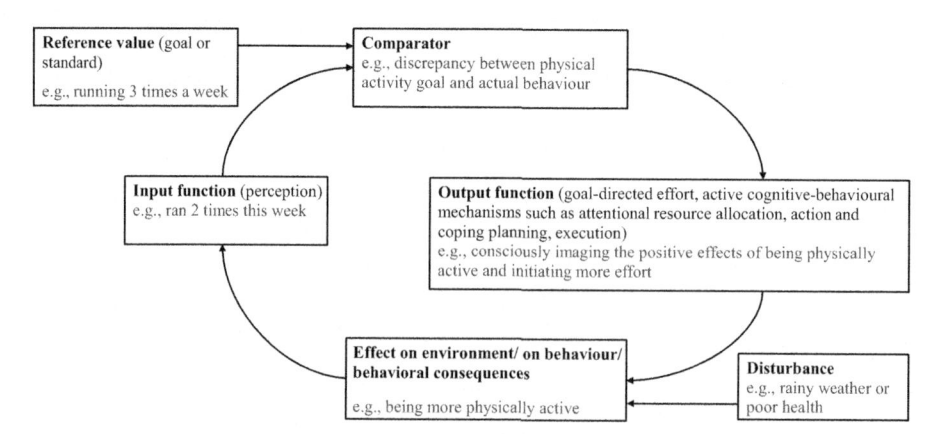

Fig. 14.1 Feedback loop with physical activity-related examples (Modified after Carver and Scheier 2002, p. 305)

the perception of the difference of one time exercising activates him/her to begin another session (monitoring and feedback). External factors or disturbances, which might come into play, can influence the performance (e.g., bad mood or physical exhaustion or conflicting goals and behaviours). Supporting the assumptions of the Control Theory empirically, Prestwich et al. (2016) found that fostering all three key techniques of the Control Theory together—goal setting, self-monitoring, and feedback—resulted in increased PA levels as compared with a goal-setting-only condition and a self-monitoring plus goal-setting condition.

Many other behaviour change theories such as the Theory of Planned Behaviour (Ajzen 1991) or the Social Cognitive Theory (Bandura 1989) focus on motivational processes related to PA initiation whereas behavioural maintenance is often neglected (see Chap. 11 for details on other behaviour change theories; motivation for PA is discussed in Chap. 13). However, beyond motivation, self-regulation may explain why some individuals who are motivated to be physically active do not translate their intentions into subsequent PA behaviour. While some people act on their intentions (so-called inclined actors) others fail to act despite good intentions (inclined abstainers; Orbell and Sheeran 1998). The intention-behaviour gap which is the phenomenon of not acting upon one's intentions might be explained by failed self-regulation. To illustrate this, once a person is motivated and a PA goal is set, the individual moves from goal setting, which is mainly driven by norms, expectations, and perceptions to goal striving where self-regulatory processes gain importance because they make behaviour happen. Models such as the Rubicon Model of Action Phases (Heckhausen and Gollwitzer 1987), the Transtheoretical Model (Stages of Change; Prochaska and DiClemente 1992), the Health Action Process Approach, or the Reflective and Automatic Process Model (Rothman et al. 2009) propose self-regulatory strategies like self-monitoring and planning to bridge the gap between intention and actual behaviour (see Chap. 11 for details on these models).

14.3 Self-Monitoring as a Self-Regulatory Strategy

Following Carver and Scheier's Control Theory (1981, 1982), self-monitoring as a self-regulatory strategy works as input function providing information about the current state (e.g., My step count on the step counter device for today at 6 pm shows 6114 steps). In alliance with the reference value or simply the goal (e.g., I aim to walk 8000 steps a day), self-monitoring allows for evaluating whether a goal was attained (e.g., I have not yet met my goal today) so that, if necessary, the individual exerts discrepancy-reducing self-regulatory effort (e.g., After dinner I will have an additional walk; Sniehotta et al. 2006). Self-monitoring is especially useful when a new behaviour is already initiated but has not yet become a routine. Michie et al. (2013) distinguish several behaviour change techniques, which are associated with self-monitoring such as feedback and monitoring, feedback on behaviour, biofeedback, other(s) monitoring with awareness, self-monitoring of outcome of behaviour, and self-monitoring of behaviour (for further details, see Chap. 11).

When it comes to increasing PA, self-monitoring has been shown to be a promising strategy. In a correlational meta-analysis on the effectiveness of PA interventions, post hoc analyses of intervention effects indicated that interventions which contained self-monitoring were significantly more effective than interventions that did not include this technique; this was especially true when self-monitoring was combined with other self-regulatory strategies (Michie et al. 2009). This meta-analysis did not reported age group differences. This gap was filled with a meta-analysis on interventions promoting PA self-efficacy and PA behaviour in healthy older adults (60 years and older). Overall, the PA interventions included in the meta-analysis were successful in changing PA self-efficacy and PA in older adults. However, the researchers found all techniques that are based on self-regulation to have the smallest effect on PA self-efficacy and PA compared to other techniques (French et al. 2014). Self-regulatory techniques such as setting behavioural goals, prompting self-monitoring of behaviour, providing normative information, and providing feedback on performance were associated with lower levels of both PA self-efficacy and PA. Although interventions from randomised controlled trials were used in this meta-analysis, the results were derived only from correlational post hoc moderator analyses. In a third meta-analysis of 138 intervention studies, self-monitoring interventions were compared to various controls (Harkin et al. 2016). The authors subdivided self-monitoring into different dimensions that reflect different ways in which self-monitoring can be applied in interventions. In this study, self-monitoring was related to behavioural goal attainment with equally strong effects across all age groups. Further, public reporting showed larger effect sizes compared to private or not reporting, recording had larger effect sizes than non-recording, and using phones and pedometers to monitor had the largest effect sizes compared to other monitoring modes. Finally, objectively measured goal attainment was related to larger effect sizes whereas the type of reference value did not affect the effect sizes. To conclude, the meta-analytical findings suggest that self-monitoring is an effective behaviour change technique to improve PA levels in older adults, although there are differences between intervention studies and individuals.

An example study that aimed at increasing PA by means of self-monitoring is described in more detail. The researchers investigated 204 sedentary women aged 70 and older in Dundee, Scotland (McMurdo et al. 2010). The women were randomly allocated to either a six-month goal-setting intervention, a goal-setting intervention which included a pedometer to self-monitor the goal progress, or to usual care. At three-month follow-up, accelerometer assessed PA increased in both the goal setting and goal setting plus pedometer intervention, with slightly stronger effects for the latter. At six-month follow-up (attrition rate 88%), PA decreased in both intervention groups to values near baseline level. From this study, self-monitoring successfully initiated PA increase in participants, but failed to create PA habits.

14.4 Action and Coping Planning as Self-Regulatory Strategies

Planning is a strategy to ease PA goal attainment and maintenance. Gollwitzer (1993, 1999) developed the concept of planning or implementation intentions. Planning processes are supposed to help actualise goal intentions (e.g., I want to be more physically active) into subsequent behaviour (e.g., I am active). The literature differentiates between two forms of planning (Sniehotta et al. 2005). Action planning describes the process of planning in advance when, where, and how a specific behaviour will be performed (e.g., "Every day after I finish my breakfast, I will go out to the park and walk for 20 minutes."). These action plans are prospective self-regulation strategies because they combine defined responses to situations that occur in the future and they increase personal commitment. Gollwitzer (1993, 1999) describes two processes that explain their functionality. Firstly, the mental representation of an environmental cue becomes highly accessible ("Every day after breakfast"). That leads to an almost automatic identification of goal-directed action opportunities and a reduction of the likelihood that these opportunities pass by without notice. The environmental cue can be internal (e.g., feeling bored) or external (e.g., time-based at 4:30 pm or event-based after breakfast or when seeing the running shoes in the morning; Gollwitzer and Sheeran 2006). Secondly, a strong link between the environmental cue and the behavioural response ("going to the park and walk 20 minutes") is created that increases the likelihood of pursuing the goal-directed behaviour (Webb and Sheeran 2007). Therefore, once the individual encounters the pre-defined situation (a time or an event) that triggers the intended behaviour, there is no need to actively think whether or how to act because the link between environmental cue and behaviour was mentally rehearsed in advance. Thus, intended behaviour can be habitualised easier and faster in those who plan (Gollwitzer and Sheeran 2006; Orbell and Sheeran 2000; Sheeran 2002).

To ensure stable long-term behaviour in the face of obstacles, inhibitors must be anticipated and detailed plans for alternative behavioural solutions need to be developed (Schwarzer 2008). Coping planning is a barrier-focussed prospective self-regulation strategy where an individual imagines possible threats towards successful implementation of action plans and creates concrete plans to cope with the respective barriers (Kwasnicka et al. 2013; Sniehotta et al. 2005). For example, if an older adult created the action plan of going for a 20-minute walk every day after breakfast and then realises that it rains heavily, he might make use of the coping plan "If it rains after breakfast and I cannot go for my walk I will postpone it to after lunch". Although action and coping plans can be seen as two distinct self-regulatory strategies, evidence exists that their combined use yields the best behaviour change results (Bélanger-Gravel et al. 2013; Caudroit et al. 2014; Kwasnicka et al. 2013; Sniehotta et al. 2005).

Gollwitzer and Sheeran (2006) in their meta-analysis of implementation intentions discuss the mechanisms of why action and coping planning may be helpful. When initiating a new behaviour, an action plan helps to remember to act when conflicting goals or obstacles come into place. Seizing the opportunity to act might also be accelerated in individuals who have formulated a concrete plan when, where, and how to act compared to individuals who just want to act without any goal-directed planning. Another strength of an action plan is that it enables the individual to overcome the initial reluctance to act. Gollwitzer and Sheeran (2006) also refer to mechanisms that explain why and when coping plans may be helpful. If an individual is getting derailed, a coping plan shields goal striving from unwanted influences, for example, by suppressing unwanted attention and behavioural responses and blocking detrimental self-states or adverse contextual influences.

Setting up an action plan is a conscious act, which requires cognitive resources. However, although planning may be cognitively demanding, plans reduce the demand for cognitive resources in the long term because a behaviour can be habitualised and hence pursued automatically (Rothman et al. 2009; Sheeran et al. 2013). Action planning even facilitates the creation of new routines and habits. Thus, if the link between a PA cue and PA behaviour has been rehearsed in advance (Gollwitzer 1999; Sniehotta et al. 2005), planning strategies do not require a great deal of cognitive control and attention capacities. The same holds true for maintaining PA in the face of barriers. Once coping plans have been formed, no great cognitive effort to overcome barriers is needed because the response to them has been rehearsed in advance.

The taxonomy of behaviour change techniques (Michie et al. 2013) lists the following techniques as being related to goals and planning: Action planning (including implementation intentions), problem solving/coping planning, commitment, goal setting (outcome), behavioural contract, discrepancy between current behaviour and goal standard, goal setting (behaviour), review behaviour goal(s), and review of outcome goal(s) (see also Chap. 11).

The effectiveness of planning on PA and other health behaviours in the overall population is well established (Bélanger-Gravel et al. 2013; Kwasnicka et al. 2013; Michie et al. 2009; Hagger and Luszczynska 2014). A recent meta-analysis (Bélanger-Gravel et al. 2013) found solid support for the notion that planning interventions targeted at increasing PA were successful in participants from studies with a mean age between 18 and 64 years. Planning was more effective among clinical samples compared to general population samples and when coping planning was included in the intervention. Similar results were found in a meta-analysis of coping planning interventions across all age groups (Kwasnicka et al. 2013). Coping planning interventions were more effective when the formulation of coping plans was assisted rather than self-administered. Further, the combination of coping and action plans was more effective compared with interventions using action planning only.

For older adults, French et al. (2014) found that PA interventions focussing on the promotion of PA self-efficacy and PA were successful in changing these outcomes. However, further analyses revealed that all self-regulatory techniques such as setting behavioural goals and action and coping planning were associated with lower levels of both PA self-efficacy and PA compared to other techniques. A meta-analysis of correlational and experimental action and coping planning studies in PA research was conducted by Carraro and Gaudreau (2013). The authors reported mixed results concerning the role of ageing: In correlational studies, the relation of action planning and PA weakened with increasing age, which might reflect associated age-related changes in attitudes or cognitive functioning. Contrariwise, the meta-analysis revealed that the effect of action planning in experimental studies strengthened with increasing age. These findings indicate that there is a need to further investigate the effectiveness of planning interventions on PA behaviour in older people and to conduct more in-depth research exploring the mechanisms how planning interacts with ageing and for which subgroups of older adults planning is most feasible.

Two planning studies may serve as examples for the mixed results. Warner et al. (2016) investigated the effects of a PA intervention using a set of behaviour change techniques including planning delivered face-to-face in interactive group sessions in 310 older adults aged 64 years and older. The researchers found the intervention to be ineffective and hypothesised that planning strategies might not appeal to older adults because they may threaten their autonomy. Another study that explicitly focussed on age differences in the effectiveness of action and coping planning interventions to increase PA in 205 cardiac rehabilitation patients was conducted by Scholz et al. (2007). Participants were randomly allocated to an action planning condition, to an action and coping planning condition, or to a control condition. Baseline coping planning was higher in older (65–82 years) than in younger (38–54 years) and middle-aged (55–64 years) adults. At follow-up, across all age groups, the action-and-coping-planning-combined intervention group showed a significant increase in PA levels with older participants being the only age group without substantial increase in coping planning as they started on a high level. This might indicate that older adults may gain more experience with critical situations over the lifespan, which may explain their high levels of coping planning.

Taken together, there is strong evidence that planning promotes PA in general population, yet the findings regarding the effectiveness of planning interventions in older adults are rather mixed. Possible factors that may affect the effectiveness of self-regulation, related to cognition, motivation, and physical functioning (see following paragraphs), should be taken into account when approaching older populations.

14.5 Developmental Self-Regulation Theories

Self-regulatory processes are important across the lifespan. Developmental self-regulation theories propose that the relative importance of different self-regulatory processes changes with increasing age. In childhood but also in old age, control is more limited than in adulthood. The Theory of Selection, Optimisation, and Compensation (Baltes and Baltes 1990; Freund and Baltes 2007) and the Life-Span Theory of Control (Heckhausen et al. 2010) are two theories that have implications for self-regulation during the ageing process, which have also been applied in the context of PA.

The Theory of Selection, Optimisation, and Compensation is a developmental theory (Baltes and Baltes 1990; Freund and Baltes 2007), which outlines three self-regulatory processes that gain importance in old age as resources decrease and goals that were attained in younger age become harder to attain. As a person gets older, running a longer distance (e.g., five miles) may take longer or may even become impossible. The process of selection in old age refers to developing and committing to a personal goal (e.g., focussing on running five miles but disengaging from other resource-demanding goals like finishing the run in a certain time; so-called elective selection) or to adjusting the goal in response to the loss of goal-relevant means (e.g., running only one mile or walking five miles or to disengage from running completely; loss-based selection). Optimisation refers to engaging in goal-directed behaviours (e.g., putting more effort, running five miles is still possible, but it needs more resources than before). Compensation means acquiring and using alternative ways and resources to achieve a goal (e.g., using Nordic Walking sticks to manage the distance more easily).

A study conducted by Evers et al. (2012) investigated the use of the strategies of selection, optimisation, and compensation as well as the use of coping plans in older women aged 70–90 years undergoing a 26-week PA program. The researchers found that regardless of the level of coping planning, individuals with high use of selection, optimisation, and compensation showed high PA program adherence. Another study that compared a motivational and self-regulation intervention (control condition) with an intervention that additionally promoted the use of selection, optimisation, and compensation strategies (intervention condition) to increase PA in 386 older adults from 60 to 95 years of age provided further insights of the potential value of these strategies (Gellert et al. 2014). In the booklet-based intervention, participants were asked to adopt the strategies to achieve their PA goals by writing them down. Strategies were integrating PA into the personal goal hierarchy or committing to an age-appropriate subset of activity goals (selection); reformulation of activity goals after a loss (loss-based selection); acquisition and investment of goal-relevant means (optimisation); and executing the PA in a slightly different way (compensation). Allocation to the intervention condition predicted PA change from 6- to 12-month follow-up, but not from baseline to 6-month follow-up. Thus, it appears that selection, optimisation, and compensation are potentially effective in the long run.

A second developmental theory is the Life-Span Theory of Control (Heckhausen et al. 2010). According to this theory, two regulatory control processes are involved in decreasing the discrepancy between goal setting and goal attainment. Primary control is favoured throughout the lifespan yet secondary control becomes more important with increasing age. Primary control refers to engagement in goal-directed behaviour such as putting in effort to reach the PA goal. In the face of barriers to goal attainment or when goals are blocked entirely (e.g., as a result of chronic illness in old age), secondary control processes gain importance. These processes are to adjust goals in order to align them with the current competencies and capacities (e.g., disengagement from running as a goal and adjustment that walking is defined as the new goal), disengaging from blocked goals, or investing in goals that avoid further losses. Secondary control is not thought to be an alternative to or the opposite of primary control, but should enable the maximisation of primary control.

In the domain of PA, Hamm et al. (2014) investigated the relationship of primary and secondary control with accelerometer-measured PA and cardiorespiratory fitness in 107 very old adults aged 80–97 years. The researchers found primary control (invest in goal-directed means) predicted PA and cardiorespiratory fitness only in individuals with high levels of secondary control (mentally shield goals from distractions or disengage from blocked goals). The lowest levels of everyday PA and fitness were found in older adults who had high secondary but low primary control. This result underpins that both processes work in alliance and that conflicts between primary and secondary control can undermine goal attainment in older adults.

In sum, developmental self-regulatory theories such as the Theory of Selection, Optimisation and Compensation and the Life-Span Theory of Control have been applied to the field of PA and ageing and may expand the views of more general self-regulation approaches.

14.6 Age-Specific Factors Related to Self-Regulatory Strategies

Are there age-specific factors that explain why self-regulation is effective in some older adults but not in others? There are a number of possible explanations addressing self-regulation related to PA in older adults. The most prominent explanations focus on (1) cognitive control and memory deficits, (2) the adjustments to changed motives in old age, as well as (3) the demands of physical limitations.

14.7 Executive Functioning

It appears that limitations in executive functioning—that are processes involved in cognitive control of behaviour such as attention, inhibition, or memory—influence the effectiveness of self-regulatory strategies in old age with mixed findings in both directions. From pooled results of PA intervention studies, self-regulatory strategies appear to be beneficial in some meta-analyses (Carraro and Gaudreau 2013), whereas others found self-regulation not being beneficial in older adults (French et al. 2014). This might be due to the fact that self-regulatory strategies are simply too cognitively demanding for some older adults. It is well established that the ageing process is negatively associated with executive functioning (Jurado and Rosselli 2007). Executive functioning, however, is an essential requisite of successful behavioural self-regulation (Allan et al. 2011; Buckley et al. 2014; Rueda et al. 2005). For example, Daly et al. (2014) in their study of more than 4500 older adults found that changes in executive functioning predict changes in PA. Similarly, McAuley et al. (2011) reported executive functions to be important for PA adherence in older adults. These studies suggest that the decline in executive functioning during the ageing process has a profound impact on older adults' ability to effectively engage in regular PA. Further, several researchers confirmed that the quality of self-regulation depends on the quality of executive functions such as memory, attention, inhibitive control, planning, scheduling, and flexible task switching (Buckley et al. 2014; Rueda et al. 2005). An intervention study by Hall et al. (2014), for instance, found planning to be effective for enhancing PA among older adult women, and the effects were especially pronounced for those with relatively stronger executive function.

Although decline in cognitive functioning appears to be related to the declining effectiveness of self-regulation, a growing body of research provides evidence suggesting that self-regulatory planning may compensate for age-related decline in cognitive abilities such as prospective remembering to act on planned intentions (e.g., Brom and Kliegel 2014; McFarland and Glisky 2011). Gollwitzer and Sheeran (2006) outline that the initial task of setting up an action plan is cognitively demanding. However, once an action plan is formed, fewer cognitive resources are required to enact the behaviour because through the action plan an automatic activation of a behavioural response (e.g., going for a walk at 2 pm) is triggered when a certain cue occurs (e.g., clock shows it's 2 pm). Some studies indicate that individuals with executive functioning deficits tend to benefit from action planning interventions (Brom und Kliegel 2014). This compensatory effect of action planning was found in older adults with deficits in executive functioning (low frontal lobe functioning; McFarland and Glisky 2011), in patients with Korsakoff's syndrome (Altgassen et al. 2015), and in individuals with very mild Alzheimer's disease (Shelton et al. 2016). Using action planning as a compensatory strategy in older adults with deficits in executive functioning is a strategy that needs to be further investigated. More generally, the interdependence of PA self-regulation and cognitive functioning should be taken into account when approaching older adults.

14.8 Adjustments to Changed Motives in Old Age

Self-regulatory strategies may be less acceptable to older adults. This is because most self-regulatory strategies are meant to help people who have behavioural intentions to fit leisure activities such as PA into a busy and demanding schedule (Buckley et al. 2014). In older age finding an opportunity to be active might not be such an important concern because enough time is usually available (French et al. 2014). In addition, not only the need for self-regulation may change with increasing age; the motivational structure and the goal hierarchy may be subject to age-related changes as well. As a substantial body of research on goal selectivity across the lifespan suggests older adults become more interested in short-term emotional benefits, they can gain from PA which may lead to limited interest in regularly setting and monitoring goals that might bring a benefit in the far future (e.g., health benefits; Devereux-Fitzgerald et al. 2016). The Socioemotional Selectivity Theory proposes that with increasing age the perceived time perspective becomes more and more limited, and as a result a shift in goal preference from long-term self-improvement goals to present-oriented emotionally beneficial goals occurs (Carstensen, et al. 1999; Charles and Carstensen 2010). In terms of PA in older adults, Notthoff and Carstensen (2014) investigated changes in daily step count in response to positively or negatively framed messages over a 28-day period. They reported that positively framed messages were more effective in increasing step count than negatively framed messages. Similar results were reported by Freund et al. (2010), as they showed that for PA goal adherence older adults have a preference for process orientation (i.e., PA for enjoyment or PA related to social activities with friends or family) rather than for outcomes (i.e., long-term health benefits of PA). This implies that generating intentions (i.e., motivating older adults to be active) might be more crucial than supporting the enactment of PA behaviour once intentions have been formed. Following implications of the Socioemotional Selectivity Theory, for older adults planning of salient goals and goals that are emotionally beneficial becomes more relevant. Planning PA that incorporates activities in social groups or with significant others may be examples of adequate self-regulation in older age.

14.9 Physical Limitations

Chronic conditions and decreases in physical resources that are associated with increasing age might limit the effectiveness of self-regulatory strategies. This is especially the case in the oldest old as they experience the strongest physical, functional, and cognitive decline (Gerstorf and Ram 2009). Meta-analytical findings by Chase (2015) indicated that PA interventions among community-dwelling adults aged 65 and older were in general more effective among healthy cohorts compared to chronically ill ones. However, a promising example that self-regulation interventions may be beneficial despite physical limitations is the pilot randomised controlled trial by Focht et al. (2014) who recruited 80 sedentary older adults with knee osteoarthritis. The researchers conducted a self-regulation intervention that incorporated self-monitoring, group and individual goal setting, action planning, coping planning, and pain management strategies. Following the intervention, they found that objectively measured PA increased significantly more compared to a traditional group exercise condition (Focht et al. 2014). Knittle et al. (2013) reported similar results in 78 older adults with rheumatoid arthritis. A five-week self-regulation intervention to increase moderate-intensity PA yielded significant treatment effects at post-treatment and six-month follow-up in terms of number of participants who met the current PA recommendation of 30 minutes of moderate PA on at least five days per week.

Despite multiple chronic conditions or frailty in the oldest old, PA interventions have shown to be effective in slowing down the physical decline (Cameron et al. 2015). Yet, self-regulation of PA demands effort, is resource dependent, and becomes less effective as people age due to the progressing physical or cognitive deterioration (Gerstorf and Ram 2009). Coping planning on how to adjust PA goals in accordance with current capabilities and how to compensate for physical losses, for example, via social support, supportive environments or technology becomes more relevant in very old age. For example, using the internet, mobile phones, and other assistive technologies might be a viable way to deliver self-regulation interventions targeting PA in older adults (Müller and Khoo 2014; see Chap. 35).

14.10 Practical Implications

Self-regulatory strategies such as self-monitoring and planning are generally effective in changing PA levels; they are relatively simple and easy to implement in interventions across all age groups and settings. New technologies such as mobile phone applications and wearables can further expand the use of these strategies into everyday life contexts. However, empirical evidence suggests that caution should be exercised in the use of self-regulatory techniques for older adults, although there is no clear explanation why self-regulation is not always effective in this population. One explanation is that there is simply less need for self-regulation in the lives of many older adults.

The application of developmental self-regulatory strategies in older adults has the potential to improve the effectiveness of PA self-regulation in older adults. These strategies consider necessary adjustments due to various limitations (e.g., related to physical and mental decline) and due to changes in goal focus (e.g., more present-oriented) that are likely to occur as people age. The interplay between goal pursuit and goal adjustment is necessary to consider when planning PA interventions in older adults. In this context, the hierarchy of an individual's goals becomes essential. PA goals are linked to higher-order goals which are probably different in older adults (e.g., wellbeing) compared to younger people (e.g., fitness). This means that making plans for PA that are emotionally satisfying may be important to improve the effectiveness of self-regulation in old age—yet more research is needed to further underpin this recommendation. Moreover, self-regulatory strategies may be used in combination with other behaviour change techniques that are less demanding such as social reward or practical social support (cf. French et al. 2014). Cognitive and physical limitations are more prevalent in older adults and the design of self-regulation interventions should be informed by this knowledge; self-regulatory strategies may compensate for cognitive and physical impairments, but there are also clear limitations of these strategies for these older adults. Finally, older adults are not a homogeneous group, and differences increase with increasing age. Some older adults plan ahead and are even more active than many younger people while others are largely immobile and dependent.

14.11 Conclusion

Self-regulation of PA is an important control process of the individual to reach preset PA goals. Theories that contribute to the understanding of self-regulation of behaviour such as PA have been outlined with the Control

Theory being among the most prominent ones. Self-regulation strategies for increasing PA that are widely used are self-monitoring, action planning, and coping planning, which were found to be effective in changing PA in many populations. In older adults, however, the relation of self-regulation and PA increasingly interacts with individual age-related factors such as cognition, motivation, and physical functioning. Developmental theories of self-regulation explain the age-related shift from self-regulation that is focussing on goal enactment to self-regulation that primarily focusses on preventing further losses and goal disengagement. Empirical evidence on the effectiveness of PA interventions which promote self-regulatory strategies such as self-monitoring and planning revealed mixed findings indicating that these interventions may be effective in some older adults but may have limited effects in others. Further research is needed to gain insights on how older adults can benefit the most from self-regulation for PA initiation, maintenance, and relapse prevention.

Suggested Further Readings

- Baumeister, R. F., & Vohs, K. D. (Eds.). (2016). *Handbook of self-regulation. Research, theory, and application* (3rd ed.). New York: Guilford Press.
- Carver, C. S., & Scheier, M. F. (2002). Control processes and self-organization as complementary principles underlying behavior. *Personality and Social Psychology Review, 6*(4), 304–315.
- French, D. P., Olander, E. K., Chisholm, A., & Mc Sharry, J. (2014). Which behaviour change techniques are most effective at increasing older adults' self-efficacy and physical activity behaviour? A systematic review. *Annals of Behavioral Medicine, 48*(2), 225–234. https://doi.org/10.1007/s12160-014-9593-z.

References

Ajzen, I. (1991). The theory of planned behavior. *Organizational Behavior and Human Decision Processes, 50*, 179–211.

Allan, J. L., Johnston, M., & Campbell, N. (2011). Missed by an inch or a mile? Predicting the size of intention-behaviour gap from measures of executive control. *Psychology and Health, 26*(6), 635–650. https://doi.org/10.1080/08870441003681307.

Altgassen, M., Ariese, L., Wester, A. J., & Kessels, R. P. (2015). Salient cues improve prospective remembering in Korsakoff's syndrome. *British Journal of Clinical Psychology, 55*(2), 123–136. https://doi.org/10.1111/bjc.12099.

Baltes, P. B., & Baltes, M. M. (1990). Psychological perspectives on successful aging: The model of selective optimization with compensation. In P. B. Baltes & M. M. Baltes (Eds.), *Successful aging: Perspectives from the behavioral sciences* (pp. 1–34). New York: Cambridge University Press.

Bandura, A. (1989). Human agency in social cognitive theory. *American Psychologist, 44*(9), 1175–1184.

Bargh, J. A. (1990). Goal ≠ intent: Goal-directed thought and behavior are often unintentional. *Psychological Inquiry, 1*(3), 248–251.

Baumeister, R. F., & Vohs, K. D. (Eds.). (2004). *Handbook of self-regulation. Research, theory, and application*. New York: Guilford Press.

Bélanger-Gravel, A., Godin, G., & Amireault, S. (2013). A meta-analytic review of the effect of implementation intentions on physical activity. *Health Psychology Review, 7*(1), 23–54.

Brom, S. S., & Kliegel, M. (2014). Improving everyday prospective memory performance in older adults: Comparing cognitive process and strategy training. *Psychology and Aging, 29*(3), 744–755.

Buckley, J., Cohen, J. D., Kramer, A. F., McAuley, E., & Mullen, S. P. (2014). Cognitive control in the self-regulation of physical activity and sedentary behavior. *Frontiers in Human Neuroscience, 8*, 747. https://doi.org/10.3389/fnhum.2014.00747.

Cameron, I. D., Fairhall, N., Gill, L., Lockwood, K., Langron, C., Aggar, C., et al. (2015). Developing interventions for frailty. *Advances in Geriatrics*. https://doi.org/10.1155/2015/845356.

Carraro, N., & Gaudreau, P. (2013). Spontaneous and experimentally induced action planning and coping planning for physical activity: A meta-analysis. *Psychology of Sport and Exercise, 14*(2), 228–248.

Carstensen, L. L., Isaacowitz, D. M., & Charles, S. T. (1999). Taking time seriously: A theory of socioemotional selectivity. *American Psychologist, 54*(3), 165–181. https://doi.org/10.1037/0003-066X.54.3.165.

Carver, C. S., & Scheier, M. F. (1981). *Attention and self-regulation: A control-theory approach to human behavior*. New York: Springer.

Carver, C. S., & Scheier, M. F. (1982). Control theory: A useful conceptual framework for personality–social, clinical, and health psychology. *Psychological Bulletin, 92*(1), 111–135.

Carver, C. S., & Scheier, M. F. (2002). Control processes and self-organization as complementary principles underlying behavior. *Personality and Social Psychology Review, 6*(4), 304–315.

Caudroit, J., Boiché, J., & Stephan, Y. (2014). The role of action and coping planning in the relationship between intention and physical activity: A moderated mediation analysis. *Psychology and Health, 29*(7), 768–780.

Charles, S. T., & Carstensen, L. L. (2010). Social and emotional aging. *Annual Review of Psychology, 61*(1), 383–409. https://doi.org/10.1146/annurev.psych.093008.100448.

Chase, J. A. (2015). Interventions to increase physical activity among older adults: A meta-analysis. *The Gerontologist, 55*(4), 706–718. https://doi.org/10.1093/geront/gnu090.

Daly, M., McMinn, D., & Allan, J. L. (2014). A bidirectional relationship between physical activity and executive function in older adults. *Frontiers in Human Neuroscience, 8*, 1044. https://doi.org/10.3389/fnhum.2014.01044.

Devereux-Fitzgerald, A., Powell, R., Dewhurst, A., & French, D. P. (2016). The acceptability of physical activity interventions to older adults: A systematic review and meta-synthesis. *Social Science & Medicine, 158*, 14–23. https://doi.org/10.1016/j.socscimed.2016.04.006.

Evers, A., Klusmann, V., Ziegelmann, J. P., Schwarzer, R., & Heuser, I. (2012). Long-term adherence to a physical activity intervention: The role of telephone-assisted vs. self-administered coping plans and strategy use. *Psychology and Health, 27*(7), 784–797. https://doi.org/10.1080/08870446.2011.582114.

Focht, B. C., Garver, M. J., Devor, S. T., Dials, J., Lucas, A. R., Emery, C. F., et al. (2014). Group-mediated physical activity promotion and mobility in sedentary patients with knee osteoarthritis: Results from the IMPACT-pilot trial. *The Journal of Rheumatology, 41*(10), 2068–2077. https://doi.org/10.3899/jrheum.140054.

French, D. P., Olander, E. K., Chisholm, A., & Mc Sharry, J. (2014). Which behaviour change techniques are most effective at increasing older adults' self-efficacy and physical activity behaviour? A systematic review. *Annals of Behavioral Medicine, 48*(2), 225–234. https://doi.org/10.1007/s12160-014-9593-z.

Freund, A. M., & Baltes, P. B. (2007). Toward a theory of successful aging: Selection, optimization, and compensation. In R. Fernández-Ballesteros (Ed.), *Geropsychology: European perspectives for an aging world* (pp. 239–254). Ashland: Hogrefe and Huber Publishers.

Freund, A. M., Hennecke, M., & Riediger, M. (2010). Age-related differences in outcome and process goal focus. *European Journal of Developmental Psychology, 7*(2), 198–222.

Gellert, P., Ziegelmann, J. P., Krupka, S., Knoll, N., & Schwarzer, R. (2014). An age-tailored intervention sustains physical activity changes in older adults: A randomized controlled trial. *International Journal of Behavioral Medicine, 21*(3), 519–528. https://doi.org/10.1007/s12529-013-9330-1.

Gerstorf, D., & Ram, N. (2009). Limitations on the importance of self-regulation in old age. *Human Development, 52*(1), 38–43. https://doi.org/10.1159/000189214.

Gollwitzer, P. M. (1993). Goal achievement: The role of intentions. *European Review of Social Psychology, 4*(1), 141–185. https://doi.org/10.1080/14792779343000059.

Gollwitzer, P. M. (1999). Implementation intentions: Strong effects of simple plans. *American Psychologist, 54*(7), 493–503.

Gollwitzer, P. M., & Sheeran, P. (2006). Implementation intentions and goal achievement: A meta-analysis of effects and processes. *Advances in Experimental Social Psychology, 38*, 69–119. https://doi.org/10.1016/S0065-2601(06)38002-1.

Hagger, M. S., & Luszczynska, A. (2014). Implementation intention and action planning interventions in health contexts: State of the research and proposals for the way forward. *Applied Psychology: Health and Well-Being, 6*(1), 1–47. https://doi.org/10.1111/aphw.12017.

Hall, P. A., Zehr, C., Paulitzki, J., & Rhodes, R. (2014). Implementation intentions for physical activity behavior in older adult women: An examination of executive function as a moderator of treatment effects. *Annals of Behavioral Medicine, 48*(1), 130–136. https://doi.org/10.1007/s12160-013-9582-7.

Hamm, J. M., Chipperfield, J. G., Perry, R. P., Heckhausen, J., & Mackenzie, C. S. (2014). Conflicted goal engagement: Undermining physical activity and health in late life. *The Journals of Gerontology Series B: Psychological Sciences and Social Sciences, 69*(4), 533–542. https://doi.org/10.1093/geronb/gbu048.

Harkin, B., Webb, T. L., Chang, B. P., Prestwich, A., Conner, M., Kellar, I., et al. (2016). Does monitoring goal progress promote goal attainment? A meta-analysis of the experimental evidence. *Psychological Bulletin, 142*(2), 198–229. https://doi.org/10.1037/bul0000025.

Heckhausen, H., & Gollwitzer, P. M. (1987). Thought contents and cognitive functioning in motivational versus volitional states of mind. *Motivation and Emotion, 11*(2), 101–120.

Heckhausen, J., Wrosch, C., & Schulz, R. (2010). A motivational theory of life-span development. *Psychological Review, 117*(1), 32–60. https://doi.org/10.1037/a0017668.

Jurado, M. B., & Rosselli, M. (2007). The elusive nature of executive functions: A review of our current understanding. *Neuropsychology Review, 17*(3), 213–233.

Knittle, K., De Gucht, V., Hurkmans, E., Peeters, A., Ronday, K., Maes, S., & Vlieland, T. V. (2013). Targeting motivation and self-regulation to increase physical activity among patients with rheumatoid arthritis: A randomised controlled trial. *Clinical Rheumatology, 34*(2), 231–238.

Kwasnicka, D., Presseau, J., White, M., & Sniehotta, F. F. (2013). Does planning how to cope with anticipated barriers facilitate health-related behaviour change? A systematic review. *Health Psychology Review, 7*(2), 129–145. https://doi.org/10.1080/17437199.2013.766832.

McAuley, E., Mailey, E. L., Mullen, S. P., Szabo, A. N., Wójcicki, T. R., White, S. M., et al. (2011). Growth trajectories of exercise self-efficacy in older adults: Influence of measures and initial status. *Health Psychology, 30*(1), 75–83. https://doi.org/10.1037/a0021567.

McFarland, C. P., & Glisky, E. L. (2011). Implementation intentions and prospective memory among older adults: An investigation of the role of frontal lobe function. *Aging, Neuropsychology, and Cognition, 18*(6), 633–652.

McMurdo, M. E. T., Sugden, J., Argo, I., Boyle, P., Johnston, D. W., Sniehotta, F. F., & Donnan, P. T. (2010). Do pedometers increase physical activity in sedentary older women? A randomized controlled trial. *Journal of the American Geriatrics Society, 58*(11), 2099–2106. https://doi.org/10.1111/j.1532-5415.2010.03127.x.

Michie, S., Abraham, C., Whittington, C., McAteer, J., & Gupta, S. (2009). Effective techniques in healthy eating and physical activity interventions: A meta-regression. *Health Psychology, 28*(6), 690–701. https://doi.org/10.1037/a0016136.

Michie, S., Richardson, M., Johnston, M., Abraham, C., Francis, J., Hardeman, W., et al. (2013). The behavior change technique taxonomy (v1) of 93 hierarchically clustered techniques: Building an international consensus for the reporting of behavior change interventions. *Annals of Behavioral Medicine, 46*(1), 81–95. https://doi.org/10.1007/s12160-013-9486-6.

Mischel, W., Shoda, Y., & Rodriguez, M. L. (1989). Delay of gratification in children. *Science, 244*, 933–938.

Müller, A. M., & Khoo, S. (2014). Non-face-to-face physical activity interventions in older adults: A systematic review. *International Journal of Behavioral Nutrition and Physical Activity, 11*, 35. https://doi.org/10.1186/1479-5868-11-35.

Muraven, M., & Baumeister, R. F. (2000). Self-regulation and depletion of limited resources: Does self-control resemble a muscle? *Psychological Bulletin, 126*(2), 247–259.

Notthoff, N., & Carstensen, L. L. (2014). Positive messaging promotes walking in older adults. *Psychology and Aging, 29*(2), 329–341.

Orbell, S., & Sheeran, P. (1998). 'Inclined abstainers': A problem for predicting health-related behaviour. *British Journal of Social Psychology, 37*(2), 151–165.

Orbell, S., & Sheeran, P. (2000). Motivational and volitional processes in action initiation: A field study of the role of implementation intentions. *Journal of Applied Social Psychology, 30*(4), 780–797. https://doi.org/10.1111/j.1559-1816.2000.tb02823.x.

Prestwich, A., Conner, M., Hurling, R., Ayres, K., & Morris, B. (2016). An experimental test of control theory-based interventions for physical activity. *British Journal of Health Psychology, 21*(4), 812–826. https://doi.org/10.1111/bjhp.12198.

Prochaska, J. O., & DiClemente, C. C. (1992). In search of how people change. Applications to addictive behaviors. *American Psychologist, 47*(9), 1102–1114.

Rebar, A. L., Dimmock, J. A., Jackson, B., Rhodes, R. E., Kates, A., Starling, J., & Vandelanotte, C. (2016). A systematic review of the effects of non-conscious regulatory processes in physical activity. *Health Psychology Review*, 1–13. https://doi.org/10.1080/17437199.2016.1183505.

Rothman, A. J., Sheeran, P., & Wood, W. (2009). Reflective and automatic processes in the initiation and maintenance of dietary change. *Annals of Behavioral Medicine, 38*(1), 4–17.

Rueda, M. R., Posner, M. I., & Rothbart, M. K. (2005). The development of executive attention: Contributions to the emergence of self-regulation. *Developmental Neuropsychology, 28*(2), 573–594.

Scholz, U., Sniehotta, F. F., Burkert, S., & Schwarzer, R. (2007). Increasing physical exercise levels: Age-specific benefits of planning. *Journal of Aging and Health, 19*(5), 851–866.

Schwarzer, R. (2008). Modeling health behavior change: How to predict and modify the adoption and maintenance of health behaviors. *Applied Psychology, 57*(1), 1–29. https://doi.org/10.1111/j.1464-0597.2007.00325.x.

Sheeran, P. (2002). Intention-behavior relations: A conceptual and empirical review. *European Review of Social Psychology, 12*(1), 1–36. https://doi.org/10.1080/14792772143000003.

Sheeran, P., Gollwitzer, P. M., & Bargh, J. A. (2013). Nonconscious processes and health. *Health Psychology, 32*(5), 460–473. https://doi.org/10.1037/a0029203.

Shelton, J. T., Lee, J. H., Scullin, M. K., Rose, N. S., Rendell, P. G., & McDaniel, M. A. (2016). Improving prospective memory in healthy older adults and individuals with very mild Alzheimer's disease. *Journal of the American Geriatric Society, 64*(6), 1307–1312. https://doi.org/10.1111/jgs.14134.

Sniehotta, F. F., Schwarzer, R., Scholz, U., & Schüz, B. (2005). Action planning and coping planning for long-term lifestyle change: Theory and assessment. *European Journal of Social Psychology, 35*(4), 565–576.

Sniehotta, F. F., Nagy, G., Scholz, U., & Schwarzer, R. (2006). The role of action control in implementing intentions during the first weeks of behaviour change. *British Journal of Social Psychology, 45*(1), 87–106.

Warner, L. M., Wolff, J. K., Ziegelmann, J. P., Schwarzer, R., & Wurm, S. (2016). Revisiting self-regulatory techniques to promote physical activity in older adults: Null-findings from a randomised controlled trial. *Psychology and Health, 31*, 1–21. https://doi.org/10.1080/08870446.2016.1185523.

Webb, T. L., & Sheeran, P. (2007). How do implementation intentions promote goal attainment? A test of component processes. *Journal of Experimental Social Psychology, 43*(2), 295–302. https://doi.org/10.1016/j.jesp.2006.02.001.

15

Making Physical Activity Interventions Acceptable to Older People

Angela Devereux-Fitzgerald, Laura McGowan, Rachael Powell, and David P. French

15.1 Introduction

Physical activity and desire to perform physical activity decline with age (Scholes and Mindell 2013; Department for Culture 2011). This suggests that engaging in physical activity may not be a priority for, or attractive to, many older adults, that is, physical activity may have low *acceptability*. Acceptability is a key concept in the Medical Research Council (MRC) Framework for Developing and Evaluating Complex Interventions (MRC 2008). According to this Framework, it is essential for an intervention, or the behaviours promoted by an intervention, to be acceptable to the target population for that intervention to be feasible. That is, if people are not willing to engage with the intervention or the targeted behaviour, then that intervention is unlikely to result in behaviour change. Despite acceptability being central to intervention development, there has been little discussion of how to conceptualise acceptability (Sekhon et al. 2017).

One simple way of assessing whether a behaviour is acceptable is to assess the extent to which people do the behaviour without the need for an intervention. This approach has some uses, but it risks being tautologous: a behaviour is acceptable because it is commonly performed and vice versa. It may be more useful to define acceptability as the combined effect of *antecedents* of

---

A. Devereux-Fitzgerald (✉) • L. McGowan • R. Powell • D. P. French
Manchester Centre for Health Psychology, School of Health Sciences, University of Manchester, Manchester, UK

performing a behaviour, such as attitudes towards the behaviour or perceived norms regarding the behaviour: the more positive these are, the more likely a behaviour is to be performed. By targeting these antecedents there is an opportunity to increase acceptability and therefore the target behaviour.

Acceptability is often taken as indicating that people are willing to tolerate an intervention or behaviour to gain some anticipated rewards, for example, attend an unpleasant screening test to prevent the even worse prospect of cancer. Alternatively, acceptability can be thought of as those features of an intervention or behaviour that are attractive and actively sought. It will be argued below that this latter conceptualisation of acceptability is more useful when considering how best to promote the engagement of older people in physical activity.

15.2 Factors Related to Physical Activity in Older Age

There has been much research examining the correlates of physical activity in older adults, which sheds some light on the acceptability of this behaviour. Being male and of younger age are positively associated with physical activity (Koeneman et al. 2011). Adults of low socio-economic status (SES) are less likely to engage in leisure time physical activity than those of high SES (Hallal et al. 2012). Having a history of engaging in physical activity, being generally more active, having greater functional abilities in daily life, and having a healthy weight are all positively associated with being more physically active in older age (Koeneman et al. 2011). Reporting health and other benefits of being physically active is positively associated with physical activity in older adults (Koeneman et al. 2011). Higher self-efficacy, the belief that one is capable of carrying out a behaviour (Bandura 1977), is also associated with physical activity (Koeneman et al. 2011) in line with Rothman's (2000) theory (see below). (See Chaps. 11 and 12 for details of Social Cognitive Theory and self-efficacy.)

A systematic review identified differences between determinants of initiation of physical activity and determinants of maintenance of physical activity in older adults (van Stralen et al. 2009). Given this, a different approach may need to be taken to encourage those who are already physically active to maintain their activity throughout older age, as opposed to that needed to encourage inactive older adults to become more physically active.

Social support has been associated with both the initiation and maintenance of physical activity, but the source of such support was crucial for the latter (van Stralen et al. 2009). Support from healthcare providers was negatively associated with maintaining physical activity in older adults who have been regularly active for at least six months, perhaps suggesting that active older adults find engaging in physical activity for health reasons to be unacceptable, or else maintenance requires different kinds of support to that offered by healthcare providers. By contrast, social support from sports instructors and group members/sports partners was positively associated with maintaining physical activity, highlighting the importance of the social connection and perhaps also the relevance of the source of support. Those within the individual's physical activity context may be better able to give individualised support as they are likely to be more aware of what the person is achieving and their context. Perceived barriers to being physically active were negatively associated with maintenance but not initiation of physical activity in older adults (van Stralen et al. 2009). It may be that direct experience of undertaking physical activity leads to an increased awareness of the barriers.

In summary, being healthier, higher SES, having a history of physical activity, confidence in ability, and belief in benefits of physical activity are associated with higher activity in older age. Different approaches may be needed to encourage uptake and maintenance of physical activity, with support from relevant professionals and peers having a positive impact.

15.3 Exploring Acceptability of Physical Activity

Much research aimed at identifying what makes physical activity acceptable to older people has focussed on the barriers and facilitators of engaging in physical activity. A recent synthesis of 132 studies identified issues such as social influences, physical limitations, competing priorities, access difficulties, personal benefits, and motivation and beliefs as barriers or facilitators to physical activity (Franco et al. 2015). Although useful, the scope of this review was very broad as it included both clinical and non-clinical populations aged over 65 years and covered all forms of physical activity. As noted in Chap. 1, the diverse abilities and preferences of older people need to be considered when conducting research with, and delivering interventions to, this population.

The forms of physical activity that are acceptable to clinical and non-clinical populations may differ. Although most older people have at least one chronic condition, clinical populations that are defined by a particular condition are likely to have more barriers to overcome. This is especially true for those who often attend healthcare appointments, are hospitalised or live in a care facility, and who therefore may lack the autonomy to participate in their preferred activities. Further, some clinical populations may be motivated to become more physically active in order to recover from an operation or illness, or to prevent complications from their chronic condition, whereas other clinical populations may face barriers due to chronic pain or physiological deconditioning. It is therefore important to consider whether different factors affect the acceptability of physical activity to clinical and non-clinical populations.

The umbrella term "physical activity" describes a wide variety of behaviours. Physical activity guidelines distinguish between vigorous-, moderate-, and light-intensity activity and sedentary behaviours. Intensity refers to how hard an individual has to work to achieve the behaviour (World Health Organisation (WHO) 2010) and as such, individual perceptions of the forms of physical activity within these categories can vary. Also, although brisk walking, gardening, yoga, golf, and ballroom dancing may constitute moderate physical activity to most, it is likely that they will differ in acceptability to a specific older adult. The context of the activity can also affect acceptability, for example, brisk walking by oneself may be unacceptable to an individual, whereas brisk walking with other people in a scenic location may be more acceptable. Hence, one must also be careful to consider whether the precise behaviour in a particular context is acceptable or not, and not assume that all behaviours of similar intensity are equally acceptable.

Thus, acceptability of physical activity is likely to be determined by more than simple barriers and facilitators. It is important to consider individuals' health status, the context and setting of activity, and the meaning of an activity to an individual.

15.4 Qualitative Studies of Acceptability of Physical Activity to Older People

Given the limitations of a simple count of facilitators and barriers across diverse populations and behaviours, a more nuanced understanding of facilitators and barriers may be obtained through qualitative research. The qualitative literature on the experiences of non-clinical samples of older adults (>65 years) who had recently participated in a physical activity intervention has been systematically reviewed and meta-synthesised (Devereux-Fitzgerald et al. 2016). The meta-synthesis resulted in a model of acceptability of

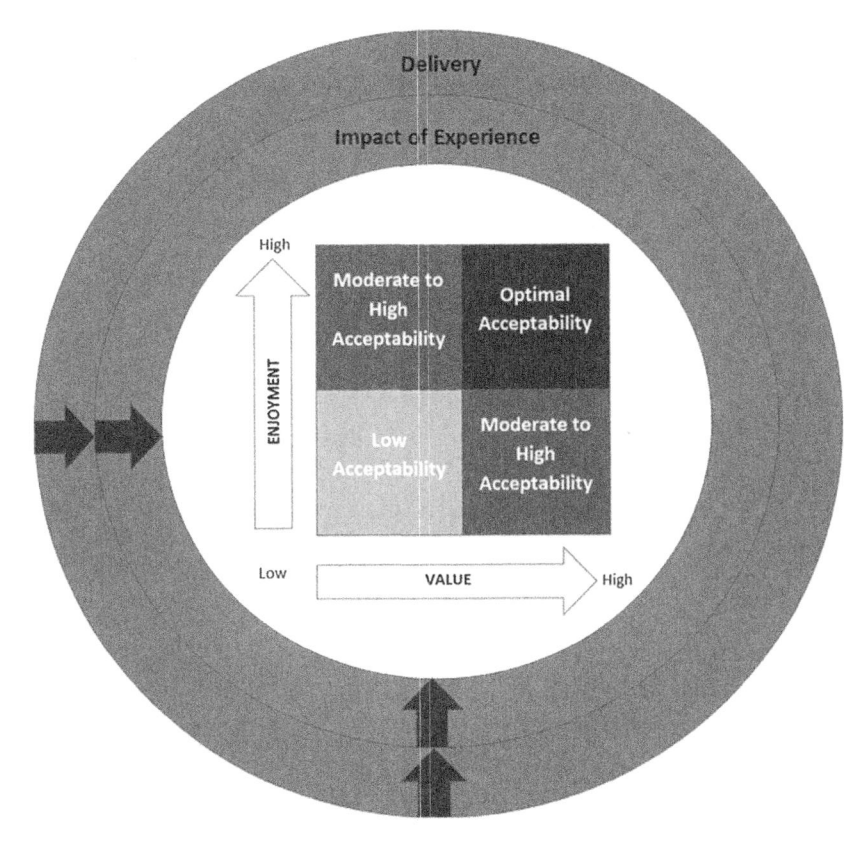

Fig. 15.1 Dynamic model of older adults' acceptability of physical activity interventions

interventions (see Fig. 15.1) that highlights four interrelated factors. These were the enjoyment older adults experience whilst being physically active, the perceived value they place on being physically active, the impact of first-hand experience, and the delivery of interventions (in terms of pace, language, style, setting, etc.).

Enjoyment was the key factor regarding acceptability of these interventions for older adults. Enjoyment of social contact was considered particularly rewarding and seemed to influence engagement with the intervention and physical activity itself, as well as maintenance of activity after the intervention ceased. The perceived value that older adults placed on physical activity was increased when they attributed positive short-term functional and psychosocial outcomes to physical activity. This suggests that it may be more acceptable to promote physical activity to older adults on the basis of it being an enjoyable social activity that produces positive, relevant short-term benefits, as opposed to focussing on the benefits of physical activity for long-term health.

The Devereux-Fitzgerald et al. (2016) review only covered older adults with recent experience of a physical activity intervention. Those who were willing to take part in such interventions may have been more open to increasing activity than might be typical of older people. Another meta-synthesis focussed on studies involving older adults (>65 years) who were not involved in physical activity interventions or programmes and who therefore could be inactive and/or disinclined to be physically active (McGowan et al. 2017). McGowan et al. (2017) found that many older adults did not distinguish between "physical activity" and "exercise". Thus, researchers are often talking at crossed purposes with older people, as researchers typically consider "physical activity" to be a broad class of activities that includes lifestyle physical activity as well as "exercise", that is, structured repetitive movement undertaken for its own sake. Possibly for this reason, many older adults questioned the relevance of physical activity for themselves as an older person.

Many inactive older people did not consider physical activity as a purposeful activity in its own right acceptable (McGowan et al. 2017). Instead, they saw physical activity as something they might engage in as a by-product of other activities, such as household chores and maintenance, shopping, gardening, and care of grandchildren and pets. Their main concern was being mobile enough to fulfil their daily needs in the community, which they saw as appropriate physical activity for their age. This was in line with their self-perception as an ageing member of society, where family roles and maintaining social connectedness took priority, and structured physical activity was seen as incompatible with ageing and therefore irrelevant to them. Many inactive older adults were aware of increasing physical limitations and this reduced their confidence to engage in physical activity, even though they wished to retain their functional capacity and independence.

McGowan et al. (2017) found that most research focussed on moderate-vigorous physical activity, perhaps as this is the main focus of physical activity guidelines (WHO 2010). However, older adults may consider this level of physical activity to be more suitable for younger than older people, which may explain why the desire to perform "physical activity" declines with age (Department for Culture 2011).

Light-intensity activities, such as slow walking or light housework, do not currently count towards the health-enhancing recommended levels of moderate and vigorous activities for older adults (WHO 2010). Despite this, they are still important as they can break up periods of sedentary behaviour, and reductions in sedentariness and small increases in low levels of physical activity can considerably reduce mortality in older adult populations (Hupin et al. 2015). Promoting such light-intensity activities could foster greater acceptability of physical activity in people who feel unable to engage in higher-intensity physical activity: "Encouraging baseline activities helps build a culture where physical activity in general is the social norm" (US Department of Health and Human Services 2008 p. 3).

15.5 Effectiveness of Interventions to Increase Physical Activity in Older People

Having identified what older adults consider to be acceptable about physical activity, it is useful to contrast this with the contents of interventions to promote physical activity. There is often a stark mismatch between what people want from such interventions (e.g. fun and social contact) and what is provided.

The specific components of interventions to increase physical activity can be characterised using standardised taxonomies of behaviour change techniques (BCTs), such as that of Michie et al. (2013). (See Chap. 11 for details of BCT taxonomies.) Many BCTs involve people trying to self-regulate their own behaviour in the same way that a heating system regulates temperature. Such BCTs might involve people assessing their current behaviour, setting behavioural goals, making plans regarding how to bring about these goals, monitoring their progress towards such goals or receiving feedback on progress, and adjusting their goals where appropriate. Such BCTs are generally effective for increasing physical activity in younger adults (see Williams and French 2011 for a systematic review). However, physical activity interventions based on self-regulatory approaches appear to be less effective for older adults (French et al. 2014). This may be because self-regulatory techniques are less acceptable to older people.

French et al. (2014) also found interventions including the BCT *Feedback on performance* to be less effective at increasing physical activity levels and surmised that this may be due to the demoralising effect of being made aware of physical limitations in older age. However, another review found that the only effective BCT in physical activity interventions for older adults was the self-regulatory BCT *Feedback* (either of their own data or of discrepancies between their data and their goals; O'Brien et al. 2015). These differences may be due to French et al. (2014) being focussed on interventions to increase physical activity, whereas O'Brien et al. (2015) focussed on maintenance of physical activity. There were also differences in participant age ranges: 60–84 years (French et al. 2014) and 55–70 years (O'Brien et al. 2015). Including more middle-aged adults and excluding many older adults may have masked self-regulatory issues within the latter older adult population (see Chap. 14 for details of self-regulation).

There are many possible explanations for the assumption that self-regulatory techniques could be less effective in older populations. For example, one self-regulation BCT is *Prompting self-monitoring*, whereby participants keep a record of their behaviour through diaries or pedometers. This BCT is predominantly used in interventions to assist people in identifying when they are achieving a level of physical activity that maps onto WHO guidelines. Such a BCT may not be acceptable to many older adults as they are more concerned with finding physical activities which they find enjoyable and achieving social goals rather than reaching particular fitness goals or meeting guidelines (Kassavou et al. 2014, 2015).

One reason why self-regulatory techniques may be less acceptable for older adults is provided by the Socioemotional Selectivity Theory (SST; Carstensen et al. 1999). According to SST, those nearing the end of life, whether through natural ageing or through life-limiting illnesses, display different motivational patterns to those with more time left to live and are more concerned with maintaining emotional balance in the present than risking this balance by processing possible negative information (Löckenhoff and Carstensen 2004). This tendency towards positive feelings in the present may impact on behaviour change interventions, particularly if negative risk-related health information is part of the intervention or if challenging activity goals are recommended to avoid negative health states. This is supported by O'Brien et al.'s (2015) finding that physical activity interventions which included the BCT *Information on consequences of behaviour to the individual* were less effective. A more positive approach when promoting physical activity to older adults may help in acceptability of physical activity through decreasing the need to process negative information. This could be achieved through focussing on *relevant* benefits such as increased mobility and better sleep rather than health risks, and focussing on immediate gains such as opportunities for social connection rather than future health gains. The latter may be particularly important to older adults with little or no social network, as social support is acknowledged to have a positive impact on physical and mental health (Uchino 2006).

According to SST, present-oriented goals are prioritised by older adults over future-oriented goals (Löckenhoff and Carstensen 2004). This could explain a lack of motivation in many older adults to improve long-term health, particularly the older old. As self-regulatory BCTs seek to translate an individual's motivation into action (Gollwitzer and Sheeran 2006), a possible lack of long-term health motivation in older people may deem the use of such BCTs less relevant. Further examples of irrelevance in physical activity interventions for older adult populations could simply be where planning aspects deal primarily with fitting physical activity into a busy work schedule, or feedback being related to increasing performance levels (French et al. 2014). Framing goals and feedback in terms of how older people wish to benefit from physical activity and how they feel in themselves on becoming active may be more acceptable than performance-based goals and feedback, and may also increase the perceived value of being physically active.

Another reason why self-regulatory BCTs may be less intrinsically acceptable relates to executive functioning: the cognitive processes such as working memory, planning, and organisation which facilitate self-regulatory behavioural processes (Hofmann et al. 2012; see Chap. 14 for discussion on memory skills, self-regulation, and planning). Executive functioning decreases with age (De Luca and Leventer 2008), and cognitive decline could render the more complex processes required with some BCTs (e.g. goal setting, comparing behaviour against a goal, and making plans to address discrepancies) too cognitively demanding for some older adults. Allan et al. (2013) found that the formation of action plans only predicted improvements in a health-related behaviour (snacking) when participants had a high level of planning skill, a key component of executive function (Allain et al. 2005).

Caution is however needed when interpreting the mixed results of the French et al. (2014) and O'Brien et al. (2015) reviews, as acknowledged by the authors themselves. The nature of the interventions, where multiple BCTs are used in conjunction, could obfuscate the true effectiveness of individual BCTs, as could differences in the delivery of interventions. Effective BCTs could be cancelled out by being used alongside ineffective BCTs, or a BCT with negligible effect could be seen to be more efficacious if paired with an effective BCT. Lack of information in some primary studies may have led to insufficient data for coding purposes. Furthermore, effectiveness based on both self-reported and objectively measured outcome measures could skew the findings, as the former may be inaccurate or swayed by social desirability (O'Brien et al. 2015).

15.6 Practical Implications for Promotion and Maintenance of Physical Activity

It is important to determine optimal approaches to encouraging physical activity in older adults, as techniques developed with younger adults appear to be less effective for many older people. Facilitating initial engagement in physical activity and maintaining physical activity both need to be addressed. As noted above, different approaches may be required for different groups, for example, those who are relatively healthy, but underactive or sedentary, and those who have specific health issues to take into consideration. Therefore, this section will look firstly at implications for promotion of physical activity in older people generally, then focus more on promotion for those with health issues, before considering implications for maintenance.

15.6.1 Promoting Initiation of Physical Activity to Older People in General

Social Interaction In general, promoting interventions on the basis of social benefits is recommended, as retaining social connectedness is something older people value as part of their self-identity within the wider society (McGowan et al. 2017). Promoting the social aspect of programmes, and following this up by encouraging socialisation within programmes, may be particularly beneficial for isolated individuals or those experiencing a transition, such as retirement or bereavement. High enjoyment of social outcomes can override apathy or antipathy towards physical activity itself, and the social bonds formed whilst engaging in physical activity can strengthen the perceived obligation towards the group—a motivating factor in itself (Devereux-Fitzgerald et al. 2016). Social interaction is related to enjoyment, a key factor in acceptability.

Physical Activity as a Solo Pursuit Whilst the majority of older adults seem to enjoy group-based physical activities for the social contact, some older adults prefer physical activity as a solitary pursuit either because they dislike group activities in general or because they enjoy exercise in its own right and perceive benefit from being able to focus on it (Devereux-Fitzgerald et al. 2017). Some may see home-based physical activity as more convenient or a simple way to supplement their external physical activities. For those who do not value exercise in its own right, activities such as active travel, gardening, DIY, and strenuous housework tasks may be more acceptable (McGowan et al. 2017). Actively promoting such home-based activities may increase acceptability of physical activity in this group as these tasks may have a higher perceived value than organised exercise.

Self-Efficacy When delivering physical activity classes, great care should be given to promote self-efficacy, given its importance in bringing about increased physical activity in older adults (see Chap. 12 for discussion on self-efficacy). Seeing peers successfully perform physical activity may increase self-efficacy through role modelling, and promoting situations where the individual is likely to succeed is likely to enhance self-efficacy (Bandura 1998). Focussing on aspects of biological decline without taking into account the increased experience and knowledge which may well offset such decline, or measuring themselves against younger (or fitter) adults instead of their peers, can result in lower perceptions of self-efficacy (Bandura 1994).

Intensity of Activity Promotion of light activity levels and reducing sedentary behaviour may be more acceptable than attempting to increase moderate or vigorous activity levels for older adults who do not see physical activity as relevant or purposeful in their stage of life (McGowan et al. 2017). Activity promotion could also encourage physical activity as a by-product of attainment of purposeful goals, for example, shopping could incorporate a walk to the shops instead of using transport. As some benefit is preferable to none, reducing sedentariness in older adults could also be worthwhile. Incorporating light physical activity into typically sedentary activities (e.g. regular taster sessions at coffee mornings) is acceptable (Devereux et al. 2016) and it may be worthwhile trying this at other sedentary activity groups (e.g. bingo, crafts).

Pacing In exercise classes, older people should be encouraged to go at their own pace, but they should also be supported to increase intensity or duration when they are able to do more. This is a very important aspect of delivering physical activity, as older people may have self-limiting expectations which need to be addressed sensitively (Devereux-Fitzgerald et al. 2016). In many classes, there will be a mix of those with and without functional limitations. Delivering physical activities that can meet the needs of a mixed group (e.g. easy circuit training, walking groups) may be optimal if funding is tight, rather than providing physical activities which exclude by perceived ability (e.g. a complex dance class) or a perceived lack of benefits to many (e.g. a seated-only exercise class; Devereux-Fitzgerald et al. in preparation).

Empowering As older adults value retaining a sense of control over their lives, physical activity interventions should aim to empower participants, through greater choice of activities, and greater participant input into the delivery or development within programmes (McGowan et al. 2017). Also, as autonomy is valued, providing more publicly available resources such as benches, public toilets, and safe walking environments allows older adults to engage in physical activity on their own terms, increasing their independence in the community. Providing such resources also facilitates walking as transport, an acceptable physical activity for many older adults (McGowan et al. 2017).

Dispelling Misconceptions and Managing Expectations Prior to engaging in any physical activity in their current physical state, older adults may not know what to expect in terms of what they can achieve or what benefits they may receive. These uncertainties could act as barriers to attempting new physical activities. Face-to-face recruitment where knowledgeable professionals can give advice (e.g. at taster sessions) may help to dispel misconceptions about capabilities and allow older adults to feel safe enough to take part, particularly for novel physical activities or after changes in ability (Devereux-Fitzgerald et al. 2016). Having experienced physical activity, older adults may then perceive barriers they were previously unaware could exist, such as muscle aches at the start of a programme or travel difficulties. This shows the need to normalise sensations experienced when becoming more active and so allay fears of physical activity being harmful (Devereux-Fitzgerald et al. 2016). It would be helpful for instructors running such classes to be aware of these issues and handle them sensitively and appropriately.

Perceptions of Ageing At a societal level, it would be helpful to challenge the negative perceptions and attitudes society holds towards the ageing population with respect to physical activity. McGowan et al. (2017) have shown that many older adults do not see physical activity as relevant to their self-identity (see Chap. 13 for more detail on self-identity and self-perceptions of ageing). Given this, addressing self-perception of older people within society may be useful, to create a new social norm of activity in older age. This could be facilitated through a national campaign, similar to the "This Girl Can" campaign developed by Sport England (2015), which celebrated women's participation in sport through posters and television adverts. A similar campaign promoting physically active older adults as the norm could increase the salience of the idea that all older people can participate in some form of physical activity and reap the benefits of increased social connections and uplifted mood, whatever their physical ability (McGowan et al. 2017).

15.6.2 Promoting Initiation of Physical Activity for Health Reasons

Assistance from Healthcare Professionals The recommendations above are particularly applicable to older adults without significant health problems, but other issues may apply for some older adults with chronic conditions. Both chronic illness and depression are negatively associated with being physically active (Koeneman et al. 2011). Depression particularly has been negatively associated with engagement in recreational physical activities outside the home (Pritchard et al. 2015). Depression can lead to social isolation, which is also linked with low SES (Pinquart and Sorensen 2001). Deprivation in turn has been linked to higher levels of impaired mobility in older adults and a reduced tendency to leave the home (Fox et al. 2011). Inactive older adults experiencing health conditions may be more receptive than healthy older adults to receiving counselling by healthcare professionals on increasing their physical activity (Weiss et al. 2012). Therefore, older people with health issues may benefit from assistance to undertake physical activity from their healthcare provider (e.g. prescribed subsidised/free physical activity). This could be particularly helpful for those with limited resources such as older people living in low SES environments.

Self-Management of Chronic Conditions For older adults with long-term conditions it may be pertinent to raise awareness of the role of physical activity in the management of chronic disease (e.g. Chodzko-Zajko et al. 2009). Many older adults with chronic conditions perceive themselves as particularly vulnerable to limitations of the ageing body, which in turn inhibits rather than promotes engagement in physical activity (McGowan et al. 2017). Relating the relevance of appropriate, manageable physical activities to achievable improvements in *their daily experience* of managing their condition (rather than numbers on a medical measure) may increase the acceptability of physical activity (Devereux-Fitzgerald et al. 2016). Functional programmes which teach balance and strength training within the context of everyday activities have been found to be effective in such older adults (Clemson et al. 2012).

Maintaining Independence Inactive older adults may have limited physical ability or be completely sedentary and may not be attracted to engaging in physical activity as a leisure pursuit (McGowan et al. 2017). Some however may be willing to engage in a physical activity programme specifically designed to increase their mobility or retain their ability to carry out the day-to-day activities required to support their independence. Focussing on independence may increase physical activity acceptability as independence has high perceived value.

15.6.3 Promoting Maintenance of Physical Activity Throughout Older Age

Long-Term Thinking Promotion of physical activity should not stop with older adults engaging in a short-term programme or intervention. For example, many "exercise on referral" schemes help older adults develop a pattern of attending the gym or exercise classes, but financial support for these is often time-limited, resulting in dropout at the end of this subsidised period (Campbell et al. 2015). Physical activity promotion should address both initial and maintained engagement in activity by considering ongoing motivations for adherence to a more physically active lifestyle and delivering programmes which have longevity.

Maintaining Social Networks Using existing community-based physical activity and social programmes rather than research/medical facilities to implement interventions allows for a longer-term approach to physical activity provision and encourages continuation of the social network formed. This may encourage maintenance after an intervention ends, and also removes transitional barriers post intervention, as older adults can continue their physical activity in an already familiar, acceptable setting (Devereux-Fitzgerald et al. 2016). A central motivation for many older people in taking up new forms of physical activity is enjoyment of the social aspects (Devereux-Fitzgerald et al. 2016), so ensuring this is satisfied is a key consideration in developing new interventions or services which will effectively retain members. If interventions are developed in line with older people's needs and values, it is more likely that their goals will be fulfilled which can facilitate maintenance of the behaviour (Kassavou et al. 2015). For example, older people taking part in walking groups are primarily looking for social contact; hence, those who were most satisfied with the social contact they experienced were most likely to maintain their attendance (Kassavou et al. 2014). These findings fit well with Rothman's (2000) hypothesis that a key determinant of maintenance is satisfaction with the anticipated outcomes of a new behaviour.

Independent Physical Activity Similar physical improvements to health have been found in home-based and externally based programmes, but adherence to the programme and long-term maintenance of physical activity can be better for individuals who perform physical activity at home (Ashworth et al. 2005). Home-based physical activity may be more acceptable and easier to maintain for those who have problems accessing external physical activities, whether this is due to lack of mobility, confidence, or resources. Encouraging older adults to incorporate some form of physical activity around their routine daily activities may be more acceptable, particularly to those who may see organised exercise as not applicable to them (Clemson et al. 2012). However, all older adults could benefit from this apparent ease of maintenance with home-based activity, and those who attend classes could be encouraged to engage in supplemental physical activity at home by group leaders.

Valued Benefits in Daily Life Helping older adults to relate their increased physical activity to tangible benefits (e.g. improved function, increased capabilities, increased mobility, better sleep, better mood, more confidence) may increase the value of maintaining engagement in physical activity, increase self-efficacy for further physical activities, and address misconceptions about loss of function being inevitable in ageing (Devereux-Fitzgerald et al. 2016). Relating this maintenance or improvement of physical function to valued issues, such as independence or being able to safely look after grandchildren, may help to increase motivation to maintain a physically active lifestyle, as these are perhaps more personally relevant than abstract health measures and have a higher perceived value (Devereux-Fitzgerald et al. 2016). Highlighting such relationships may also reduce the perception of family roles as competing commitments and instead increase the level of priority given to maintaining physical activity as it can aid them in meeting family responsibilities

(McGowan et al. 2017). This may be especially important as competing commitments, particularly related to caregiving and family, are often cited as the reason for dropping out of exercise programmes in later life.

Habit Formation Another important aspect of maintenance of physical activity in older age is habit formation. Habits are formed through repetition of behaviours in association with cues, creating automaticity around the behaviour when the cue is present, thereby requiring less mental capacity to initiate the behaviour (Gardner et al. 2012). Being able to rely on an activity taking place at the same time and place and with the same people, each day or week, can help with this habit formation and so services need to provide consistency and continuity of long-term community programmes, rather than short-term interventions (Devereux-Fitzgerald et al. 2017). This can reduce the effort required to engage in the activity and thereby assist with the maintenance of a physically active lifestyle.

15.7 Future Research Needed

There are a number of gaps in the evidence that it would be useful for future research to address. Little qualitative research on acceptability of physical activity interventions is based on low SES populations. Low SES older adults are less likely to engage in leisure time physical activity (Hallal et al. 2012), and exploring the reasons for this further may yield new insights into acceptability. It is currently unclear if lower engagement in physical activity is associated with barriers related to low income or to more environmental issues of low SES adults living in physical settings where they feel less safe outside of the home. Qualitative research is also needed to explore older adults' experiences of using different BCTs within physical activity interventions to establish how to optimise acceptability.

Further research on the benefits and perceptions of lower-intensity physical activity is required from the perspective of older adults themselves and also from professionals engaged with older adults and policymakers. If promotion of lower-intensity day-to-day physical activity is more acceptable, it may be more easily maintained, leading to higher general levels of physical activity. More research is needed to develop activities and programmes which would match older people's values and goals, and this may involve interventions or services that are not badged as physical activity, for example, community gardening or history walks. Research into the acceptability of incorporating low-intensity physical activity into social programmes may also be fruitful. It is important for future research to discern the extent to which reducing sedentary behaviour can act as a gateway to increasing physical activity in this population.

There is a particular dearth of research on the acceptability of interventions to reduce sedentariness in older people. It is unclear how older adults conceptualise the differences between reducing sedentariness and increasing physical activity, and what older adults' views are on decreasing the overall amount of their sedentary behaviour or breaking up long periods of sedentariness. Research is needed to identify what factors predict sedentariness and what forms of non-sedentary behaviours and modes of intervention delivery older adults would find most acceptable to reduce sedentariness.

15.8 Conclusion

Promotion of physical activity in older adults should focus on enjoyment, social interaction, and activities perceived to be of value to older adults. Ideally, interventions should be community based so that the social bonds created can continue post-intervention and there are no transitional barriers to be overcome. Short-term functional and psychosocial benefits of being physically active should be promoted, with individuals encouraged to note their own progress so that they can see the difference they are making to themselves, for themselves. Such increased awareness of real-life benefits may promote maintenance of a physically active lifestyle. Giving older adults more control over programme content and delivery could create autonomy and ownership and encourage the social bond of a group, all factors which could help older adults maintain their physical activity. Promoting physically active older adults as the norm using peer role models, and including lower-intensity activities, could show that all older adults can do something to increase their levels of activity and reap the health, functional, and psychosocial benefits.

Suggested Further Reading
- Devereux-Fitzgerald, A., Powell, R., Dewhurst, A., & French, D. P. (2016). The acceptability of physical activity interventions to older adults: A systematic review and meta-synthesis. *Social Science & Medicine, 158,* 14–23.
- McGowan, L., Devereux-Fitzgerald, A., Powell, R., & French, D. P. (2017). How acceptable do older adults find the concept of being physically active? A systematic review and meta-synthesis. *International Review of Sport and Exercise Psychology.* http://doi.org/10.1080/1750984X.2016.1272705.

References

Allain, P., Nicoleau, S., Pinon, K., Etcharry-Bouyx, F., Barré, J., Berrut, G., Dubas, F., & Le Gall, D. (2005). Executive functioning in normal aging: A study of action planning using the Zoo Map Test. *Brain and Cognition, 57*(1), 4–7.

Allan, J. L., Sniehotta, F. F., & Johnston, M. (2013). The best laid plans: Planning skill determines the effectiveness of action plans and implementation intentions. *Annals of Behavioral Medicine, 46*(1), 114–120.

Ashworth, N. L., Chad, K. E., Harrison, E. L., Reeder, B. A., & Marshall, S. C. (2005). Home versus center based physical activity programs in older adults. *Cochrane Database of Systematic Reviews, 1*, CD004017.

Bandura, A. (1977). Self-efficacy: Toward a unifying theory of behavioral change. *Psychological Review, 84*(2), 191–215.

Bandura, A. (1994). Self-efficacy. In V. S. Ramachaudran (Ed.), *Encyclopedia of human behavior* (Vol. 4, pp. 71–81). New York: Academic Press.

Bandura, A. (1998). Health promotion from the perspective of social cognitive theory. *Psychology and Health, 13*, 623–649.

Campbell, F., Holmes, M., Everson-Hock, E., Davis, S., Woods, H. B., Anokye, N., Tappenden, P., & Kaltenthaler, E. (2015). A systematic review and economic evaluation of exercise referral schemes in primary care: A short report. *Health Technology Assessment, 19*(60), 1–110. issn:1366-5278

Carstensen, C. E., Isaacowitz, D. M., & Charles, S. T. (1999). Taking time seriously: A theory of socioemotional selectivity. *American Psychologist, 54*(3), 165–181.

Chodzko-Zajko, W., Schwingel, A., & Park, C. H. (2009). Successful aging: The role of physical activity. *American Journal of Lifestyle Medicine, 3*(1), 20–28.

Clemson, L., Fiatarone Singh, M. A., Bundy, A., Cumming, R. G., Manollaras, K., O'Loughlin, P., et al. (2012). Integration of balance and strength training into daily life activity to reduce rate of falls in older people (the LiFE study): Randomised parallel trial. *British Medical Journal, 345*, e4547.

De Luca, C. R., & Leventer, R. J. (2008). Developmental trajectories of executive functions across the lifespan. In P. Anderson, V. Anderson, & R. Jacobs (Eds.), *Executive functions and the frontal lobes: A lifespan perspective* (pp. 3–21). Washington, DC: Taylor & Francis.

Department for Culture. (2011). Adult participation in sport: Analysis of the taking part survey. https://www.gov.uk/government/uploads/system/uploads/attachment_data/file/137986/tp-adult-participation-sport-analysis.pdf. Accessed 10 July 2015.

Devereux-Fitzgerald, A., Powell, R., Dewhurst, A., & French, D. P. (2016). The acceptability of physical activity interventions to older adults: A systematic review and meta-synthesis. *Social Science & Medicine, 158*, 14–23.

Devereux-Fitzgerald, A., Powell, R., & French, D. P. (2017). Conflating time and energy: Views from older adults in lower socioeconomic status areas on physical activity. *Journal of Aging and Physical Activity.* https://doi.org/10.1123/japa.2017-0283

Devereux-Fitzgerald, A., Powell, R., & French, D. P. (in preparation). Older adults' acceptability of being physically active: Views from older people and providers of physical activity in low socioeconomic areas.

Fox, K. R., Hillsdon, M., Sharp, D., Cooper, A. R., Coulson, J. C., Davis, M., et al. (2011). Neighbourhood deprivation and physical activity in UK older adults. *Health & Place, 17*, 633–640.

Franco, M. R., Tong, A., Howard, K., Sherrington, C., Ferreira, P. H., Pinto, R. Z., & Ferreira, M. L. (2015). Older people's perspectives on participation in physical activity: A systematic review and thematic synthesis of qualitative literature. *British Journal of Sports Medicine, 49*, 1268. https://doi.org/10.1136/bjsports-2014-094015.

French, D. P., Olander, E. K., Chisolm, A., & McSharry, J. (2014). Which behaviour change techniques are most effective at increasing older adults' self-efficacy and physical activity behaviour? A systematic review. *Annals of Behavioral Medicine, 48*(2), 225–234.

Gardner, B., Lally, P., & Wardle, J. (2012). Making health habitual: The psychology of 'habit-formation' and general practice. *British Journal of General Practice, 62*(605), 664–666.

Gollwitzer, P. M., & Sheeran, P. (2006). Implementation intentions and goal achievement: A meta-analysis of effects and processes. *Advances in Experimental Social Psychology, 38*, 69–119.

Hallal, P. C., Andersen, L. B., Bull, F., Guthold, R., Haskell, W., & Ekelund, U. (2012). Global physical activity levels: Surveillance progress, pitfalls, and prospects. *The Lancet, 380*, 247–257.

Hofmann, W., Schmeichel, B. J., & Baddeley, A. D. (2012). Executive functions and self-regulation. *Trends in Cognitive Sciences, 16*(3), 174–180.

Hupin, D., Roche, F., Gremeaux, V., Chatard, J. C., Oriol, M., Gaspoz, J. M., Barthélémy, J. C., & Edouard, P. (2015). Even a low-dose of moderate-to-vigorous physical activity reduces mortality by 22% in adults aged ≥ 60 years: A systematic review and meta-analysis. *British Journal of Sports Medicine, 49*(19), 1262–1267.

Kassavou, A., Turner, A., Hamborg, T., & French, D. P. (2014). Predicting maintenance of attendance at walking groups: Testing constructs from three leading maintenance theories. *Health Psychology, 33*, 752–756.

Kassavou, A., Turner, A., & French, D. P. (2015). The role of walkers' needs and expectations in supporting maintenance of attendance at walking groups: A longitudinal multi-perspective study of walkers and walk group leaders. *PLoS One, 10*(3), e0118754.

Koeneman, M. A., Verheijden, M. W., Chinapaw, M. J. M., & Hopman-Rock, M. (2011). Determinants of physical activity and exercise in healthy older adults: A systematic review. *International Journal of Behavioral Nutrition and Physical Activity, 8*, 142–156.

Löckenhoff, C. E., & Carstensen, L. L. (2004). Socioemotional selectivity theory, aging and health: The increasingly delicate balance between regulating emotions and making tough choices. *Journal of Personality, 72*(6), 1395–1424.

McGowan, L., Devereux-Fitzgerald, A., Powell, R., & French, D. P. (2017). How acceptable do older adults find the concept of being physically active? A systematic review and meta-synthesis. *International Review of Sport and Exercise Psychology*. https://doi.org/10.1080/1750984X.2016.1272705.

Michie, S., Richardson, M., Johnston, M., Abraham, C., Francis, J., Hardeman, W., Eccles, M. P., Cane, J., & Wood, C. E. (2013). The behavior change technique taxonomy (v1) of 93 hierarchically clustered techniques: Building an international consensus for the reporting of behavior change interventions. *Annals of Behavioral Medicine, 46*(1), 81–95. https://doi.org/10.1007/s12160-013-9486-6.

MRC Health Services and Public Health Research Board. (2008). Developing and evaluating complex interventions: New guidance. Retrieved July 9, 2016, from http://www.mrc.ac.uk/Utilities/Documentrecord/index.htm?d=MRC004871

O'Brien, N., McDonald, S., Araújo-Soares, V., Lara, J., Errington, L., Godfrey, A., Meyer, T. D., Rochester, L., Mathers, J. C., White, M., & Sniehotta, F. F. (2015). The features of interventions associated with long-term effectiveness of physical activity interventions in adults aged 55 to 70 years: A systematic review and meta-analysis. *Health Psychology Review, 9*(4), 417–433.

Pinquart, M., & Sorensen, S. (2001). Influences on loneliness in older adults: A meta-analysis. *Basic and Applied Social Psychology, 23*(4), 245–266.

Pritchard, E., Barker, A., Day, L., Clemson, L., Brown, T., & Haines, T. (2015). Factors impacting the household and recreation participation of older adults living in the community. *Disability and Rehabilitation, 37*(1), 56–63.

Rothman, A. J. (2000). Toward a theory-based analysis of behavioral maintenance. *Health Psychology, 19*(Supplement 1), 64–69.

Scholes, S., & Mindell, J. (2013). Physical activity in adults. In R. Craig & J. Mindell (Eds.), *Health survey for England 2012* (Vol. 1, Ch 2, pp. 1–49). London: Health and Social Care Information Centre.

Sekhon, M., Cartwright, M., & Francis, J. J. (2017). Acceptability of healthcare interventions: An overview of reviews and development of a theoretical framework. *BMC Health Services Research, 17*, 88. https://doi.org/10.1186/s12913-017-2031-8.

Sport England. (2015). This girl can. Retrieved September 1, 2016, from http://www.sportengland.org/our-work/national-work/this-girl-can/

Uchino, B. (2006). Social support and health: A review of physiological processes potentially underlying links to disease outcomes. *Journal of Behavioral Medicine, 29*(4), 377–387.

US Department of Health and Human Services. (2008). Physical activity guidelines for Americans. Retrieved August 8, 2016, from http://www.health.gov/paguidelines/guidelines/default.aspx

Van Stralen, M. M., De Vries, H., Mudde, A. N., Bolman, C., & Lechner, L. (2009). Determinants of physical activity among older adults: A literature review. *Health Psychology Review, 3*(2), 147–207.

Weiss, D. R., Wolfson, C., Yaffe, M. J., Shrier, I., & Puts, M. T. E. (2012). Physician counseling of older adults about physical activity: The importance of context. *American Journal of Health Promotion, 27*(2), 71–74.

Williams, S., & French, D. P. (2011). What are the most effective intervention techniques for changing physical activity self-efficacy and physical activity behaviour – And are they the same? *Health Education Research, 26*(2), 308–322.

World Health Organization. (2010). *Global recommendations on physical activity for health*. Geneva: WHO Press.

Section 4

Implementation of Physical Activities for Older People

Anna Barker

The first two sections demonstrate *why* we need to promote physical activity in older people (Section 1) and *what* types of programmes and initiatives can be used to achieve this (Section 2). Section 3 starts the *how* learnings by reviewing the psychological theory underpinning behaviour change with a focus on the perspective of the older person. The information presented in the chapters included in this section extends this to elaborate on *how* to effectively implement physical activity programmes for older people. Specifically, this section details the opportunities, barriers, and enablers to implementing physical activity programmes for older people and considers these from the individual, organisational, and environmental perspectives. Each chapter presents known implementation issues and concludes by outlining practical tips designed to address known barriers and harness identified enablers drawing on the learnings from the field of implementation science. As such, this section provides critical links between the theory of physical inactivity consequences and efficacy of activity programmes by focussing on strategies to promote the successful programme implementation.

Chapter 16 focusses on the role of social support in promoting physical activity among older people. It highlights the benefits that informal social networks play in facilitating older people to be physically active. Integrating appropriate social support networks, considering the role of ageism and ageist

A. Barker (✉)
School of Public Health and Preventive Medicine, Monash University, Melbourne, VIC, Australia

language, and paying careful attention to the social environment should be considered when designing physical activity interventions for older people.

Chapter 17 provides an overview of the influence the exercise instructor plays in encouraging older people's participation in physical activity sessions. It discusses the attributes of instructors and how they can influence motivation to do home-based and class-based physical activity. Personal attributes of the instructor, such as leadership and conscientiousness, and learnt skills, such as goal setting and engaging social activity, are important in supporting older people to engage. The instructors' training, skills, and personal attributes are important to whether they can deliver a successful programme which engages the older adult population.

Chapter 18 takes us to the long-term care setting where older people are typically more sedentary and frailer than those living in the broader community. These characteristics along with the environment—both from a physical and organisational perspective—present additional barriers to the implementation of physical activity programmes raised by prior chapters. The chapter outlines strategies for promoting physical activity that take into account frailty, multiple co-morbidities, and cognitive impairment to optimise inclusion and participation. Importantly, it highlights that older people who are frail or who have cognitive impairment can benefit from being more physically active. Strategies such as integration of physical activity into existing care routines to increase frequency of delivery are identified as important.

Chapter 19 focusses on implementation of physical activity programmes for older people while in hospital. The research literature relating to the functional consequences of bed rest and factors influencing activity levels of older people in hospital are reviewed, extending the information presented in Chap. 10. This chapter shares some themes with information presented in Chap. 18, for example, high levels of sedentary behaviour, cognitive impairment, and frailty amongst older people in hospital and also the need to integrate programmes and initiatives into existing care workflows to optimise delivery. Barriers to physical activity at the level of the hospital system, staff, and the older person are discussed along with key strategies to address them. Key strategies include tailoring programmes to individuals and adopting a multi-faceted approach (e.g. patient, staff and family education, and environmental modifications) to optimise effectiveness.

Chapter 20 compliments concepts presented in Chaps. 18 and 19 on the implementation of physical activity programmes in long-term care and hospital settings where there is a high prevalence of physical impairment amongst older people in these settings. Chapter 20 explores implementation issues specific to physical activity programmes targeted to people with early signs of physical frailty living in the community. The chapter identifies older people's perceptions about appropriateness of exercise for them, compromised health, transport issues, and a lack of social support, progress recognition, and long-term maintenance strategies as key barriers to participation in physical activity programmes. Working in multidisciplinary teams, adopting social marketing principles, focussing on social and purposeful activities, and focussing on supporting participants to maintain physical activity in the long term are promising implementation strategies for community programmes targeting older people with early signs of frailty.

Successful physical activity programmes are underpinned by a matrix of individual, contextual, and organisational factors that moderate their uptake and sustained use. Programme implementation must consider these moderators to ensure outcomes and impacts are optimised. Even if a programme has demonstrated high levels of efficacy in clinical trials and is replicated precisely in practice, if the implementation strategy does not appropriately consider and address implementation moderators, the programme may fail and be ineffective, yielding little or no improvement in intended outcomes and impacts. Programmes do not implement themselves. Therefore, of equal importance to deciding *what* programme will be implemented is determining *how* best to implement it.

Collectively, the chapters in this section provide a critical and comprehensive review of the evidence on the challenges for implementing physical activity programmes in a variety of settings and for a range of older people. The practical implementation tips included in each chapter represent a best evidence synthesis augmented by the extensive hands-on experience of the authors in the implementation of physical activity programmes in real-life settings. Consistent themes across chapters are the need to work in multidisciplinary teams, adopting social marketing principles in programme promotion, focussing on social and purposeful activities, and tailoring programmes to individual needs. Effectively engaging with support networks was also raised as an essential ingredient for successful implementation be it peers, staff who care for older people in long-term care facilities and hospitals, or their family and carers. Implementation strategies need to consider both the initial start-up and adoption stages and the ongoing and sustained programme delivery and individual participation. Indeed, a key challenge facing policymakers and programme developers is finding strategies that attract older adults to participate in physical activity programmes and keep them attending. In conclusion, it's not just *what* you do that counts with physical activity programmes, but *how* you do it is of critical importance.

16

Social Relationships and Promoting Physical Activity Among Older People

Diane E. Whaley

16.1 Social Relationships and Promoting Physical Activity in Older People

Our relationships with others are central to our life story. Whether it is friendships, romantic relationships, family members, neighbours, co-workers, or even strangers, our lives revolve around our relationships with others (Whitbourne and Whitbourne 2014). We give and receive support from others, and support influences how we feel about ourselves, what we think and do. With regard to physical activity in older people, social relationships with family, friends, community members, and medical professionals have the potential to encourage the initiation and maintenance of physical activity (Franke et al. 2013; Wilson and Spink 2009). Interventions targeting social support to increase physical activity can be extremely effective (Greaves et al. 2011). Despite this, we do not know enough about *how* social ties influence behaviour, nor do we thoroughly understand how the sources (e.g., who provides social support) and types (e.g., informational, emotional) can be combined to maximise benefits (Thoits 2011).

A potential missing link to utilising social support optimally is an understanding of how social relationships change over the life span (Whaley 2016). Adult development theory suggests there are important differences in how

D. E. Whaley (✉)
Educational Psychology/Applied Developmental Science Program,
University of Virginia, Charlottesville, VA, USA

adults relate to, learn from, and choose their social partners. These differences can have direct implications for the choices older adults make. Importantly, failure to recognise what sort of relationships adults prioritise, as well as the goals for those relationships, could lead us down a path to planning programmes that are not attractive to older adults.

Rook (2000) describes the changes in older adult social relationships in terms of two key components: 1. the underlying motivations for social contact and 2. changes that result from the loss of social ties, with the resulting compensation for such losses (p. 173). Central to this discussion will be Carstensen and her colleague's socioemotional selectivity theory (e.g., Carstensen 1998; Carstensen et al. 1999; English and Carstensen 2014). We will also attempt to debunk some stereotypes about the social lives of older adults, such as the inevitability of social isolation (Cornwell et al. 2008), and discuss how stereotypes of aging impact older adult behaviour (Ory et al. 2003). We will focus on the resilience and capacity of older adults; as Zimmermann and Grebe (2014) suggest, older adults often retain a positive outlook on life, even in difficult circumstances. They label this outlook "senior coolness"; the goal here is to understand how we might facilitate this mindset in order to optimise physical activity in older adults. Existing interventions that promote physical activity will then be reviewed, with particular attention to social approaches (e.g., Heath et al. 2012). The chapter concludes with strategies that best represent the convergence of theory and research around adult development and best practices in using the social environment to optimise physical activity in older people.

16.1.1 What Do We Know About Social Relationships in Older Adults?

A dependable finding in the adult development literature is that the number of social contacts diminishes with age (Rook 2000). The reason for this has been the subject of much debate. Early explanations ranged from the phenomenon being a way for older adults to intentionally distance themselves from society as a way to prepare for death (e.g., disengagement theory; Cumming and Henry 1961), to a product of an ageist society that rejects older persons, thus forcing the older adult into fewer social contacts (e.g., activity theory; Maddox 1963). These views of decline in social activity as either involuntary (activity theory) or maladaptive (disengagement) would imply increasing social networks may not be useful (activity theory) and that providing opportunities to increase social interaction should result in more social contacts (activity theory). However, that oversimplifies a more complex social world. Although there is no doubt stereotypes of ageing impact older adult behaviour (a point we will return to shortly), more recent research on this topic has evolved to one where the choice of social contact is seen as voluntary and *adaptive*, led by the work of Laura Carstensen and her colleagues (Carstensen 1998; Carstensen et al. 1999).

According to Carstensen's socioemotional selectivity theory, motives for social relationships change over the lifetime. Carstensen posits three psychological goals for social contact: 1. acquiring information, 2. the development and maintenance of self-concept, and 3. the regulation of emotion (Carstensen 1998; Rook 2000). When we perceive a great deal of time left in our lives (that is, when we are young and in good health), relationships serve an important informational function; we gather information from others in order to learn and grow (English and Carstensen 2014; Whaley 2016). Given this goal, a larger circle of support is likely to provide the information we desire, and relationships are likely to provide a wide range of information. As our anticipated time left diminishes (through advancing age or severe illness), the primary goal of relationships is not so much about information gathering but instead emotional regulation, particularly satisfaction; adults look for people who will make them feel better (Whitbourne and Whitbourne 2014). In fact, older people prune those relationships that do not contribute to emotional needs (English and Carstensen 2014), purposefully decreasing the size of their social network, while increasing the importance of remaining relationships.

With regard to self-concept (i.e., the individual as known to the individual; Markus and Herzog 1992), early in life social contacts help the individual form and elaborate the view an individual has of him or herself. In adulthood, social interaction serves to reinforce one's self-concept, and this is best done by close social relationships, like family and friends (Rook 2000). According to socioemotional selectivity theory, not only do the goals for social interaction change as we age, but the *size* of one's social network may not be as critical as *who* occupies the network and *what* type of support they provide. There is substantial support for socioemotional selectivity theory (e.g., English and Carstensen 2014; Sims et al. 2015), but it does not tell the whole story of social relationships in older adulthood.

A criticism of research about the social lives of older adults is that many conclusions are based on assumptions or small samples. In an attempt to rectify this, Cornwell et al. (2008), using a large, nationally representative sample, examined the social connectedness of older adults living in the United States. Age was negatively related to network size, closeness to network members, and number of non-primary (non-familial) group ties. However, age was positively related to frequency of socialising with neighbours, religious participation, and volunteering. Although the authors suggest their findings call into question socioemotional selectivity theory's premise that close social ties are key in older adulthood, it is important to consider that at advanced age, older adults have likely lost a number of their close social ties (e.g., spouse, life-long friends). Recall that Rook (2000) viewed social relationships as constituting both changes in the underlying motives for social contact, *and* changes that result in losses in one's social world. In fact, substituting close social ties is a prime example of the adaptability and resilience consistently seen in older adults. Older people may, as socioemotional selectivity theory predicts, *prefer* close social ties, but, in the absence of that possibility, are willing and able to reach out and establish new ties.

Replacing social ties with individuals who provide new sources of emotional support is not inconsistent with socioemotional selectivity theory. Cornwell et al. (2008) found older adults with fewer network members in their households tended to interact with neighbours more frequently. They conclude the phenomenon of older adults' greater involvement in activities like civic engagement is "not an outcome of generational differences…but an effort to regain control over their social environments" (Cornwell et al., p. 200). Older adults purposefully negotiate changes in their lives to optimise their emotional experience. Social relationships play a significant role in this process, with an emphasis on the type of support offered by those important to the individual. Of course, these compensatory strategies are not always successful (Rook 2000). It is important to understand how social relationships influence behaviour if we are to design effective physical activity interventions.

Thoits (2011) proposed a number of mechanisms through which social support and social relationships may impact physical and psychological health. She concludes two broad types of support—emotional sustenance and active coping assistance—provided by significant others and experientially similar others, best represent this mechanism. Her conclusions can help guide the planning of physical activity interventions most likely to effectively utilise social support. In short, the nature of the social tie, as well as the type of support provided, is key to enhancing well-being. For example, significant others (grown children, spouse, close friends) would be appropriate sources for providing emotional support for physical activity as well as instrumental assistance (e.g., transportation). Similar others (fellow widows/widowers, church members, neighbours) can provide empathy (e.g., understand the difficulties of being active in older adulthood), act as role models for physical pursuits, and inspire hope. However, Thoits (2011) warns, "deliberate helpfulness can cause recipients of social support to feel indebted, unjustly over rewarded, too dependent, over controlled, or incompetent in the eyes of support providers" (p. 151). She suggests the best support is invisible, defined as that which is unsolicited and subtly supplied. This is an area much in need of additional research; clearly, we need to understand who can provide the critical types of social support needed to engage in and sustain physical activity over time. It is equally important to recognise actions perceived as controlling older adults can have the opposite effect.

It seems appropriate here to include mention of stereotypes about aging and the effects these may have on older people's physical activity. Ageism is inherent in our language and in our culture, norms, and everyday interactions, both explicit and implicit (Gendron et al. 2015; Levy 2009). The stereotype content model (Fiske et al. 2002) explains how stereotypes consist of two dimensions—warmth and competence. Older adults are typically characterised as warm but incompetent, such as the "adorable (but helpless)" older person. Gendron et al., in a study that coded the language of students involved in an older adult mentoring programme, reported 12% of the tweets sent from students were discriminatory, ranging from assumptions and judgements—"older people don't have many opportunities for touch, so give hugs!", to old as negative—"the youngest senior I've ever met", to internalised ageism—"there is still so much to learn, even at my age". It is important to note that although some of these tweets sound positive, they convey messages that old age is different, wrong, or something to be avoided. Ageism is so pervasive, it becomes internalised in many older adults. One result of this internalised ageism is the tendency for an older adult to define herself separate from what would be perceived as the "out group" (Gendron et al. 2015; Whaley and Ebbeck 2002). For example, Whaley and Ebbeck (2002), in a study examining exercise identity in older adults, consistently found that older adults, when asked explicitly to define what it meant to be "old", found ways to exclude themselves from the "old" category, instead giving examples of how they were "not old" because of their activity status (e.g., "I think I'd feel older if I didn't go to this exercise class").

Older adults with a positive view of aging participate in physical activity more often (Wurm et al. 2010). Endorsement of ageing stereotypes, negative attitudes toward one's own aging, and low physical self-worth is associated with a decrease in physical activity (Emile et al. 2014). Emile et al. examined French adults 60–93 years of age on their views of ageing, the stereotypes they held about older people and physical activity, their physical self-worth, their implicit theories of ability (e.g., entity, or fixed view of ability, vs. an incremental, or growth view; see Dweck 1986), and their perceived level of physical activity. Among their findings, openness to experience was a predictor of positive attitude toward one's own ageing, suggesting it helps the individual to fight negative stereotypes of old age. This study contributes to our understanding of the role of stereotypes in impacting physical activity, but much remains unknown. For instance, although Ory et al. (2003) proposed challenging ageing stereotypes could increase the effectiveness of health promotion programmes, little research has been conducted in this area. As a first step, we move now to examine what we know "works" with regard to interventions that increase physical activity, focusing specifically on the social context.

16.1.2 The Evidence for Social Factors Promoting Physical Activity

In a systematic "review of reviews" of intervention components, Greaves et al. (2011) concluded that engaging social support was one of several causal factors that promoted change in physical activity. They specified interventions could be delivered in a wide range of settings (home, workplace), by a wide range of people with appropriate training (doctors, exercise specialists, lay people), but others important to the exerciser should provide social support. Similarly, Heath et al. (2012) reviewed physical activity interventions from around the world, concluding (among other strategies) initiatives that increase social support for physical activity within communities, specific neighbourhoods, and worksites promote physical activity. Finally, Bauman et al. (2012) synthesised physical activity correlates (factors associated with physical activity), concluding that ecological models that include interpersonal (social support, social norms) and social environmental (behavioural modelling, neighbourhood walkability) factors are important determinants of physical activity.

There is strong evidence the social environment plays a significant role in physical activity behaviour. McNeill et al. (2006) identified five social environment dimensions: social support and social networks, socioeconomic position and income inequality, racial discrimination, social cohesion and social capital, and neighbourhood factors. They stress most of these dimensions are modifiable, although each has its own mechanisms that are critical to understand in order to design optimal interventions. For example, interventions that focus on increasing access to physical activity opportunities must also focus on racial discrimination, since these issues are highly correlated. Recently, in a review of the cultural influences on exercise participation and fall prevention, Jang et al. (2016) concluded that to be effective, programmes must be culturally appropriate and utilise the positive influences of social support to optimise effect. Community-based participation effectively increases exercise rates across all racial and ethnic groups (Correa-de-Araujo 2015). However, physical activity rates differ along race, class, and gender lines, so our interventions need to take these factors into account. Social support and social networks, according to McNeill et al. (2006), increase physical activity by establishing social norms that constrain or enable health-promoting behaviours. For example, engaging in physical activity with others provides role modelling, information about effective ways to be active, and verbal encouragement from similar others. Social networks can also provide a sense of attachment and connectedness to one another, resulting in sharing of resources that support physical activity. This might come in the form of shared transportation, or even sharing caregiving responsibilities among group members.

16.1.3 Physical Activity Interventions Specific to Older Adults

For the most part, the review papers summarised above looked at physical activity interventions targeted across the entire adult developmental period. Additional important details of social relationships and physical activity specific to older adulthood are reported in the following studies and show the complexity inherent in investigating social support in this population. Martinez Del Castillo et al. (2010) interviewed 603 older adults (65 and older) in the Madrid, Spain, region. They explored the relationship between early life physical activity experiences and later life physical activity, as well as factors that influenced physical activity in old age (social class, occupation) and the impact agents of socialisation (spouse, children, friends) have on levels of physical activity. Although most people who were active early in life were more likely to be active in older adulthood, this was not the case for all individuals. In fact, some older individuals who were sedentary in their younger years had, in their later years, incorporated physical activity into their lifestyles. In examining this group, they concluded these older adults found themselves in new environments that socialised them toward physical activity. Examples include social support from friends to join a walking group and local opportunities for activities like gardening. Importantly, active older adults reported above-average social support and encouragement, especially from grown children and friends, and to a lesser extent spouse and neighbours. The company of family and friends was also associated with higher rates of walking, as well as more moderate to vigorous physical activity, in Brazilian older adults (Böhm et al. 2016). Importantly, "joint practice" (i.e., walking or exercising with another) had the biggest impact on physical activity behaviour, but it was the least reported type of social support received.

Wilson and Spink (2009) examined if older women's activity preferences (active alone, with others, no preference) impacted *how* others influenced them. Older females who preferred to be active with others were influenced by modelling and compliance/conformity from friends (e.g., request to be active or pressure to be active due to group membership). Friends were the only significant other who influenced behaviour (not family or healthcare providers). The authors suggest this may have been due to the high number (64%) of single women in the study and needs further investigation. But again, it points to the resilience and adaptability of older people. In this case, single women, without a spouse or possibly grown children, embrace other sources of support meaningful to them. Finally, Franke et al. (2013), in a qualitative study examining the "secrets of highly active adults", found social connections, or the presence of relationships with friends, neighbours, and institutions, facilitated physical activity. Access to physical activity opportunities was key and consistent with other studies showing physical activity to be a medium for socialising and enjoying time with friends. For example, Kohn et al. (2016) found participants were motivated to join an exercise programme because of the expected physical benefits and the social environment afforded by the group class.

A few studies have directly manipulated social interaction as a way of increasing physical activity. Pierre et al. (2015) designed an exercise programme based on social cognitive theory, with the goal of increasing self-efficacy for exercise and social support. They used peers and student trainers (experts), finding both were equally effective in fostering social support in the new exercisers. In a study of diabetic middle-aged and older adults, Beverly and Wray (2010) found spouses to be a powerful source of support for each other's exercise behaviour; themes of "collective support", "collective motivation", and "collective responsibility" provided strong evidence that interventions can be created that capitalise on this sense of collective efficacy. In a study that examined the perspective of exercise instructors of older adults (Hawley-Hague et al. 2016), the instructors maintained that peers "were ultimately the most important promoter of classes and the main way of recruiting new participants to classes" (p. 125).

As evidenced by these examples, a range of people can provide social support to older exercisers. In some studies, family members (adult children or spouses) are critical; in others, friends and neighbours are the primary influence. But consistently, when individuals are provided meaningful sources of social support, older exercisers seem to take advantage of that opportunity, including spouses, peers, and even younger people perceived to be experts. Who delivers support isn't the whole story. Research in this area does provide some important clues. In a recent study examining the US National Health and Nutrition Examination Survey (NHANES) data from 1999 to 2006, older adults who perceived themselves as high in received emotional social support had a 41% greater chance of meeting US physical activity guidelines. However, the only significant source of such support was from friends (Loprinzi and Joyner 2016). In another large-scale study from Brazil (Oliveira et al. 2011), the type of social support provided, rather than the source of social support, was examined. Several types of social support were identified (emotional, informational, and material); but social support was particularly critical for initial engagement in physical activity rather than maintenance. As this study examined adult workers, results should be interpreted with caution. Based on developmental theory, we cannot say with certainty these same relationships hold for older adults, as having left the work force will likely change one's sources of social support. In a study of middle- to older men in the UK (Kosteli et al. 2016), physical activity was viewed as a "key part of their social life"; having an exercise partner was considered an enabler, while not having one was a barrier to exercise. What we can conclude from these studies is that *who* provides social support, the *type* of social support provided, and the *personal characteristics* of the exerciser (age, gender, work status, activity experience) interact. Understanding the specific nature of these interactions is important for maximising physical activity behaviour in older adults. As researchers and practitioners, it is critical we find the right combinations that yield the best results for new and continuing physical activity behaviours.

There is also theoretical support for this interplay between components of social support and physical activity. In a discussion of conceptual frameworks that link social and built environments with physical activity, Li (2012) includes social cognitive theory (Bandura 2001), the social ecological model (King et al. 2002), and the sociological concepts of social cohesion and social capital (Kawachi and Berkman 2000). Each approach points out the need for examining multiple perspectives to understand a behaviour as complex as initial and continued participation in physical activity. We next turn our attention to the built environment to examine how this variable may influence social relationships and physical activity.

16.1.4 The Social Environment and Physical Activity

Oliveira et al. (2011) examined social support and physical activity in Brazilian adults and concluded "maintenance of leisure-time physical activity must be associated with other factors beyond the individual's level of social support, such as a suitable environment…" (p. 77). Contextual factors, including the social context, have been extensively studied as they apply to older adult exercise. As discussed previously, McNeill et al. (2006) identified five dimensions of the social environment (social support, socioeconomic position, racial discrimination, social cohesion/social capital, and neighbourhood factors). Here, we more closely examine neighbourhood factors and their role in facilitating or inhibiting social support. McNeill et al. further divide the influence of neighbourhoods into two categories: 1. the impact of the physical environment and 2. the social aspects of neighbourhoods.

Much of the literature examining older adults and neighbourhoods has focused on walking as the primary mode of physical activity. Aspects of the physical environment are commonly implicated in older adults' health and activity behaviour (Carlson et al. 2012; Maisel 2016; Notthoff and Carstensen 2015; Yen et al. 2009). For example, Notthoff and Carstensen (2015) examined the relationship between walkable neighbourhoods and effective motivational messages in a sample of low-income US residents. Walkability assessment included components like mixed use of the environment, density, pedestrian infrastructure, safety, and crime. When perceived walkability was high, residents walked more after viewing positive messages (e.g., messages about the benefits of exercise) than viewing negative (messages about the potential negative consequences of not walking). Residents who perceived their neighbourhood as low on walkability increased their walking regardless of the valence of the message. While this may seem to be a somewhat surprising finding, the authors note the sensibility in such a response. That is, for those who have barriers that must be overcome to walk, to do so demands problem-solving and deliberative processing. Since older people are more likely to pursue goals about satisfaction and meaning (consistent with socioemotional selectivity theory; Carstensen 1998), the tone of the message may not be as important for this group as with younger exercisers or for older people with less barriers to their walking. However, Maisel (2016) found higher street connectivity, less traffic, and higher perceived safety from crime were associated with higher rates of walking, regardless of neighbourhood type (rural, urban, suburban). The presence of green space has also been associated with social support, with less perceived green space associated with increased feelings of loneliness and a perceived shortage of social support in Dutch adults (Maas et al. 2009). From these studies we conclude that aspects of the neighbourhood itself is an important piece of the physical activity puzzle, and understanding that environment is key to constructing effective messages to promote physical activity.

In addition to the actual physical environment, Van Cauwenberg et al. (2014) examined the perceived social environment and its association with walking for transportation in a large study (51,000) of Belgian older adults (65 and over). Results indicated higher frequency of contacts with neighbours and greater perceived social support from neighbours were positively related to walking rates. Additionally, higher numbers of immigrants residing in the neighbourhood (postulated to relate to the vibrant social life of migrant communities or, alternatively, the loss of connection within a neighbourhood that encourages the residents to go elsewhere) was also positively related to walking rates. Greater neighbourhood involvement, greater participation in community events, and more volunteering were also positively related to daily walking for transportation. The authors concluded that it is critical to include interpersonal relationships, place attachment, and formal community engagement as factors related to older adults' physical activity. Mahmood et al. (2012), in a qualitative investigation of older adults in Vancouver, Canada, and Portland, Oregon, USA, also found support for the importance of social aspects of the environment. In particular, themes of feeling safe, comfort in movement, existence of community-based programmes, peer support, and intergenerational/volunteer activities, all helped foster everyday and intentional physical activity.

Carlson et al. (2012) concluded there appears to be a "synergistic interaction between the built environment and psychosocial factors in explaining physical activity among older adults" (p. 68). However, according to McNeill et al. (2006), few studies have evaluated the social aspects of neighbourhoods, particularly as it relates to physical activity. Van Cauwenberg et al. (2014) did find a relationship between frequency of contacts with neighbours and physical activity behaviour, but more research is needed in this area. Such an effort will require the combined efforts of community planners, government officials, and the residents themselves. This is an issue that warrants repeating; in order to increase physical activity through social relationships, it is imperative older adults be included in the process. Studies that have included the voices of older adults (e.g., Beverly and Wray 2010; Franke et al. 2013; Hawley-Hague et al. 2016; Mahmood et al. 2012) have added to our understanding of older people's lived experience rather than relying on other's perceptions of that reality.

16.1.5 Blending Developmental Theory and Physical Activity Research: Practical Implications for Promoting Physical Activity

From this overview of developmental concepts and research on physical activity in older adult populations, three interconnected themes focusing on social support, ageism, and the social environment are evident (see Table 16.1). First, an understanding of *who* older adults associate with and are influenced by, as well as the *type* of social support provided, are important components of the physical activity puzzle. Understanding the goals for social contact, as well as the flexibility possible in the relationships of older adults, can help us to better plan exercise programmes and interventions. Second, an awareness of pervasive *ageism*, in our language and in our actions, is important if we are to optimise physical activity in this population. Much of this ageism is implicit; therefore, making it visible will be the first step. Third, the *places* available to older adults for physical activity, that

Table 16.1 Summary of major themes and strategies for maximising physical activity through social interactions

Themes	Strategies
Understanding the 'who' and 'how' of social support	Recognise developmental reasons for social contacts
	Encourage peer modelling using "experientially similar" others ("champions")
	Educate family members and facilitate intergenerational exercise programmes
	Provide opportunities for active volunteering
	Engage in routine emotional (empathy for overcoming physical activity barriers), informational (facts regarding physical activity), and instrumental (transportation) support
Countering ageism	Be aware of ageist language, even that which seems "warm"
	Focus on what older people *can do* rather than deficits
	Recognise the adaptability and resilience of older people
	Actively debunk myths of ageing (e.g., inability to learn new things) and seek opportunities to foster positive images of ageing
Optimising the social environment	Strive for culturally appropriate activities
	Consider the objective physical environment and the perceived environment
	Enlist community members to better understand physical activity barriers
	Use positive messages to encourage physical activity
	Develop community-based programmes that foster shared identities and cooperation among residents

is, the social environment, must be carefully considered to increase the low numbers of older adults who are physically active. Each of these themes will be discussed, with an eye toward an integrative approach.

Although the overall number of social contacts diminish with age, Carstensen et al. (1999) have shown how this is a voluntary, adaptive process. Cornwell et al. (2008) found frequency of contact with neighbours increased with age, and Thoits (2011) proposed "experientially similar" others were key to understanding social relationships in older adults. While research links family members and close friends to physical activity behaviour (Böhm et al. 2016; Loprinzi and Joyner 2016; Martinez del Castillo et al. 2010), older adults are able to adapt to changing situations caused by moving or death of friends and loved ones (Pierre et al. 2015). Thoits differentiates between primary groups (family, relatives, and friends) and secondary groups (community members, religious organisations).

Optimally, physical activity programmes should target primary groups, as these are most likely to provide the emotional sustenance older adults are looking for (Thoits 2011). Intergenerational programmes, as suggested by Mahmood et al. (2012), could be one way to bring families together to support each other in physical activity programmes. Families are likely to benefit from educational programmes that help them become advocates for physical activity (Greaves et al. 2011; Heath et al. 2012), while avoiding the mistake of "deliberate helpfulness" (Thoits 2011) that is more likely to cause the older adult to feel overcontrolled and dependent. Adult children should see their role as encouraging, not pressuring, and choices to be active should be made jointly, not mandated or prescribed. Another strategy consistent with theory would be the use of physical activity "champions"; role models who can motivate like-others to become active (Franke et al. 2013; Hawley-Hague et al. 2016; Pierre et al. 2015). Finally, creating systems that encourage exercise buddies, enabling "joint practice" (Böhm et al. 2016), can increase adherence to physical activity, such as what Beverly and Wray (2010) found with spouses participating together in their exercise programme.

Perhaps as importantly, research on older adult physical activity has been slow to embrace ageism as a specific barrier to physical activity. As Gendron et al. (2015) showed, often ageist remarks can be quite subtle and even warm (e.g., the "sweet old lady"); however, such statements can render the older person powerless, incompetent, or make them feel incapable. Ory et al. (2003) provide examples from Rowe and Kahn's (1998) MacArthur Foundation of Successful Ageing report to illustrate this point. Myths such as, "you can't teach an old dog new tricks" and "the secret to successful ageing is to choose your parents wisely" imply an inability to change and adapt with age, myths that have been thoroughly debunked empirically.

A strength-based approach, focusing on the abilities of older adults, is one way to counter ageist stereotypes. Given older adults hold these ageist beliefs (Emile et al. 2014), it is doubly important for "experts" (medical, exercise, or otherwise) to provide counter narratives to those myths. With regard to the examples above, the evidence is clear that people can adopt new behaviours well into older adulthood, and genetic factors play a relatively small role in later health; social and behavioural factors are far more relevant (Ory et al. 2003). As suggested above, using peer role models can help older adults see themselves as capable and are consistent with social cognitive theory (Bandura 2001) and adult development theory (Rook 2000). As evidenced in the study by Whaley and Ebbeck (2002), many older adults are looking for a way to exclude themselves from the "old" category; clearly, participation in a physical activity programme can be such a qualifier, as being able to say one is "still moving" or "physically inclined" would not be consistent with a more negative view of aging. Cultivating a positive view of ageing has been shown to increase walking in older adults (Wurm et al. 2010); thus, this is a strategy deserving of more attention and further investigation.

With regard to physical contexts, it is vital that spaces are both available and welcoming (Maisel 2016; McNeill et al. 2006) and that spaces are considered safe and walkable (Carlson et al. 2012; Notthoff and Carstensen 2015; Van Cauwenberg et al. 2014). But given a neighbourhood, what makes for a positive perception, or a high level of walkability? Infrastructure aspects include having sufficient lighting, unobstructed walking paths, and high street connectivity (i.e., ease of travel between two points). Just as important, though, are the perceptions of walkability, perceived safety, and someone to walk with (Maisel 2016). Li (2012) stresses the importance of fostering social cohesion with a community by increasing civil engagement, participation, and cooperation between residents. Consistent with this idea, neighbourhood or community-based programmes that incorporate physical activity (e.g., political canvassing, clean up campaigns) would make sense and have been shown to be an effective strategy across racial and ethnic groups (Correa de Araujo 2015). Optimally, programme planning would engage community members early on. For example, if a given community perceives a safety issue, it is important for them to define what safety means. Lighting, fear of crime, weather-related concerns, or lack of sidewalks could all fall under this heading, and each would require a different strategy to overcome. Interventions will serve the community best if they are targeted, intentional, and multifaceted.

16.1.6 Final Thoughts

This chapter has argued for closer attention to adult development theory, for recognising and avoiding stereotypical assumptions related to ageism, and for a deeper investigation of contexts that promote physical activity in older adults. A better understanding of the lived experience of older adults, particularly as it relates to social relationships, has the potential to improve physical activity programme design and implementation. The goal should be to embrace a positive, developmental approach where the resilience and abilities of older people are celebrated. Engaging older adults in the process is an important step in providing programmes that best meet those needs, with the ultimate goal of providing opportunities to live healthier, richer lives.

Suggested Further Reading

- English, T., & Carstensen, L. L. (2014). Selective narrowing of social networks across adulthood is associated with improved emotional experience in daily life. *International Journal of Behavioral Development, 38*, 195–202. https://doi.org/10.1177/0165025.13515404.
- Franke, T., Tong, C., Ashe, M. C., McKay, H., & Sims-Gould, J. (2013). The secrets of highly active older adults. *Journal of Aging Studies, 27*(4), 398–409. https://doi.org/10.1016/j.jaging.2013.09.003.
- Thoits, P. A. (2011). Mechanisms linking social ties and support to physical and mental health. *Journal of Health and Social Behavior, 52*(2), 145–161. https://doi.org/10.1177/0022146510395592.

References

Bandura, A. (2001). Social cognitive theory: An agentic perspective. *Annual Review of Psychology, 52*, 1–26.

Bauman, A. E., Reis, R. S., Sallis, J. F., Wells, J. C., Loos, R. J., & Martin, B. W. (2012). Correlates of physical activity: Why are some people physically active and others not? *The Lancet, 380*(9838), 258–271. https://doi.org/10.1016/S0140-6736(12)60735-1.

Beverly, E. A., & Wray, L. A. (2010). The role of collective efficacy in exercise adherence: A qualitative study of spousal support and type 2 diabetes management. *Health Education Research, 25*, 211–223. https://doi.org/10.1093/her/cyn032.

Böhm, A. W., Mielke, G. I., da Cruz, M. F., Ramires, V. V., & Wehrmeister, F. C. (2016). Social support and leisure-time physical activity among the elderly: A population-based study. *Journal of Physical Activity and Health, 13*, 599–605. https://doi.org/10.1123/jpah.2015-0277.

Carlson, J. A., Sallis, J. F., Conway, T. L., Saelens, B. E., Frank, L. D., Kerr, J., et al. (2012). Interactions between psychosocial and built environment factors in explaining older adults' physical activity. *Preventive Medicine, 54*, 68–73. https://doi.org/10.1016/j.ypmed.2011.10.004.

Carstensen, L. L. (1998). A life-span approach to social motivation. In J. Heckhausen & C. Dweck (Eds.), *Motivation and self-regulation across the life span* (pp. 341–364). New York: Cambridge University Press.

Carstensen, L. L., Isaacowitz, D., & Charles, S. T. (1999). Taking time seriously: A theory of socioemotional selectivity. *American Psychologist, 54*, 165–181.

Cornwell, B., Laumann, E. O., & Schumm, L. P. (2008). The social connectedness of older adults: A national profile. *American Sociological Review, 73*(2), 185–203. https://doi.org/10.1177/000312240807300201.

Correa-de-Araujo, R. (2015). Cultural considerations for exercise in older adults. In G. M. Sullivan & A. K. Pomidor (Eds.), *Exercise for aging adults* (pp. 85–96). Springer. https://doi.org/10.1007/978-3-319-16095-5.

Cumming, E., & Henry, H. W. (1961). *Growing old: The process of disengagement*. New York: Basic Books.

Dweck, C. S. (1986). Motivational processes affecting learning. *American Psychologist, 41*, 1040e1048. https://doi.org/10.1037/003-066x.41.10.1040.

Emile, M., Chalabaev, A., Stephan, Y., Corrion, K., & d'Arripe-Longueville, F. (2014). Aging stereotypes and active lifestyle: Personal correlates of stereotype internalization and relationships with level of physical activity among older adults. *Psychology of Sport and Exercise, 15*(2), 198–204. https://doi.org/10.1016/j.psychsport.2013.11.002.

English, T., & Carstensen, L. L. (2014). Selective narrowing of social networks across adulthood is associated with improved emotional experience in daily life. *International Journal of Behavioral Development, 38*, 195–202. https://doi.org/10.1177/0165025.13515404.

Fiske, S. T., Cuddy, A. J. C., Glick, P., & Xu, J. (2002). A model of (often mixed) stereotype content: Competence and warmth respectively follow from perceived status and competition. *Journal of Personality and Social Psychology, 82*, 878–902. https://doi.org/10.1037//0022-3514.82.6.878.

Franke, T., Tong, C., Ashe, M. C., McKay, H., & Sims-Gould, J. (2013). The secrets of highly active older adults. *Journal of Aging Studies, 27*(4), 398–409. https://doi.org/10.1016/j.jaging.2013.09.003.

Gendron, T. L., Welleford, E. A., Inker, J., & White, J. T. (2015). The language of ageism: Why we need to use words carefully. *The Gerontologist*, 1–10. https://doi.org/10.1093/geront/gnv066.

Greaves, C. J., Sheppard, K. E., Abraham, C., Hardeman, W., Roden, M., & Evans, P. H., et al. (2011). *BMC Public Health, 11*, 119. http://www.biomedcentral.com/1471-2458/11/119

Hawley-Hague, H., Horne, M., Skelton, D. A., & Todd, C. (2016). Older adults' uptake and adherence to exercise classes: Instructors' perspectives. *Journal of Aging and Physical Activity, 24*(1), 119–128. https://doi.org/10.1123/japa.2014-0108.

Heath, G. W., Parra, D. C., Sarmiento, O. L., Andersen, L. B., Owen, N., Goenka, S., et al. (2012). Evidence-based intervention in physical activity: Lessons from around the world. *The Lancet, 380*(9838), 272–281. https://doi.org/10.1016/S0140-6736(12)60816-2.

Jang, H., Clemson, L., Lovarini, M., Willis, K., Lord, S. R., & Sherrington, C. (2016). Cultural influences on exercise participation and fall prevention: A systematic review and narrative synthesis. *Disability and Rehabilitation, 38*(8), 724–732. https://doi.org/10.3109/09638288.2015.1061606.

Kawachi, I., & Berkman, L. F. (2000). Social cohesion, social capital, and health. In L. Berkman & I. Kawachi (Eds.), *Social epidemiology* (pp. 174–190). New York: Oxford University Press.

King, A. C., Stokols, D., Talen, E., Brassington, G. S., & Killingsworth, R. (2002). Theoretical approaches to the promotion of physical activity: Forging a transdisciplinary paradigm. *American Journal of Preventive Medicine, 23*, 15–25.

Kohn, M., Belza, B., Petrescu-Prahova, M., & Miyawaki, C. E. (2016). Beyond strength: Participant perspectives on the benefits of an older adult exercise program. *Health Education & Behavior, 43*, 305–312. https://doi.org/10.1177/1090198115599985.

Kosteli, M., Williams, S. E., & Cumming, J. (2016). Investigating the psychosocial determinants of physical activity in older adults: A qualitative approach. *Psychology & Health, 31*, 730–749. https://doi.org/10.1080/08870446.2016.1143943.

Levy, B. (2009). Stereotype embodiment a psychosocial approach to aging. *Current Directions in Psychological Science, 18*, 332–336. https://doi.org/10.1111/j.1467-8721.2009.01662.x.

Li, F. (2012). Influences of social and built environments on physical activity in middle-aged and older adults. In A. L. Meyer & T. P. Gullotta (Eds.), *Physical activity across the lifespan: Prevention and treatment for health and well-being* (pp. 65–80). New York: Springer.

Loprinzi, P. D., & Joyner, C. (2016). Source and size of emotional and financial-related social support network on physical activity behavior among older adults. *Journal of Physical Activity & Health, 13*, 776–779. https://doi.org/10.1123/jpah.2015-0629.

Maas, J., van Dillen, S. M. E., Verheij, R. A., & Groenewegen, P. P. (2009). Social contacts as a possible mechanism behind the relation between green space and health. *Health & Place, 15*(2), 586–595. https://doi.org/10.1016/j.healthplace.2008.09.006.

Maddox, G. L. (1963). Activity and morale: A longitudinal study of selected elderly subjects. *Social Forces, 42*, 195–204.

Mahmood, A., Chaudhury, H., Michael, Y. L., Campo, M., Hay, K., & Sarte, A. (2012). A photovoice documentation of the role of neighborhood physical and social environments in older adults' physical activity in two metropolitan areas in North America. *Social Science & Medicine, 74*, 1180–1192. https://doi.org/10.1016/socscimed.2011.12.039.

Maisel, J. L. (2016). Impact of older adults' neighborhood perceptions on walking behavior. *Journal of Aging and Physical Activity, 24*, 247–255. https://doi.org/10.1123/japa.2014-0278.

Markus, H. R., & Herzog, A. R. (1992). The role of the self-concept in aging. In K. W. Shaie & M. P. Lawton (Eds.), *Annual review of gerontology and geriatrics* (Vol. 11, pp. 110–143). New York: Springer.

Martinez del Castillo, J., Jimenez-Beatty Navarro, J. E., Graupera Sanz, J. L., Martin Rodriguez, J., Campos Izquierdo, A., & Del Hierro Pines, D. (2010). Being physically active in old age: Relationships with being active earlier in life, social status, and agents of socialization. *Ageing and Society, 30*, 1097–1113. https://doi.org/10.1017/S0144686X10000358.

McNeill, L. H., Kreuter, M. W., & Subramanian, S. V. (2006). Social environment and physical activity: A review of concepts and evidence. *Social Science & Medicine, 63*(4), 1011–1022. https://doi.org/10.1016/j.socscimed.2006.03.012.

Notthoff, N., & Carstensen, L. L. (2015). Promoting walking in older adults: Perceived neighborhood walkability influences the effectiveness of motivational messages. *Journal of Health Psychology*, 1–10. Advance on-line publication. https://doi.org/10.1177/1359105315616470.

Oliveira, A. J., Lopes, C. S., Ponce de Leon, A. C., Rostila, M., Griep, R. H., Werneck, G. L., & Faerstein, E. (2011). Social support and leisure-time physical activity: Longitudinal evidence from the Brazilian Pro-Saude cohort study. *International Journal of Behavioral Nutrition and Physical Activity, 8*, 77. Retrieved from http://www.ijbnpa.org/content/8/1/77. https://doi.org/10.1186/1479-5868-8-77.

Ory, M., Kinney Hoffman, M., Hawkins, M., Sanner, B., & Mockenhaupt, R. (2003). Challenging aging stereotypes: Strategies for creating a more active society. *American Journal of Preventive Medicine, 25*(3, Supplement 2), 164–171. https://doi.org/10.1016/S0749-3797(03)00181-8.

Pierre, J., Gammage, K. L., Lamarche, L., Adkin, A. L. (2015). "You got a friend in me": The effects of an exercise intervention on peer and expert social support in older adults. Proceedings of the SCAPPS 2015 annual conference. *Journal of Exercise, Movement, and Sport, 47*. Abstract retrieved from http://jps.library.utoronto.ca/index.php/jems/article/view/25440

Rook, K. S. (2000). The evolution of social relationships in later adulthood. In S. H. Qualls & N. Abeles (Eds.), *Psychology and the aging revolution: How we adapt to longer life* (pp. 173–191). Washington, DC: American Psychological Association.

Rowe, J. W., & Kahn, R. L. (1998). *Successful aging*. New York: Pantheon Books.

Sims, T., Hogan, C. L., & Carstensen, L. L. (2015). Selectivity as an emotion regulation strategy: Lessons from older adults. *Current Opinion in Psychology, 3*, 80–84. https://doi.org/10.1016/j.copsyc.2015.02.012.

Thoits, P. A. (2011). Mechanisms linking social ties and support to physical and mental health. *Journal of Health and Social Behavior, 52*(2), 145–161. https://doi.org/10.1177/0022146510395592.

Van Cauwenberg, J., De Donder, L., Clarys, P., De Bourdeaudhuij, I., Buffel, T., De Witte, N., Dury, S., Verte, D., & Deforche, B. (2014). Relationships between the perceived neighborhood social environment and walking for transportation among older adults. *Social Science and Medicine, 104*, 23–30. https://doi.org/10.1016/j.socscimed.2013.12.016.

Whaley, D. E. (2016, Summer). Physical activity for social engagement in older Americans. *Elevate Health: A quarterly research digest of the President's Council on Fitness, Sports, & Nutrition, 17*. http://www.fitness.gov/pdfs/2016-summer_elevate_health.pdf

Whaley, D. E., & Ebbeck, V. (2002). Self-schemata and exercise identity in older adults. *Journal of Aging and Physical Activity, 10*, 245–259.

Whitbourne, S. K., & Whitbourne, S. B. (2014). *Adult development and aging: Biopsychosocial perspectives* (5th ed.). Hoboken: Wiley.

Wilson, K. S., & Spink, K. S. (2009). Social influence and physical activity in older females: Does activity preference matter? *Psychology of Sport and Exercise, 10*(4), 481–488. https://doi.org/10.1016/jpsychsport.2009.01.002.

Wurm, S., Tomasik, M. J., & Tesch-Romer, C. (2010). On the importance of a positive view on ageing for physical exercise among middle-aged and older adults: Cross-sectional and longitudinal findings. *Psychological Health, 25*, 25–42. https://doi.org/10.1080/08870440802311314.

Yen, I. H., Michael, Y. L., & Perdue, L. (2009). Neighborhood environment in studies of health of older adults: A systematic review. *American Journal of Preventive Medicine, 37*(5), 455–463. https://doi.org/10.1016/j.amepre.2009.06.022.

Zimmermann, H.-P., & Grebe, H. (2014). "Senior coolness": Living well as an attitude in later life. *Journal of Aging Studies, 28*, 22–34. https://doi.org/10.1016/j.jaging.2013.11.002.

17

The Role of the Instructor in Exercise and Physical Activity Programmes for Older People

Helen Hawley-Hague, Bob Laventure, and Dawn A. Skelton

17.1 Introduction

This chapter will provide an overview of the influence the exercise instructor plays in encouraging older peoples' participation in formal exercise programmes and physical activity both in groups and one to one in peoples' homes. We outline the instructors' main role when working with older people, their role within wider services and exercise pathways (particularly related to older people with health conditions), and the key evidence base for their role and influence on participation including evidence gaps. We also identify the important attributes of an exercise instructor and make practical recommendations for encouraging motivation, uptake, and retention to exercise and physical activity.

An exercise instructor is someone who delivers a programme of exercise to either a group of people or one-to-one instruction to individuals. In this chapter,

---

H. Hawley-Hague (✉)
Division of Nursing, Midwifery and Social Work, School of Health Sciences, Manchester Academic Health Science Centre, Faculty of Biology, Medicine and Health, University of Manchester, Manchester, UK

B. Laventure
Consultant in Physical Activity, Ageing and Health, Amble, Northumberland, UK

D. A. Skelton
School of Health and Life Sciences, Institute for Applied Health Research, Glasgow Caledonian University, Glasgow, UK

we mainly discuss the role of the instructor in relation to formal exercise programmes rather than physical activity programmes as this is where most research evidence lies.

Exercise instructors deliver programmes which help older people to maintain good health and well-being and prevent ill-health. Whichever setting they work in (e.g. hospital, community health services, community leisure service, or long-term care), they have to engage and work with a variety of professionals and organisations. As a team, they need to motivate older people to take up and maintain an exercise programme. They also need to be cognisant of the support strategies and activity approach for each individual, in order to improve outcomes. Even when working with relatively healthy older people, exercise instructors need to be adequately trained to adapt the programme to issues related to ageing (see suggested reading for how this can be done in practice). There has been a growth in advanced training to deliver specific evidence-based programmes for specific conditions which commonly occur in older people. Examples include falls prevention, stroke, Parkinson's, cancer, cardiovascular disease, and chronic obstructive pulmonary disease (Register of Exercise Professionals 2016). Exercise instructors are increasingly being engaged to offer exercise programmes to patients post-rehabilitation (Best et al. 2010; Hawley-Hague et al. 2017; Saunders et al. 2016). Their role in delivering exercise to older people is important to ensure programmes are evidence-based exercise and maintain outcomes following rehabilitation (Gillespie et al. 2012). For example, falls rehabilitation in the National Health Service (NHS) in the UK normally offer between 6 and 12 weeks (Royal College of Physicians 2012), yet 50 hours is an effective dose (Sherrington et al. 2016). This makes the provision of follow-on classes by instructors essential.

17.2 The Evidence Base on an Instructors' Role in Promoting Uptake and Retention to Exercise and Physical Activity

There is considerable evidence regarding the effectiveness of exercise and physical activity for older people for improving physical, mental and social well-being (Department of Health 2011; Spirduso et al. 2005). However, physical activity levels remain low (Agency for Health Care Research and Quality 2002; Townsend et al. 2015) and retention to exercise programmes is poor, whether they are general exercise (Jancey et al. 2007), disease-specific or health-related programmes (Royal College of Physicians 2012; Voglar et al. 2012). In the following sections, we explore the evidence base around how instructors' actions and approach can influence older peoples' participation in exercise and physical activity. We also discuss the skills and personal attributes associated with improved participation.

17.2.1 Attributes of the Individual Instructor

17.2.1.1 Leadership Style

Leadership is the instructors' interaction with the participant when teaching the programme. It can be defined as 'a process of social influence in which one person is able to enlist the aid and support of others in the accomplishment of a common task' (Chemers et al. 2000). When an instructor works with older people, they must coach, guide, and support them to carry out exercise or activity that satisfies the individuals' personal needs and goals. In a group setting, instructors need to enable all participants to contribute to attaining the group goal (e.g. cohesiveness and positive outcomes). To achieve this, they must understand the abilities, values, motives, and personalities of the exercise participants so that they can provide the most effective support. Creating a sense of group confidence, coherence, and empowerment through successful leadership encourages each group member to participate (Chemers et al. 2000; Marzano 2007).

Estabrooks et al. (2004) describe exercise instructor leadership as 'the most important determinant of participation in physical activity groups'. However, it is difficult to establish what particular aspects of leadership are important from an older person's perspective. There are several studies with younger populations where the leadership of the programme has been enhanced to explore its effects on attendance. In a study by Fox et al. (2000) this is described as including encouragement, social interaction, and positive performance feedback. The exercise environment was also altered to ensure that it was more relaxed, interactive, and motivating, something the exercise instructor has a key role in facilitating. In other studies, the exploration of the exercise instructors' leadership role is grounded in psychological theory and characterised by the provision of autonomy support, structure, and interpersonal involvement (Edmunds et al. 2008). This approach is taken from Social Determination Theory (see Chap. 13). An instructor who provides support for a participant to be autonomous does this by acknowledging the exercisers' feelings and perspectives; encouraging choice and initiative; and identifying, nurturing, and developing their interests and goals (Black and Deci 2000; Reeve 2002). They provide structure by giving clear guidance, outlining their expectations clearly and consistently, and they give responsive, person-centred feedback (Reeve 2002). The instructor is seen to display interpersonal involvement when they show feelings of warmth and care towards the participant, such as calling them when they miss a session to enquire after their well-being (Reeve et al. 2004). Edmunds et al. (2008) adopted this approach in an exercise programme with younger female participants and compared it to a programme where the same instructor delivered with their usual style. Attendance was significantly higher in the group with enhanced Social Determination Theory-based leadership. There are no known studies where this has been carried out for older people, but we explore the different characteristics and different aspects of leadership style within the exercise and physical activity literature in this area.

17.2.1.2 Personality

There are few studies which examine the personality traits of exercise instructors in relation to the delivery of exercise and physical activity programmes to older people. One exploratory study confirmed that there is a relationship between the instructors' personality and older peoples' exercise class attendance (weekly) and retention (Hawley-Hague et al. 2014), and that this endures over time. The study used the Big Five personality traits (Digman 1990):

- *Extraversion* which includes traits such as being talkative, energetic, and assertive.
- *Agreeableness* which includes traits such as being sympathetic, kind, and affectionate.
- *Conscientiousness* which includes being organised, thorough, planning, goal setting and outcome orientated.
- *Emotional stability* which includes being calm and relaxed.
- *Intellect* which includes being imaginative and insightful.

Instructors with very strong extravert, agreeable, and intellectual personality traits had poorer class attendance. On the other hand, instructors with a stronger conscientiousness trait were found to have better attendance and retention to their exercise classes. Factors associated with conscientiousness, such as goal setting and being organised, may relate to person-centred delivery and therefore meeting expectations in older participants (Hawley-Hague et al. 2014). When interviewing instructors who teach older people, they report that they believe it is their personality and enthusiasm for what they are doing, which can make a difference to the success of the class (Hawley-Hague et al. 2016). In an unpublished piece of work that triangulated instructors and participants views by the main author, there was agreement that skills, knowledge, and a sense of warmth and enthusiasm was important for building group cohesion and supporting adherence.

17.2.2 Factors That Make for Better Participation in Programmes (Predominantly Community Based)

Research suggests that instructors' qualifications, training, and experience are important attributes for older people and encourage uptake and retention (Hawley-Hague et al. 2016; McPhate et al. 2016). Skills learnt on the job and from other instructors also play a key part in the success of an instructor. Older peoples' social support networks, fostered by the instructor, may also be key.

17.2.2.1 Qualifications and Training

Qualifications and training are important when working with an older population. Older people are at increased risk of chronic disease, and long-term conditions can negatively impact on their ability to carry out physical activities. Despite this, we know little of how an instructor's skills and qualifications impact on older peoples' perceptions of the programme they receive or their retention to it. Qualitative studies with exercise instructors who deliver community-based exercise classes to older people suggest older people believe it is important that the instructor is appropriately qualified. Other studies also suggest that a qualified instructor is trusted by older people (Hawley-Hague et al. 2016; Dinan et al. 2006). A review by Franco et al. (2015) reported that in 40 (30%) studies, participants believed that the quality of exercise instructors influenced physical activity behaviour. They also reported that exercises that were tailored to the participant's physical capacity and individual needs were appreciated. These skills are partly acquired through training and are more likely to ensure appropriate delivery and progression of exercises. According to exercise instructors, appropriate qualifications and training strengthen participants' belief that they will achieve the outcomes that they desire (Hawley-Hague et al. 2016). This is especially important when the instructor is trained to deliver proven, evidence-based programmes. When older people are referred from a health professional, this also helps them to feel confident that the instructor is appropriately trained and delivering an evidence-based programme (Hawley-Hague et al. 2016, 2017).

Hawley-Hague et al. (2016) found that qualified instructors believed that advanced practical training and teaching experience was essential for delivery which engaged participants. Instructor education, training, and qualifications in physical activity and ageing relate to their beliefs about older peoples' participation in exercise classes (Hawley et al. 2012). Instructors with condition-specific qualifications (e.g. balance and strength for frailer, older participants at risk of falls, cardiac rehabilitation training) expressed more positive attitudes about exercise that was predominantly standing. This shows their understanding of the need to encourage older people to carry out weight-bearing exercise for maximum benefits, and the experience of these benefits is important for participant satisfaction. They also discussed carrying out assessments, for example, Timed up and Go Test (Podsiadlo and Richardson 1991), which enabled them to tailor their exercises and reassess participants to show them their improvement (Hawley-Hague et al. 2016, 2017). These instructors suggested that advanced qualifications and experience of delivery gave increased confidence. This confidence then translated into increased participant confidence and higher levels of retention to the programme (Hawley-Hague et al. 2016). This exploratory work indicates that advanced older adult exercise training is particularly important for work with participants with specific conditions and follow-up to rehabilitation by health services (Hawley-Hague et al. 2017). Focusing on safety, injury prevention, and a reduction in the risk of pain and discomfort is related to a reduction in participant dropout (De Groot and Fagerstrom 2011). We would argue this can only be achieved when the instructor has adequate training and experience.

There is some evidence that instructors undertaking motivational training (based on behaviour change theory), which includes developing skills for motivating older participants to exercise, for example, goal setting, risk identification and solutions to barriers (see Chap. 11) appear to achieve better participation in exercise programmes. In one study, instructors with motivational training (Hawley-Hague et al. 2014) had participants who attended more frequently than instructors without motivational training, particularly in the first three months of follow-up (behaviour is often established in the first six months of carrying it out). This is often the period when the instructor can play a key role in assisting older people to transition to maintenance of regular activity (Hawley-Hague et al. 2014).

17.2.2.2 Experience

The strongest evidence emerging relates to the experience of the instructor in motivating older people to uptake and maintain participation in exercise programmes (Dinan et al. 2006; Hawley-Hague et al. 2014, 2016; Seguin et al. 2010). However, it is difficult to specify which aspects of experience enable instructors to support participants successfully. As already highlighted, qualitative work with instructors indicates that if they feel confident about their own skills, this has a positive impact on both participation and the outcomes achieved with their participants (Hawley-Hague et al. 2012, 2014, 2016). Skills and associated confidence are not necessarily developed through training alone. They can be developed and refined over time through practice and through observation of others. Practice and observation should include different types of groups and populations such as different clinical conditions, long-term care settings, and community settings. It is possible that instructors with experience are more able to support their participants and increase their self-efficacy (see Chap. 12). Participant self-efficacy related to health improvement and function relate to older peoples' retention to classes (Hickey et al. 1995; Williams and Lord 1995; Sjosten et al. 2007).

17.2.3 Skills (Often Developed Through Training and Experience)

The skill set built up by an instructor over time is thought to be key in both uptake and retention to exercise and physical activity programmes (Laventure and Skelton 2007; Stewart et al. 2006).

17.2.3.1 Listening and Engaging

Instructors themselves have said that the way that they describe their exercise programmes is important to uptake, and it must fit with older peoples' perceptions of their own identities. They should use positive language around healthy active ageing rather than focusing on preventing the negative aspects of ageing (Hawley-Hague et al. 2016; Help the Aged 2005). Being able to listen to and talk to that person and then reach out to them and understand what would motivate them to participate is an important skill and requires the instructor to spend time with participants. Instructors believe emphasising the health benefits of exercise, providing free sample sessions, and encouraging potential participants to come and watch a class were important to participant uptake (Hawley-Hague et al. 2016). These factors are likely to be important for increasing self-efficacy. Listening to participants and understanding their thoughts, beliefs, and barriers and being responsive where possible (both in relation to the programme and externally) as they continue the class are also important for long-term retention (Hawley-Hague et al. 2016).

17.2.3.2 Meeting Expectations Through Goal Setting, Assessment and Person-Centred Delivery

The support offered by the instructor in the initial sessions (which were seen by older people as the most difficult) helps participants grow in confidence and fitness (Fox et al. 2007). Stathi et al. (2010) found that if older people feel empowered to improve their own functional performance in both everyday life and the exercise programme, they are more likely to continue. Instructors' have also suggested that participants continued to participate because their outcome expectations were met (Hawley-Hague et al. 2016). The instructors used their knowledge of the participant, (developed through initial discussion and regular assessment of both function and motivation) and their goals to improve delivery. They emphasised improvements and benefits (partly through re-assessment of function and motivation at regular intervals), ensuring realistic goals were set and that expectations were met. It was a real skill to achieve this in a group setting. Goal setting was an important skill, whether it was done formally or informally and one which could be developed through motivational training. It is important that goals are relevant to the individual and jointly agreed between the instructor and participant. Instructors then focused on delivery that was person-centred (e.g. considering different levels of cognition, previous experience, gender, life stage, physical, and psychological function, motives), tailored, and offered progression to meet those individual needs (Hawley-Hague et al. 2016). Instructors found that actively facilitating discussion within the group reinforced older peoples' positive outcomes and led to increased satisfaction with the class and higher retention levels (Hawley-Hague et al. 2016). Other studies have also found that feedback provided by instructors helped participants to assess their progress and served as a motivator to continue with the programme (Chiang et al. 2008; Dunlop and Beauchamp

2013). Encouraging self-monitoring outside of contact with the instructor (exercise diary, pedometers, smartphone apps) may be another way that instructors can motivate participants (Chase 2013; Nicklas et al. 2014). Instructors need to ensure these support strategies (which can often be mapped to behaviour change techniques) are tailored and personalised. Behaviour change techniques that work with younger people are not always effective with older people (French et al. 2014). For example, older people are less interested in behaviour change techniques which focus on self-monitoring and feedback on performance compared with other age groups and are more responsive to techniques which emphasise enjoyment and social opportunities.

17.2.3.3 Demonstrate a Sense of Care

Qualitative research suggests that instructors need to show a sense of care. This is important in encouraging older people to participate in exercise in the long term, ensuring they come back to the programme after a lapse in attendance. Sensitivity, kindness, and compassion are important attributes (McPhate et al. 2016). Reaching beyond the class (e.g. social engagements outside of class, phone calls to check a participant is okay) to engage with older people is perceived as important by both instructors and their participants (Chiang et al. 2008; Dinan et al. 2006; Hawley-Hague et al. 2016; Stathi et al. 2010).

17.2.3.4 Social Support

Different types of social support have been found to relate to older people's participation in exercise and physical activity programmes (Farrance et al. 2016; Franco et al. 2015; Hawley-Hague et al. 2014; also see Chap. 16). Instructors have the potential to engage with these influences to promote uptake and retention (Hawley-Hague et al. 2016, McPhate et al. 2016), even if it is just to sit and have tea afterwards with the group to foster group cohesion.

17.2.3.5 Develop Group Cohesion

Several studies have identified that instructors play a role in the cohesion within the exercise group and that group cohesion fosters both attendance and retention in activity programmes for older people (Hawley-Hague et al. 2014; Estabrooks et al. 2004). In addition, Loughead and Carron found that participants were more likely to feel cohesion with the class if the leader was interactive (2004). However, some studies suggest that group cohesion could be a participation barrier as well as a motivator to some older people, with new participants finding an already-established exercise or physical activity group intimidating (Costello et al. 2011; Franco et al. 2015). Therefore, the instructor again plays a role in making new participants feel that they are part of the group and able to successfully participate in activities (Hawley-Hague et al. 2016).

17.2.3.6 Utilise Health Professional Referral/Support

Several studies have emphasised the importance of health professional referral in promoting uptake and retention to exercise and physical activity programmes, particularly where they have a health or self-management emphasis. There is evidence that if a health professional recommends a programme, then follows this up with regular feedback and encouragement, he/she will help to build the participant's confidence and re-affirm positive beliefs about the importance and value of exercise (Grossman and Stewart 2003; Hawley-Hague et al. 2016; Schutzer and Graves 2004). Communication between health professionals and exercise instructors is of paramount importance to ensure the instructor knows what stage the participant is at in their exercise journey. Communication about details of conditions and medications when referred from primary care is important. Instructors need to have an active role in engaging with health professionals (Hawley-Hague et al. 2016, 2017).

17.2.3.7 Utilise Peers

There is evidence that peer support, both outside and within exercise and physical activity programmes, can enhance participation in exercise and physical activity programmes (Dorgo et al. 2011; Laventure et al. 2008; Stewart et al. 2006). Instructors have said that peers were ultimately the most important promoters of exercise programmes and the main way of recruiting new participants (Hawley-Hague et al. 2016). This could include 'modelling behaviour', where peers provide a positive role model. Instructors suggested that if they ensured their current participants were satisfied with the programme, this led to them sharing their experiences with others.

In referral-only (condition-specific) programmes, peer promotion was not as prominent but could still be a factor in older peoples' motivation to attend (Hawley-Hague et al. 2016).

17.2.4 Different Settings

17.2.4.1 Long-Term Care Settings

There is evidence around what factors influence older peoples' uptake and retention to exercise programmes in care homes, including adequate staffing levels, funding, and the use of volunteers (Benjamin et al. 2009; Finnegan et al. 2015). However, evidence looking at the role of the instructor is sparse. Social engagement is an important factor related to older peoples' retention to exercise in low-level residential care, mirroring community-based literature (Guerin et al. 2008; Ingrid and Marsella 2008; Weeks et al. 2008). However, none of the factors (social engagement, chronic conditions, depression, demographic factors, fear of falling, activity co-ordinator) that were explored in Finnegan and colleagues' study (2015) were predictive of attendance and retention in care homes (Chap. 18). This could be due to the specific cohort or measurement issues. In this study, the role of the instructor was not specifically examined, but other qualitative literature has identified staff support as important (Guerin et al. 2008). In Hawley-Hague et al.'s (2016) study, exercise instructors identified care home staff as 'gatekeepers' to residents' participation. Their role in bringing people to sessions within the care home (in time for class, etc.) was often interrupted by the formal care they were providing. They found care staff would bring different residents every week and could interrupt the programme, as formal care was seen as the priority (see Chap. 18 for further information).

In Stathi and Simey's study (2007), exercise participants within the care home reported negative experiences in previous settings, where some exercise instructors were unprofessional and did not identify their needs or abilities. Participants reported that this exposed them to unnecessary risks and made them anxious about participating in the programme within the home. However, once the programme started, they felt different about the exercise instructor who delivered it and reported that the instructor's knowledge and experience would be difficult to replace. Mirroring the community-based exercise literature; residents felt that they were given self-efficacy and confidence in their body as a result of confidence in the instructor. The instructor enabled them to feel less concerned about performing new exercises, and they felt that exercises were carefully chosen for them. The professional help and psychological support of the exercise specialist appear to be a critical factor for the success of an exercise programme in a nursing home environment. Stathi and Simey (2007) suggest that instructors who demonstrate their exercise knowledge, specifically for frail people, might help participants feel safe and be willing to perform activities that they thought were beyond them. This care home had both engaged and motivated management and staff. Therefore, although there is only sparse evidence around the role of the instructor, it is important that exercise instructors work closely with managers, staff, and possibly even family members to ensure long-term sustainability for the programme.

Finally, a Swedish study (Lindelöf et al. 2017) examining the views of older residents living with dementia found that the residents spoke about how supervised exercise (by trained instructors) in small groups created safety, coherence, and encouraged them to continue. The authors also interviewed therapist instructors (Fjellman-Wiklund et al. 2016) delivering the high-intensity exercise to residents; they spoke about continuously developing their own learning in an iterative process (experience). They built on previous knowledge to communicate with residents and staff and tailored the exercise in relation to each individual at that time point (experience). They also described the importance of using group members and the room to create interplay between exercise and social interaction.

17.2.4.2 Home-Based Exercise

Evidence suggests retention is higher with supervised and group programmes than home-based exercise (Picorelli et al. 2014; Nyman and Victor 2012). Evidence related to home-based exercise is mostly from studies in specific conditions. While similar factors to group exercise (person-centred delivery, social support) have been identified as important for participation, there is little reference to the exercise instructor/therapist (Picorelli et al. 2014; Simek et al. 2012). Social support is a very dominant motivator within group-based exercise (Hawley-Hague et al. 2016), whereas for home-based exercise, social support is less important (Hawley 2009). However, there is some evidence supporting the benefits (in terms of motivation) related to regular contact by the therapist/instructor (Hawley 2009).

17.2.4.3 Acute Settings

There is little evidence around the instructor (or in this setting, the therapist's) role in uptake and retention in hospital-based exercise programmes (day hospital or wards). Certainly we know that the therapist can play an important role in encouraging individuals to maintain their rehabilitation programme by working closely with follow-on programmes delivered by community-based therapy services or instructor-led community programmes (Hawley 2009). The delivery of the same evidence-based programme between rehabilitation and community helps to encourage retention and confidence for the participant (Hawley-Hague et al. 2017).

17.3 Gaps in the Evidence Base and Further Research Required

Further work is required to understand the different ways in which instructors influence older people to participate in exercise and physical activity and how this changes over time (from uptake to long-term maintenance). It would be useful to establish a menu of support options which may change as participants' needs and preferences change. Our knowledge also needs to be expanded about how this influence changes in different environments/settings (acute, long-term care, community) and actions the instructor needs to take for a successful programme in practice. In particular, do leadership and skills need to be tailored to different settings and participant groups?

There has, to our knowledge, been no real work comparing the instructors' differing role in promoting and delivering a formalised exercise programme with the role of walk leaders/less-structured physical activity and the delivery of home exercise to older people. However, indications from systematic reviews suggest a commonality of factors. These include providing a sense of care, a person-centred, tailored, and individualised delivery, and engaging with significant others. However, it would be useful to know if leadership styles, personality traits, or experience are similar in those successfully leading physical activity options wider than group exercise.

17.4 Key Practical Recommendations

There are some key practical recommendations for exercise instructors that arise from the literature. Instructors should consider the following when engaging older people and encouraging them to take up and then adhere to an exercise or physical activity programme.

17.4.1 Communicating with Potential Participants

Instructors should try where possible to communicate directly with potential participants through phone calls (where it is a referral based system or they receive an enquiry), demonstrations, or free tasters. This will increase the likelihood of a participant attending and will build their self-efficacy. It gives the older person a chance to discuss, see, or experience the content of the programme and understand that it will be tailored to their needs.

17.4.2 Communication with Others

Communicating effectively with different organisations that act as gatekeepers to activity for older people promotes the older person's confidence to participate and continue with exercise. Working with health professionals (both in primary care, community service, and acute services) can ensure that there is continuity in delivery (transfer from rehabilitation to community classes). Health professionals can signpost/refer to a programme and ensure participants are safe to exercise.

Local councils, social care providers, commissioners of health services (either private insurance or state health care), and charitable and private organisations can support instructors to set up classes and provide training and venues for them to deliver in. This provides a framework for them to ensure that their programmes are effective in supporting older people to achieve their outcomes and goals. Commissioners of health and social care services can fund programmes, dictate type of delivery, level of training required, and standards and reporting on participant outcomes, all important for participant motivation. Family and friends provide important physical support (e.g. transport to venues) as well as increasing confidence and self-efficacy, providing encouragement and motivation.

17.4.3 Assessments

We recommend that instructors carry out regular assessments of their participants. This enables the instructor to tailor the programme so that the participant can achieve the maximum gains and also enables re-assessment, which can help to highlight to the participant the improvements they have made. Assessment every 12 weeks is a good timescale to see improvements. It is important to reassure participants that sometimes staying the same or even reducing the rate of decline is still an achievement. This assessment may be motivational (see Chap. 11) and also functional, for example, Timed Up and Go (Podsiadlo and Richardson 1991), or Berg balance scale (Berg et al. 1992).

17.4.4 Goal Setting

Goal setting can also be linked to assessments, and whether done informally by asking older people about their aspirations or whether done in a formal way (see Eccelstone and Jones 2004), it is important and has been linked to participants' outcome expectations (Hawley-Hague et al. 2016). Tailoring the intervention and feedback that is given to a participant to ensure it meets their individual goals will improve motivation to attend a programme. Instructors should consider going on motivational training (preferably specifically related to exercise) and consider discussing participants' aspirations both in the short and the long term (see Chaps. 11 and 13 and further reading below).

17.4.5 Feedback

Receiving feedback from the instructor on progress is essential to motivation to continue and can also relate to self-monitoring. Within a group setting, encouraging feedback amongst the group can increase self-efficacy and re-affirm participants' beliefs in their progress. This can be done in person, or there are an increasing number of smartphone applications being developed that provide real-time feedback on both exercise behaviour and achievement of goals (see Chaps. 15 and 35).

17.4.6 Social Engagement/Support from Group

Research suggests older people appreciate being 'part of something' bigger. Instructors can play an important role in facilitating a supportive group environment, by ensuring no one feels excluded and that everyone can participate. They can also provide opportunities for interaction outside of a class environment (such as showcase events, or social events) and develop group cohesion with a group name/identity or social media presence.

17.4.7 Show Care

Instructors need to show compassion and care within sessions and between sessions (such as calling the participant if they are unwell). This supports participants to feel that they can attend again if they lapse or are unable to attend on a given week due to ill health or caring responsibilities.

17.5 Conclusion

With an increasing ageing population, a rise in chronic conditions, and increased strain on health and social care service, exercise instructors have an important role to play in encouraging older people's participation in physical activity and exercise. There is increased emphasis now on delivering evidence-based provision for a range of conditions (e.g. stroke, cardiovascular disease, falls, cancer, Parkinson's, dementia) as well as preventative community-based programmes. Instructors, whether delivering as part of a clinical therapist role or in the community/long term care, need to consider the different services and individuals who they must engage with to provide maximum support to participants. The instructors training, skills, and personal attributes are important to whether they can deliver a successful programme which engages the older adult population.

Suggested Further Reading
- Eccelstone, N. A., & Jones, J. C. (2004). International curriculum guidelines for preparing physical activity instructors of older adults, in collaboration with the aging and life course, World Health Organization. *Journal of Aging and Physical Activity,* 12, 467–479.

- Jones, J., & Rose, D. (eds.). (2005). *Physical activity instruction of older adults* (pp 192–210). Champaign: Human Kinetics. isbn: 0736045139.
- Laventure, R., & Skelton, D. A. (2007). Breaking down the barriers: Strategies to motivate the older client to begin and sustain exercise participation. *Fitness Professionals,* 42–43.

References

Agency for Health Care Research and Quality. (2002). Centers for Disease Control and Prevention. Physical activity and older Americans. Benefits and Strategies. http://www.ahrq.gov/ppip/activity.htm

Benjamin, K., Edwards, N., & Caswell, W. (2009). Factors influencing the physical activity of older adults in long-term care: Administrators' perspectives. *Journal of Aging and Physical Activity, 17*(2), 181–195.

Berg, K. O., Wood-Dauphinée, S. L., Williams, J. I., & Maki, B. (1992). Measuring balance in the elderly: Validation of an instrument. *Canadian Journal of Public Health, 83*(S2), S7–S11.

Best, C., van Wijck, F., Dinan-Young, S., Dennis, J., Smith, M., Fraser, H., Donaghy, M., & Mead, G. (2010). *Best practice guidance for the development of exercise after stroke services in community settings*. https://www.scribd.com/document/73480314/Exercise-After-Stroke-Guidelines

Black, A. E., & Deci, E. L. (2000). The effects of instructors' support and students' autonomous motivation on learning organic chemistry: A self-determination theory perspective. *Science Education, 84*, 740–756.

Chase, J. D. (2013). Physical activity interventions among older adults: A literature review. *Research and Theory in Nursing Practice, 27*(1), 53–80.

Chemers, M. M., Watson, C. B., & May, S. T. (2000). Dispositional affect and leadership effectives: A comparison of self-esteem, optimism and efficacy. *Personal and Social Psychology Bulletin, 26*(3), 267–277.

Chiang, K., Seman, L., Belza, B., & Hsin-Chun Tsai, J. (2008). "It is our exercise family": Experiences of ethnic older adults in a group-based exercise program. *Preventing Chronic Diseas, 5,* A05–A05.

Costello, E., Kafchinski, M., Vrazel, J., & Sullivan, P. (2011). Motivators, barriers, and beliefs regarding physical activity in an older adult population. *Journal of Geriatric Physical Therapy, 34,* 138–147.

De Groot, G. C. L., & Fagerstom, L. (2011). Older adults' motivating factors and barriers to exercise to prevent falls. *Scandinavian Journal of Occupational Therapy, 18,* 153–160.

Department of Health. (2011). Start active, stay active. UK physical activity guidelines: Older adults (65+ years). Crown copyright. https://www.gov.uk/government/uploads/system/uploads/attachment_data/file/213741/dh_128146.pdf

Digman, J. M. (1990). Personality structure: Emergence of the five-factor model. *Annual Review of Psychology, 41*, 417–440.

Dinan, S., Lenihan, P., Tenn, T., & Iliffe, S. (2006). Is the promotion of physical activity in vulnerable older people feasible and effective in general practice? *British Journal of General Practice, 56*, 791–793.

Dorgo, S., King, G. A., Bader, J. O., & Limon, J. S. (2011). Comparing the effectiveness of peer mentoring and student mentoring in a 35-week fitness program for older adults. *Archives of Gerontology and Geriatrics, 52*(3), 344–349.

Dunlop, W. L., & Beauchamp, M. R. (2013). Birds of a feather stay active together: A case study of an all-male older adult exercise program. *Journal of Aging and Physical Activity, 21*(2), 222–232.

Eccelstone, N. A., & Jones, J. C. (2004). International curriculum guidelines for preparing physical activity instructors of older adults, in collaboration with the aging and life course, World Health Organization. *Journal of Aging and Physical Activity, 12*, 467–479.

Edmunds, J., Ntoumanis, N., & Duda, J. L. (2008). Testing a self-determination theory-based teaching style intervention in the exercise domain. *European Journal of Social Psychology, 38*, 375–388.

Estabrooks, P. A., Munroe, K. J., Fox, E. H., Gyurcsik, N. C., Hill, J. L., Lyon, R., Rosenkranz, S., & Shannon, V. R. (2004). Leadership in physical activity groups for older adults: A qualitative analysis. *Journal of Aging and Physical Activity, 12*, 232–245.

Farrance, C., Tsofliou, F., & Clark, C. (2016). Adherence to community based group exercise interventions for older people: A mixed-methods systematic review. *Preventive Medicine, 87*, 155–166.

Finnegan, S., Bruce, J., Lamb, S. E., & Griffiths, F. (2015). Predictors of attendance to group exercise: A cohort study of older adults in long-term care facilities. *BMC Geriatrics, 15*, 37.

Fjellman-Wiklund, A., Nordin, E., Skelton, D. A., & Lundin-Olsson, L. (2016). Reach the person behind the dementia – Physical therapists' reflections and strategies when composing physical training. *PLoS One, 11*(12), e0166686.

Fox, L. D., Rejeski, W. J., & Gauvin, L. (2000). Effects of leadership style and group dynamics on enjoyment of physical activity. *American Journal of Health Promotion, 14*(5), 277–283.

Fox, K. R., Stathi, A., Mckenna, J., & Davis, M. G. (2007). Physical activity and mental well-being in older people participating in the better ageing project. *European Journal of Applied Physiology, 100*, 591–602.

Franco, M. R., Tong, A., Howard, K., Sherrington, C., Ferreira, P. H., Pinto, R. Z., & Ferraira, M. L. (2015). Older people's perspectives on participation in physical activity: A systematic review and thematic synthesis of qualitative literature. *British Journal of Sports Medicine, 0*, 1–9.

French, D. P., Olander, E. K., Chisholm, A., & McSharry, J. (2014). Which behaviour change techniques are most effective at increasing older adults' self-efficacy and physical activity behaviour? A systematic review. *Annals of Behavioural Medicine, 48,* 225–234.

Gillespie, L. D., Robertson, M. C., Gillespie, W. J., Sherrington, C., Gates, S., Clemson, L. M., & Lamb, S. E. (2012). Interventions for preventing falls in older people living in the community. *Cochrane Database of Systematic Reviews, 9,* CD007146.

Grossman, M. D., & Stewart, A. L. (2003). 'You aren't going to get better by just sitting around': Physical activity perceptions, motivations, and barriers in adults 75 years of age or older. *American Journal of Geriatric Cardiology, 12,* 33–37.

Guerin, M., Mackintosh, S., & Fryer, C. (2008). Exercise class participation among residents in low-level residential aged care could be enhanced: A qualitative study. *The Australian Journal of Physiotherapy, 54*(2), 111–117.

Hawley, H. (2009). Older adults' perspectives on home exercise after falls rehabilitation – An exploratory study. *Health Education Journal, 68*(3), 207–218.

Hawley, H., Skelton, D. A., Campbell, M., & Todd, C. (2012). Are attitudes of exercise instructors who work with older adults influenced by their training and personal characteristics? *Journal of Aging and Physical Activity, 20,* 47–63.

Hawley-Hague, H., Horne, M., Campbell, M., Demack, S., Skelton, D. A., & Todd, C. (2014). Multiple levels of influence on older adults' attendance and adherence to community exercise classes. *The Gerontologist, 54*(4), 599–610.

Hawley-Hague, H., Horne, M., Skelton, D. A., & Todd, C. (2016). Older adults take up and adherence to exercise classes: Instructors' perspectives. *Journal of Ageing and Physical Activity, 24,* 119–128.

Hawley-Hague, H., Roden, A., & Abbott, J. (2017). The evaluation of a strength and balance exercise program for falls prevention in community primary care. *Disability and Rehabilitation, 33*(8), 611–621.

Help the Aged. (2005). *Don't mention the F word encouraging positive attitudes to falls prevention in later life.* London: Help the Aged.

Hickey, T., Wolf, F. M., Robins, L. S., Wagner, M. B., & Harik, W. (1995). Physical activity training for functional mobility in older persons. *Journal of Applied Gerontology, 14,* 357–371.

Ingrid, B., & Marsella, A. (2008). Factors influencing exercise participation by clients in long-term care. *Perspectives, 32*(4), 5–11.

Jancey, J., Lee, A., Howat, P., Clarke, A., Wang, K., & Shilton, T. (2007). Reducing attrition in physical activity programs for older adults. *Journal of Aging and Physical Activity, 15,* 152–165.

Laventure, R., & Skelton, D. A. (2007). Breaking down the barriers: Strategies to motivate the older client to begin and sustain exercise participation. *Fitness Professionals,* 42–43. http://www.laterlifetraining.co.uk/wp-content/uploads/2010/12/Breaking-down-the-barriers-Laventure-and-Skelton-FitPro-2008.pdf

Laventure, R. M. E., Dinan, S. M., & Skelton, D. A. (2008). Someone like me: Increasing participation in physical activity among seniors with senior peer health motivators. *Journal of Aging and Physical Activity, 16*(Suppl), S76–S77.

Lindelöf, N., Lundin-Olsson, L., Skelton, D. A., Lundman, B., & Rosendahl, E. (2017). Experiences of older people living with dementia participating in high-intensity functional exercise in residential care facilities: "While it is tough, it's useful". *PLOS One, 12*(11). https://doi.org/10.1371/journal.pone.0188225

Loughead, T. M., & Carron, A. V. (2004). The mediating role of cohesion in the leader behaviour-satisfaction relationship. *Psychology of Sport and Exercise, 5*, 355–371.

Marzano, R. J. (2007). *The art & science of teaching: A comprehensive framework for effective instruction*. Association for Supervision & Curriculum Development (ASCD). isbn:97801-4166-0571.

McPhate, L., Simek, E. M., Haines, T. P., Hill, K. D., Finch, C. F., & Day, L. (2016). "Are your clients having fun?" The implications of respondents' preferences for the delivery of group exercise programs for falls prevention. *Journal of Aging and Physical Activity, 24*(1), 129–138.

Nicklas, B. J., Gaukstern, J. E., Beavers, K. M., Newman, J. C., Leng, X., & Rejeski, J. W. (2014). Self-monitoring of spontaneous physical activity and sedentary behavior to prevent weight regain in older adults. *Journal of Aging and Physical Activity, 24*, 129–138.

Nyman, S. R., & Victor, C. R. (2012). Older people's participation in and engagement with falls prevention interventions in community settings: An augment to the Cochrane systematic review. *Age and Ageing, 41*(1), 16–23.

Picorelli, A. M. A., Souza, L., Pereira, M., Pereira, D. S., Felı́cio, D., & Sherrington, C. (2014). Adherence to exercise programs for older people is influenced by program characteristics and personal factors: A systematic review. *Journal of Physiotherapy, 60*, 151–156.

Podsiadlo, D., & Richardson, S. (1991). The timed "Up & Go": A test of basic functional mobility for frail elderly persons. *Journal of the American Geriatric Society, 39*(2), 142–148.

Reeve, J. (2002). Self-determination theory applied to educational settings. In E. L. Deci & R. M. Ryan (Eds.), *Handbook of self-determination research* (pp. 183–203). Rochester: University of Rochester Press.

Reeve, J., Jang, H., Carrell, D., Jeon, S., & Barch, J. (2004). Enhancing students engagement by increasing teachers autonomy support. *Motivation and Emotion, 28*, 147–169.

Register of Exercise Professionals. (2016). *REPs categories*. http://www.exerciseregister.org/about-reps/reps-categories

Royal College of Physicians. (2012). *Older people's experiences of therapeutic exercise as part of a falls prevention service-patient and public involvement*. London: RCP.

Saunders, D., van Wijck, F., Townley, B., Skelton, D. A., Fitzsimons, C., & Mead, G. (2016). The BASES expert statement on fitness, physical activity and exercise after stroke. *The Sport and Exercise Scientist, 49*, 22–23.

Schutzer, K., & Graves, S. (2004). Barriers and motivations to exercise in older adults. *Preventive Medicine, 39*, 1056–1061.

Seguin, R. A., Economos, C. D., Palombo, R., Hyatt, R., Kuder, J., & Nelson, M. E. (2010). Strength training and older women: A cross-sectional study examining factors related to exercise adherence. *Journal of Aging and Physical Activity, 18*(2), 201–218.

Sherrington, C., Michaleff, Z. A., Fairhall, N., Paul, S. S., Whitney, J., Cumming, R. G., Herbert, R. D., Close, J. C. T., & Lord, S. R. (2016). Exercise to prevent falls in older adults: An updated systematic review and meta-analysis. *British Journal of Sports Medicine, pii*, bjsports-2016-096547.

Simek, E. M., McPhate, L., & Haines, T. P. (2012). Adherence to and efficacy of home exercise programs to prevent falls: A systematic review and meta-analysis of the impact of exercise program characteristics. *Preventive Medicine, 55*, 262–275.

Sjôsten, N. M., Salonoja, M., Piirtola, M., Vahlberg, T. J., Isoaho, R., Hyttinen, H. K., Aarnio, P. T., & Kivela, S. L. (2007). A multifactorial fall prevention programme in the community-dwelling aged: Predictors of adherence. *European Journal of Public Health, 17*, 464–468.

Spirduso, W., Francis, K., & MacRae, P. (2005). *Physical dimensions of ageing*. Champaign: Human Kinetics.

Stathi, A., & Simey, P. (2007). Quality of life in the fourth age: Exercise experiences of nursing home residents. *Journal of Aging and Physical Activity, 15*(3), 272–286.

Stathi, A., Mckenna, J., & Fox, K. R. (2010). Processes associated with participation and adherence to a 12-month exercise program for adults aged 70 and older. *Journal of Health Psychology, 15*(6), 1–10.

Stewart, A. L., Gillis, D., Grossman, M., Castrillo, M., Pruitt, L., McLellan, B., & Sperber, N. (2006). Diffusing a research-based physical activity promotion program for seniors into diverse communities: CHAMPS III. *Prevention of Chronic Disease, 3*(2), A51.

Townsend, N., Wickramasinghe, K., Williams, J., Bhatnagar, P., & Rayner, M. (2015). *Physical activity statistics*. London: British Heart Foundation.

Voglar, C. M., Menant, J. C., Sherrington, C., Ogle, S. J., & Lord, S. R. (2012). Evidence of detraining after 12-week home-based exercise programs designed to reduce fall-risk factors in older people recently discharged from hospital. *Archives of Physical Medicine and Rehabilitation, 93*(10), 1685–1691.

Weeks, L. E., Profit, S., Campbell, B., Graham, H., Chircop, A., & Sheppard-LeMoine, D. (2008). Participation in physical activity: Influences reported by seniors in the community and in long-term care facilities. *Journal of Gerontological Nursing, 34*(7), 36–43.

Williams, P., & Lord, S. (1995). Predictors of adherence to a structured exercise program for older women. *Psychology and Aging, 10*, 617–624.

18

Promoting Physical Activity Among Older People in Long-Term Care Environments

Julie Whitney

18.1 Introduction

This chapter starts by describing the long-term care (LTC) population. It then discusses what is known about activity in this population and the benefits of increasing activity. Finally, barriers and enablers to activity will be discussed as will strategies to implement activity in this setting.

The US government describes LTC as "a range of services and supports you may need to meet your personal care needs", implying that these services could also be delivered in a person's own home (US Department of Health and Human Services 2017). However, for the purposes of this chapter, LTC will be defined as a facility that provides permanent accommodation as well as the necessary care services within the same location. The term LTC covers a wide range of facilities ranging from accommodation where residents live in their own self-contained apartments with carers providing assistance with some activities of daily living to settings where residents with many healthcare needs require full-time qualified nursing care. In different parts of the world, these facilities may have different names. These include assisted living, hostel care or residential care homes for those requiring a lower level of support and nursing home or long stay hospital for those requiring full time healthcare in addition to care services. Facilities or units may specialise in specific conditions such as dementia. The heterogeneity of what might be described as LTC throughout the world means that it is necessary to interpret the evidence on

---

J. Whitney (✉)
Clinical Age Research Unit, King's College Hospital, Cheyne Wing, London, UK

© The Author(s) 2018
S. R. Nyman et al. (eds.), *The Palgrave Handbook of Ageing and Physical Activity Promotion*, https://doi.org/10.1007/978-3-319-71291-8_18

physical activity within the context of the study population. A trial that is effective in an assisted living unit may not be generalisable to a nursing home setting.

Optimising physical activity in the LTC setting is important. The fundamental principles are the same as other settings but in this population, there are some specific features that are unique and require special consideration. Those living in the LTC setting are likely to present with frailty, multiple medical conditions and/or cognitive impairment which require interventions to be flexible and individually tailored. Attitudes among residents and staff towards physical activity may be unique to this setting where an approach "to provide care" and "be cared for" negates an emphasis on promoting activity.

18.2 The Long-Term Care Population

Gordon et al. (2014) analysed the health status of people living in UK nursing and residential homes. Most residents were female (83%) and they had a mean age of 85. In this survey of 277 residents, 16% died during the 6-month follow-up period. There was a significant burden of ill health with a mean of 6.2 conditions per person that required a mean of 8 different medications. A median Barthel score of 9/20 indicated that most residents had a large degree of functional impairment and a median Mini Mental State Examination (MMSE) of 13/30 indicated that cognitive impairment was common. Sixty-six percent of this cohort exhibited what the authors described as "challenging behaviour". Only 14% were found to have normal nutritional status with 30% being clinically malnourished. Those living in residential care were generally better in all categories than those living in facilities where 24/7 nursing care was provided.

The picture this paints is important when considering physical activity interventions. Many of these issues may impact on the ability to remain physically active. Difficulties walking and/or rising from a chair and the resulting dependency is likely to limit the amount of time spent being active, as activity will be dependent on the availability of carers to assist. However, it also highlights the importance of promoting simple forms of physical activity that residents can perform independently. For example, moving the arms and legs whilst seated. Multi-morbidity including conditions such as osteoarthritis or stroke may cause difficulties with movement, fatigue or pain which may result in more sedentary behaviour. Up to half of older people living in LTC are fearful of falling, another common cause of activity restriction (Lach and Parsons 2013). Malnourishment contributes to sarcopenia and subsequent reduced functional capacity (Senior et al. 2015). The prevalence of cognitive impairment and related behaviours may impact on activity levels and participation in interventions. Pharmaceutical management of behavioural and psychological symptoms associated with dementia using psychotropic medication may also increase sedentary behaviour due to drowsiness.

There have been a few small studies measuring activity levels in this setting. Barber et al. (2015) measured 33 residents using activity monitors and found that on average residents were sedentary for 79% of the day. Buckinx et al. (2017) recorded a median of 1300 steps per day in 27 nursing home residents. In a similar study, in 43 residents, we found that a median of 22 hours of the day were spent sitting or lying down and a median of 2000 steps taken per day (Whitney et al. 2011). While there is no accepted figure for healthy older people with step counts ranging from 2000 to 9000 (Tudor-Locke et al. 2009), the findings in the LTC population are at the lower end of this spectrum. Measuring step counts in a population where a significant proportion are not ambulant may not be the optimal method for capturing physical activity levels and further research is required. These very low levels of physical activity compound many of the conditions described above, resulting in functional decline, muscle wasting and weakness (Buckinx et al. 2017), as well as possible negative effects on cognition and mood.

18.3 What Are the Effects of Physical Activity Interventions in the Long-Term Care Setting?

Physical activity interventions tested in trials have included both structured exercise and methods to increase activity within daily routines (Benjamin et al. 2011). A literature search for interventions including physical activity or exercise in LTC identified more than 50 randomised or quasi-randomised controlled trials. Most of these trials investigated structured exercise and used physical performance measures rather than activity monitoring to evaluate effect. Fewer trials investigated changing models of care or the environment to increase routine physical activity.

18.3.1 Structured Exercise Interventions

Most of the trials investigating structured exercise in LTC included small numbers of participants (fewer than 100 residents) and were of moderate quality in terms of study design and reporting (Crocker et al. 2013). Generally, structured exercise tested in this setting involved group-based interventions undertaken on average 3 times a week for 30–45 minutes and delivered by either exercise professionals such as physiotherapists or by care staff (Shakeel et al. 2015). Structured exercise programmes tested in LTC have included: Tai Chi (Cheng et al. 2014; Choi et al. 2005; Lee et al. 2009), resistance training (Bruunsgaard et al. 2004; Damush and Damush 1999; Fien et al. 2016), functional task training (Rosendahl et al. 2006), strength and balance training (Cheung et al. 2008; Dorner et al. 2007; Faber et al. 2006), multiple component (including a combination of two or more of the following: strength and balance, function, flexibility or endurance exercise) (Lazowski et al. 1999; Meuleman et al. 2000; Rolland et al. 2007; Schoenfelder and Rubenstein 2004) and dance (da Silva Borges et al. 2014; Vankova et al. 2014).

18.3.1.1 Effects of Structured Exercise on Physical Activity Levels

Despite many of the interventions tested in the LTC population stating an aim of improving physical activity, few trials of structured exercise have specifically measured this. There was a significant increase in activity counts using integrated monitors worn for 72 hours following a 10-week strength-training programme (Fiatarone et al. 1994). However, no change in activity levels were found following a 12-week walking intervention (MacRae et al. 1996). After a three-month individually tailored programme of physical and daily activity delivered by a physiotherapist and occupational therapist, activity levels improved (Grönstedt et al. 2013), but this effect was not sustained a further three months after the intervention ended (Frändin et al. 2016) A recent novel intervention, a giant board game which required participants to perform exercises to participate in the game, resulted in increases in steps taken. The board game was tested on a small sample (intervention group $n = 10$) who were cognitively intact (MMSE = 27) but shows promise as an engaging way of improving activity and encouraging independence in exercise resulting in a more sustainable approach (Mouton et al. 2017).

18.3.1.2 Other Effects of Structured Exercise

More trials have focused on the effect of structured exercise on physical performance such as balance (Cheung et al. 2008; Choi et al. 2005; de Bruin and Murer 2007; Faber et al. 2006; Lazowski et al. 1999; Rosendahl et al. 2006;

Telenius et al. 2015), walking ability (Baum et al. 2003; Cheung et al. 2008; Choi et al. 2005; Franzke et al. 2015; Rolland et al. 2007; Rosendahl et al. 2006) and muscle strength (Bruunsgaard et al. 2004; Damush and Damush 1999; Fien et al. 2016; Franzke et al. 2015; Lazowski et al. 1999; McMurdo and Rennie 1993; Meuleman et al. 2000) with mixed results. Participating in structured exercise appears to result in small but significant improvements in functional ability (Barreto Pde et al. 2016; Crocker et al. 2013). However, it is important not to overstate this effect as some large-scale trials found no changes in function, physical performance or other outcome measures (Kerse et al. 2008; Underwood et al. 2013). There is currently no evidence that exercise prevents falls in this population (Sherrington et al. 2016) and limited evidence for effects on behaviour (Telenius et al. 2015), cognition (Cichocki et al. 2015; Mulrow et al. 1994) and quality of life. A meta-analysis found some evidence that structured exercise may have a beneficial effect on mood (Barreto Pde et al. 2015).

The reasons for the mixed results in the literature are likely to be due to differences in trial populations in the extent of the prevalence of physical and cognitive frailty. It also may reflect different interventions tested, approaches to optimising uptake and participation and engaging with LTC staff. These differences are likely to have resulted in variability in the dose of exercise administered. Since optimising dose is important, barriers and enablers of uptake and adherence will be discussed in more detail in the section on implications for practice.

18.3.2 Interventions to Increase Routine Activity

18.3.2.1 Increasing Activity when Toileting

Alessi et al. (1999) carried out a small randomised controlled trial (RCT) ($N = 29$) where every two hours when residents were approached for toileting, they were also encouraged to do either upper or lower limb exercises, stand up and sit down or walk. The emphasis was on getting out and staying out of the bed during the day. After 14 weeks, there were no between-group differences in physical activity, but the intervention group slept better at night and were less agitated in the day. Looking more closely at the data, activity levels did increase in the intervention group, but it is likely that it did not reach statistical significance due to the small sample size. When the same intervention was tested in a larger RCT ($N = 107$) significant improvements in strength, endurance and continence were observed in the intervention group after eight weeks. However, no measure of physical activity was collected (Ouslander et al. 2005).

A similar intervention tested in a RCT including 256 LTC residents resulted in higher activity levels and significant improvements in measures of strength, walking and continence (Schnelle et al. 2002). This intervention involved frequent input from research staff throughout the day, on a two-hourly basis to encourage continence and activity. Implementation was good with most sessions involving an element of physical activity in addition to toileting. The key to adherence in these trials seems to have been that compared to a structured exercise programme, sessions were more frequent but shorter in duration and due to the functional nature of the activity, less likely to be perceived as exercise.

18.3.2.2 Goal Setting and Staff Training

Several large trials have investigated the approach of increasing activity levels through training LTC staff in resident assessment and goal setting aiming to increase activity levels. Two studies used goal setting in conjunction with changes in the environment to encourage activity and greater involvement in everyday function (Galik et al. 2014; Sackley et al. 2006). Galik et al. (2014) tested an intervention called the function-focused care for 103 cognitively impaired nursing home residents (FFC-CI). The aim of FFC-CI was to maximise the amount of independent functional activity incorporated into the everyday lives of the residents. The programme involved environmental modifications such as creating pleasant walking areas and access to outdoors, a 30-minute staff and family training about the importance of activity, working with a trained research nurse to set person-centred activity goals and ongoing motivation and monitoring of staff to promote activity rather than focus on completing care tasks. This final component was achieved through newsletters, awards for staff "caught in the act" promoting activity and the use of activity champions. This intervention, which was provided for residents with MMSE < 15/30, resulted in significantly increased activity and fewer falls during follow-up.

Resnick et al. (2009) tested a six-week staff training programme to improve knowledge and understanding of rehabilitation philosophy followed by support from a research nurse to develop individual resident goals around incorporating activity into everyday function. Activity levels were not reported; however, on average participants in this intervention who spent 70 minutes a day for 12 months involved in rehabilitation activities, improved in gait and balance measures but grip strength, quality of life and self-efficacy did not change.

Two large cluster randomised controlled trials (N = 149 (Peri et al. 2008) and N = 682 (Kerse et al. 2008)) involving nursing assessment and goal setting aimed at increasing activity levels, while not measuring activity, found negligible benefits in terms of function (Peri et al. 2008), no effect on falls (Kerse et al. 2008; Peri et al. 2008) and lower mood in those in the intervention group who were cognitively impaired (Kerse et al. 2008). Adherence to these latter trials was modest with Kerse et al. (2008) reporting 45% doing none or few of their exercises and Peri et al. (2008) reporting that half the participants exercised only once a day rather than the suggested two times. The fact that falls were unchanged by these interventions may be a positive finding. Increasing activity levels increases the exposure to falling and therefore could result in more falls. However, no firm conclusions can be made without both activity and falls data.

The outcomes from interventions aimed at increasing routine activity suggest that there is potential for incorporating increased physical activity into usual care routines. Importantly, goal setting and educational interventions only result in clinically meaningful changes in activity if care staff are supported and motivated to make this happen with the right training, supervision, feedback and physical environment.

18.3.3 Barriers and Enablers to Implementing Activity Interventions in LTC

18.3.3.1 Residents

There are several reasons why residents of LTC are motivated to remain active. These include a desire to return home, to maintain some level of functional independence, to help lift their mood and to fill empty time (Chen and Li 2014). Previous experience and attitudes towards exercise have a very strong bearing on the likelihood of continuing to remain active with those who have a positive attitude and good earlier life experiences of exercise being more likely to exercise in LTC (Chen and Li 2014; Phillips and Flesner 2013; Weeks et al. 2008).

Residents generally see physical activity as a good thing that will benefit their health and well-being. The main barrier to participation is lack of diversity of exercise on offer. Benjamin et al. (2011) conducted focus groups on residents' views of exercise. Residents felt a variety of options available was very important in that if a programme did not appeal to them, they would be put off participating. They thought that exercise that was insufficiently challenging, boring or designed for "other patient groups" such as those with dementia was also a barrier to uptake.

Finally, in mobility-limited older adults with multiple comorbidities, adverse events that limit participation in exercise are common (Hinrichs et al. 2015) and include musculoskeletal disorders, injury due to falling and exacerbations of respiratory conditions.

18.3.3.2 Staff

Institutional routines can be limiting if residents and carers must adhere to strict timetables to ensure that personal and healthcare tasks are completed in a timely fashion (Benjamin et al. 2011). Care staff may also have the attitude that their own role is to look after and care for residents' which may be perceived contradictory to increasing activity levels. There is evidence that nursing staff tend to "take-over" tasks from residents rather than enable or supervise the resident to complete the task themselves (den Ouden et al. 2017). Most physiotherapists (71%) working in LTC questioned by Baert et al. (2015), believed that exercise was useful in this setting to enable residents to maintain independence, reduce the risk of falls, reduce pain and to provide an opportunity to socialise. They also identified barriers which included the impact of frailty, multi-morbidity, passivity from residents and difficult resident behaviours. In a similar study, the same authors questioned LTC administrators about the importance of physical activity interventions in their own organisations. Again, administrators were motivated to organise activity interventions by the perceived health benefits and the prospect of improved social interaction. Administrators thought that residents would not be keen to take part in exercise and were also concerned that exercise would increase the risk of falls. They also mentioned that other care tasks tend to take priority over physical activity (Baert et al. 2016).

18.3.3.3 Environment and Culture

The LTC environment can create a barrier preventing activity due to lack of designated exercise areas, poor access to the outdoors and lack of space (Benjamin et al. 2011). In an observational study comparing two residential care facilities, three environmental themes were identified that enabled more activity: open or automatic doors, accessible outdoor footpaths with the opportunity to integrate with the wider community (i.e. watch children playing) and sufficient space in communal and bedroom areas (Nordin et al. 2016). Implicit social norms may influence levels of activity. A group of residents who were shown photographs and text about physically active peers in a newsletter expressed greater intention to be active than another group who looked at pictures not involving activity (Koeneman et al. 2017). This suggests that a home where activity is not encouraged or engaged in will perpetuate inactivity as normative behaviour.

18.4 Implications for Practice

The following recommendations for implementing physical activity interventions in LTC have been made based on research evidence where it is available but also drawing on experience where evidence is lacking.

In 2016, recommendations were made from a task force on physical activity and exercise in LTC (Barreto Pde et al. 2016). They were made on the basis of an update of the Cochrane review 2013 (Crocker et al. 2013) and expert opinion. Barreto Pde et al. (2016) recommendations have been incorporated into this chapter's focus not only on what type of activity should be provided but also factors required to address barriers and optimise uptake and participation. These are summarised in Fig. 18.1.

18.4.1 What Type of Physical Activity Is Recommended?

18.4.1.1 Structured Exercise Interventions

Those who are able should participate in resistance training exercise as part of a multi-component programme lasting 30–45 minutes, 2–3 times per week (Barreto Pde et al. 2016).

How to Implement Resistance Training

- Use elastic bands or simple strap-on weights to provide resistance.
- Resistance can be applied when practising functional activities by using the weight of the body (i.e. sit-to-stand practice or heel-raise exercises).

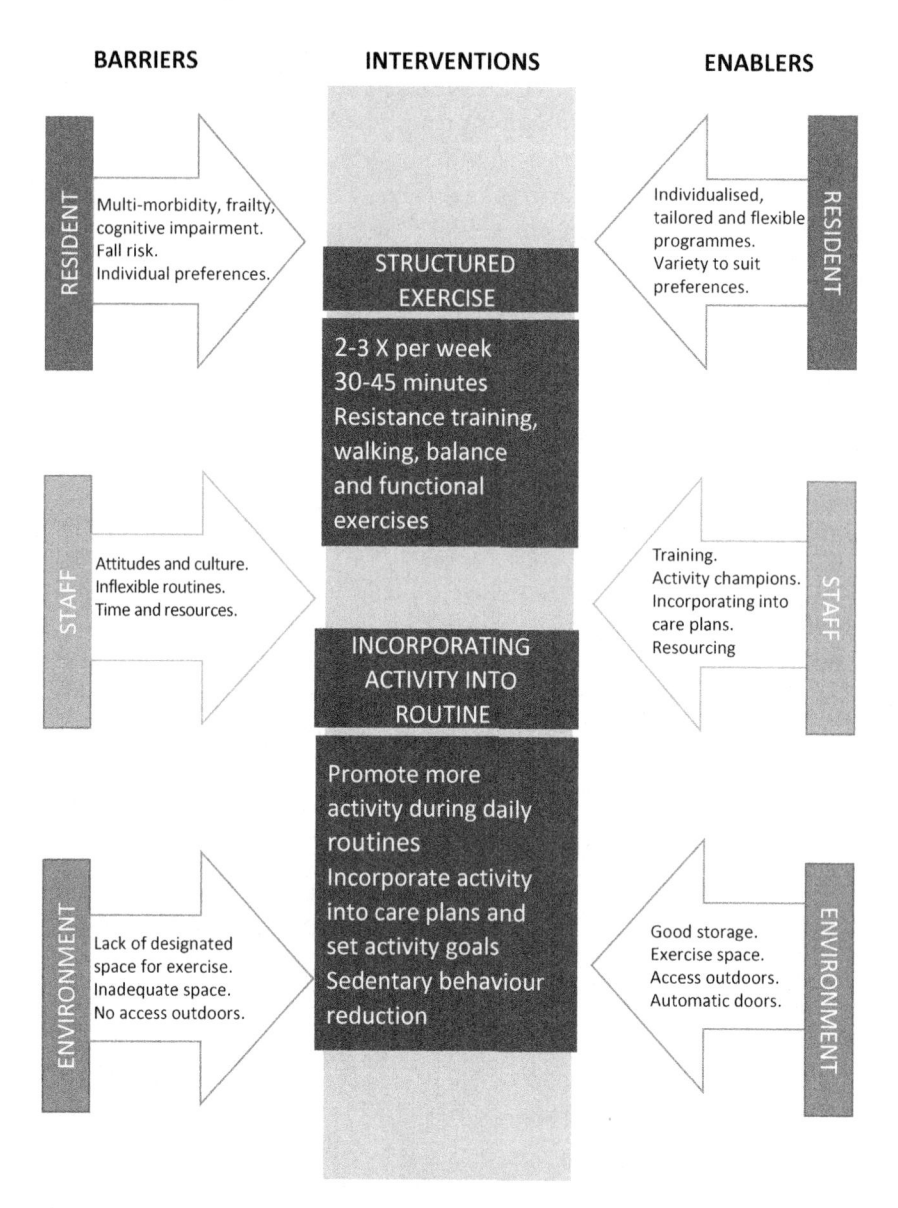

Fig. 18.1 Recommended activity interventions in LTC with barriers and enablers

BARRIERS

RESIDENT: Multi-morbidity, frailty, cognitive impairment. Fall risk. Individual preferences.

STAFF: Attitudes and culture. Inflexible routines. Time and resources.

ENVIRONMENT: Lack of designated space for exercise. Inadequate space. No access outdoors.

INTERVENTIONS

STRUCTURED EXERCISE
2-3 X per week
30-45 minutes
Resistance training, walking, balance and functional exercises

INCORPORATING ACTIVITY INTO ROUTINE

Promote more activity during daily routines
Incorporate activity into care plans and set activity goals
Sedentary behaviour reduction

ENABLERS

RESIDENT: Individualised, tailored and flexible programmes. Variety to suit preferences.

STAFF: Training. Activity champions. Incorporating into care plans. Resourcing

ENVIRONMENT: Good storage. Exercise space. Access outdoors. Automatic doors.

- Those prescribing and supervising resistance training require appropriate training.
- Avoid using very heavy loads to train muscles in this population as the resulting muscle soreness and stiffness may reduce adherence.
- Moderate intensity using 1–2 sets of 13–15 repetitions is recommended.
- Ensure 48 hours between sessions.
- Activity programmes should be ongoing.

For those who are ambulant, walking, balance training and functional activities should also be part of a multi-component exercise programme.

How to Implement Balance, Walking and Functional Exercise

- Undertake activities that increase the amount and frequency of walking such as walking groups or access to outdoor space.
- Modify the environment to accommodate safer walking.
- Encouragement from care staff to walk rather than use a wheelchair.
- Balance exercise should be individually tailored to ensure that it provides a challenge to balance without increasing the risk of falls.
- Exercises that challenge balance should be performed where possible standing up and could include Tai Chi or dance.
- Those delivering balance training exercise should be appropriately trained.

For those who are non-ambulant, consider chair- or bed-based exercises. Not all trials have required participants to be mobile with some including wheelchair propelling (Mulrow et al. 1994; Ouslander et al. 2005) or using seated-exercise programmes (Baum et al. 2003) as part of the intervention.

How to Promote Activity in Those Who Are Non-ambulant

- Exercises can be performed in a bed or a chair.
- Practice wheelchair propulsion and manoeuvring.

18.4.1.2 Incorporating More Activity into Daily Routines

Incorporating activity into everyday routines shows promise as a way of promoting increased activity in this population. Methods to increase activity in routines might include establishing exercise and activity in care plans, goal setting, encouraging families to help with activity, training for LTC staff, introducing "activity" champions and modifying the environment and care routines to encourage more activity.

How to Implement Enhanced Routine Activity

- Create environments that encourage safe activity—spaces without clutter, access to handrails, floor surfaces that are not shiny or distracting and automatic doors.
- Develop interesting walking choices including outdoor paths or routes that provide things to look at and motivation to get up. If possible design outdoor areas to optimise integration with wider community.
- Instead of focusing on task-based care, ensure care staff are trained and empowered to engage and enable residents to be as active as possible (i.e. to walk instead of push in a chair or to stand up to help with personal care rather than being dressed in bed).
- Develop a philosophy of care where activity is part of the care plan where care staff aim for a role of enablement and supervision.
- To incorporate frequent bursts of short duration activity into daily routines (i.e. every two hours encourage movement as part of a toileting programme).

18.5 How to Address Barriers to Participation

18.5.1 Resident

18.5.1.1 Frailty and Multi-morbidity

Interventions should be tailored to account for multiple comorbidities and frailty as these are common in the LTC population. Care should be taken that when increasing activity levels, there is not an increase in falls and injuries as a result. This can be done by judicious tailoring of programmes, assessing and modifying the environment, providing appropriate supervision and addressing all possible fall risk factors. Careful tailoring of exercise and having a flexible programme that can be modified after breaks due to illness or injury is required. The fatigue associated with frailty may discourage participation in physical activity, but since exercise interventions can be beneficial even in frail populations, fatigue should be addressed through individual tailoring and pacing and "little but often" dosing of activity (Theou et al. 2011).

Addressing Frailty and Multi-morbidity

- Schedule frequent opportunities to engage so that if sessions are missed due to ill health, it is still possible to achieve an adequate dose of activity.
- Ensure that programmes have built-in capacity to tailor intensity during recovery from illness or injury.
- Optimise management of medical conditions and pain control.
- Review and address modifiable fall risk factors and ensure adequate supervision.
- For those who fatigue easily, offer frequent but short duration exercise sessions.
- Carefully tailor exercise to ensure that it is challenging but not prohibitively difficult.

18.5.1.2 Cognitive Impairment

There is good evidence that those at various stages of cognitive impairment can participate in physical activity (Heyn et al. 2004). Most effective structured exercise programmes in LTC didn't exclude on the basis of cognitive impairment but did expect participants to be able to follow simple instructions. Those who are unable to follow simple instructions might still benefit from enhancing activity as part of daily routines. Methods of delivery may need to be modified. For example, more supervision could be required to ensure participants remember how to perform exercises safely and correctly and different methods of communication may need to be used with more emphasis on demonstrating (non-verbal) rather than describing (verbal).

Addressing Cognitive Impairment

- Those who can follow simple instructions should be able to participate in structured exercise classes but supervision levels might need to be higher to ensure safety.
- Participation can be enhanced by using simple verbal instructions, demonstrating or mirroring the exercise and establishing routine exercises which can be learnt by rote, tapping into procedural motor learning.

18.5.1.3 Variety and Person-Centred Approach

Activity interventions should consider individual preferences and a range of options should be available to do this. Residents are put off when there is inadequate variety to meet their differing tastes and capabilities. Not all residents find exercising in groups enjoyable while for others the social element of group is a vital factor in uptake and participation. Activity interventions should be tailored and progressive to neither be too challenging nor understimulating. Without addressing these issues, and aiming for a truly person-centred individualised approach to activity, it is unlikely that residents will engage and participate to achieve an adequate activity dose.

Providing Person-Centred Activity Options

- Provide different options so that exercise can be undertaken in a group format or individually.
- Consider the supervision requirements for a group to be safe. This would depend on the intensity of the exercise and the abilities of the participants. A group that involves lots of standing up and moving around may require a higher ratio of staff to participants to prevent falls.
- Adapt the level of challenge depending on participants' physical and cognitive abilities.
- Offer a variety of ways to achieve activity. This could range from dance and Tai Chi sessions to chair-based exercise.
- Provide opportunities for individual exercise sessions. The support required should be individually tailored ranging from providing a suitable space for someone to exercise alone to one-to-one supervision for all activity.

18.5.2 Staff and Environment

There are two key staffing-related barriers that need to be addressed. The first is attitudes and the culture relating to activity and the second is around ensuring that staff delivering interventions are adequately trained.

Staff training alone is unlikely to change attitudes to activity without a change in the culture of the home. Any change in culture needs to involve staff at all levels from managers to care staff. For this culture change to happen, activity must be given the same priority as other areas of care planning such as skin care and nutrition. In addition, an organisational change to shift the focus from scheduled task completion to encouraging optimal involvement in daily routines is required. For example, if a resident needs to be in the dining room for a meal, a task-based approach would be to transport the resident in the quickest possible manner which might mean using a wheelchair. Walking part of the way to the dining room might take longer but would increase activity levels and may also provide meaningful occupation for the resident. This approach comes with resource implications.

Good leadership and appointing activity champions is one way of disseminating a change of culture around activity. Use of newsletters and "caught in the act" awards may also be useful (Galik et al. 2014).

There is evidence that exercise and activity interventions can be delivered in LTC both by exercise professionals such as therapists or by trained LTC staff. There are advantages and disadvantages of both. Some residents may be more motivated to work with external "professionals" while others may be more comfortable exercising with staff that they know and trust. It is important that those responsible for delivering interventions are appropriately trained to ensure that exercise is performed effectively and safely. To be effective and acceptable to participants, exercise must be challenging and individually tailored. However, if it is too challenging, it could result in falls, fractures and other adverse events. Communicating how to exercise safely and effectively to those with cognitive impairment requires specific skills in both verbal and non-verbal methods.

Addressing Barriers to Activity Relating to Staffing

- Incorporating increased activity into usual care requires additional resources to be effective (i.e. a carer to resident ratio of 1:5 was required to deliver a continence and exercise programme (Schnelle et al. 2002) and a similar programme was found to cost three times more than usual care costs due to additional staff time required (Ouslander et al. 2005).
- Having staff who are well known to residents can be a significant motivation (Benjamin et al. 2011).
- Using volunteers or family members to support physical activity could be one way of providing opportunities when resources are limited. More research is needed to determine if this is safe and effective.
- Staff prescribing and delivering interventions should be appropriately trained.

To address the built environment, it is recommended that where possible, homes are set up with activity in mind. Optimal designs include a designated space for structured exercise, plenty of storage space to prevent corridors and rooms being cluttered and difficult to negotiate, automatic opening doors and access to the outdoors, particularly if it can encompass links with the wider community. Other important aspects of the environment include good lighting and temperature control, flooring which is not shiny or distracting (ideally plain carpet or if hard floor surface, a matt effect) and easily accessible handrails and walking aids. Having an environment where activity is part of everyday normal routine may positively influence residents' attitudes to activity (Koeneman et al. 2017).

18.6 Conclusion

There is insufficient evidence to support a single optimal type of intervention but structured multi-component exercise programmes and interventions aimed at increasing routine activity are safe and well tolerated. In many cases, the between-group differences in trials examined demonstrated that activity interventions slowed down a decline rather than improving performance and where longer-term follow-up has been conducted, any immediate benefits were lost once an activity programme stopped. Therefore, maintaining good participation is vital and programmes should be ongoing. Addressing resident, staff, environmental and cultural barriers is paramount to the success of any activity strategy.

Suggested Further Reading

- Barreto Pde, S., Morley, J. E., Chodzko-Zajko, W., K, H. P., Weening-Djiksterhuis, E., Rodriguez-Manas, L., et al. (2016). Recommendations on physical activity and exercise for older adults living in long-term care facilities: A taskforce report. *Journal of the American Medical Directors Association, 17*(5), 381–392.
- Care inspectorate – Scotland. Care about physical activity project. http://www.careinspectorate.com/index.php/meet-sid/9-professional/2615-care-about-physical-activity
- Shakeel, S., Newhouse, I., Malik, A., & Heckman, G. (2015). Identifying feasible physical Activity Programs for Long-Term Care Homes in the Ontario Context. *Canadian Geriatrics Journal, 18*(2), 73–104.

References

Alessi, C. A., Yoon, E. J., Schnelle, J. F., Al-Samarrai, N. R., & Cruise, P. A. (1999). A randomized trial of a combined physical activity and environmental intervention in nursing home residents: Do sleep and agitation improve? *Journal of the American Geriatrics Society, 47*(7), 784–791.

Baert, V., Gorus, E., Guldemont, N., De Coster, S., & Bautmans, I. (2015). Physiotherapists' perceived motivators and barriers for organizing physical activity for older long-term care facility residents. *Journal of the American Medical Directors Association, 16*(5), 371–379. https://doi.org/10.1016/j.jamda.2014.12.010.

Baert, V., Gorus, E., Calleeuw, K., De Backer, W., & Bautmans, I. (2016). An administrator's perspective on the organization of physical activity for older adults in long-term care facilities. *Journal of the American Medical Directors Association, 17*(1), 75–84. https://doi.org/10.1016/j.jamda.2015.08.011.

Barber, S. E., Forster, A., & Birch, K. M. (2015). Levels and patterns of daily physical activity and sedentary behavior measured objectively in older care home residents in the United Kingdom. *Journal of Aging and Physical Activity, 23*(1), 133–143. https://doi.org/10.1123/japa.2013-0091.

Barreto Pde, S., Demougeot, L., Pillard, F., Lapeyre-Mestre, M., & Rolland, Y. (2015). Exercise training for managing behavioral and psychological symptoms in people with dementia: A systematic review and meta-analysis. *Ageing Research Reviews, 24*(Pt B), 274–285. https://doi.org/10.1016/j.arr.2015.09.001.

Baum, E. E., Jarjoura, D., Polen, A. E., Faur, D., & Rutecki, G. (2003). Effectiveness of a group exercise program in a long-term care facility: A randomized pilot trial. *Journal of the American Medical Directors Association, 4*(2), 74–80. https://doi.org/10.1097/01.JAM.0000053513.24044.6C.

Benjamin, K., Edwards, N., Guitard, P., Murray, M. A., Caswell, W., & Perrier, M. J. (2011). Factors that influence physical activity in long-term care: Perspectives of residents, staff, and significant others. *Canadian Journal on Aging, 30*(2), 247–258. https://doi.org/10.1017/S0714980811000080.

Bruunsgaard, H., Bjerregaard, E., Schroll, M., & Pedersen, B. K. (2004). Muscle strength after resistance training is inversely correlated with baseline levels of soluble tumor necrosis factor receptors in the oldest old. *Journal of the American Geriatrics Society, 52*(2), 237–241.

Buckinx, F., Mouton, A., Reginster, J. Y., Croisier, J. L., Dardenne, N., Beaudart, C., et al. (2017). Relationship between ambulatory physical activity assessed by activity trackers and physical frailty among nursing home residents. *Gait & Posture, 54*, 56–61. https://doi.org/10.1016/j.gaitpost.2017.02.010.

Chen, Y.-M., & Li, Y.-P. (2014). Motivators for physical activity among ambulatory nursing home older residents. *The Scientific World Journal, 2014*, 7. https://doi.org/10.1155/2014/329397.

Cheng, S. T., Chow, P. K., Song, Y. Q., Yu, E. C., Chan, A. C., Lee, T. M., et al. (2014). Mental and physical activities delay cognitive decline in older persons with dementia. *American Journal of Geriatric Psychiatry, 22*(1), 63–74. https://doi.org/10.1016/j.jagp.2013.01.060.

Cheung, K. K. W., Au, K. Y., Lam, W. W. S., & Jones, A. Y. M. (2008). Effects of a structured exercise programme on functional balance in visually impaired elderly living in a residential setting. *Hong Kong Physiotherapy Journal, 26*(1), 45–50. https://doi.org/10.1016/S1013-7025(09)70007-7.

Choi, J. H., Moon, J. S., & Song, R. (2005). Effects of Sun-style Tai Chi exercise on physical fitness and fall prevention in fall-prone older adults. *Journal of Advanced Nursing, 51*(2), 150–157. https://doi.org/10.1111/j.1365-2648.2005.03480.x.

Cichocki, M., Quehenberger, V., Zeiler, M., Adamcik, T., Manousek, M., Stamm, T., et al. (2015). Effectiveness of a low-threshold physical activity intervention in residential aged care – Results of a randomized controlled trial. *Clinical Interventions in Aging, 10*, 885–895. https://doi.org/10.2147/CIA.S79360.

Crocker, T., Forster, A., Young, J., Brown, L., Ozer, S., Smith, J., et al. (2013). Physical rehabilitation for older people in long-term care. *Cochrane Database of Systematic Reviews, 2*, CD004294. https://doi.org/10.1002/14651858.CD004294.pub3.

da Silva Borges, E. G., de Souza Vale, R. G., Cader, S. A., Leal, S., Miguel, F., Pernambuco, C. S., et al. (2014). Postural balance and falls in elderly nursing home residents enrolled in a ballroom dancing program. *Archives of Gerontology and Geriatrics, 59*(2), 312–316. https://doi.org/10.1016/j.archger.2014.03.013.

Damush, T. M., & Damush, J. G., Jr. (1999). The effects of strength training on strength and health-related quality of life in older adult women. *Gerontologist, 39*(6), 705–710.

de Bruin, E. D., & Murer, K. (2007). Effect of additional functional exercises on balance in elderly people. *Clinical Rehabilitation, 21*(2), 112–121. https://doi.org/10.1177/0269215506070144.

de Souto Barreto, P., Morley, J. E., Chodzko-Zajko, W., Pitkala, K. H., Weening-Djiksterhuis, E., Rodriguez-Manas, L., et al. (2016). Recommendations on physical activity and exercise for older adults living in long-term care facilities: A taskforce report. *Journal of the American Medical Directors Association, 17*(5), 381–392. https://doi.org/10.1016/j.jamda.2016.01.021.

den Ouden, M., Kuk, N. O., Zwakhalen, S. M. G., Bleijlevens, M. H. C., Meijers, J. M. M., & Hamers, J. P. H. (2017). The role of nursing staff in the activities of daily living of nursing home residents. *Geriatric Nursing, 38*(3), 225–230. https://doi.org/10.1016/j.gerinurse.2016.11.002.

Dorner, T., Kranz, A., Zettl-Wiedner, K., Ludwig, C., Rieder, A., & Gisinger, C. (2007). The effect of structured strength and balance training on cognitive function in frail, cognitive impaired elderly long-term care residents. *Aging Clinical and Experimental Research, 19*(5), 400–405.

Faber, M. J., Bosscher, R. J., Chin, A. P. M. J., & van Wieringen, P. C. (2006). Effects of exercise programs on falls and mobility in frail and pre-frail older adults: A multicenter randomized controlled trial. *Archives of Physical and Medical Rehabilitation, 87*(7), 885–896. https://doi.org/10.1016/j.apmr.2006.04.005.

Fiatarone, M. A., O'Neill, E. F., Ryan, N. D., Clements, K. M., Solares, G. R., Nelson, M. E., et al. (1994). Exercise training and nutritional supplementation for physical frailty in very elderly people. *New England Journal of Medicine, 330*(25), 1769–1775. https://doi.org/10.1056/NEJM199406233302501.

Fien, S., Henwood, T., Climstein, M., & Keogh, J. W. (2016). Feasibility and benefits of group-based exercise in residential aged care adults: A pilot study for the GrACE programme. *PeerJ, 4*, e2018. https://doi.org/10.7717/peerj.2018.

Frändin, K., Grönstedt, H., Helbostad, J. L., Bergland, A., Andresen, M., Puggaard, L., et al. (2016). Long-term effects of individually tailored physical training and activity on physical function, well-being and cognition in Scandinavian nursing home residents: A randomized controlled trial. *Gerontology, 62*(6), 571–580.

Franzke, B., Halper, B., Hofmann, M., Oesen, S., Pierson, B., Cremer, A., et al. (2015). The effect of six months of elastic band resistance training, nutritional supplementation or cognitive training on chromosomal damage in institutionalized elderly. *Experimental Gerontology, 65*, 16–22. https://doi.org/10.1016/j.exger.2015.03.001.

Galik, E., Resnick, B., Hammersla, M., & Brightwater, J. (2014). Optimizing function and physical activity among nursing home residents with dementia: Testing the impact of function-focused care. *Gerontologist, 54*(6), 930–943. https://doi.org/10.1093/geront/gnt108.

Gordon, A. L., Franklin, M., Bradshaw, L., Logan, P., Elliott, R., & Gladman, J. R. (2014). Health status of UK care home residents: A cohort study. *Age and Ageing, 43*(1), 97–103. https://doi.org/10.1093/ageing/aft077.

Grönstedt, H., Frändin, K., Bergland, A., Helbostad, J. L., Granbo, R., Puggaard, L., et al. (2013). Effects of individually tailored physical and daily activities in nursing home residents on activities of daily living, physical performance and physical activity level: A randomized controlled trial. *Gerontology, 59*(3), 220–229.

Heyn, P., Abreu, B. C., & Ottenbacher, K. J. (2004). The effects of exercise training on elderly persons with cognitive impairment and dementia: A meta-analysis. *Archives of Physical Medicine and Rehabilitation, 85*(10), 1694–1704.

Hinrichs, T., Bucker, B., Wilm, S., Klaassen-Mielke, R., Brach, M., Platen, P., et al. (2015). Adverse events in mobility-limited and chronically ill elderly adults participating in an exercise intervention study supported by general practitioner practices. *Journal of the American Geriatrics Society, 63*(2), 258–269. https://doi.org/10.1111/jgs.13253.

Kerse, N., Peri, K., Robinson, E., Wilkinson, T., von Randow, M., Kiata, L., et al. (2008). Does a functional activity programme improve function, quality of life, and falls for residents in long term care? Cluster randomised controlled trial. *BMJ, 337*, a1445. https://doi.org/10.1136/bmj.a1445.

Koeneman, M. A., Chorus, A., Hopman-Rock, M., & Chinapaw, M. J. M. (2017). A novel method to promote physical activity among older adults in residential care: An exploratory field study on implicit social norms. *BMC Geriatrics, 17*, 8. https://doi.org/10.1186/s12877-016-0394-z.

Lach, H. W., & Parsons, J. L. (2013). Impact of fear of falling in long term care: An integrative review. *Journal of the American Medical Directors Association, 14*(8), 573–577. https://doi.org/10.1016/j.jamda.2013.02.019.

Lazowski, D. A., Ecclestone, N. A., Myers, A. M., Paterson, D. H., Tudor-Locke, C., Fitzgerald, C., et al. (1999). A randomized outcome evaluation of group exercise programs in long-term care institutions. *Journals of Gerontology Series A: Biological Sciences and Medical Sciences, 54*(12), M621–M628.

Lee, L. Y., Lee, D. T., & Woo, J. (2009). Tai Chi and health-related quality of life in nursing home residents. *Journal of Nursing Scholarship, 41*(1), 35–43. https://doi.org/10.1111/j.1547-5069.2009.01249.x.

MacRae, P. G., Asplund, L. A., Schnelle, J. F., Ouslander, J. G., Abrahamse, A., & Morris, C. (1996). A walking program for nursing home residents: Effects on walk endurance, physical activity, mobility, and quality of life. *Journal of the American Geriatrics Society, 44*(2), 175–180. https://doi.org/10.1111/j.1532-5415.1996.tb02435.x.

McMurdo, M. E., & Rennie, L. (1993). A controlled trial of exercise by residents of old people's homes. *Age and Ageing, 22*(1), 11–15.

Meuleman, J. R., Brechue, W. F., Kubilis, P. S., & Lowenthal, D. T. (2000). Exercise training in the debilitated aged: Strength and functional outcomes. *Archives of Physical and Medical Rehabilitation, 81*(3), 312–318.

Mouton, A., Gillet, N., Mouton, F., Van Kann, D., Bruyère, O., Cloes, M., & Buckinx, F. (2017). Effects of a giant exercising board game intervention on ambulatory physical activity among nursing home residents: A preliminary study. *Clinical Interventions in Aging, 12*, 847–858. https://doi.org/10.2147/CIA.S134760.

Mulrow, C. D., Gerety, M. B., Kanten, D., Cornell, J. E., DeNino, L. A., Chiodo, L., et al. (1994). A randomized trial of physical rehabilitation for very frail nursing home residents. *JAMA, 271*(7), 519–524.

Nordin, S., McKee, K., Wallinder, M., von Koch, L., Wijk, H., & Elf, M. (2016). The physical environment, activity and interaction in residential care facilities for older people: A comparative case study. *Scandinavian Journal of Caring Sciences*. https://doi.org/10.1111/scs.12391.

Ouslander, J. G., Griffiths, P., McConnell, E., Riolo, L., & Schnelle, J. (2005). Functional incidental training: Applicability and feasibility in the veterans affairs nursing home patient population. *Journal of the American Medical Directors Association, 6*(2), 121–127. https://doi.org/10.1016/j.jamda.2005.01.004.

Peri, K., Kerse, N., Robinson, E., Parsons, M., Parsons, J., & Latham, N. (2008). Does functionally based activity make a difference to health status and mobility? A randomised controlled trial in residential care facilities (The Promoting

Independent Living Study; PILS). *Age and Ageing, 37*(1), 57–63. https://doi.org/10.1093/ageing/afm135.

Phillips, L., & Flesner, M. (2013). Perspectives and experiences related to physical activity of elders in long-term-care settings. *Journal of Aging and Physical Activity, 21*(1), 33–50. https://doi.org/10.1123/japa.21.1.33.

Resnick, B., Gruber-Baldini, A. L., Zimmerman, S., Galik, E., Pretzer-Aboff, I., Russ, K., et al. (2009). Nursing home resident outcomes from the Res-Care intervention. *Journal of the American Geriatrics Society, 57*(7), 1156–1165. https://doi.org/10.1111/j.1532-5415.2009.02327.x.

Rolland, Y., Pillard, F., Klapouszczak, A., Reynish, E., Thomas, D., Andrieu, S., et al. (2007). Exercise program for nursing home residents with Alzheimer's disease: A 1-year randomized, controlled trial. *Journal of the American Geriatrics Society, 55*(2), 158–165. https://doi.org/10.1111/j.1532-5415.2007.01035.x.

Rosendahl, E., Lindelof, N., Littbrand, H., Yifter-Lindgren, E., Lundin-Olsson, L., Haglin, L., et al. (2006). High-intensity functional exercise program and protein-enriched energy supplement for older persons dependent in activities of daily living: A randomised controlled trial. *The Australian Journal of Physiotherapy, 52*(2), 105–113.

Sackley, C., Wade, D. T., Mant, D., Atkinson, J. C., Yudkin, P., Cardoso, K., et al. (2006). Cluster randomized pilot controlled trial of an occupational therapy intervention for residents with stroke in UK care homes. *Stroke, 37*(9), 2336–2341. https://doi.org/10.1161/01.STR.0000237124.20596.92.

Schnelle, J. F., Alessi, C. A., Simmons, S. F., Al-Samarrai, N. R., Beck, J. C., & Ouslander, J. G. (2002). Translating clinical research into practice: A randomized controlled trial of exercise and incontinence care with nursing home residents. *Journal of the American Geriatrics Society, 50*(9), 1476–1483.

Schoenfelder, D. P., & Rubenstein, L. M. (2004). An exercise program to improve fall-related outcomes in elderly nursing home residents. *Applied Nursing Research, 17*(1), 21–31.

Senior, H. E., Henwood, T. R., Beller, E. M., Mitchell, G. K., & Keogh, J. W. L. (2015). Prevalence and risk factors of sarcopenia among adults living in nursing homes. *Maturitas, 82*(4), 418–423. https://doi.org/10.1016/j.maturitas.2015.08.006.

Shakeel, S., Newhouse, I., Malik, A., & Heckman, G. (2015). Identifying feasible physical activity programs for long-term care homes in the Ontario context. *Canadian Geriatrics Journal, 18*(2), 73–104. https://doi.org/10.5770/cgj.18.158.

Sherrington, C., Michaleff, Z. A., Fairhall, N., Paul, S. S., Tiedemann, A., Whitney, J., et al. (2016). Exercise to prevent falls in older adults: An updated systematic review and meta-analysis. *British Journal of Sports Medicine.* https://doi.org/10.1136/bjsports-2016-096547.

Telenius, E. W., Engedal, K., & Bergland, A. (2015). Effect of a high-intensity exercise program on physical function and mental health in nursing home residents with dementia: An assessor blinded randomized controlled trial. *PLoS One, 10*(5), e0126102. https://doi.org/10.1371/journal.pone.0126102.

Theou, O., Stathokostas, L., Roland, K. P., Jakobi, J. M., Patterson, C., Vandervoort, A. A., & Jones, G. R. (2011). The effectiveness of exercise interventions for the management of frailty: A systematic review. *Journal of Aging Research, 2011*, 19. https://doi.org/10.4061/2011/569194

Tudor-Locke, C., Hart, T. L., & Washington, T. L. (2009). Expected values for pedometer-determined physical activity in older populations. *International Journal of Behavioral Nutrition and Physical Activity, 6*(1), 59. https://doi.org/10.1186/1479-5868-6-59.

Underwood, M., Lamb, S. E., Eldridge, S., Sheehan, B., Slowther, A. M., Spencer, A., et al. (2013). Exercise for depression in elderly residents of care homes: A cluster-randomised controlled trial. *Lancet, 382*(9886), 41–49. https://doi.org/10.1016/S0140-6736(13)60649-2.

US Department of Health and Human Services. (2017). What is long term care. Retrieved from https://longtermcare.acl.gov/the-basics/what-is-long-term-care.html

Vankova, H., Holmerova, I., Machacova, K., Volicer, L., Veleta, P., & Celko, A. M. (2014). The effect of dance on depressive symptoms in nursing home residents. *Journal of the American Medical Directors Association, 15*(8), 582–587. https://doi.org/10.1016/j.jamda.2014.04.013.

Weeks, L., Profit, S., Campbell, B., Graham, H., Chircop, A., & Sheppard-LeMoine, D. (2008). Participation in physical activity: Influences reported by seniors in the community and in long-term care facilities. *Journal of Gerontological Nursing, 34*(7), 36–43. https://doi.org/10.3928/00989134-20080701-11.

Whitney, J., Close, J., Lord, S., & Jackson, S. (2011). Do carers accurately estimate activity in care home residents? *Age and Ageing, 40*(Suppl 1), i53.

19

Promoting Physical Activity Among Older People in Hospital

Anna Barker and Sze-Ee Soh

19.1 Introduction

19.1.1 The Hospital Setting

Understanding the hospital environment provides a foundation for the design and delivery of programmes to increase the physical activity levels of older people in hospital. As presented in Section 5 of this Handbook, the physical environment can influence how physically active older people are, with certain characteristics being motivators to activity and some, barriers. The following paragraphs illustrate how this is also true in the hospital setting. In addition, the hospital environment and the characteristics of older people in hospital affect the types of physical activity programmes that can be effectively and safely delivered.

Hospitals provide medical treatment to people of all ages with a variety of health conditions. Older people commonly seek care from acute and rehabilitation hospitals. Each has different patient, staffing, and environmental profiles that have implications for promoting physical activity. Acute care hospitals typically include an emergency department and specialty units such as intensive care, cardiovascular, oncology and respiratory. They provide short-duration treatment for injury, illness, or urgent medical conditions. Treatments may include drug therapy, medical procedures and surgery. Acute care is

---

A. Barker (✉) • S.-E. Soh
School of Public Health and Preventive Medicine, Monash University, Melbourne, VIC, Australia

typically provided by medical specialists, surgeons, nurses, and diagnostic and allied health professionals. Patients can be quite unwell when admitted to acute hospitals; however, the length for stay is often less than three days (Hirshon et al. 2013). While in acute hospitals, patients often receive extensive investigations such as pathology tests, imaging and medical specialist review. These investigations can be time-consuming and place demands on the time of older people. This may result in physical activity being de-prioritised.

Inpatient rehabilitation hospitals, sometimes known as rehabilitation centres, provide longer-term care than acute hospitals. On average, patients spend more than 17 days in a rehabilitation hospital (Ottenbacher et al. 2004; Turner-Stokes 2007). Such hospitals tend to have a greater number of geriatricians and allied health professionals including dieticians and social workers when compared to acute hospitals. This reflects the rehabilitative nature of the care and highlights the opportunity for the promotion of physical activity in older patients to be multi-disciplinary. Time and space are less of an issue in this setting with patients receiving therapy four to five times per week and having access to specialised gym equipment like exercise bikes to improve their functional ability (de Morton et al. 2015). These factors may help older people to be more physically active in rehabilitation compared to acute hospitals.

19.1.2 Profile of Older People Admitted to Hospital and Their Activity Levels

Older people represent around one-third of all hospital admissions (Australian Institute of Health and Welfare 2012; Hall et al. 2010), despite representing just over a tenth of the population (Levit et al. 2009). The profile of older people in hospital is diverse, with a range of conditions and events precipitating their admission and differing levels of illness, co-morbidity, medications and social support. Each of these can impact on an older person's capacity to be physically active.

Compared to younger people, older people are more likely to have multiple chronic diseases including arthritis, stroke and dementia. Over half of Australians aged more than 65 years have arthritis, while a third of those over 85 years have a diagnosis of dementia (Australian Institute of Health and Welfare 2016). Similar figures have been reported in Europe and the United Kingdom (Gasior 2012; Mortimer and Green 2015). Older people in hospital often take more than four medications, have some difficulty walking, and a degree of malnutrition (Buurman et al. 2011). In addition, up to two-thirds have some cognitive impairment (Dewing 2001; Tolson et al. 1999). An older person may be admitted to hospital to receive therapy for an acute illness such as a urinary tract or respiratory infection. Alternatively, their admission may be a planned event to manage a pre-existing condition such as a knee replacement for osteoarthritis. Occasionally, the hospital admission may be to transition the older person from home into residential care (Naylor and Keating 2008).

The fundamental goal of hospital care is to restore people to good health. Unfortunately, in addition to the negative consequences discussed in Chap. 10, hospitalisation can also negatively affect how physically active an older person is. In clinical research, physical activity is commonly measured using pedometers or accelerometers that record steps per day or time spent in an upright position. In prior studies, the number of steps taken per day by hospitalised older people varies considerably—from 50 to 8000 steps (Agmon et al. 2017). It should be noted that the accuracy of these devices in older people in hospital is limited due to their slow walking speed (McCullagh et al. 2016). The majority of hospitalised older people are substantially less active than older adults in the community. Studies consistently report that older people in hospital take less than 1000 steps per day (Agmon et al. 2017; Fisher et al. 2016; Peiris et al. 2012). Some studies report less than 100 steps per day (Davenport et al. 2015), whereas older people living in the community take around 7000 steps per day (Tudor-Locke et al. 2011).

A similar picture of inactivity emerges when other activity measures are considered. In hospital, older people spend as little as 30 minutes a day being physically active (Ong et al. 2016). In an acute geriatric ward, they spend as little as seven minutes a day walking (Villumsen et al. 2015). This is also the case in orthopaedic populations even though they are often younger and have less co-morbidity, reflecting a high proportion of elective procedures. Older people spend 99% of their day lying or sitting while in hospital, with just 16 minutes of physical activity per day (Davenport et al. 2015).

Interestingly, there is little difference in the physical activity profile of patients across acute and rehabilitation hospitals (Astrand et al. 2016). This is despite older people in rehabilitation hospitals being more medically stable than those in acute hospitals, having greater access to resources such as physiotherapists and dedicated exercise areas such as gyms and exercise equipment. While the goal of rehabilitation is to promote independence, older people in this setting still spend less than two hours a day in an upright posture (Peiris et al. 2012). This highlights opportunity to increase the physical activity levels of older people while they are in acute and rehabilitation hospitals.

19.1.3 Functional Consequences of Reduced Physical Activity in Older People in Hospital

As discussed in Chap. 10, low levels of physical activity due to prolonged bed rest in hospital can result in a loss of muscle strength and power (Kortebein et al. 2008). This increases the risk of falls (Oliver et al. 2010). It also leads to functional decline such as decreased walking capacity (reduction in walking speed, distance and/or independence) and loss of ability to perform simple activities like showering and dressing.

Given this information on low levels of physical activity of older patients, it is not surprising that more than half of older people experience functional decline while there (Gill et al. 2010). This decline is seen as early as the second day of a hospital admission and continues after they recover from the original illness or injury precipitating their admission (Hirsch et al. 1990). People aged over 85 are most likely to develop new functional deficits during hospitalisation (Covinsky et al. 2003). Reduced physical activity and subsequent functional decline can negatively affect the older person's health and well-being both in hospital and after discharge (Boltz et al. 2012), highlighting an inactivity cascade where reduced physical activity in hospital leads to further inactivity after discharge (Nitz and Low Choy 2008).

Prolonged periods of physical inactivity in hospital is also associated with increased risk of skin injury and pressure ulcers (Lindgren et al. 2004). Similarly, the respiratory system may be compromised with the development of atelectasis, increasing the risk of complications such as hospital-acquired pneumonia (Convertino et al. 1997). Postural hypotension can develop within 72 hours of prolonged bed rest, together with reduced stroke volume and increase in resting heart rate (Convertino 1997; Convertino et al. 1982). Each of these events and physiological effects can lengthen the time the older person spends in hospital. This can have a negative effect on the older person's feelings of well-being, and also creates stress on an already overloaded health care system. Importantly, these events and physiological effects can limit an older person's ability to be physically active. For example, an older person who develops postural hypotension may feel dizzy when getting out of bed or walking. This may result in them walking less to avoid feelings of dizziness.

Being physically inactive in hospital also affects post-hospital outcomes. While most older people discharged from rehabilitation are able to walk ten meters, only a tenth walk at a speed that would enable them to cross the street safely (Gorgon et al. 2007). For one quarter of older people who experience functional decline while in hospital, this loss remains after leaving hospital

(Covinsky et al. 2003). Older people who are less physically active in hospital are at greater risk of functional decline post-hospital than those who are more active (Zisberg et al. 2015). Importantly, low levels of physical activity in hospital are associated with an increased risk of hospital readmission within one month (Fisher et al. 2016), admission to residential aged care and death, even after controlling for important confounders (Brown et al. 2004).

19.1.4 Why Older People Are Physically Inactive in Hospital

There are several factors that contribute to how active older people are while in hospital. These relate to the patient, staff, hospital system and environment. The factors are summarised in Fig. 19.1 and described in the following section.

At the patient level, observational studies have identified that lower levels of functional ability (Zisberg et al. 2011) and poor nutritional status (Izawa et al. 2014) are associated with older people being less physically active while in hospital. Qualitative studies have identified older people believing they are unwell (Holst et al. 2015), feeling fatigued (Brown et al. 2007) and impairments such as 'breathing' and 'leg' problems that limit their ability to be active in hospital (Buttery and Martin 2009). This study also reported that older patients believed they needed to rest and relax rather than be active. A common myth about hospitalisation is that people are unwell and that bed rest is important for recovery. Although bed rest may be ordered by medical staff for around one-third of older patients, there is often no documented medical indication for this suggesting factors other than medical instability are responsible for bed rest while in hospital (Brown et al. 2004). Importantly, many older people believe their activity levels while in hospital are adequate, despite substantial evidence of inactivity (Buttery and Martin 2009). If older people believe their activity levels are adequate, they are unlikely to be motivated to be more active. In addition, patients who have a fear of falling are less likely to be physically active (Holst et al. 2015).

Staff encouragement to be more active is a key facilitator to older people increasing their activity levels (Holst et al. 2015). Despite this, few patients (11%) recall being advised by clinical staff to be active (Buttery and Martin 2009). One small study reported that older people perceived useful ways to maintain functional ability while in hospital were good relationships between patients and nurses, strong basic care, appropriate assessment, and respect for level of autonomy (Lafreniere et al. 2015).

Barriers

Patients
- Reduced functional ability:
  - Muscle weakness, fatigue, pain, shortness of breath, poor nutritional status
- Beliefs:
  - Their activity levels are adequate
  - Need to relax and rest → bed rest is an important component of recovery
  - Fear of falling/injury

Staff
- Perceived lack of:
  - Time to promote/undertake physical activity with patients
  - Skills
- Beliefs:
  - Patients are reluctant and apprehensive to be more physically active
  - Fear of the patient falling and/or sustaining injury
- Little reimbursement or incentive

Organisational (Hospital)
- Organisational routines (e.g. rounds, waiting for examinations) place demands on patient time
- Availability of staff to support safe physical activity
- Lack of resources (e.g. gait aids)
- Hospital gowns or inappropriate footwear and clothing deter patients from being physically active

Environmental
- Ward characteristics (e.g. location of television, space for chairs)
- Unsafe/hazardous hospital wards
- Medical devices (e.g. intravenous drips, drains and/or catheters) restrict mobility

Strategies

Patients
- Ensure patient is medically stable
- Ensure physical activity care plans are patient centred and tailored to individuals needs
- Use positive heath messages to educate patients on the benefits of physical activity
- Promote a sense of motivation by promoting that exercise helps you feel better
- Provide falls prevention education and strategies
- Engage family, friends and carers
- Encourage patients to perform daily activities independently when safe

Staff
- Integrate physical activity reminders and strategies into usual care process
- Increase clinician's skills in designing and delivering physical activity programs
- Use motivational interviewing and goal-setting techniques to enhance patient participation
- Engage physiotherapists to ensure safe mobility
- Management should acknowledge efforts to increase physical activity

Organisational (Hospital)
- Use of education and support materials to encourage patients to be active while waiting to be reviewed by staff on ward round or to be transported for examinations
- Integrate physical activity programs/ prompts into routine care activities (e.g. admission assessments and handover)
- Provide sufficientre sources (staff and equipment), establish formal exercise programs
- Provide clothing or encourage patients to wear their own clothing

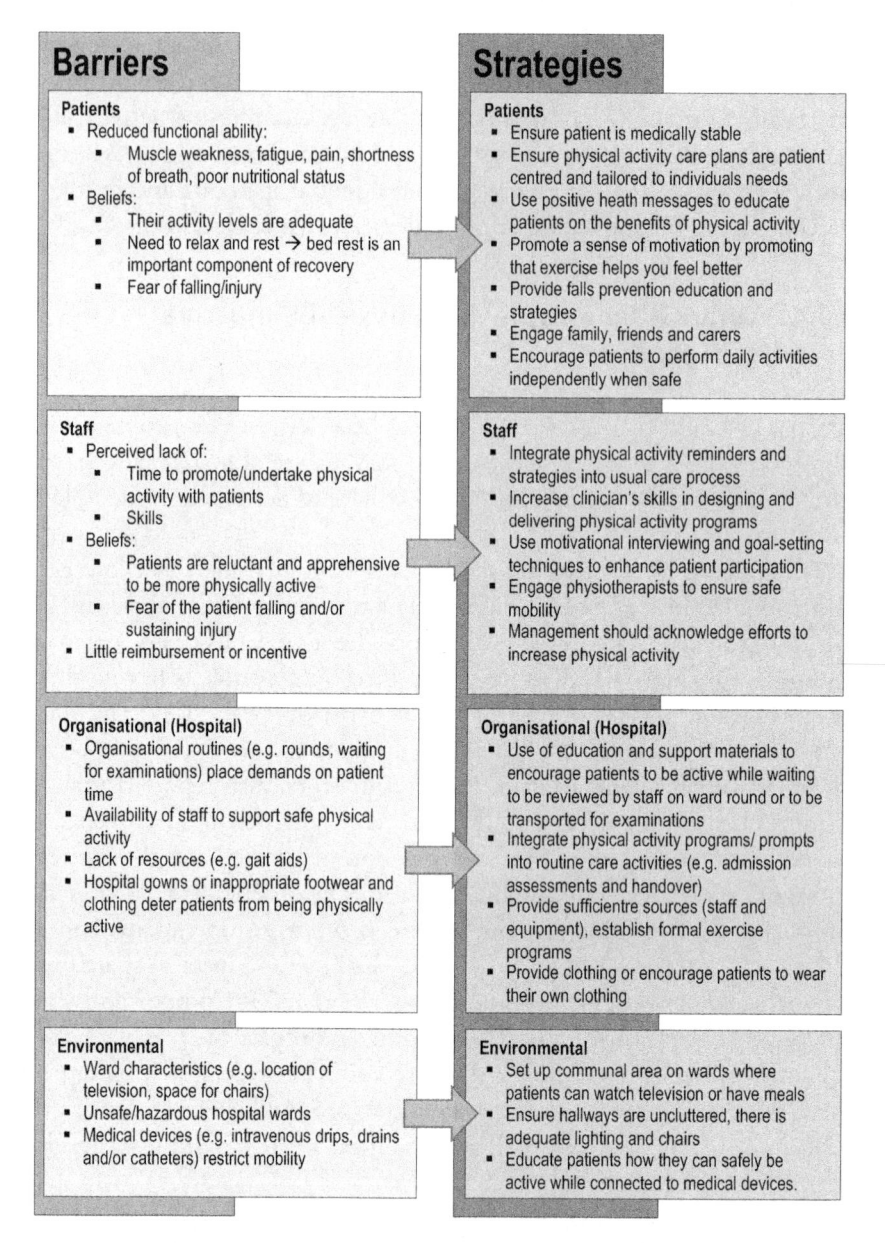

Environmental
- Set up communal area on wards where patients can watch television or have meals
- Ensure hallways are uncluttered, there is adequate lighting and chairs
- Educate patients how they can safely be active while connected to medical devices.

Fig. 19.1 Barriers to increasing older people's physical activity while in hospital and strategies to address these

While nurses are aware of the many benefits to older people of being more active while in hospital, a perceived lack of time is a common reason why they do not prescribe physical activity for them (Lamarche and Vallance 2013). Nurses also believe patients are apprehensive about being more active which is also a disincentive to encouraging activity (Lamarche and Vallance 2013). Staff are less likely to encourage older people who have a history of falls to get out of bed and be more physically active, fearing this may lead to further falls (Boltz et al. 2012). This creates a vicious cycle in which each fall causes further restriction in physical activities, which again increases the risk of falling and other adverse events associated with inactivity. Additional factors that may contribute to hospital staff being less likely to promote and support physical activity in older people include inadequate training, little reimbursement and a perceived lack of patient benefit (VanWormer et al. 2009).

At the level of the hospital system, organisational routines, availability of staff and equipment to ensure safe mobility have been identified as barriers to patients being physically active. Waiting for examinations and rounds can mean patients are reluctant to get out of bed and go for a walk as they are concerned they will miss seeing clinical staff or investigations (Holst et al. 2015). Both patients and nurses perceive a lack of nurses and physiotherapists are a barrier to older patients getting out of bed and walking more during their hospital stay (Brown et al. 2007). Hospital staff have also acknowledged that a lack of gait aids is a barrier to patients walking more (Brown et al. 2007). This study also identified that patients perceived hospital gowns as a barrier to being active because 'Gowns lead to embarrassing moments, are designed for benefit of staff, not patients' (Brown et al. 2007, p. 310). Hospital staff also believe gowns prohibit mobility: 'I think the gown exposes the patient a lot and they might feel embarrassed to go around. And outside the hospital room, nobody wants to be perceived as sick and draw attention' (Brown et al. 2007, p. 310). Within rehabilitation hospitals, staff are becoming more aware of the need to provide clothing or encourage older people to wear their own clothing as it can help to maintain their dignity and promote physical activity. However, most patients in acute hospitals continue to wear hospital gowns even though there is no medical need for them (McDonald et al. 2014).

Characteristics of the hospital ward environments such as location of the television—it is often positioned so that optimal viewing is achieved when resting in bed (Brown et al. 2007)—and a lack of chairs (Kuys et al. 2011) or space for chairs in the hospital room are also barriers to older patients getting out of bed. Additionally, some medical treatments require the use of intravenous lines and catheters that may physically restrain older people from being more active in hospitals. Patients have described being tethered to equipment: 'If the nurse unplugs the IV line, I can walk okay. If not, I can walk only as far as the line will let me.' Some patients mentioned not wanting to bother the nurses: 'I know it would be good for me, but I just don't want to impose upon them' (Despond et al. 1999).

19.1.5 Practical Tips for Increasing Physical Activity of Older People While in Hospital

This section provides practical tips and strategies for increasing the physical activity levels of older patients. These are targeted to the older person, hospital staff and the hospital system reflecting multi-factorial barriers to activity presented in the above section. Of note, there is limited evidence specifically on the effectiveness of different implementation strategies for physical activity programmes targeted to older patients. Therefore, the strategies presented are based on the clinical experience of the authors and informed by the broader evidence base related to physical activity, hospital care and implementation science (see Fig. 19.1).

1. Ensure safety

Safety should be a priority when considering ways to optimise the physical activity levels of older patients. As highlighted at the start of the chapter, older patients can be unwell, medically unstable and have physical and cognitive impairments that impact on their ability to be safely physically active. Older people may become faint or unsteady when sitting out of bed or walking, increasing their risk of falls. Adequate fall prevention measures need to be in place to reduce the risk of falls (Oliver et al. 2010). For example, check the patients' medical notes and observation chart so that you understand their current medical, physical and cognitive status. Being at an increased risk of falls does not mean a patient should rest in bed to avoid falling. It means appropriate strategies should be in place to minimise the risk of a fall. For example, ensuring appropriate footwear, gait aid and assistance are used or educating staff and family members on how they can assist the patient to walk safely. It is also important to discuss physical activity plans with the patient's care team (prior to seeing the patient) to ensure there is input about what type of activity an individual patient would benefit most from. For example, bed or chair exercises for those who are less mobile versus walking programmes for those who are more mobile. On occasions, a patient will be assessed by the care team as requiring bed rest due to medical instability (e.g., unstable angina), unknown injuries (e.g., potential unstable fractures) or post-surgery (some orthopaedic procedures). It is important to ensure that the treating medical team is supportive of the patient being physically active and that it is not unsafe for the patient to get out of bed or perform certain movements or exercises. After gaining information and input from the care team it is important to speak to the patient before getting them out of bed or a chair.

Conversation around how they are feeling, how active they have been and what their knowledge and attitudes are about being physically active will help build a relationship with the patient. This information can be used to design a physical activity programme that is safe, effective and tailored to their needs and preferences (see Chap. 15).

2. Create a culture, system and environment that promotes physical activity as the norm.

Creating a culture where getting out of bed each day while in hospital is the norm rather than the exception will assist in older people to be more active while in hospital. Encouraging family to bring in comfortable clothing and footwear for patients to wear rather than hospital gowns is also likely to promote a 'get out of bed' culture. Likewise, ensuring the physical environment is conducive to physical activity is important; for example, adequate lighting, hand rails, chairs and beds that are at an appropriate height. The bedside, bathroom and hallway should be free of clutter (Boltz et al. 2012). Strategically positioned armchairs along hallways may encourage patients to walk more because they can rest if necessary (Landefeld et al. 1995). Including magazines, newspapers or other activities on tables with chairs may also encourage patients to get out of bed to read the paper or perform other activities of interest. Another strategy is to suggest patients eat their meals in a separate area of the ward—this will not only make them more active in hospital but also allows them to socialise with other patients on the ward. Acknowledge patient and staff efforts to increase physical activity so that there is positive reinforcement of a get out of bed culture.

3. Add resources—staff, equipment and training

Providing additional resources such as extra physiotherapy on the weekends has been shown to increase the number of steps older orthopaedic patients take while in hospital (Peiris et al. 2012). In addition to physiotherapists, nursing and allied health assistants are key people to help physically, and encourage, older patients to go for a walk and perform simple exercise programmes prescribed by physiotherapists. Many older patients require a gait aid such as a walking stick or walking frame to walk safely. Patients may have their own if this is something they used prior to their hospital admission or it may be a new requirement if their functional ability has changed with recent illness. Hospitals should have sufficient gait aids for patients to use during their hospital stay. These should be easily accessible with on-ward storage and well maintained to ensure safety. Need for a gait aid should be assessed on admission to hospital and provided at admission so that safe mobility can be promoted early in the stay. Positioning the gait aid within reach may encourage patients to go for a walk and minimise their risk of falls. Providing clinical staff such as doctors, nurses and allied health professionals with specific training on how to promote physical activity may also be beneficial. A nurse-driven mobility protocol which included a formal, intensive three-day continuing education programme demonstrated improvements in their patients' functional status at discharge and a shorter length of stay (Padula et al. 2009). Similarly, education of ward and multi-disciplinary team members as part of a multi-component intervention programme resulted in improvements in functional status as measured by the modified Barthel Index (Mudge et al. 2008).

4. Create formal activity programmes

As discussed in Chap. 10, formal activity programmes such as the STRIDE walking programme increases the likelihood of older patients being discharged directly home from hospital rather than to rehabilitation or residential aged care (Hastings et al. 2014). A supervised exercise programme following lower extremity bypass surgery also showed patients were able to walk more steps daily. Of note, patients undertaking the exercise programme had a lower incidence of adverse events compared to the inactive group (Matsuo et al. 2015). Implementing a similar programme that provides supervised walking along with education about the benefits of daily walking while in hospital may be beneficial to increase the physical activity levels of older patients. Likewise, daily exercise groups that focus on high intensity functional exercise supervised either by a physiotherapist or allied health assistant may also promote physical activity and functional independence (Toots et al. 2016).

5. Integrate physical activity into usual care

One strategy for improving activity levels is for nurses and allied health staff to encourage patients to be more independent when performing activities of daily living such as walking, bathing, dressing and eating, rather than performing these tasks for the patient. This approach was adopted in a study by Boltz et al. (2012). Function-focused care is an approach whereby nurses support patients to engage in activities of daily living and physical activity with the goal of preventing functional decline. Physical activity programmes need to be well integrated into existing staff workflows so that they do not overburden staff. For example, items relating to current physical activity levels, recommendations for ways to be physically active and the benefits of doing so should be incorporated into admission assessments and patient handover. For example, staff could hand over the level of assistance a patient requires to walk or the number of times they have walked or sat out of bed in a day.

6. Use support materials

Reminders such as posters and signs promoting clinicians to discuss, encourage and integrate strategies into care plans may help to increase activity levels of older patients (Mudge et al. 2008). Additionally, providing simple education materials to older people and their families and carers that promote the benefits of physical activity as well as reminders to be active may motivate them to be active while in hospital. For example, a poster that has a phrase like 'a short walk a day shortens the hospital stay' could be placed in a patient's bedroom. In addition, a handout of bedside exercises could be provided to encourage patients to be active whilst waiting for ward rounds or transport for tests or imaging. These materials should be tailored appropriately to the intended audience.

7. Start early in the hospital stay, don't forget the weekends and adopt a little and often approach!

As functional decline begins soon after admission, it is important to screen older people when they are admitted to hospital so an appropriate care plan can be implemented to promote their physical activity. It is well-established that patients are less active on weekends (Davenport et al. 2015). Thus, there is a need for staff to encourage patients to continue being active every day of the week, including weekends, while in hospital. Providing an exercise programme that patients can complete on their own is important because even simple bed or chair exercises can reduce loss of muscle strength in older people. Additionally, keeping sessions short may minimise fatigue and optimise adherence—taking a short walk is less daunting than doing 20 minutes of exercises. Given their low physical activity levels in hospital, any amount of activity will be more beneficial than simply resting in bed.

8. Physical activity is everyone's business and champions are required

Engage the family, carers and support people in the promotion of physical activity. Clinical staff should communicate with patients, their family and carers about the benefits of, and expectations and opportunities for, older people to be physically active while in hospital. Due to their ability to observe and guide patients 24 hours a day, nurses play a key role in promoting older people to be physically active in hospital. This is particularly important in the acute hospitals where the length of stay is short. If nurses do not promote physical activity, patients may remain inactive as they may not be seen by therapy staff if admitted after hours or over the weekend. However, promoting physical activity during a hospital admission should be a priority for all clinical staff including doctors, allied health professionals such as dieticians and podiatrists and patient care assistants. Clinical staff should identify those most at risk of functional decline, assess their individual needs and based on these, multi-professional interventions implemented. All clinical staff also need to encourage patients to be more physically active. This could be as simple as encouraging them to sit out of bed instead of resting in bed or taking them for a walk on the ward.

9. Ensure physical activity care plans are patient-centred, positively framed and reviewed and updated regularly

As noted earlier, the profile of older patients is diverse. One single approach to optimising physical activity will not meet the needs of all older patients. Programmes may require adaptation to address specific underlying conditions, for example, stroke, lower-limb arthroplasty or chronic obstructive pulmonary disease. In addition to the tailoring to clinical needs, programmes should be tailored to the preferences and interests of the individual. Programmes that are patient-centred—aligned with an individual's interests and goals—are more likely to promote participation. It may be beneficial for staff to ask the patient about their hobbies and interests so that they can design activity programmes that align with these. The use of motivational interviewing and goal-setting techniques can also help optimise participation in physical activity programmes (see Section 3 of this Handbook).

Clinical staff should help patients to identify physical activity goals, barriers and enablers. Regular progress checks should be scheduled to provide feedback, ensure activities are appropriate and maintain older people's motivation to continue to be active. Framing messages about being physically active as positive rather than negative is likely to achieve greater uptake. Promoting that exercise can enhance well-being and recovery motivates older people to be more active while in hospital (So and Pierluissi 2012). For example, when encouraging older patients to get out of bed or go for a walk, using positive frames such as 'you will feel more energised and keep your legs strong' rather than negative risk frames like 'you are more likely to get a pressure sore or chest infection if you stay in bed' are likely to motivate older patients to be more active.

10. Make it social

For many older patients, adding a social component to physical activity will enhance uptake. For example, assisting a small number of patients to walk to a communal area so they can have morning tea together may be more enticing than simply encouraging them to get out of bed and go for a walk without purpose.

19.1.6 Increasing Physical Activity Levels in Older Patients: Learnings from the Field of Implementation Science

The introduction of effective physical activity interventions in hospitals is a complex process. The section below adds depth to the above discussion by reviewing knowledge from the field of implementation science about the successful implementation of health programmes in clinical settings such as hospitals.

Grol and colleagues have identified three stages to consider when introducing a new health programme into clinical practice (Cosby 2006). There needs to be a decision to work with an intervention (the adoption stage), deliver it as intended (the implementation stage) and continue to use it over a longer period of time (the continuation stage). These stages require changes in organisation, patient and professional behaviour.

At the adoption stage, a critical first step is to identify a champion who will take a leadership role in designing and implementing the physical activity programme. Key activities of the champion at this stage include stakeholder engagement, establishment of a working group, gaining information about the local problem and establishing potential programme components that align with local needs and resources. It is important to build an alliance among key stakeholders who will be involved with or affected by the programme delivery within the adoption stage. This includes nursing, medical and allied health staff and, importantly, older patients. The adoption stage should facilitate the development of shared understandings about the local problem of inactivity of older patients and create local solutions. Understanding the local problem might involve activities such as audits of time patients spend sitting out of bed and number of walks undertaken each day. Environmental audits to identify hazards and facilitators to patient mobility and access to equipment should be undertaken. Talking to patients, staff and families about their perceptions of the value of, and barriers to physical activity amongst older patients will help in designing strategies tailored to the local problem of inactivity. The working group should identify what will work best for the team, ward, unit or hospital, and opportunities to integrate the programme within existing care processes. Resources such as staff and patient education materials and tools and processes for audits, reminders and feedback will need to be developed and, ideally, pilot-tested to ensure optimum usability.

At the implementation stage, physical activity programmes are delivered as part of usual care. This may involve staff training and education regarding the new process, modification of patient documentation such as assessments and care plans, modification of the ward environment, and installation of equipment and support materials such as reminder posters. As part of this stage, it is important to gain feedback from the patients, their family and hospital staff on their views on the programme's effectiveness and perceived success of the implementation. This may lead to further programme refinement and implementation strategies.

In the continuation stage, it is important to create formal processes that ensure the programme is sustained over time. This includes integration of programme components and outcomes into hospital systems so that the physical activity programme becomes part of the hospital's core business and culture.

19.2 Conclusion

A variety of factors relating to patients, clinical staff, the hospital system and environment influence how physically active an older person is when in hospital. Despite an abundance of evidence of very low levels of physical activity amongst older patients, there is limited evidence to support interventions for increasing physical activity. Little is also known about the potential benefits this may have for the older person, hospital staff and the health care system. However, the strategies and practical tips presented in this chapter build on learnings from research evidence and the authors' clinical experience, representing a best-evidence synthesis of strategies to promote physical activity in older patients. Best practice hospital care should strive to promote the physical activity of older people to minimise the risk of functional decline and the negative effects outlined at the beginning of this chapter. Strategies to promote physical activity in hospitalised older adults include: comprehensive assessment of physical, psychosocial, cognitive and functional status at admission; staff encouraging patients to get out of bed and perform everyday activities like walking, showering and dressing during their admission; implementation of structured exercise and walking programmes; ensuring access to gait aids, appropriate clothing and footwear to encourage mobility and use of environmental enhancements such as handrails, chairs and uncluttered hallways. Importantly, safety must be considered and promoted while encouraging independence and mobility, to ensure that older people do not fall or experience other adverse events as a result of inappropriate activity. Programmes should be tailored to the individual needs and preferences of each older person to optimise participation.

Suggested Further Reading

- Brown, C. J., Williams, B. R., Woodby, L. L., Davis, L. L., & Allman, R. M. (2007). Barriers to mobility during hospitalization from the perspectives of older patients and their nurses and physicians. *Journal of Hospital Medicine, 2*(5), 305–313. doi: https://doi.org/10.1002/jhm.209.
- Grol, R., & Grimshaw, J. (2003). From best evidence to best practice: Effective implementation of change in patients' care. *The Lancet, 362*(9391), 1225–1230.
- Tucker, S. J., & Carr, L. J. (2016). Translating physical activity evidence to hospital settings: A call for culture change. *Clinical Nurse Specialist, 30*(4), 208–215.

References

Agmon, M., Zisberg, A., Gil, E., Rand, D., Gur-Yaish, N., & Azriel, M. (2017). Association between 900 steps a day and functional decline in older hospitalized patients. *JAMA Internal Medicine, 177*(2), 272–274.

Astrand, A., Saxin, C., Sjoholm, A., Skarin, M., Linden, T., Stoker, A., et al. (2016). Poststroke physical activity levels no higher in rehabilitation than in the acute hospital. *Journal of Stroke and Cerebrovascular Diseases, 25*(4), 938–945. https://doi.org/10.1016/j.jstrokecerebrovasdis.2015.12.046.

Australian Institute of Health and Welfare. (2012). Australian Hospital Statistics 2010–11. Health services series no. 43. Cat. no. HSE 117. Retrieved from Canberra.

Australian Institute of Health and Welfare. (2016). *Australia's health 2016*. Australia's health series no. 15. Cat. no. AUS 199. Canberra: AIHW.

Boltz, M., Resnick, B., Capezuti, E., Shuluk, J., & Secic, M. (2012). Functional decline in hospitalized older adults: Can nursing make a difference? *Geriatric Nursing, 33*(4), 272–279. https://doi.org/10.1016/j.gerinurse.2012.01.008.

Brown, C. J., Friedkin, R. J., & Inouye, S. K. (2004). Prevalence and outcomes of low mobility in hospitalized older patients. *Journal of the American Geriatrics Society, 52*(8), 1263–1270. https://doi.org/10.1111/j.1532-5415.2004.52354.x.

Brown, C. J., Williams, B. R., Woodby, L. L., Davis, L. L., & Allman, R. M. (2007). Barriers to mobility during hospitalization from the perspectives of older patients and their nurses and physicians. *Journal of Hospital Medicine, 2*(5), 305–313. https://doi.org/10.1002/jhm.209.

Buttery, A. K., & Martin, F. C. (2009). Knowledge, attitudes and intentions about participation in physical activity of older post-acute hospital inpatients. *Physiotherapy, 95*(3), 192–198. https://doi.org/10.1016/j.physio.2009.03.002.

Buurman, B. M., Hoogerduijn, J. G., de Haan, R. J., Abu-Hanna, A., Lagaay, A. M., Verhaar, H. J., et al. (2011). Geriatric conditions in acutely hospitalized older patients: Prevalence and one-year survival and functional decline. *PLoS One, 6*(11), e26951. https://doi.org/10.1371/journal.pone.0026951.

Convertino, V. A. (1997). Cardiovascular consequences of bed rest: Effect on maximal oxygen uptake. *Medicine and Science in Sports and Exercise, 29*(2), 191.

Convertino, V., Hung, J., Goldwater, D., & Debusk, R. F. (1982). Cardiovascular responses to exercise in middle-aged men after 10 days of bedrest. *Circulation, 65*(1), 134.

Convertino, V. A., Bloomfield, S. A., & Greenleaf, J. E. (1997). An overview of the issues: Physiological effects of bed rest and restricted physical activity. *Medicine and Science in Sports and Exercise, 29*(2), 187.

Cosby, J. L. (2006). *Improving patient care: The implementation of change in clinical practice*. Elsevier: BMJ Publishing Group.

Covinsky, K. E., Palmer, R. M., Fortinsky, R. H., Counsell, S. R., Stewart, A. L., Kresevic, D., et al. (2003). Loss of independence in activities of daily living in older adults hospitalized with medical illnesses: Increased vulnerability with age. *Journal of the American Geriatrics Society, 51*(4), 451–458.

Davenport, S. J., Arnold, M., Hua, C., Schenck, A., Batten, S., & Taylor, N. F. (2015). Physical activity levels during acute inpatient admission after hip fracture are very low. *Physiotherapy Research International, 20*(3), 174–181.

de Morton, N. A., Nolan, J., O'Brien, M., Thomas, S., Govier, A., Sherwell, K., et al. (2015). A head-to-head comparison of the de Morton mobility index (DEMMI) and elderly mobility scale (EMS) in an older acute medical population. *Disability and Rehabilitation, 37*(20), 1881. https://doi.org/10.3109/09638288.2014.982832.

Despond, O., Buchser, E., Sprunger, A. L., & Sloutkis, D. (1999). Influence of patient's dressing on spontaneous physical activity and length of hospital stay in surgical patients. *Sozial-und Präventivmedizin, 44*(1), 8–13.

Dewing, J. (2001). Care for older people with a dementia in acute hospital settings. *Nursing Older People, 13*(3), 18–20. PubMed PMID: 12008241.

Fisher, S. R., Graham, J. E., Ottenbacher, K. J., Deer, R., & Ostir, G. V. (2016). Inpatient walking activity to predict readmission in older adults. *Archives of Physical Medicine and Rehabilitation, 97*(9 Suppl), S226–S231. https://doi.org/10.1016/j.apmr.2015.09.029.

Gasior, K. (2012). In R. Rodrigues, M. Huber, & G. Lamura (Eds.), *Facts and figures on healthy ageing and long-term care, Europe and North America, Occasional reports series 8*. Vienna: European Centre.

Gill, T. M., Allore, H. G., Gahbauer, E. A., & Murphy, T. E. (2010). Change in disability after hospitalization or restricted activity in older persons. *JAMA, 304*(17), 1919–1928. https://doi.org/10.1001/jama.2010.1568.

Gorgon, E., Said, C., & Galea, M. (2007). Mobility on discharge from an aged care unit. *Physiotherapy Research International, 12*(2), 72.

Hall, M. J., DeFrances, C. J., Williams, S. N., Golosinskiy, A., & Schwartzman, A. (2010). National Hospital Discharge Survey: 2007 summary. *National Health Statistics Reports, 29*(1–20), 24.

Hastings, S. N., Sloane, R., Morey, M. C., Pavon, J. M., & Hoenig, H. (2014). Assisted early mobility for hospitalized older veterans: Preliminary data from the STRIDE program. *Journal of the American Geriatrics Society, 62*(11), 2180–2184. https://doi.org/10.1111/jgs.13095.

Hirsch, C. H., Sommers, L., Olsen, A., Mullen, L., & Winograd, C. H. (1990). The natural history of functional morbidity in hospitalized older patients. *Journal of the American Geriatrics Society, 38*(12), 1296–1303. https://doi.org/10.1111/j.1532-5415.1990.tb03451.x.

Hirshon, J. M., Risko, N., Calvello, E. J. B., de Ramirez, S. S., Narayan, M., Theodosis, C., & Oneill, J. (2013). Health systems and services: The role of acute care. (Perspectives). *Bulletin of the World Health Organization, 91*(5), 386.

Holst, M., Hansen, P. L., Pedersen, L. A., Paulsen, S., Valentinsen, C. D., & Kohler, M. (2015). Physical activity in hospitalised elderly medical patients: How active are they, and what motivates to physical activity. *Journal of Aging Research and Clinical Practice, 4*(2), 116–123.

Izawa, K. P., Watanabe, S., Oka, K., Osada, N., Omiya, K., Brubaker, P. H., & Shimizu, H. (2014). Differences in daily in-hospital physical activity and geriatric nutritional risk index in older cardiac inpatients: Preliminary results. *Aging Clinical and Experimental Research, 26*(6), 599–605. https://doi.org/10.1007/s40520-014-0233-z.

Kortebein, P., Symons, T. B., Ferrando, A., Paddon-Jones, D., Ronsen, O., Protas, E., et al. (2008). Functional impact of 10 days of bed rest in healthy older adults. *The Journals of Gerontology Series A: Biological Sciences and Medical Sciences, 63*(10), 1076–1081.

Kuys, S. S., Dolecka, U. E., & Morrison, C. A. (2011). Appropriate seating for medical patients: An audit. *Australian Health Review, 35*(3), 316–319. https://doi.org/10.1071/AH10943.

Lafreniere, S., Folch, N., Dubois, S., Bedard, L., & Ducharme, F. (2015). Strategies used by older patients to prevent functional decline during hospitalization. *Clinical Nursing Research.* https://doi.org/10.1177/1054773815601392.

Lamarche, K., & Vallance, J. (2013). Prescription for physical activity a survey of Canadian nurse practitioners. *The Canadian Nurse, 109*(8), 22–26.

Landefeld, C. S., Palmer, R. M., Kresevic, D. M., Fortinsky, R. H., & Kowal, J. (1995). A randomized trial of care in a hospital medical unit especially designed to improve the functional outcomes of acutely ill older patients. *New England Journal of Medicine, 332*(20), 1338–1344. https://doi.org/10.1056/Nejm199505183322006.

Levit, K., Wier, L., Stranges, E., Ryan, K., & Elixhauser, A. (2009). HCUP facts and figures: Statistics on hospital-based Care in the United States, 2007. Retrieved from http://www.hcup-us.ahrq.gov/reports.jsp

Lindgren, M., Unosson, M., Fredrikson, M., & Ek, A. C. (2004). Immobility – A major risk factor for development of pressure ulcers among adult hospitalized patients: A prospective study. *Scandinavian Journal of Caring Sciences, 18*(1), 57–64. https://doi.org/10.1046/j.0283-9318.2003.00250.x.

Matsuo, T., Sakaguchi, T., Ishida, A., Yuguchi, S., Saito, K., Nakajima, M., et al. (2015). Effect of in-hospital physical activity on cardiovascular prognosis in lower extremity bypass for claudication. *Journal of Physical Therapy Science, 27*(6), 1855–1859. https://doi.org/10.1589/jpts.27.1855.

McCullagh, R., Brady, N. M., Dillon, C., Horgan, N. F., & Timmons, S. (2016). A review of the accuracy and utility of motion sensors to measure physical activity of frail, older hospitalized patients. *Journal of Aging and Physical Activity, 24*(3), 465–475. https://doi.org/10.1123/japa.2014-0190.

McDonald, E. G., Dounaevskaia, V., & Lee, T. C. (2014). Inpatient attire: An opportunity to improve the patient experience. *JAMA Internal Medicine, 174*(11), 1865. https://doi.org/10.1001/jamainternmed.2014.4513.

Mortimer, J., & Green, M. (2015, October). *The health and care of older people in England 2015.* Age UK.

Mudge, A. M., Giebel, A. J., Mgt, M. A., & Cutler, A. J. (2008). Exercising body and mind: An integrated approach to functional independence in hospitalized older people. *Journal of the American Geriatrics Society, 56*(4), 630–635. https://doi.org/10.1111/j.1532-5415.2007.01607.x.

Naylor, M., & Keating, S. A. (2008). Transitional care: Moving patients from one care setting to another. *The American Journal of Nursing, 108*(9 Suppl), 58–63. https://doi.org/10.1097/01.NAJ.0000336420.34946.3a.

Nitz, J. C., & Low Choy, N. (2008). Falling is not just for older women: Support for pre-emptive prevention intervention before 60. *Climacteric, 11*(6), 461–466. https://doi.org/10.1080/13697130802398517.

Oliver, D., Healey, F., & Haines, T. P. (2010). Preventing falls and fall-related injuries in hospitals. *Clinics in Geriatric Medicine, 26*(4), 645–692. https://doi.org/10.1016/j.cger.2010.06.005.

Ong, T., Anand, V., Tan, W., Watson, A., & Sahota, O. (2016). Physical activity study of older people in hospital: A cross-sectional analysis using accelerometers. *European Geriatric Medicine, 7*(1), 55–56. https://doi.org/10.1016/j.eurger.2015.10.008.

Ottenbacher, K. J., Smith, P. M., Illig, S. B., Linn, R. T., Ostir, G. V., & Granger, C. V. (2004). Trends in length of stay, living setting, functional outcome, and mortality following medical rehabilitation. *JAMA, 292*(14), 1687.

Padula, C. A., Hughes, C., & Baumhover, L. (2009). Impact of a nurse-driven mobility protocol on functional decline in hospitalized older adults. *Journal of Nursing Care Quality, 24*(4), 325–331. https://doi.org/10.1097/NCQ.0b013e3181a4f79b.

Peiris, C. L., Taylor, N. F., & Shields, N. (2012). Additional Saturday allied health services increase habitual physical activity among patients receiving inpatient rehabilitation for lower limb orthopedic conditions: A randomized controlled trial. *Archives of Physical Medicine and Rehabilitation, 93*(8), 1365–1370. https://doi.org/10.1016/j.apmr.2012.03.004.

So, C., & Pierluissi, E. (2012). Attitudes and expectations regarding exercise in the hospital of hospitalized older adults: A qualitative study. *Journal of the American Geriatrics Society, 60*(4), 713–718. https://doi.org/10.1111/j.1532-5415.2012.03900.x.

Tolson, D., Smith, M., & Knight, P. (1999). An investigation of the components of best nursing practice in the care of acutely ill hospitalized older patients with coincidental dementia: A multi-method design. *Journal of Advanced Nursing, 30*(5), 1127–1136. PubMed PMID: 10564412.

Toots, A., Littbrand, H., Lindelöf, N., Wiklund, R., Holmberg, H., Nordström, P., et al. (2016). Effects of a high-intensity functional exercise program on dependence in activities of daily living and balance in older adults with dementia. *Journal of the American Geriatrics Society, 64*(1), 55–64. https://doi.org/10.1111/jgs.13880.

Tudor-Locke, C., Craig, C. L., Aoyagi, Y., Bell, R. C., Croteau, K. A., De Bourdeaudhuij, I., et al. (2011). How many steps/day are enough? For older adults and special populations. *The International Journal of Behavioral Nutrition and Physical Activity, 8*, 80–80. https://doi.org/10.1186/1479-5868-8-80.

Turner-Stokes, L. (2007). Cost-efficiency of longer-stay rehabilitation programmes: Can they provide value for money. *Brain Injury, 21*(10), 1015–1021. https://doi.org/10.1080/02699050701591445.

VanWormer, J. J., Pronk, N. P., & Kroeninger, G. J. (2009). Clinical counseling for physical activity: Translation of a systematic review into care recommendations. *Diabetes Spectrum, 22*(1), 48–55.

Villumsen, M., Jorgensen, M. G., Andreasen, J., Rathleff, M. S., & Molgaard, C. M. (2015). Very low levels of physical activity in older patients during hospitalization at an acute geriatric Ward: A prospective cohort study. *Journal of Aging and Physical Activity, 23*(4), 542–549. https://doi.org/10.1123/japa.2014-0115.

Zisberg, A., Shadmi, E., Sinoff, G., Gur-Yaish, N., Srulovici, E., & Admi, H. (2011). Low mobility during hospitalization and functional decline in older adults. *Journal of the American Geriatrics Society, 59*(2), 266–273. https://doi.org/10.1111/j.1532-5415.2010.03276.x.

Zisberg, A., Shadmi, E., Gur-Yaish, N., Tonkikh, O., & Sinoff, G. (2015). Hospital-associated functional decline: The role of hospitalization processes beyond individual risk factors. *Journal of the American Geriatrics Society, 63*(1), 55–62. https://doi.org/10.1111/jgs.13193.

20

Implementing Physical Activity Programmes for Community-Dwelling Older People with Early Signs of Physical Frailty

Afroditi Stathi, Max Western, Jolanthe de Koning, Oliver Perkin, and Janet Withall

20.1 Introduction

Frailty and associated comorbidities compromise quality of life for older adults and contribute major societal costs, directly to people who live with frailty, to friends and family providing care and losing productivity, and to the health and social care services (Clegg et al. 2013; National Centre for Social Research 2010). In a US-wide sample, 15.3% of >65-year-olds were recognised as frail; however, a third of adults aged 85–89 years and 38% of people over the age of 90 were classified as frail (Bandeen-Roche et al. 2015). The English Longitudinal Study of Ageing observed a 14% prevalence of frailty (Gale et al. 2015). Adults aged over 75 years accounted for 60% of hospital admissions, despite representing only 43% of the over 65-year-old population. Worldwide, 11% of people over the age of 65 meet frailty criteria (Ward 2013), while 42% are estimated to have mild frailty or pre-frailty (Collard et al. 2012).

The Cardiovascular Health Study-Frailty Phenotype proposes five criteria for defining frailty including unintentional weight loss, self-reported exhaustion, weakness (measured by grip strength), slow walking speed, or low physical activity (Fried et al. 2001). People are classified as non-frail if they meet no criteria, pre-frail if they meet one or two criteria, and frail if they meet three

A. Stathi (✉) • M. Western • J. de Koning • O. Perkin • J. Withall
Department for Health, University of Bath, Bath, UK

or more criteria. Just moving from pre-frail to frail incurs substantial health and social care costs, highlighting the importance of implementation of preventive strategies to delay, or in some cases reverse, the transition into full frailty (Bock et al. 2016). This is particularly important as in the UK spending on healthcare is projected to see the largest rise of all elements of age-related spending, rising from 6.8% to 9.1% of GDP between 2016–2017 and 2061–2062 (Silcock and Sinclair 2012). Physical frailty as defined by Fried et al. (2001) is a medical syndrome with numerous causes that can result in functional decline, increased dependence, and/or death (Morley et al. 2013). Crucially, there is considerable evidence that physical features of frailty such as reduced muscular strength or endurance can be reversed, or at least the progression of these frailty indicators can be slowed, by undertaking an appropriate exercise programme (Giné-Garriga et al. 2014; Pahor et al. 2014).

20.2 Challenges of Implementing Physical Activity Programmes for People with Early Signs of Physical Frailty

The evidence base supports the beneficial effects of physical activity in older adults with early signs of physical frailty although some uncertainty exists regarding the optimal type and dose (Chase et al. 2017; Giné-Garriga et al. 2014). However, older adults do not engage in community exercise programmes in significant numbers (Chatfield et al. 2005; Harris and Dyson 2001).

A recent systematic review of the challenges of recruiting and retaining frail older adults defined frail people as a population with reduced reserves and resistance to stressors, and thus at increased risk of falls, disability, hospitalisation, and institutionalisation (Provencher et al. 2014). The 15 studies included focussed on the challenges and strategies pertaining to recruitment and retention but did not target people with dementia or cancer or those residing in nursing homes. Of the 15 studies, only 3 were rated as having good methodological quality. Few studies compared the impact of specific challenges and strategies on recruitment of participants. As a result, there is only limited evidence as to how different barriers affect engagement and dropout of frail older adults and how these issues can best be addressed.

The evidence is clearly limited and is mainly based on findings from English-speaking countries. The available data suggests that there are specific challenges in engaging frailer older adults in physical activity, while there are some approaches which may be effective (Harris and Dyson 2001; Provencher et al. 2014). The following section summarises barriers to physical activity that are commonly cited by those exhibiting early signs of frailty.

20.2.1 The Perception That 'I Am Not Frail'

Often older people do not consider themselves to be frail or understand exactly what the word means, while some actively dislike the term (Ipsos MORI 2014). Therefore, recruitment materials and approaches should avoid this term and instead adopt a positive message approach and provide alternative means by which participants can self-identify as suitable for the programme (Harris and Dyson 2001). More acceptable mechanisms for identifying frailty could include asking older adults to assess how difficult they find completing activities of daily living.

20.2.2 The Perception That 'I Am Too Old'

A lack of perceived benefits or an underestimation of the potential positive effects of physical activity has been shown to deter people from taking part in tailored exercise programmes (Provencher et al. 2014). Attitudes such as 'I am too old' or 'my family will think I'm crazy' reflect a lack of self-efficacy, negative social influences, and an overestimation of the effort and risk involved (Hawley-Hague et al. 2016). When promoting physical activity to older adults, it may be beneficial to address this issue when advertising programmes and directly tackle it during the first contact. Clear, straightforward education regarding the benefits, effort, and risks involved could influence engagement, while using case studies featuring 'people like me' could be powerful (Freiberger et al. 2016).

20.2.3 The Perception That 'I'm Not the Sporty Type'

A recent review synthesised ten qualitative studies which assessed the acceptability of physical activity to older adults who were living independently. A significant finding was that older adults considered physical activity to be a by-product of engaging in other activities. They walked in order to access local amenities, shop, and visit friends and family. The physical activity involved tended not to be their prime purpose. This was associated with their view of themselves as 'old', that physical activity was not relevant to them and that other priorities, especially their family, took precedence (McGowan et al. 2017).

Older adults, particularly those 70 and older, did not grow up in an era when exercise was regarded as a leisure activity; rather it was a by-product of a physical job. This may explain why few older people see physical activity as a pleasurable pastime and most activity they undertake is a means to an end (Craig et al. 2009; Davis et al. 2011). Historically, one of the main reasons cited by middle aged to older adults as to why they are not active for health is because they are not the 'sporty' type (Allied Dunbar 1992). This identifying as a non-active person is partly related to the association of physical activity with a level of sporting prowess that they don't possess. This perception of increased activity as too demanding and requiring of skills and know-how they don't have is a substantial barrier to increased activity (Stathi et al. 2014). With only limited, if any, experience of physical activity programmes, these attitudes and beliefs go unchallenged and often prevent engagement. Methods of tackling this issue include programmes designed to increase incidental, lifestyle activity, avoidance of terms such as sport, exercise, and even physical activity in recruitment materials and provision of taster sessions (McGowan et al. 2017; Withall et al. 2016).

20.2.4 The Perception That 'It Is Not Safe for Me'

Fear of falling has been strongly associated with diminished function (Malini et al. 2016; Rochat et al. 2010). It is a factor that influences activity levels across older groups and is likely to be particularly relevant in frail older adults. A decline in strength, coordination, and balance often reduces confidence and increases fear of injury and falling when exercising (Stathi et al. 2014). A study that considered the impact of threat appraisal (fear of falling, its consequences, and perceived risk) and of coping appraisal (benefits and appropriateness of the programme) found intention to exercise to be more closely related to coping appraisal than to threat appraisal (Yardley et al. 2006). Coping appraisal included the belief in the benefits of exercise, a positive social identity, and the perception that family, friends, and doctors would be supportive of exercise participation. This supports the potential power of influencing positive beliefs about exercising amongst not only frail older adults but also amongst their support networks.

Many older adults believe that as they age they should start to take it easy rather than doing more. They often believe that their incidental activity (gardening, housework, shopping, etc.) constitutes sufficient exercise (Stathi et al. 2014). The feeling that exercise is unsafe can be exacerbated by the fact that it can result in sweating, increased heart and breathing rates, and potentially pain and muscle soreness. Fear that these effects are damaging health and increasing risks can be a profound barrier to engagement (Stathi et al. 2014).

20.2.5 Professionals' and Social Network's Concerns About Risk of Exercising

Support networks can provide both positive and negative influences. Cited barriers to exercising often include the concerns and attitudes of nurses and GPs who are unsure of the risks of exercising for older adults. Particularly in the case of patients they consider to be frail, this may lead to their voicing concerns about potential injury, which naturally acts as a powerful deterrent (Freiberger et al. 2016). It is therefore important, where possible, to involve medical personnel in session recruitment and participation support and to provide them with specific education on the benefits of exercise for their older patients, across the frailty spectrum. Similarly, concerned friends and family members can easily discourage participation, so they need to be educated regarding not only the potential benefits but also the positive influence they can have (Provencher et al. 2014). Intervention providers and session leaders can negatively impact engagement if there is a reticence about including people with chronic disease or people who appear to be frail. Specialist training and education can tackle this. Exercise instructors need to be knowledgeable and experienced in the challenges and complexity of working with older participants, how to cope with the impact of common chronic diseases and frailty, and when exercising is contraindicated. In this way the programme will be run safely, and both instructor and participants will be confident and reassured (see Chap. 17).

20.2.6 Transport Issues

Issues of transport are particularly relevant to uptake and participation in community programmes. Infrequent, unreliable, and difficult to access public transport is commonly cited by older adults as negatively impacting their ability to be generally physically active (to get out and about) and to access physical activity sessions in particular (Stathi et al. 2012). With increasing inability to walk far and the resulting difficulty of using public transport, accessing a community programme can appear impossible to frailer adults (Provencher et al. 2014). Techniques that address this are engagement with community transport providers, volunteer drivers, lift-sharing schemes, and engaging family and friends to provide support. Addressing this problem and potential solutions in recruitment materials could positively impact recruitment. It could prevent older adults from immediately ruling themselves out of any community programme because they feel it is inaccessible. The challenge is then to manage a reliable, consistent transport solution within the auspices of programme delivery. An alternative approach is to focus on home exercise programs where barriers such as lack of transport, confidence, and time have less impact. Participation in home exercise programmes can be low. However, a study looking at home exercising in relation to falls prevention concluded that participation was positively affected by the inclusion of balance exercises or increased walking, home visit or telephone support, and physiotherapist-led delivery (Simek et al. 2015).

20.2.7 Compromised Health as a Barrier to Regular Commitment

Older people regularly cite health issues as their main barrier to becoming more active (Schutzer and Graves 2004). Qualitative findings show health problems (pain, functional limitations, loss of strength, and energy) have the most influence on older adults' physical activity decisions (Stathi et al. 2012). In particular, health issues reduce uptake of physical activity by frailer adults and are common causes of dropping out (Provencher et al. 2014). Promising strategies include being flexible about time and place, although this may not always be practical; reminder phone calls to discuss strategies to work around health issues; and cue cards to remind participants of session times. Being clear at the point of uptake that it is acceptable to miss sessions in the case of health issues or medical appointments, and actively supporting participants to return to the programme after illness, is also important. Even with discontinuity of attendance, participants still benefit from physical activity programmes (Cesari et al. 2015; Phillips et al. 2010). In fact participants can be motivated by the persistence of less functional participants and benefit from witnessing that people can reinitiate participation after significant health problems (Rejeski et al. 2013).

20.2.8 Lack of Social Support

A lack of social support to be active negatively affects participation. Many older adults prefer to engage in physical activity with others (Dye and Wilcox 2006). Not having a friend or relative to attend with can make participation less likely (Annear et al. 2009; Withall et al. 2016). People are particularly anxious about attending alone, joining a pre-existing group where they don't know anyone and not being socially accepted by the group (Graham and Connelly 2013; Janssen and Stube 2014). Programmes adopting a peer supporter or buddying model offering support to attend sessions show some potential (Withall et al. 2016).

Older adults report the importance of short-term, rather than long-term, benefits. Factors such as enjoyment and socialising are programme elements repeatedly reported as having a positive influence on uptake and participation (McPhate et al. 2016). Frail older adults participate more in programmes with enjoyable and sociable aspects (Rejeski et al. 2013). The LIFE study found the social environment was valued independently of the physical activity aspects of the programme and positively impacted attendance. This indicates community programmes should consider how to proactively facilitate social interaction, build group cohesion, and maximise enjoyment. These are too important to be just accidental by-products and should be a key focus of programme development (Gateway to Research 2015).

20.2.9 A Lack of Progress Recognition

Session leader training can neglect the importance of reflecting on participants' success and celebrating their progress. Training programmes should emphasise the importance of observing and celebrating participant success to underline the positive outcomes of their attendance so the group becomes a means of instilling pride in accomplishments (Rejeski et al. 2013). These include a focus on their perception of functional improvement and health benefit (Cesari et al. 2015), so the participant is motivated to maintain session attendance as they recognise the benefits they are feeling in their daily life.

In general, factors discussed above in relation to uptake also impact participant engagement with community programmes (Provencher et al. 2014; Stathi et al. 2010). A review of 20 quantitative studies reported lower levels of participation in group-based interventions that lasted 20 weeks or longer, had two or fewer sessions per week, or incorporated a flexibility component (McPhate et al. 2013). A review of 132 qualitative studies reported six major themes affected participation: social influences (pleasurable socialising, social anxiety, social support, and encouragement); physical limitations, pain, and fear of falling; other priorities; accessibility and affordability; benefits of increased activity (improved physical function, health, self-confidence, and mental well-being); and motivation and beliefs (Franco et al. 2015). A further review identified similar themes with the addition of empowering/energising effects and the impact of instructor behaviour (Farrance et al. 2016).

20.3 Characteristics of Promising Physical Activity Programmes for People with Early Signs of Physical Frailty

20.3.1 Range of Types of Exercise

As is often the case when promoting and implementing physical activity programmes in any setting, there is not a one-size-fits-all approach for community-dwelling individuals with early signs of frailty (Chase 2013). Current recommendations for adults over 65 stress the importance of accumulating a minimum of 150 minutes of moderate to vigorous physical activity and incorporate exercises to improve balance and muscle strength on two days a week (World Health Organisation 2010). This recommendation is a challenging target for many older adults especially those with early signs of frailty.

However, given their existing low levels of activity and physical function, doing more regardless of current activity level provides important physical and mental health benefits for all older adults. Moving towards the recommended amounts of activity should always receive priority over pushing too hard too early, particularly in older adults with early signs of physical frailty. Programmes that include a range of exercise modalities (i.e. aerobic, strength, flexibility, and balance) can target the various physiological factors contributing to frailty and are therefore recommended (Chodzko-Zajko et al. 2009; Theou et al. 2011).

A key aim of any exercise programme for individuals with early signs of frailty is to help them maintain independence and community engagement (Giné-Garriga et al. 2014). Thus, to prevent or even reverse the onset of mobility problems, programmes should put a lot of emphasis on lower body activities and the promotion of walking (Chou et al. 2012). Examples of lower body activities could be body weight strengthening of major muscle groups such as stepping up onto a raised surface, or repeatedly standing up from a chair, and balance and flexibility activities such as walking sideways or backwards, stretching, Pilates, and Tai Chi (Elsawy and Higgins 2010). Even if a programme doesn't incorporate structured walking activities, it should be designed to actively promote walking and support participants' confidence to do so (Bauman et al. 2016). Finally, an important characteristic of the exercise plan for individuals in this target group is that it should be progressive in nature (Peterson and Gordon 2011). There is evidence that older adults are generally novices or avoiders of structured exercise, so allowing participants to familiarise and build up their strength and fitness over time will enhance their self-efficacy and ensure the safe uptake of new, health-harnessing physical activity (Rejeski et al. 2007).

20.3.2 Tailoring Content

To change physical activity behaviour itself and understand properly the components that are effective in improving physical function in pre-frail older adults, it is important that a programme is grounded in behavioural science (Chase et al. 2017; Gardner et al. 2017). One prominent feature of successful exercise programmes in older adults is the importance of tailoring the content to the participants within a group. Individuals within a programme can have highly varied profiles in terms of age, frailty status, and associated physical issues or health concerns (Picorelli et al. 2014). Similarly, even if when the physical function level of two adults is similar, their existing levels of physical activity may be different. Concerted efforts to adapt an activity programme to the ability of a given individual should be made and could involve modifying the dose, frequency, or intensity of an exercise (de Labra et al. 2015). It is important to be realistic about the capability of participants and not to expect all members of a group-based programme to progress at the same rate (Hobbs et al. 2013). In this instance, allowances should be made so as to keep all participants fully engaged and not feel like they are holding others, or being held, back. Strategies to overcome this might be the promotion of personal targets and an emphasis on 'more-than-before' rather than any specified numbers for all to hit. A useful way of allowing individuals to progress at their own pace in a group setting is to incorporate portable, easy-to-use equipment such ankle weights or resistance bands for individuals to use at their leisure (Thomas et al. 2010). In addition to addressing physical capability, programmes should also tailor their content to combat individual psychosocial differences in motivation, goals, interests, and levels of social interaction and barriers (Costello et al. 2011; Baert et al. 2011).

20.3.3 Supporting Engagement with Community- and Home-Based Initiatives

When designing and implementing any physical activity programme for older adults, it is imperative to make it as engaging as possible. Programme participation is central to success and the long-term maintenance of any physical outcomes (Picorelli et al. 2014). Making physical activity programmes highly varied, progressive, and tailored will inherently be more appealing; however, there are a number of other ways that can support sustained attendance. Group-based programmes can offer additional enjoyment and social well-being benefits (Franco et al. 2015). Where possible, once- or twice-weekly group-based exercise sessions at local leisure centres or community spaces such as village halls or churches in areas with good social transport links should be promoted (King 2001). Undertaking a programme in an age-appropriate, convenient, and enjoyable fashion is also important when engaging older adults who report aversion to 'exercise centres' (Olanrewaju et al. 2016). Thus, marketing a physical activity programme should emphasise the social benefits and community engagement rather than exercise per se as this may be more motivating to this particular demographic. Alternatively, home-based programmes afford an opportunity to overcome logistical barriers and can be effective at improving mobility in pre-frail older adults (Faber et al. 2006; Fairhall et al. 2013). The individually tailored, progressive strength, balance, and walking Otago programme is one such intervention that has been shown to be effective in preventing falls and reducing mortality risk (Thomas et al. 2010). However, assuring participation in home-based initiatives, once unsupervised, could be challenging albeit improved via regular check-ups during home visits or via telephone contact that enable regular feedback on progress (Simek et al. 2012).

20.3.4 Targeting Maintenance of Physical Activity Beyond a Specific Programme

The ageing process means any improvements made by older adults in terms of their physiology would reverse should the exercises cease (Perkin et al. 2016). It is therefore imperative to provide individuals with as many of the necessary tools to sustain their increased physical activity and exercise regime during their time in a programme. Firstly, it is important to educate participants as to the benefits and risks of being physically active so they rationalise sustaining a physically active lifestyle beyond just being involved with a programme

(Gardner et al. 2017). Moreover, older adults should be supported to develop the skills and confidence to undertake the exercises they complete at home in their own time, and encouraged to do so while participating in a structured, group-based programme (Bauman et al. 2016). Therein lies another reason to ensure exercise programmes are simple and do not require specialist equipment. Older adults should be encouraged to get out and about more while the programme is underway as frequent active trips are associated with increased physical function and contribute towards meeting the aerobic activity target of 150 minutes (Jacobs et al. 2008). A useful way of supporting participants' maintenance of aerobic physical activity is by providing them with tools for self-monitoring and helping them set personal targets (Hobbs et al. 2013). A cheap and easy-to-use tool in this context is the pedometer that provides feedback on the numbers of steps one takes a day. These are particularly appropriate for older adults given their penchant for walking above other modes of active transport (Davis et al. 2011). An additional method to support prolonged physical activity is to create awareness of local opportunities for exercise, be it similar programmes at local leisure centres or even alternative community classes that are active by nature such as dance.

20.3.5 Making the Programme Cost-Effective

One of the most convenient ways to sustain individuals' engagement with physical activity is to maintain the delivery of community-based physical activity programmes. A major issue with many physical activity programmes is that they are either funded to run for a finite period of time or they cease running due to financial constraints that organisations delivering these initiatives face. There are a few steps one could take to encourage the more successful initiatives to be adopted by local authorities or commercial enterprises and kept running. First, an inevitable key concern is the cost of running a physical activity programme and how cost-effective the programme is. Frailty and a lack of physical activity for older adults can incur major healthcare costs; however, the governmental budgets for preventive public health initiatives are low, and programmes need to keep the staffing and resource costs low to be sustainable (Buckinx et al. 2015). Not relying on expensive specialist equipment, engaging peer-support and volunteers to help run programmes, and maximising benefit by promoting daily physical activity alongside structured exercise programme sessions are all ways costs can be minimised. To maximise the effectiveness of the programme, it is useful to seek feedback and involve participants in any efforts to reshape and refine it to optimise the content so it is enjoyable, engaging, and sustainable (Bethancourt et al. 2014).

20.3.6 Employing Social Marketing Principles for Effective Recruitment

Physical activity programmes struggle to engage older adults, particularly those with early signs of physical frailty, from ethnic minorities and lower socio-economic groups. One evidence-based approach to effective recruitment is social marketing which applies commercial marketing concepts and techniques to achieve health-related behavioural goals aiming to improve health and reduce health inequalities (National Social Marketing Centre for Excellence 2005). Social marketing has much in common with the marketing techniques used by large commercial companies. However, rather than selling a product, the social marketer seeks to affect behaviour change amongst the target group that leads to an improvement in their health, which then ultimately benefits society as a whole (Andreasen 1994). There are a number of key elements to the approach:

(1) Consumer research

An insight into why older adults don't currently engage with physical activity programmes is essential to tackling the issue. Without this understanding, it is unlikely we will effectively tackle the barriers to participation. Consumer research will always reveal different 'market segments' within the target group. As discussed earlier in this chapter, some people may feel they are 'not the sporty type'. Some may lack confidence to attend an unfamiliar group or doubt their capabilities. Others may consider they are already sufficiently active. These barriers affect people in entirely different ways and it is not possible for one marketing approach to effectively tackle all of these barriers. Viewing each of these groups as a different segment allows for a targeted approach that can address each specific barrier directly and simply (Stathi et al. 2014).

(2) Product development

Once an understanding of the target group has been established, it becomes easier to deliver a product (programme) that is as likely as possible to be appealing and so lead to good levels of participation. The programme should be built around the preferences of the market segment and so will deliver preferred session timing, an accessible venue, and the desired benefits while tackling the identified barriers.

(3) Framing the message

Once the target group has been defined and the programme developed, the promotional campaign is created. Its two essential elements are the message content itself and how it is delivered to the target group. The message content should be clear, straightforward, and consistent. It is vital to include what motivates the target group. Just stressing the potential, long-term health benefits has limited impact on older people's behaviour today. Emphasising important benefits such as enjoyment and socialising opportunities can be more effective as these deliver a more immediate 'payback'.

(4) Delivery mechanisms

Delivering the message effectively to the target group is crucial if behaviour change is to occur. Research in the commercial field indicates multiple exposures are required before people remember they have seen a promotional message and consider acting on it. Community-based programmes with small budgets often struggle to deliver these repeated exposures which impact levels of engagement (see Table 11 in Stathi et al. 2014 for guidance on the use of promotional tools).

20.4 Implications for Policy and Practice

Many experts would argue initiatives that are successful in helping older adults improve or sustain physical activity and physical function into older age could offer one of the best value buys in public health today.

The greatest challenge facing policymakers and programme developers lies with finding strategies that attract older adults with early signs of physical frailty to activity initiatives and keep them attending. Ideally these strategies should also promote ongoing involvement with local community initiatives. Breaking the spiral of decline characterised by loss of physical and cognitive function, loss of capacity to independently manage daily tasks, reductions in social interaction, and capacity to contribute to community is fundamental to healthy ageing.

Table 20.1 Key areas for successful implementation of physical activity programmes

What to consider	How to approach it
Involve a multidisciplinary interdisciplinary team in your programme development	Local authority coordinators, policymakers, academics, charitable trusts, industry, service providers, and service users all have important perspectives to offer. Public involvement in local decision-making process can take the form of consultation or collaboration involving active, ongoing partnership with members of the public
Employ social marketing principles to promote your programme	Engage with people with expertise in social marketing when developing promotional tools. Use clear, specific, and positively framed messages. Highlight the benefits that your target group values most. Capitalise on the power of word of mouth but also invest in available community and healthcare structures
Focus on social benefits and enjoyment rather than health messages to attract participants	The health message is oversold. Highlight the social benefits, focus on activities that are fun and purposeful, and engage people in ways ensuring that their opinion matters
Include a diverse range of exercise in your programmes and where safe to do so always promote walking and daily active living	Supporting people to walk more in their neighbourhoods and focussing on lower body activities such as strengthening of major muscle groups with use of portable, easy-to-use equipment such as resistance bands or ankle weights are strategies for effective implementation
Focus on gradual progress based on your participants' initial functional ability levels	Embrace the wide range of functional ability levels amongst your participants and support them in setting achievable, personally set goals. Assess their readiness to change and help them to build competence and confidence based on their individual needs
Help your participants identify their real level of physical competence and how best to improve it	Explore the reasons for the potential discrepancy between what participants think they are capable of doing and what they actually can do. Agree on an action plan that is based on their real ability to perform certain activities
Start with maintenance in mind	Make sure that your programme prepares participants for maintenance of physical activity in the long term. Actively support participants in engaging with other community initiatives. While benefiting from attending a specific programme, ensure that participants do not become dependent on that programme. Consider a variety of contexts promoting home-based and facility-based exercise listening to people's preferences

(continued)

Table 20.1 (continued)

What to consider	How to approach it
Make sure that your programme is cost-effective	Not relying on expensive equipment, engaging peer-support and volunteers to help run the programme, and inviting programme participants to act as programme ambassadors and actively promote the programme within their social networks are some strategies to keep the costs low
Know what the successful elements of your programme are	Incorporate behavioural science in your programme content development. Strategies such instructing people to perform activities safely and correctly, teaching them to self-monitor their performance, providing them with regular feedback, and enhancing social contact within and outside the programme have been found to work in programmes targeting older adults. Engage with behavioural scientists in developing the right set of techniques for your programme and ensure your exercise leaders are trained in using them correctly focussing on the power of communication skills
Provide evidence that your programme works	Programme planning and evaluation need to go hand in hand. Even with a limited budget, make sure that you collect basic audit data (e.g. participant characteristics, attendance rates, adherence to the programme), cost data (e.g. staffing, training, facilities), process data (participants and staff perceptions on what works), and change data (e.g. do participants increase what is set as the main outcome of your programme? (e.g. physical function or physical activity))

To be successful, implementation of physical activity programmes should target people with early signs of physical frailty, utilise promising practices, and invest in testing new and innovative ways to overcome personal, social, and environmental challenges. Table 20.1 provides a list of key areas for consideration and ways to approach them.

20.5 Conclusions

During old age, there is a population-wide transition from independence to frailty, mobility-related disability, and high demand for health and support services. Successful implementation of community programmes which target people with early signs of frailty is compromised by several uptake and participation barriers including people's perceptions about appropriateness of exercise for them, lack of social support, compromised health, transport issues, social network's concerns about safety of exercising, lack of progress recognition, and lack of long-term maintenance strategies. Working in multidisciplinary teams, adopting social marketing principles in programme promotion, focussing on social and purposeful activities, tailoring programmes to an individual's needs, developing multicomponent programmes, ensuring programmes are feasible and cost-effective, and focussing on supporting participants to maintain physical activity in the long term are promising strategies for successful implementation of community programmes targeting older people with early signs of frailty.

Further Reading

- Rejeski, W. J., Axtell, R., Fielding, R., Katula, J., King, A. C., Manini, T. M., et al. (2013). Promoting physical activity for elders with compromised function: The lifestyle interventions and independence for elders (LIFE) study physical activity intervention. *Clinical Interventions in Aging, 8*, 1119–1131.
- Stathi, A., Fox, K., Withall, J., Bentley, G., & Thompson, J. L. (2014). Promoting physical activity in older adults: A guide for local decision makers. From http://ageactionalliance.org/wordpress/wp-content/uploads/2014/03/AVONet-report-2014-March.pdf
- National Obesity Observatory. (2012). Standard evaluation framework for physical activity interventions. Available at http://www.noo.org.uk/uploads/doc/vid_16722_SEF_PA.pdf

References

Andreasen, A. R. (1994). Social marketing: Its definition and domain. *Journal of Public Policy & Marketing, 13*, 108–114.

Annear, M. J., Cushman, G., & Gidlow, B. (2009). Leisure time physical activity differences among older adults from diverse socioeconomic neighborhoods. *Health & Place, 15*(2), 482–490.

Baert, V., Gorus, E., Mets, T., Geerts, C., & Bautmans, I. (2011). Motivators and barriers for physical activity in the oldest old: A systematic review. *Ageing Research Reviews, 10*(4), 464–474.

Bandeen-Roche, K., Seplaki, C. L., Huang, J., Buta, B., Kalyani, R. R., Varadhan, R., et al. (2015). Frailty in older adults: A nationally representative profile in the United States. *The Journals of Gerontology Series A: Biological Sciences and Medical Sciences, 70*(11), 1427–1434.

Bauman, A., Merom, D., Bull, F. C., Buchner, D. M., & Singh, M. A. F. (2016). Updating the evidence for physical activity: Summative reviews of the epidemiological evidence, prevalence, and interventions to promote "active aging". *The Gerontologist, 56*(Suppl 2), S268–S280.

Bethancourt, H. J., Rosenberg, D. E., Beatty, T., & Arterburn, D. E. (2014). Barriers to and facilitators of physical activity program use among older adults. *Clinical Medicine & Research, 12*(1–2), 10–20.

Bock, J.-O., König, H.-H., Brenner, H., Haefeli, W. E., Quinzler, R., Matschinger, H., et al. (2016). Associations of frailty with health care costs – Results of the ESTHER cohort study. *BMC Health Services Research, 16*(1), 128.

Buckinx, F., Rolland, Y., Reginster, J.-Y., Ricour, C., Petermans, J., & Bruyère, O. (2015). Burden of frailty in the elderly population: Perspectives for a public health challenge. *Archives of Public Health, 73*(1), 19.

Cesari, M., Vellas, B., Hsu, F.-C., Newman, A. B., Doss, H., King, A. C., et al. (2015). A physical activity intervention to treat the frailty syndrome in older persons—Results from the LIFE-P study. *The Journals of Gerontology Series A: Biological Sciences and Medical Sciences, 70*(2), 216–222.

Chase, J. D. (2013). Physical activity interventions among older adults: A literature review. *Research and Theory for Nursing Practice, 27*(1), 53–80.

Chase, J. D., Phillips, L. J., & Brown, M. (2017). Physical activity intervention effects on physical function among community-dwelling older adults: A systematic review and meta-analysis. *Journal of Aging and Physical Activity, 25*, 149–170.

Chatfield, M. D., Brayne, C. E., & Matthews, F. E. (2005). A systematic literature review of attrition between waves in longitudinal studies in the elderly shows a consistent pattern of dropout between differing studies. *Journal of Clinical Epidemiology, 58*(1), 13–19.

Chodzko-Zajko, W. J., Proctor, D. N., Fiatarone Singh, M. A., Minson, C. T., Nigg, C. R., Salem, G. J., et al. (2009). Exercise and physical activity for older adults: American College of Sports Medicine position stand. *Medicine and Science in Sports and Exercise, 41*(7), 1510–1530.

Chou, C.-H., Hwang, C.-L., & Wu, Y.-T. (2012). Effect of exercise on physical function, daily living activities, and quality of life in the frail older adults: A meta-analysis. *Archives of Physical Medicine and Rehabilitation, 93*(2), 237–244.

Clegg, A., Young, J., Iliffe, S., Rikkert, M. O., & Rockwood, K. (2013). Frailty in elderly people. *Lancet, 381*(9868), 752–762.

Collard, R. M., Boter, H., Schoevers, R. A., & Oude Voshaar, R. C. (2012). Prevalence of frailty in community-dwelling older persons: A systematic review. *Journal of the American Geriatric Society, 60*(8), 1487–1492.

Costello, E., Kafchinski, M., Vrazel, J., & Sullivan, P. (2011). Motivators, barriers, and beliefs regarding physical activity in an older adult population. *Journal of Geriatric Physical Therapy, 34*(3), 138–147.

Craig, R., Mindell, J., & Hirani, V. (2009). Health Survey for England 2008: Physical activity and fitness. Retrieved from http://www.ic.nhs.uk/webfiles/publications/HSE/HSE08/HSE_08_Summary_of_key_findings.pdf (summary) or http://www.ic.nhs.uk/cmsincludes/_process_document.asp?sPublicationID=1257511982491&sDocID=5956 (full survey, volume 1), or http://www.ic.nhs.uk/cmsincludes/_process_document.asp?sPublicationID=1257511982491&sDocID=5957 (full survey, volume 2). General access: http://www.ic.nhs.uk/statistics-and-data-collections/health-and-lifestyles-related-surveys/health-survey-for-england/health-survey-for-england--2008-physical-activity-and-fitness

Davis, M. G., Fox, K. R., Hillsdon, M., Coulson, J. C., Sharp, D. J., Stathi, A., et al. (2011). Getting out and about in older adults: The nature of daily trips and their association with objectively-assessed physical activity. *International Journal of Behavioral Nutrition and Physical Activity, 8*, 116–125.

de Labra, C., Guimaraes-Pinheiro, C., Maseda, A., Lorenzo, T., & Millán-Calenti, J. C. (2015). Effects of physical exercise interventions in frail older adults: A systematic review of randomized controlled trials. *BMC Geriatrics, 15*(1), 1.

Dunbar, A. (1992). *Allied Dunbar National Fitness Survey: Main findings: A report on activity patterns and fitness levels.* London: Sports Council and Health Education Authority.

Dye, C. J., & Wilcox, S. (2006). Beliefs of low-income and rural older women regarding physical activity: You have to want to make your life better. *Women & Health, 43*(1), 115–134.

Elsawy, B., & Higgins, K. E. (2010). Physical activity guidelines for older adults. *American Family Physician, 81*(1), 55–59.

Faber, M. J., Bosscher, R. J., Paw, M. J. C. A., & van Wieringen, P. C. (2006). Effects of exercise programs on falls and mobility in frail and pre-frail older adults: A multicenter randomized controlled trial. *Archives of Physical Medicine and Rehabilitation, 87*(7), 885–896.

Fairhall, N., Sherrington, C., Lord, S. R., Kurrle, S. E., Langron, C., Lockwood, K., et al. (2013). Effect of a multifactorial, interdisciplinary intervention on risk factors for falls and fall rate in frail older people: A randomised controlled trial. *Age and Ageing, 43*(5), 616–622.

Farrance, C., Tsofliou, F., & Clark, C. (2016). Adherence to community based group exercise interventions for older people: A mixed-methods systematic review. *Preventive Medicine, 87*, 155–166.

Franco, M. R., Tong, A., Howard, K., Sherrington, C., Ferreira, P. H., Pinto, R. Z., et al. (2015). Older people's perspectives on participation in physical activity: A systematic review and thematic synthesis of qualitative literature. *British Journal of Sports Medicine.* https://doi.org/10.1136/bjsports-2014-094015.

Freiberger, E., Kemmler, W., Siegrist, M., & Sieber, C. (2016). Frailty and exercise interventions. *Zeitschrift für Gerontologie und Geriatrie, 7*, 1–6.

Fried, L. P., Tangen, C. M., Walston, J., Newman, A., Hirsch, C., Gottdiener, J., et al. (2001). Frailty in older adults: Evidence for a phenotype. *The Journals of Gerontology. Series A, Biological Sciences and Medical Sciences, 56*, M146–M156.

Gale, C. R., Cooper, C., & Aihie Sayer, A. (2015). Prevalence of frailty and disability: Findings from the English longitudinal study of ageing. *Age and Ageing, 44*(1), 162–165.

Gardner, B., Jovicic, A., Belk, C., Kharicha, K., Iliffe, S., Manthorpe, J., et al. (2017). Specifying the content of home-based health behaviour change interventions for older people with frailty or at risk of frailty: An exploratory systematic review. *BMJ Open, 7*(2). https://doi.org/10.1136/bmjopen-2016-014127.

Gateway to Research. (2015). The Avon network for the promotion of active ageing in the community. From http://gtr.rcuk.ac.uk/project/D2AC5A4B-6E17-4C5F-9304-B2F9798DC988

Giné-Garriga, M., Roqué-Fíguls, M., Coll-Planas, L., Sitja-Rabert, M., & Salvà, A. (2014). Physical exercise interventions for improving performance-based measures of physical function in community-dwelling, frail older adults: A systematic review and meta-analysis. *Archives of Physical Medicine and Rehabilitation, 95*(4), 753–769. e753.

Graham, L. J., & Connelly, D. M. (2013). "Any movement at all is exercise": A focused ethnography of rural community-dwelling older adults' perceptions and experiences of exercise as self-care. *Physiotherapy Canada, 65*(4), 333–341.

Harris, R., & Dyson, E. (2001). Recruitment of frail older people to research: Lessons learnt through experience. *Journal of Advanced Nursing, 36*(5), 643–651.

Hawley-Hague, H., Horne, M., Skelton, D. A., & Todd, C. (2016). Older adults' uptake and adherence to exercise classes: Instructors' perspectives. *Journal of Aging and Physical Activity, 24*(1), 119–128.

Hobbs, N., Godfrey, A., Lara, J., Errington, L., Meyer, T. D., Rochester, L., et al. (2013). Are behavioral interventions effective in increasing physical activity at 12 to 36 months in adults aged 55 to 70 years? A systematic review and meta-analysis. *BMC Medicine, 11*, 75.

Ipsos MORI. (2014). Understanding the lives of older people living with frailty: A qualitative investigation. Retrieved November 18, 2016, from http://www.ageuk.org.uk/Documents/EN-GB/For-professionals/Research/Living_with_frailty.pdf?dtrk=true

Jacobs, J. M., Cohen, A., Hammerman-Rozenberg, R., Azoulay, D., Maaravi, Y., & Stessman, J. (2008). Going outdoors daily predicts long-term functional and health benefits among ambulatory older people. *Journal of Aging and Health, 20*(3), 259–272.

Janssen, S. L., & Stube, J. E. (2014). Older adults' perceptions of physical activity: A qualitative study. *Occupational Therapy International, 21*(2), 53–62.

King, A. C. (2001). Interventions to promote physical activity by older adults. *The Journals of Gerontology Series A: Biological Sciences and Medical Sciences, 56*(Supplement 2), 36–46.

Malini, F. M., Lourenço, R. A., & Lopes, C. S. (2016). Prevalence of fear of falling in older adults, and its associations with clinical, functional and psychosocial factors: The frailty in Brazilian older people-Rio de Janeiro study. *Geriatrics & Gerontology International, 16*(3), 336–344.

McGowan, L. J., Devereux-Fitzgerald, A., Powell, R., & French, D. P. (2017). How acceptable do older adults find the concept of being physically active? A systematic review and meta-synthesis. *International Review of Sport and Exercise Psychology*, 1–24. https://doi.org/10.1080/1750984X.2016.1272705

McPhate, L., Simek, E. M., & Haines, T. P. (2013). Program-related factors are associated with adherence to group exercise interventions for the prevention of falls: A systematic review. *Journal of Physiotherapy, 59*(2), 81–92.

McPhate, L., Simek, E. M., Haines, T. P., Hill, K. D., Finch, C. F., & Day, L. (2016). "Are your clients having fun?" The implications of respondents' preferences for the delivery of group exercise programs for falls prevention. *Journal of Aging and Physical Activity, 24*(1), 129–138.

Morley, J. E., Vellas, B., van Kan, G. A., Anker, S. D., Bauer, J. M., Bernabei, R., et al. (2013). Frailty consensus: A call to action. *Journal of the American Medical Directors Association, 14*(6), 392–397.

National Centre for Social Research. (2010). *Health Survey for England, 2001* (3rd ed.). UK Data Service. University College London. Department of Epidemiology and Public Health. SN: 4628, https://doi.org/10.5255/UKDA-SN-4628-1.

National Social Marketing Centre for Excellence. (2005). *Social marketing pocket guide*. London: National Social Marketing Centre for Excellence.

Olanrewaju, O., Kelly, S., Cowan, A., Brayne, C., & Lafortune, L. (2016). Physical activity in community dwelling older people: A systematic review of reviews of interventions and context. *PLoS One, 11*(12), e0168614.

Pahor, M., Guralnik, J. M., Ambrosius, W. T., Blair, S., Bonds, D. E., Church, T. S., et al. (2014). Effect of structured physical activity on prevention of major mobility disability in older adults: The LIFE study randomized clinical trial. *The Journal of the American Medical Association, 311*(23), 2387–2396.

Perkin, O., McGuigan, P., Thompson, D., & Stokes, K. (2016). A reduced activity model: A relevant tool for the study of ageing muscle. *Biogerontology, 17*, 435–447.

Peterson, M. D., & Gordon, P. M. (2011). Resistance exercise for the aging adult: Clinical implications and prescription guidelines. *American Journal of Medicine, 124*(3), 194–198.

Phillips, E. M., Katula, J., Miller, M. E., Walkup, M. P., Brach, J. S., King, A. C., et al. (2010). Interruption of physical activity because of illness in the lifestyle interventions and independence for elders pilot trial. *Journal of Aging and Physical Activity, 18*(1), 61–74.

Picorelli, A. M. A., Pereira, L. S. M., Pereira, D. S., Felício, D., & Sherrington, C. (2014). Adherence to exercise programs for older people is influenced by program characteristics and personal factors: A systematic review. *Journal of Physiotherapy, 60*(3), 151–156.

Provencher, V., Mortenson, B., Tanguay-Garneau, L., Bélanger, K., & Dagenais, M. (2014). Challenges and strategies pertaining to recruitment and retention of frail elderly in research studies: A systematic review. *Archives of Gerontology and Geriatrics, 59*, 18–24.

Rejeski, W. J., Miller, M. E., King, A. C., Studenski, S. A., Katula, J. A., Fielding, R. A., et al. (2007). Predictors of adherence to physical activity in the lifestyle interventions and independence for elders pilot study (LIFE-P). *Clinical Interventions in Aging, 2*(3), 485–494.

Rejeski, W. J., Axtell, R., Fielding, R., Katula, J., King, A. C., Manini, T. M., et al. (2013). Promoting physical activity for elders with compromised function: The lifestyle interventions and independence for elders (LIFE) study physical activity intervention. *Clinical Interventions in Aging, 8*, 1119–1131.

Rochat, S., Büla, C. J., Martin, E., Seematter-Bagnoud, L., Karmaniola, A., Aminian, K., et al. (2010). What is the relationship between fear of falling and gait in well-functioning older persons aged 65 to 70 years? *Archives of Physical Medicine and Rehabilitation, 91*(6), 879–884.

Schutzer, K. A., & Graves, B. S. (2004). Barriers and motivations to exercise in older adults. *Preventive Medicine, 39*(5), 1056–1061.

Silcock, D., & Sinclair, D. (2012). *The cost of our ageing society*. London: ILC-UK.

Simek, E. M., McPhate, L., & Haines, T. P. (2012). Adherence to and efficacy of home exercise programs to prevent falls: A systematic review and meta-analysis of the impact of exercise program characteristics. *Preventive Medicine, 55*(4), 262–275.

Simek, E. M., McPhate, L., Hill, K. D., Finch, C. F., Day, L., & Haines, T. P. (2015). What are the characteristics of home exercise programs that older adults prefer?: A cross-sectional study. *American Journal of Physical Medicine & Rehabilitation, 94*(7), 508–521.

Stathi, A., McKenna, J., & Fox, K. R. (2010). Processes associated with participation and adherence to a 12-month exercise programme for adults aged 70 and older. *Journal of Health Psychology, 15*(6), 838–847.

Stathi, A., Gilbert, H., Fox, K. R., Coulson, J. C., Davis, M. G., & Thompson, J. L. (2012). Determinants of neighborhood activity of adults age 70 and over: A mixed-methods study. *Journal of Aging and Physical Activity, 20*(2), 148–170.

Stathi, A., Fox, K., Withall, J., Bentley, G., & Thompson, J. L. (2014). Promoting physical activity in older adults: A guide for local decision makers. From http://ageactionalliance.org/wordpress/wp-content/uploads/2014/03/AVONet-report-2014-March.pdf

Theou, O., Stathokostas, L., Roland, K. P., Jakobi, J. M., Patterson, C., Vandervoort, A. A., et al. (2011). The effectiveness of exercise interventions for the management of frailty: A systematic review. *Journal of Aging Research, 2011*, 569194.

Thomas, S., Mackintosh, S., & Halbert, J. (2010). Does the 'Otago exercise programme' reduce mortality and falls in older adults?: A systematic review and meta-analysis. *Age and Ageing, 39*(6), 681–687.

Ward, R. A. (2013). Change in perceived age in middle and later life. *The International Journal of Aging and Human Development, 76*(3), 251–267.

Withall, J., Thompson, J., Fox, K., Davis, M., Gray, S., de Koning, J., et al. (2016). Participant and public involvement in refining a peer-volunteering active aging intervention: Project ACE (active, connected, engaged). *The Gerontologist*. pii: gnw148. https://doi.org/10.1093/geront/gnw148.

World Health Organisation. (2010). Physical activity and older adults: Recommended levels of physical activity for adults aged 65 and above. Available at http://www.who.int/dietphysicalactivity/factsheet_olderadults/en/

Yardley, L., Donovan-Hall, M., Francis, K., & Todd, C. (2006). Older people's views of advice about falls prevention: A qualitative study. *Health Education Research, 21*(4), 508–517.

Section 5

Physical Environmental Factors and Physical Activity Among Older People

Charles Musselwhite

Traditionally, ageing people were seen to be strongly influenced by the environment within which they lived, worked, and interacted, encapsulated by approaches such as 'environmental press' or 'person-environment reactivity' (Lawton and Nahemow 1973). Research and theory now suggests older people are more actively engaged with their environment, that the process is dynamic, two-way, and ever changing. With roots in environmental psychology, cultural geography, and sociology, the examination of the relationship between older people and their environment is termed 'environmental gerontology' or sometimes the 'ecology of ageing' (Wahl and Lang 2006; Wahl and Oswald 2010). Environments and ageing are multidisciplinary in nature, utilising theoretical perspectives from psychology, sociology, architecture, human geography, urban studies, planning, and occupational therapy.

This section examines structural environmental factors that influence and are influenced by older people in relation to their physical activity, drawing on theory and research from environmental gerontology. These physical environmental factors can be defined in many different ways. A widespread theoretical direction suggests environmental constriction occurs in later life, so that people's interaction with the outside world reduces in nature. This results in the immediate microscopic nature of the environment becoming more important: the room, the home, the street, and the neighbourhood over the wider

---

C. Musselwhite (✉)
Centre for Innovative Ageing, Swansea University, UK

community, national, or international perspective. Similarly, the importance of the environmental fit approach (Lawton and Nahemow 1979), where there is equilibrium between the affordance of the environment and the ability of the person to use the environment, cannot be overlooked in terms of its influence on research questions and on policy and practice. These approaches, although pervasive and dynamic in nature, still somewhat see the older person as being in deficit, something to be corrected or facilitated.

Thin et al. (Chap. 21) and Van Cauwenberg et al. (Chap. 22) highlight theoretical approaches that can help both classify different physical and social structures that influence the older person and suggest how a dynamic relationship with such structures might work. One of the most commonly used approaches, for example, is the interactionist socioecological approach with its origins in Bronfenbrenner's (1979) concentric model of human development that has been adapted for ageing contexts previously, for example, rural ageing (Keating and Phillips 2008) and mobility and built environment contexts (Ormerod et al. 2015). This approach highlights the importance of interactions with different layers of the environment, with the person at the centre surrounded by concentric rings of social, built, and cultural environments. Thin et al. (Chap. 21) remind us, despite its use in defining different environments, the complexity of the different structures involved means it is hard to examine the theory in relation to robust evidence and even harder to use the model to enact behaviour change. More recently there has been a move towards co-design of environments with older people themselves at the heart of the change. As Thin et al. (Chap. 21) note, this is useful in identifying parts of the environment most pertinent to needs and interests of the individual and gives people a stake in their environment, making people feel they are truly able to enact change.

Thin et al. (Chap. 21) and Van Cauwenberg et al. (Chap. 22) both highlight the plethora of research that suggests how important the natural environment is in terms of both promoting physical activity and fostering positive mental health. Roe and Roe (Chap. 24) highlight natural environments as restorative in nature, in which such environments restore older people's mental health and wellbeing. It seems there is a quick win here for planners designing villages, towns, and cities; keep them green! However, it is important to note that not everyone can access green space; there may simply be a lack of green space available and accessible. Musselwhite (Chap. 25) suggests that sometimes well-designed grey space (town or industrial space) can be as important as green space for people who have always lived in such areas, and Ashe (Chap. 23) shows how important a well-designed indoor environment is to promoting health and wellbeing.

The importance of building physical activity into daily activity and routine of older people is noted throughout this section. In addition to access on foot to parks and public open spaces, access to local shops, services, public transit, and recreational facilities are paramount for promoting physical activity among older adults. As Van Cauwenberg et al. (Chap. 22) and Musselwhite (Chap. 25) note, walking to these places needs to be on dedicated well-maintained pathways away from traffic that feel safe and are attractive in nature. The importance of the aesthetic is often underestimated with the dominance of providing a merely functional environment. Yet growing evidence suggests desirability of the environment is every bit as important as functionality in motivating people to be physically active (see Musselwhite, Chap. 25).

In relation to the complexity of interactionist or ecological approaches, there is a word of caution stressed here for people reading this section to be wary of what exactly the research is saying. As Thin et al. (Chap. 21.) note, the factors that promote or inhibit physical activity are complex, long term, and highly uncertain. Nevertheless, research methodology can often oversimplify such relationships, and there are times when inferring causes from correlations erroneously overemphasise the cause-and-effect relationship. What results is a much more deterministic outcome for something that is actually interactionist.

Overall, the collection of chapters in this section stress the importance of the physical environment in motivating and sustaining physical activity in later life. It is imperative that designers and planners get the built environment right, both inside and out, including accessibility between home, neighbourhood, and the wider community. There is a call throughout all chapters for a more robust evidence base, to examine which elements of the environment have most effect on physical activity, in order to aid planning and promote cost-effective interventions. Policies to promote physical activity need to do so across the life course. In particular, it is essential to integrate health into the design and building of our neighbourhoods, streets, buildings, and homes.

References

Bronfenbrenner, U. (1979). *Ecology of human development*. Cambridge, MA: Harvard University Press.

Keating, N., & Phillips, J. E. (2008). A critical human ecology perspective on rural ageing. In N. Keating (Ed.). *Rural ageing: A good place to grow old?* (pp. 1–10). Bristol: Policy Press.

Lawton, M. P., & Nahemow, L. (1973). Ecology and aging process. In

C. Eisdorfer & M. P. Lawton (Eds.). *The psychology of adult development and aging* (pp. 619–674). Washington, DC: American Psychological Association.

Ormerod, M., Newton, R., Philips, J., Musselwhite, C., McGee, S., & Russell, R. (2015). *How can transport provision and associated built environment infrastructure be enhanced and developed to support the mobility needs of individuals as they age?* Future of an ageing population: Evidence review Foresight, Government Office for Science, London.

Wahl, H.-W., & Lang, F. (2006). Psychological aging. A contextual view. In P. M. Conn (Ed.). *Handbook of models for human aging* (pp. 881–895). Amsterdam: Elsevier.

Wahl, H.-W., & Oswald, F. (2010). Environmental perspectives on ageing. In D. Dannefer & C. Phillipson (Eds.). *The Sage handbook of social gerontology* (pp. 111–124). London: Sage.

21

Outdoor Mobility and Promoting Physical Activity Among Older People

Neil Thin, Katherine Brookfield, and Iain Scott

21.1 Introduction: Understanding Needs, Objectives, and Evidence

It is widely agreed that regular outdoor physical activity (PA) is beneficial; that too many people, especially older adults, are living relatively 'inactive' indoor lifestyles; and that achieving optimal levels of outdoor PA becomes increasingly difficult and risky as people get older. We also know that environmental and physical conditions influence the frequency, experiential qualities, and wellbeing outcomes of outdoor PA. Although it is commonly found that there is no systematic correlation between activity levels and specific environmental features in older adults (Van Cauwenberg et al. 2011), there is some evidence that specific everyday physical attributes of outdoor environments such as surfaces, rails benches, and toilets are particularly crucial as enablers or inhibitors for this population (Brookfield et al. 2017).

Increasingly, these beliefs are 'evidence-based' (Cama 2009; Mccullough 2010; Cooper Marcus and Sachs 2014), following increased public interest and research output on outdoor activity promotion. Further public investments

N. Thin (✉)
School of Social Political Sciences, University of Edinburgh, Edinburgh, UK

K. Brookfield
Environment Department, University of York, York, UK

I. Scott
Edinburgh College of Art, University of Edinburgh, Edinburgh, UK

© The Author(s) 2018
S. R. Nyman et al. (eds.), *The Palgrave Handbook of Ageing and Physical Activity Promotion*, https://doi.org/10.1007/978-3-319-71291-8_21

will demand more evidence, so we emphasise here the approaches and methods required to produce genuinely useful and persuasive evidence. Note that 'evidence' includes not only factual empirical information but also causal theories of which there are two main varieties: *theories of maintenance* (how do situations persist, how do individuals, institutions, and facilities keep going?) and *theories of change* (how do situations worsen or improve, and how can they be deliberately improved?). With epidemic health and mental health problems being attributed to inactivity worldwide, pressure is mounting to find better ways of persuading and enabling people to take advantage of the many benefits that outdoor PA offers.

We review here the opportunities, benefits, and risks of outdoor PA and recommend some analytical tools to support research, monitoring, and promotion. We emphasise that every individual interacts with environments in their own way and that one-way 'deterministic' assumptions about environmental influence are misleading. Simplified generalisations can provide helpful pointers to the benefits that environmental features tend to afford. But each environmental characteristic only achieves its influence via situation-specific and individual-specific interactions and subsequent appreciations. We recommend an *interactionist* socio-ecological approach, promoting careful consideration of how characteristics become 'affordances' which are then used and appreciated, resulting in benefits and in sustainable use and support for those characteristics (Gibson 1977).

'Mobility' (self-transport, getting about) and 'physical activity' (PA: using energy to move the body, including both deliberate structured 'exercise' and unstructured activities) are distinct but overlapping concepts that relate to aspects of life that are crucial for wellbeing. Since this chapter is about outdoor PA which requires mobility, we'll treat the two as much the same although the physical inhibitors and enablers of self-transport may be different from those that influence activities in place. Designed or modifiable features of built and 'natural' environments can facilitate or hinder outdoor PA, in particular, among older people. Physical, cognitive, and sensory impairments tend to increase with age, but late life offers new opportunities for enjoyment of outdoor PA. We also introduce the rationale for collaborative and inclusive research and design approaches to some of the debates and practical challenges involved in promoting outdoor PA among older people.

Most research and most policies promoting outdoor activities have been in middle- to high-income countries, in which the situations and trends outlined in Table 5.1 can be expected.

This attempt to simplify and universalise our arguments doesn't imply that we don't appreciate the many important diversities in socio-economic,

Table 5.1 Global trends and typical situations relevant to outdoor PA

Issues	Situations, trends, implications for research and planning
Demography	The numbers and proportion of older people in the population are increasing sharply (hence, new research and new approaches must be anticipated in rapidly changing demographies)
Residence and land use	Many older people live and conduct most of their PA in urban or suburban environments that are to a significant extent 'built' though not necessarily 'designed', and hence can be changed to improve wellbeing (Plouffe and Kalache 2011)
Transport mobility and PA	Although most older people are considerably more transport-mobile than their parents and grandparents were, most could improve their wellbeing and longevity prospects through enhanced PA
Wellbeing	Late-life flourishing has become an expectation for billions of people worldwide (hence, it's not all about the quantity and the instrumental benefits of physical activities but also about their quality and intrinsic enjoyability) (Pike 2011)
Gender	Older women outnumber men, but are at every age less physically active then men are, especially outdoors (hence, researchers and planners must consider gender and women-specific issues) (Shephard 2001; Lee 2005)
Walking	For most older people, walking (for errands, for pleasure, or for health) is by far the most important and common form of outdoor PA, with most immediate potential for enhancement (Bélanger et al. 2011)
Public and private outdoor space	There is potential in private, institutional, and open-access public space for environmental enhancements that could foster better quantity and quality of PA, but the design opportunities and contextual issues in each of these are different

cultural, and personal factors that impact on the potential enhancement of outdoor PA. For example, cultural beliefs of the safety, dignity, and capabilities of older people in outdoor settings vary widely worldwide and have crucial influence on PA levels.

21.2 Life After One Direction: Deterministic Versus Interactionist Accounts of Environmental Causation

The phrase 'environmental influences' (or 'impacts' or 'determinants') is commonly assumed to refer to one-directional influences of physical things on people. Such assumptions ignore the fact that other people, and the cultural norms and institutions associated with them, are the most salient environmental influences on people's thoughts, feelings, and activity choices. So physical determinism isn't a realistic way of understanding human behaviour and outcomes. 'Environment' has also become a non-neutral term that is commonly associated with problems and pathologies (see, e.g., Pacyna and Pacyna 2016). And since 'health' has been similarly pathologised, the whole field of 'environmental health' is distortive, combining unrealistic environmental and medical physicalism and pathologism. These powerful influences on public thought must be resisted with *aspirational* and *interactionist* approaches to outdoor PA.

The terms 'ecology' and 'ecosystem services' are associated with more neutral and realistically interactionist and diachronic understanding of mutual adjustments between people (or other species) and their environments. The factors that promote or inhibit outdoor PA are complex, long-term, and highly uncertain. Rather than pretending that these complexities and uncertainties don't exist, explicitly interactionist causal modelling can help promote intelligent conversations that improve the quality of plans and outcomes.

We are all prone to wrongly inferring causes from correlations. Research on outdoor PA is rife with correlational findings that are misrepresented as evidence of one-directional causal effects and with unwarranted prediction of benefits on the strength of data from cross-sectional studies (e.g., Guite et al. 2006; Wilson et al. 2011; for a more honest review of the limitations of correlational studies, see Craig et al. 2002). Since we can't shut down our hardwired causal inferencing, we must make conscious efforts to keep considering multiple plausible cause-effect relationships (Dilnot and Blastland 2008, p. 111).

Accounts of how patterns of health-related behaviour come about fall somewhere on a continuum between *determinism* and *interactionism*. Any account of causality is deterministic if it emphasises one very strong and usually one-directional causal explanation. Thus *architectural determinism, technical determinism,* and *sartorial determinism* are views that buildings, technology, or clothing, respectively, make people behave in particular ways. *Physical determinism* (or geographical determinism or—less aptly—environmental determinism) is a broader concept referring to causal assumptions that behaviour or wellbeing outcomes are shaped by physical surroundings in general. *Biological determinism* assumes that a person's biology determines their destiny. *Medical determinism* assumes that health is caused by medical interventions. Marxists favour *material determinism*, believing that society is shaped by control of the physical means of production—for example, that PA habits are shaped by the macroeconomic structures which determine where people live, their transport use, and their income.

Other kinds of nonphysical determinism are worth considering too. *Cultural determinism* emphasises collectively learned and transmitted knowledge as the key shaper of human preferences and behaviour. A variant is *linguistic determinism*, emphasising how language shapes thought and hence behaviour. The labelling of spaces as 'parks', 'play areas', and 'walkways' may influence actual uses of those spaces. *Social determinism* refers to relationships and institutions as causes of character and behaviour. Club membership might be the key determinant of a form of outdoor exercise. *Psychological determinism* (or internalism) is the belief (all-pervasive in the 'self-help' industries) that the mind is the most powerful and independent factor influencing life outcomes. Texts on emotion regulation tend to ignore or downplay the important roles of mobility and environmental engagements and influences. Instead, they focus mainly on mental and psychosocial adjustments (Baumeister and Vohs 2004; Nyklíček et al. 2010). Even in the 'environment' section of Brandstatter and Eliasz's key text on 'ecological' approaches to emotion regulation (2001), the emphasis is on other people and social situations, rather than the built or natural environment.

Interactionist (or 'ecological', or 'holistic') accounts, by contrast, pursue a more complex appreciation of causality by exploring multiple interactions between many factors. Instead of highlighting a single determinative factor, interactionists consider lots of plausibly significant factors and then explore repetitive interactions among several of these components over time. For example, a 'psychosocial' causal model might focus mainly on interactions between mental processing and social relationships and structures. A more complex 'biopsychosocial' model (Engel 1977; Melchert 2014), which underpins the World Health Organisation's (2002) International Classification of Functioning, Disability and Health (or ICF) framework, or a 'socio-ecological' (Bronfenbrenner 1979; McLeroy et al. 1988) approach, might add in further elements such as technology, the built environment, and the 'natural' environment (and even 'nature' has nearly always already been subjected to thousands or millions of years of interactions with humans, including deliberate or non-deliberate modification).

Interactionists accept that determinist accounts can sometimes usefully highlight strong causal factors (e.g., that green parks promote sport and leisure exercise, that urban sprawl inhibits walking, and that socio-economic class has a massive influence on health outcomes). But determinism is 'tendentious' if it forces us to neglect other important causal factors. It can be damaging if it encourages top-down *social engineering* approaches to change that neglect or downplay the importance of personal and collective *agency* (or free will) in overcoming obstacles to make improvements. For example, provision of leisure facilities and walking routes doesn't in itself make people use those facilities.

Common sense may tell us to provide more parks and pedestrian infrastructure to improve public health, and usually those assumptions are valid. But if so, we don't need unscientific use of tendentious research to support those decisions. If we want our plans to be evidence-based, we'll need more complex causal models that consider multiple causal pathways. And if we want to make plausible causal inferences from research evidence, we can't make do with simple cross-sectional studies that just show correlations between factors at one given time. We'll need before-and-after controlled experimental studies, observations of 'natural experiments', or longitudinal 'panel study' research that explores how outcomes change as the likely causal factors change over time—for example, whether people become more active after moving to a more 'walkable' neighbourhood. Even longitudinal studies don't prove that a before-and-after correlation is an 'effect', they simply make those causal beliefs more plausible. Perhaps people move to 'walkable' neighbourhoods and become more active due to cultural influences—maybe the built environment is less significant than such studies indicate. Qualitative humanistic enquiry can help us appreciate what people themselves believe to be the causes and effects of their activities. But this, too, is prone to false beliefs for the same reason that people are hard-wired to want to find causal patterns in their observations.

As well as mapping out distinct categories involved in interactions (mind, body, society, environment, etc.), it often also helps to map out different levels of analysis from micro to macro. Probably the most influential version of this approach is Bronfenbrenner's (1979) socio-ecological modelling approach, originally developed to explore the socio-economic factors influencing child development. This takes 'environment' very literally as a set of concentric circles revealing patterns of influence on the individual at 'microsystem' levels (family, friends, local organisations), then 'mesosystem' (connections to wider social contexts), 'exosystem' (workplaces, social services), up to 'macrosystem' (cultural systems and political ideologies).

A different but similarly pragmatic approach is the 'life-space mobility' model which has been informatively used to assess older people's mobility within six concentric circles: bedroom, patio, yard, neighbourhood, out of neighbourhood, and out of town, asking people which circle they have reached in the past week and complementing this with information on health, cognitive functioning, and social life (Barnes et al. 2007).

21.3 Characteristics, Affordances, and Appreciation of Outdoor Spaces: The 'Person-Environment Fit'

'Outdoors' is a negative category. It requires an excursion, which could be to the garden, the street, or some remote mountain wilderness. Apart from exposure to an open sky, 'outdoors' specifies no positive features such as 'contact with nature' or 'green open space' or even 'public area'. Yet outdoor and indoor PAs are associated with very different motivations, benefits, and risks. Promoters and evaluators of outdoor PA need to know where people go, what they encounter there, what they do, how they experience it, and whether the effects are sustained or moderated through savouring, relating, or remembering. It also helps to know about interactions between the components: for example, the mood benefits of a relaxing park walk may be undone by the return walk through busy streets (Gee and Takeuchi 2004; Aspinall et al. 2015).

Outdoor environments can be analysed, evaluated, and mapped according to their objective physical *characteristics*, their *affordances* (the opportunities or threats they provide—Gibson 1977, 1986), and the subjective *appreciation* or perception of these characteristics and affordances (Hartig et al. 2010). For example, people living beside a busy street and a grassy park (objective characteristics) might have different abilities to negotiate the busy street, use the shops, and take exercise in the park (affordances), and they might have different perceptions of these features—some might appreciate the shopping opportunities and find the street convivial but feel unsafe in the park, others might hate the street and fear the traffic but feel relaxed and safe in the park. Information on characteristics can be gathered simply by observing, but qualitative and participatory learning strategies are needed to understand how these manifest as affordances and the extent to which they are appreciated or perceived.

These affordances and perceptions are moderated by further factors such as clothing, prosthetics, upbringing, age, gender and cultural norms, all of which have strong influences on the relevance of environmental characteristics to the likelihood that PA will happen and whether it will have good outcomes. If a park is objectively safe (crime-free and lacking in physical hazards) and has facilities like benches, bins, toilets, and play areas, it is likely to afford conviviality—regular social usage by lots of people. For some, this may encourage the perception that it's a great place for exercise. Others may feel their preferred activities are inhibited because they don't like being seen doing yoga or because dogs prevent them from relaxing while jogging.

The affordances that environmental characteristics present to people are moderated by people's preferences and capabilities. These in turn influence how people use and experience various features of the environments they interact with, which makes it more or less likely that people enjoy and savour experiences and relate them to other people. All of these factors influence the ways in which people benefit or fail to benefit, which then results in positive or negative feedback shaping people's motivation to use those environments again, or to enhance them in some way, or to encourage others to use them. Appreciation and benefit overlap, since appreciation reflects the intrinsic value of an activity—for example, 'fun' PA may be better for wellbeing than more rigorous 'exercise' (Downward and Dawson 2015).

Rather than assuming that environmental characteristics influence people in simple ways, it is more helpful to consider interactive relations between characteristics, capabilities, and people's minds. Since the 1970s, variants of the term 'person-environment fit' have been used as a general rubric for considering environment-person interactions (French et al. 1974). One highly influential variant has been a very simple socio-ecological modelling tool for comparing degrees of 'environmental press' (an obscure metaphor for environmental influence) in relation to people's competence (Lawton and Nahemow 1973). The rationale is that 'adaptive' behaviour is only likely when there is a reasonable balance or harmony between people's abilities and the relevant characteristics of their environment. Another influential model has been the 'rainbow model' for analysing factors influencing health (Dahlgren and Whitehead 1991) (see Chap. 1). Though helpful (e.g., it has informed the structure of this book), this model omits psychological causation, thus severely limiting its usefulness for interactionist mapping. One further ecological model (Sallis et al. 2006), which helpfully analyses the different ecologies of four domains of active living (active transport, and physical activities that are recreational, work-related, or household-related), will be reviewed in Chap. 22.

21.4 Biophilia, Nature Deficit and 'Mismatch' Theories, and Salutogenic/Therapeutic Environments

In 1984, Harvard biologist Edward Wilson proposed the so-called biophilia hypothesis, which quickly became a key concept for environmental psychology (Wilson 1984; Kellert and Wilson 1993). Despite Wilson's careless labelling (it wasn't about 'loving life', and there was no 'hypothesis'), this concept has proved extremely generative. Researchers and planners use it to explain why so many people say they feel better after spending time in 'natural' outdoor environments. Users of the biophilia concept tend to ignore the fact that there are lots of species and lots of 'natural' environmental characteristics people fear and dislike (for a good critique, see Joye and de Block 2011). Promoting naïve appreciation of 'nature' (e.g., see Beatley 2011; Kaplan and Kaplan 1989; Kellert 2005, 2012) without due consideration of many of the natural harms that urban hygiene has long sought to eradicate, they conveniently forget that there are lots of non-living features of natural environments (clouds, smells, sounds, rocky mountains) and lots of non-natural features of outdoor environments (beautiful buildings, interesting streets) that people love.

Despite its conceptual and terminological shortcomings, biophilia discourse (along with associated 'nature-relatedness' and 'nature-deficit' concepts) has been helpful in popularising attention to the ways in which our emotional responses to environments are influenced not just by our upbringing, background, and current personal preferences but also by deeply ingrained innate preferences that humanity developed over millions of years of savannah evolution (Louv 2011; Ruso et al. 2003).

More practical than generalised rhetoric about biophilia and nature deficits is to assess people's responses to various natural features of their environments. For example, the 'nature relatedness scale' is a simple tool for assessing the affective, cognitive, and experiential aspects of individuals' connection to nature (Nisbet et al. 2009). The more versatile concept of 'topophilia' (Tuan 1974) has been used to assess attraction to four aspects of environments—*ecodiversity*, *synesthetic tendency* (mixing sensory experiences), *cognitive challenge*, and *familiarity* (Ogunseitan 2005)—all of which could be practically relevant in people's prospects for benefiting from outdoor exercise.

21.5 Collaborative Research, Co-design, and the Co-production of Wellbeing

Designing and planning for enhanced outdoor PA needs to be *socially inclusive*. Older people and their preferences must be included in the research and design process, making sure that they have an effective voice that influences outcomes. Everyone's options to use public spaces are mediated through other people: social space must be socially and sociably designed. A lot of older people's outdoor physical activity does, of course, take place not in open-access public space but in domestic gardens or in private institutional spaces such as clubs and care homes. Nonetheless, most outdoor space is significantly more 'social' than indoor domestic space, since it involves a greater degree of exposure to other people.

Planning of multi-user, multi-use public goods also needs to be *holistic*: without ruling out the roles of sectoral specialists such as health planners and architects, the planning process overall must be comprehensive and interdisciplinary, paying integrated attention to the complex interactions among the many physical, sociocultural, and psychological factors that are relevant to the challenges and intended outcomes. A surprisingly neglected and important feature for older people, for example, is access to toilets near outdoor exercise areas (Greed 2003).

Most outdoor environments that humans use have multiple functions and diverse stakeholders. Participatory co-design approaches can ensure optimal compromises and win-win solutions to the diverse needs of different users. Older people are, most obviously, sources of wisdom concerning the preferences and needs of older users. But also, since they have lived through more life stages and have often witnessed a diversity of environments and social change over a longer period of time, they are an important source of wisdom for all users.

21.6 Outdoor Social Environments: Conviviality, Loneliness, and Fear

The planning concept of 'social capital', perhaps better described by less instrumentalist terms like 'sociability' or 'conviviality', was revived in Jane Jacobs' *Death and Life of Great American Cities* (1961), and again in William Whyte's influential book *The Social Life of Small Urban Spaces* (1980) which highlighted the dimension of soft 'social life' in outdoor public space. But

Whyte ignored the specific needs and preferences of older people. For example, when he noted that the benefits of street congestion or untidiness caused by vendors and entertainers outweigh the costs, he might also have recognised older people's need for relatively quiet and safe social spaces.

More recently, various arguments about the public space needs of older people have been put forward, with Low et al. (2005) generalising that conviviality is of prime importance for everyone even if this means sacrificing some safety, whereas Holland et al. (2007) argued for parks with seating, lighting, and toilets and quiet seating spaces away from highly active children (see also Ward Thompson and Travlou 2007). Ivory et al. (2015) conducted focus group research on neighbourhoods and outdoor PA and found that social connection and mental restoration were more salient than the 'health' motivations for outdoor PA. Given widespread concerns about epidemic levels of loneliness and social isolation worldwide (Victor et al. 2009), and the health consequences of this, (Holwerda et al. 2014), it seems likely that the benefits of sociable contact are everywhere going to be a core factor in the promotion of outdoor PA.

More generally, research on the sociability of neighbourhoods has demonstrated that this has crucial influence on people's motivation to go outdoors whether for exercise or not (for an excellent overview, see Shaftoe 2008). Cattell et al. (2008) showed ample evidence that the benefits of public spaces go beyond natural or aesthetic criteria to include the relaxation afforded by places deemed suitable for social interaction, showing that the health-giving properties of neighbourhoods depend on them being actively used.

Most research on outdoor PA is about how people respond to physical features of the environment, and too little looks at sociability. For many people who venture outdoors, the most salient and beneficial feature of outdoor environments is other people. When we approach the world on foot, a richer diversity of social and recreational opportunities present themselves (Gehl 2010). For the millions of older people who live alone, it is the conviviality of outdoor environments, from high streets to parks to town squares, that offers most motivation to go out (Brookfield and Mead 2016). For many outdoor exercisers, much of the benefit derives from convivial group exercise or from friendly, nonthreatening encounters with other people. Conversely, for those who live in neighbourhoods that they perceive as unsafe or threatening, trips out of the home can be limited.

Social analysis helps us recognise the various social characteristics, affordances, and perceptions of culturally specific, outdoor social environments. Physical characteristics serve as indicators of social quality, which influences perceptions often at subliminal levels. So apart from their functions as physical affordances for human activities, outdoor environmental features also have important symbolic importance to people. They provide culturally shared as well as personally idiosyncratic indicators of the state of society or the state of the world more generally. Thus, for example, the sight of broken windows, a messy street, or litter-strewn park can signify general social decline; dog mess on pathways can signify untrustworthiness; and security cameras can indicate crime (Brookfield et al. 2017). Well-tended public gardens can symbolise public safety but on the other hand can be interpreted as an indication that a park isn't meant for sport or exercise. Well-designed civic space can generate attachments not just to the spaces themselves but to the sense of society that they engender in their users. Occasional pieces of public exercise equipment can indicate that an area is deemed suitable for PA.

Historical information notices can convey a sense of cultural depth and interest that may encourage older people to walk to an area and pause there. Fences and high walls can indicate—perhaps unintentionally—that visitors are unwelcome. Scottish walkers, for example, benefit from probably the world's most sophisticated and walker-friendly legal protection of both the 'right of way' and the 'right to roam', yet most people will only exercise those rights if encouraged by suitable signage. A small number of confident and mainly upper-middle-class people reap the huge benefits of being free to walk or run on the country's beautiful golf courses, yet most people are unaware of this affordance.

Another important relevance of social environment to outdoor PA is the subliminal influence of observing other people. Just about everything that matters to humans—good or bad—is socially contagious. So when people venture outdoors, they are constantly picking up other people's habits. For example, in some countries it is still not the 'done thing' for women or older people to go out running. This acts as an implicit rule perpetuated mainly by visual confirmation. As has been amply demonstrated in cities in most parts of the world, once a critical mass of publicly visible outdoor exercise groups have contradicted this cultural norm, public outdoor exercise becomes something for everyone.

21.7 Bringing Outdoor Environments Indoors: Prospects for Virtual Simulation

People have always included elements of the outdoor world inside their homes, and city and garden designers have always ensured that city dwellers enjoy selected elements and reminders of the countryside. With major new developments in opportunities for virtual simulation, the forms of these outside-inside echoes are changing. And, just as real face-to-face social interactions and real-world social institutions have provided inspiration for virtual adaptations of these in online relationships, networks, and organisations based in social media, so too can outdoor activities inspire a radically new, adapted set of indoor simulations that benefit generations to come.

As with online sociality, there are of course risks that virtual enjoyment of pseudo-outdoors may prove harmful in some ways. But these threats offer no excuse for ignoring the many potential benefits and for seeking ways in which outdoor 'real' and indoor 'virtual' experiences can synergise rather than being in competition. A worryingly large number of people are described as 'housebound'. Older adults spend more time in the home than any other age group and may be particularly likely to become 'housebound'. Population ageing may mean, then, that the number of housebound individuals will rise steeply. Although there is ample sporadic research and practical guidance on dealing with the many challenges of indoor care and self-care, there has not yet been any single book or article devoted to systematic analysis of how people become housebound, what it means, and what can be done about it.

Since most older people clearly state preferences for frequently getting out and about, it is reasonably safe to assume that increases in the housebound population represent a severe threat to wellbeing, not least in terms of the probable impact on rates of PA. While we must continue with sincere efforts to facilitate good outdoor experiences for older people, we should also consider prospects for 'bringing the outside in'—that is, using new virtual technologies to enable housebound people to use simulation to enjoy at least some of the benefits of outdoor experience (Levi and Kocher 1999), while also investigating opportunities to design homes that provide more opportunities for individuals to participate in low to moderate PA indoors (Brookfield et al. 2015) (see Chap. 23).

In just a few decades, people's ability to simulate outdoor experiences within their homes has expanded massively. For thousands of years, architects and home designers have used plants, light, animal pets, and water features to bring some of the aesthetic thrills of outdoor life into the home. Only in the past century have most humans gained the ability to using artificial lighting to simulate daylight indoors. Today, billions of people already use video and audio to provide the sights and sounds of outdoor life. Buildings and spaces which actively employ technology as a way of accessing more fully the natural world around them are becoming more common. Susan Collins is an artist and academic who works with electronic media, exploring their relationship with architectural spaces and their surrounding environment. (http://susan-collins.net). Much of the research on the environmental psychology of outdoor activities, ironically, has been conducted indoors using simulation technologies (Mayer et al. 2008; Ulrich 1984). Now, new lighting systems simulate morning and evening light; alarm clocks simulate morning birdsong; robots are already allowing millions of housebound elderly people a simulation of interaction with animals; public and private gyms and swimming pools simulate desirable features of outdoor environments such as mountain views, bubbly rock pools, hills, rivers, and waves.

The next mass-scale transformation will be when virtual reality devices become widely used to provide much more realistic environmental simulations. 'Experience machine' pseudo-experiences may not appeal to everyone, and if some people may reduce their wellbeing by lazily substituted vicarious nature for the real thing (Kellert 2005). Some research evidence has unsurprisingly confirmed that real natural walks and views are more beneficial to wellbeing than video substitutes (Mayer et al. 2008). Nonetheless, it is not hard to imagine how nature simulations could radically improve life for people who are housebound, and that they are likely to have mass appeal to frail elderly people who gain the benefits of simulated outdoor activity with much less risk of injury.

21.8 Implications for Policy and Practice

This prospect has three main kinds of relevance for those who take a professional interest in outdoor PA. Firstly, promoters of outdoor PA must recognise that new opportunities to simulate outdoor experiences will reduce incentives to go outdoors. Secondly, more positively, since indoor simulations will be based on understandings of benefits from genuine outdoor experiences, there will be new opportunities for lessons from outdoor PA to enhance the lives of everyone, including housebound people. Thirdly, indoor simulations can be used to prepare people better for outdoor experiences, which may be especially helpful for those who are afraid to go out, and to identify appropriate outdoor environments for individuals to visit. For example, already

Google Earth simulation is commonly used as part of advance preparation for exploring routes on which there is a risk of getting lost while Google Street view has been used to assess the 'walkability' of urban walking routes frequented by older adults (Brookfield and Tilley 2016).

21.9 Conclusions

Promoters of older people's health need to highlight complementarities and differences between the benefits of outdoor and indoor PA. While it is tempting to use simple deterministic models of environmental effects on people, it is crucial for planners to appreciate complex interactions between mind, body, society, and environment. To understand the benefits and risks of outdoor PA also requires participatory co-design involving older people. It is also crucial to recognise that every sociocultural situation has different implications for the benefits and risks of outdoor PA and that nearly all planning situations will for the foreseeable future be subject to rapid demographic, technical, and socio-economic change. Hence, planners need socio-ecological evidence and analysis, and plans, facilities, and services need to be a flexible as possible.

Suggested Further Reading

- Barton, J., Bragg, R., Wood, C., & Pretty, J. (2016). *Green exercise: Linking nature, health and well-being.* London: Routledge.
- Giles-Corti, B., et al. (2015). The influence of urban design and planning on physical activity. In H. Barton et al. (Eds.), *The Routledge handbook of planning for health and well-being* (pp. 121–135). London: Routledge.

References

Aspinall, P., Mavros, R., Coyne, R., & Roe, J. (2015). The urban brain: Analysing outdoor physical activity with mobile EEG. *British Journal of Sports Medicine, 49*, 272–276.

Barnes, L. L., et al. (2007). Correlates of life space in a volunteer cohort of older adults. *Experimental Aging Research, 33*, 77–93.

Baumeister, R. F., & Vohs, K. D. (Eds.). (2004). *Handbook of self-regulation: Research, theory, and applications.* New York: Guilford Press.

Beatley, T. (2011). *Biophilic cities: Integrating nature into urban design and planning*. Washington, DC: Island Press.

Bélanger, M., Townsend, N., & Foster, C. (2011). Age-related differences in physical activity profiles of English adults. *Preventive Medicine, 52*(3–4), 247–249.

Brandstatter, H., & Eliasz, A. (Eds.). (2001). *Persons, situations, and emotions: An ecological approach*. Oxford: Oxford University Press.

Bronfenbrenner, U. (1979). *The ecology of human development: Experiments by nature and design*. Cambridge, MA: Harvard University Press.

Brookfield, K., & Mead, G. (2016). Physical environments and community reintegration post stroke: Qualitative insights from stroke clubs. *Disability & Society, 31*, 1013–1029.

Brookfield, K., & Tilley, S. (2016). Using virtual street audits to understand the walkability of older adults route choices by gender and age. *International Journal of Environmental Research and Public Health, 13*, 1061.

Brookfield, K., Fitzsimons, C., Scott, I., Mead, G., Starr, J., Thin, N., Tinker, A., & Ward Thompson, C. (2015). The home as enabler of more active lifestyles among older people. *Building Research & Information, 43*, 616–630.

Brookfield, K., Ward Thompson, K., & Scott, I. (2017). The uncommon impact of common environmental details on walking in older adults. *International Journal of Environmental Research and Public Health., 14*(2), 190.

Cama, R. (2009). *Evidence-based healthcare design*. Hoboken: Wiley.

Cattell, V., Dines, N., Gesler, W., & Curtis, S. (2008). Mingling, observing, and lingering: Everyday public spaces and their implications for well-being and social relations. *Health & Place, 14*, 544–561.

Cooper Marcus, C., & Sachs, N. A. (2014). *Therapeutic landscapes: An evidence-based approach to designing healing gardens and restorative outdoor spaces*. Hoboken: Wiley.

Craig, C. L., Brownson, R. C., Cragg, S. E., & Dunn, A. L. (2002). Exploring the effect of the environment on physical activity: A study examining walking to work. *American Journal of Preventive Medicine, 23*, 36–41.

Dahlgren, G., & Whitehead, M. (1991). *Policies and strategies to promote social equity in health*. Stockholm: Institute for Futures Studies.

Dilnot, A., & Blastland, M. (2008). *The tiger that isn't: Seeing through a world of numbers*. London: Profile Books.

Downward, P., & Dawson, P. (2015). Is it pleasure or health from leisure that we benefit from most? An analysis of well-being alternatives and implications for policy. *Social Indicators Research, 126*(1), 443–465.

Engel, G. L. (1977). The need for a new medical model: A challenge for biomedicine. *Science, 196*, 129–136.

French, J. R., Rodgers, W., & Cobb, S. (1974). Adjustment as person-environment fit. In G. V. Coelho, D. A. Hamburg, & J. E. Adams (Eds.), *Coping and adaptation*. New York: Basic Books.

Gee, G., & Takeuchi, D. (2004). Traffic stress, vehicular burden and well-being: A multilevel analysis. *Social Science and Medicine, 59*, 405–414.

Gehl, J. (2010). *Cities for people.* Washington, DC: Island Press.

Gibson, J. J. (1977). The theory of affordances. In R. Shaw & J. Bransford (Eds.), *Perceiving, acting, and knowing.* Mahwah: Erlbaum.

Gibson, J. J. (1986). *The ecological approach to visual perception.* Boston: Houghton Mifflin.

Greed, C. (2003). *Inclusive urban design: Public toilets.* Amsterdam: Architectural Press.

Guite, H. F., Clark, C., & Ackrill, G. (2006). The impact of the physical and urban environment on mental well-being. *Public Health, 120*, 1117–1126.

Hartig, T., et al. (2010). Health benefits of nature experience: Psychological, social and cultural processes. In K. Nilsson et al. (Eds.), *Forest, trees and human health* (pp. 127–168). Dordrecht: Springer.

Holland, C., Clark, A., Katz, J., & Peace, S. (2007). *Social interactions in urban public places.* Bristol: Policy Press.

Holwerda, J. T., et al. (2014). Feelings of loneliness, but not social isolation, predict dementia onset. *Journal of Neurology, Neuro-surgery & Psychiatry, 85*(2), 135–142.

Ivory, V. C., et al. (2015). What shape is your neighbourhood? Investigating the micro geographies of physical activity. *Social Science & Medicine, 133*, 313–321.

Jacobs, J. (1961). *The death and life of great American cities.* London: Penguin.

Joye, Y., & De Block, A. (2011). 'Nature and I are two': A critical examination of the biophilia hypothesis. *Environmental Values, 20*(2), 189–215.

Kaplan, R., & Kaplan, S. (1989). *The experience of nature: A psychological perspective.* Cambridge: Cambridge University Press.

Kellert, S. R. (2005). *Building for life: Designing and understanding the human-nature connection.* Washington, DC: Island Press.

Kellert, S. (2012). *Birthright: People and nature in the modern world.* New Haven: Yale University Press.

Kellert, S. R., & Wilson, E. O. (Eds.). (1993). *The biophilia hypothesis.* Washington, DC: Island Press.

Lawton, M. P., & Nahemow, L. (1973). Ecology and the aging process. In C. L. Eisdorfer (Ed.), *Psychology of adult development and aging.* Washington, DC: American Psychological Association.

Lee, Y.-S. (2005). Gender differences in physical activity and walking among older adults. *Journal of Women & Aging, 17*(1–2), 55–70.

Levi, D., & Kocher, S. (1999). Virtual nature: The future effects of information technology on our relationship to nature. *Environment and Nature, 31*(2), 203–226.

Louv, R. (2011). *The nature principle: Human restoration and the end of nature-deficit disorder.* Chapel Hill: Algonquin Books.

Low, S., Taplin, D., & Scheld, S. (2005). *Rethinking urban parks: Public space and cultural diversity.* Austin: University of Texas Press.

Mayer, F. S., Bruehlman-Senecal, E., & Dolliver, K. (2008). Why is nature beneficial? the role of connectedness to nature. *Environment and Behavior, 22*(28), 13–15.

Mccullough, C. S. (2010). *Evidence-based design for healthcare facilities.* Indianapolis: Sigma Theta Tau International.

McLeroy, K. R., Bibeau, D., Steckler, A., & Glanz, K. (1988). An ecological perspective on health promotion programs. *Health Education Quarterly, 15,* 351–377.

Melchert, T. P. (2014). *Biopsychosocial practice: A science-based framework for behavioral health care.* Washington, DC: American Psychological Association.

Nisbet, E. K., Zelenski, J. M., & Murphy, S. A. (2009). The nature relatedness scale: Linking individuals connection with nature to environmental concern and behavior. *Environment and Behavior, 41*(5), 715–740.

Nyklíček, I., Vingerhoets, A., & Zeelenberg, A. (Eds.). (2010). *Emotion regulation and wellbeing.* Dordrecht: Springer.

Ogunseitan, O. A. (2005). Topophilia and the quality of life. *Environmental Health Perspectives, 113*(2), 143–148.

Pacyna, J. M., & Pacyna, E. G. (2016). *Environmental determinants of human health.* Cham: Springer.

Pike, E. C. J. (2011). Growing old (dis)gracefully? The gender/aging/ exercise nexus. In E. Kennedy & P. Markula (Eds.), *Women and exercise: The body, health and consumerism* (pp. 180–196). London: Routledge.

Plouffe, L., & Kalache, A. (2011). Towards global age-friendly cities: Determining urban features that promote active aging. *Journal of Urban Health, 87*(5), 733–739.

Ruso, B., Renninger, L., & Atzwanger, K. (2003). Human habitat preferences: A generative territory for evolutionary aesthetics research. In E. Voland & L. Grammer (Eds.), *Evolutionary aesthetics* (pp. 279–294). Dordrecht: Springer.

Sallis, J., et al. (2006). An ecological approach to creating active living communities. *Annual Review of Public Health, 27,* 297–322.

Shaftoe, H. (2008). *Convivial urban spaces: Creating effective public spaces.* London: Earthscan.

Shephard, R. J. (2001). *Gender, physical activity, and aging.* Boca Raton: CRC Press.

Tuan, Y.-F. (1974). *Topophilia: A study of environmental perception, attitudes, and values.* New York: Columbia University Press.

Ulrich, R. (1984). View through a window may influence recovery from surgery. *Science, 224*(4647), 420–421.

Van Cauwenberg, J., et al. (2011). Relationship between the physical environment and physical activity in older adults: A systematic review. *Health & Place, 17,* 458–469.

Victor, C., Scambler, S., & Bond, J. (2009). *The social world of older people: Understanding loneliness and social isolation in later life.* London: Routledge.

Ward Thompson, C., & Travlou, P. (2007). *Open space: People space*. London: Taylor and Francis.

Whyte, W. H. (1980). *The social life of small urban spaces*. Washington, DC: Conservation Foundation.

Wilson, E. O. (1984). *Biophilia: The human bond with other species*. Cambridge, MA: Harvard University Press.

Wilson, L.-A. M., et al. (2011). The association between objectively measured neighborhood features and walking in middle-aged adults. *American Journal of Health Promotion, 25*(4), e12–e21.

World Health Organisation. (2002). *Towards a common language for functioning, disability and health (ICF)*. Geneva: World Health Organisation.

22

Physical Environments That Promote Physical Activity Among Older People

Jelle Van Cauwenberg, Andrea Nathan, Benedicte Deforche, Anthony Barnett, David Barnett, and Ester Cerin

22.1 Introduction

The promotion of physical activity (PA) across the lifespan can be facilitated or hindered by the physical environments surrounding us (Sallis et al. 2006). As functional capacity declines, older adults may be particularly sensitive to physical environmental barriers restricting PA (Forsyth et al. 2009). The importance of designing community spaces to support active living among older adults is well-established as evidenced by the recent emergence of urban design principles aimed at stimulating PA in this demographic (e.g., World Health Organisation's (WHO) *Age-friendly Cities* (WHO 2007) and 8-80 Cities (8 80 Cities 2016)). In this chapter, we refer to the physical environment as the characteristics of the physical context in which people spend their time (e.g.,

---

The original version of this chapter was revised. Authors' affiliations were incorrect. The chapter has been updated with the correct affiliation of the authors. An erratum to this chapter can be found at https://doi.org/10.1007/978-3-319-71291-8_36

J. Van Cauwenberg (✉)
Department of Public Health, Ghent University, Ghent, Belgium

Research Foundation Flanders, Brussels, Belgium

B. Deforche
Department of Public Health, Ghent University, Ghent, Belgium

A. Nathan • A. Barnett • D. Barnett • E. Cerin
Institute for Health and Ageing, Australian Catholic University, Melbourne, VIC, Australia

© The Author(s) 2018
S. R. Nyman et al. (eds.), *The Palgrave Handbook of Ageing and Physical Activity Promotion*, https://doi.org/10.1007/978-3-319-71291-8_22

neighbourhoods and streets), including aspects of urban design (e.g., residential density), traffic (e.g., density and speed), distance to and design of venues for PA (e.g., parks and public open spaces), crime, and safety (Davison and Lawson 2006). We are focusing on physical characteristics of where people live, which are governed by planning and government policy and, hence, are amenable to change. The aim of this chapter is to provide a critical overview of key conceptual and theoretical frameworks underpinning the importance of the environment and critically review the available evidence about the relationships between aspects of the physical environment and older adults' PA.

22.2 Theoretical Underpinnings

22.2.1 The Socio-ecological Model of Active Living

The majority of research on physical environmental correlates of older adults' PA uses the socio-ecological model of active living proposed by Sallis et al. (2006) as a theoretical background. As described in Chap. 1, socio-ecological theory posits that PA is determined by complex interrelationships between individuals and their surrounding social, physical, and policy environments (Stokols 1996). The socio-ecological model of active living describes four domains of active living: active transportation (e.g., walking/cycling to a shop), recreational PA (e.g., going for a walk in a park, engaging in a particular sport), work-related PA (e.g., walking as part of volunteer work), and household-related PA (e.g., cleaning, gardening). In this chapter we will focus on active transportation and recreational PA, since PA in these domains can be expected to be more strongly influenced by older adults' surrounding neighbourhood environments than in-home or workplace-related PA. A key premise of the model is that physical environmental correlates influence PA in a domain-specific manner. For example, easy access to shops and services is hypothesised to be particularly relevant for active transportation and less so for recreational PA.

22.2.2 Objective Versus Subjective Measures of the Physical Environment

Pikora et al. (2003) developed a framework that classifies physical environmental factors into four different features: destination (e.g., shops, services, parks, and public transit), functional (e.g., street connectivity, pedestrian infrastructure), safety (e.g., traffic safety, safety from crime), and aesthetic (e.g., cleanliness, greenery, pollution). Physical environmental factors can be measured objectively or subjectively (by means of perceptions). Objective measures aim to capture a physical environmental factor as it is in reality without subjective interpretation. Objective measures can be obtained from geographic databases (e.g., cadastral plans providing information about land use or census data providing information about population density) and can be combined using Geographic Information Systems (GIS). Researchers can also collect objective environmental data by means of auditing. When auditing, researchers scan a predefined area (e.g., a street segment) and rate several environmental characteristics using a predefined checklist. Audit tools to objectively assess physical environmental factors related to older adults' PA have been developed in the United States of America (USA) (Cain et al. 2014), Hong Kong (Cerin et al. 2011), and the Netherlands (Etman et al. 2014). Perceptions of the physical environment are measured by questionnaires. A frequently used questionnaire is the Neighbourhood Environment Walkability Scale (NEWS) (Cerin et al. 2009; Saelens et al. 2003) which consists of 67 items grouped into eight multi-item subscales. An extensive overview of objective and subjective measures can be found on the website of the Active Living Research program: http://activelivingresearch.org/toolsandresources/toolsandmeasures.

Objective and subjective neighbourhood measures capture different aspects of the physical environment and are independently related to physical and social functioning in older adults (Weden et al. 2008). How older adults perceive the neighbourhood environment may be more closely linked to their PA behaviours than the 'real' objective environment (Wen et al. 2006). Differences arise in how people experience the same environment because perceptions may be influenced by past experiences, demographic differences, and physical and cognitive functioning. For example, one study found that older adults perceived pedestrian-friendly environmental features (i.e., presence of sidewalks and nearby shopping areas) to be less prevalent in their neighbourhood than younger adults (Cao et al. 2010).

An important issue in research concerned with environment-PA relationships is the way we define a neighbourhood, that is, the scale used to measure physical environmental factors. Neighbourhood definitions may differ based on the study objectives or data availability (Roux 2001). For example, when examining environmental perceptions, participants may interpret and use their own definition of neighbourhood. However, to enable standardisation and comparability across studies, the NEWS instructs participants to consider the area within a 10–15-minute walk from their home as their neighbourhood. When studying objective environmental data (e.g., residential density or number of violent crimes), neighbourhoods are represented by the administrative units at which the data are available (e.g., statistical sectors, postcodes) or by straight-line or street-network buffers (typically ranging from 250 to 1600 m). There is currently no consensus on how to best define an older adults' neighbourhood.

22.2.3 Interactions: The Core of Socio-ecological Models

Interactions between the different levels of influence (i.e., individual and social, physical and policy environmental factors) are at the core of socio-ecological models (Sallis et al. 2006). This implies that a certain physical environmental factor may neither influence PA in all individuals nor in all social, physical, and policy environments.

As described in the previous chapter, the interplay between person and environment is also recognised in prominent environmental gerontology theories (Lawton and Simon 1968). The impact of the environment on older adults may be even more pronounced because of their increased susceptibility and vulnerability to physical environmental barriers compared with younger age groups (Iwarsson 2005). But at the same time, it is also recognised that environmental features conducive to functioning may act as environmental buoys (Satariano 2006). An environmental buoy is defined as a facilitating aspect of the environment that supports a person's activities despite the presence of functional limitations (Spivock et al. 2008). Examples of environmental buoys for active living include the quality of pedestrian infrastructure (e.g., high-quality walking path surface and the presence of benches for rests while out walking), adaptation of signage (e.g., sufficient time provided at pedestrian crossings to walk across the road), and accessibility of elements surrounding pedestrian networks (e.g., destinations to walk to and public transport options). As such, the environment may influence participation in PA more strongly among older adults with functional impairments compared to functionally fit older adults or younger populations (Barnett et al. 2016; Cao et al. 2010; Shigematsu et al. 2009). For example, sidewalk or pavement evenness may be relevant to promote transportation walking among older adults with mobility impairments but not among functionally fit older adults. Environment-PA relationships may also differ according to gender and educational level. A handful of studies have found stronger associations between environmental attributes and PA outcomes among women and the less-educated, though for the most part findings have been inconsistent (Cerin et al. 2014; Van Cauwenberg et al. 2012a).

While some environmental factors may be differentially related to PA according to individual characteristics, others may influence PA only in the presence of other physical environmental factors. For example, sidewalk evenness may promote transportation walking in neighbourhoods with easy access to local shops and services, but not in areas with poor access. Such interactions between physical environmental factors are described in Alfonzo's Hierarchy of Walking Needs (2005). Four hierarchical walking needs were identified: (1) accessibility (e.g., access to local shops and services); (2) safety from crime (e.g., surveillance, hiding places); (3) comfort (e.g., sidewalk evenness, separation from traffic, benches); and (4) pleasurability (e.g., vegetation, historic elements). Alfonzo hypothesised that a lower-order need (e.g., comfort) would not influence walking if a higher-order need (e.g., accessibility) is not satisfied. Research has only begun to unravel such interaction effects between environmental factors (Ding and Gebel 2012) and more research into these is needed to find out which environmental attributes relate to PA under which environmental circumstances.

22.3 Empirical Evidence About the Relationships Between Physical Environmental Factors and Older Adults' Transportation and Recreational PA

This section will critically review quantitative and qualitative research findings about the physical environmental factors relating to older adults' transportation and recreational PA. It should be noted at this stage that the quantitative evidence base is mainly cross-sectional. Therefore, it is impossible to confidently predict how physical environmental factors will influence age-related declines in PA or how environmental modifications will change older adults' PA levels. We discuss qualitative findings to obtain insights into older adults' perspectives and how and why physical environmental factors influence their PA behaviours (Sallis et al. 2006).

22.3.1 Destination Features

22.3.1.1 Walkability

Walkability is a composite environmental measure combining multiple aspects of community design. It is derived using GIS and usually includes measures of residential density, land use mix, and street connectivity (Frank et al. 2010). Residential density refers to the number of residences or dwellings relative to a given residential land area (Transportation Research Board 2005). Land use describes areas of land that have been zoned for specific purposes (e.g., residential or retail). Land use mix refers to the diversity of different land uses or destinations within an area. Having a variety of land uses means that people live closer to destinations used for activities, which provides the opportunity to walk or cycle. Intersection density measures the connectivity of the street network, represented by the ratio between the number of true intersections (three or more legs) to a given land area (Frank et al. 2010). Higher intersection density is associated with more direct travel paths between destinations that are closer to the Euclidean ('as the crow flies') distance between destinations and offers a greater number of alternative routes from one destination to another (Transportation Research Board 2005). To calculate the walkability index, measures of residential density, land use mix, and street connectivity are standardised and summed (Frank et al. 2010).

Strong and consistent evidence supports the importance of walkability for older adults' active travel behaviour. Positive associations of walkability with older adults' walking for transport have been found across the world (King et al. 2011; Nathan et al. 2014; Van Holle et al. 2014). In the USA, older adults living in more walkable neighbourhoods reported an average of 38.1 minutes per week of walking or cycling for errands compared to 6.7 minutes per week among those living in less walkable neighbourhoods. These findings are in line with findings among adults across the world (De Sa and Ardern 2014; Owen et al. 2007; Sallis et al. 2009; Sundquist et al. 2011; Van Dyck et al. 2010). While walkability can be anticipated to be especially relevant for older adults' transportation walking, some studies also found walkability to be positively related to recreational walking (Berke et al. 2007; Carlson et al. 2012).

22.3.1.2 Residential Density

Higher levels of residential density provide a reliable source of customers for local businesses and public transit, making shops and services economically viable and resulting in a greater variety of destinations within a more compact area. In turn, this may also increase the feasibility of more frequent public transport services. Residential density has been positively associated with walking for transport in Belgium (Van Cauwenberg et al. 2012a), Hong Kong (Cerin et al. 2014), Singapore (Nyunt et al. 2015), the USA (Shigematsu et al. 2009), and Eastern Europe (Pelclová et al. 2012). A 12-country study among adults, reported a curvilinear relationship between residential density and walking for transport, with a positive relationship observed when residential density was low to medium and no relationship when residential density was high (Kerr et al. 2016). A multi-country study covering the complete range of residential densities could confirm whether residential density also relates to older adults' walking for transport in a curvilinear fashion. However, studies in very dense regions (e.g., Hong Kong) have already reported positive relationships between residential density and older adults' walking for transport (Cerin et al. 2014). Possibly, older adults' walking for transport is more strongly related to residential density in comparison to younger adults. Residential density appeared to be unrelated to older adults' recreational PA (Barnett et al. 2016; Cerin et al. 2013d; Ding et al. 2014b; Inoue et al. 2011; Kolbe-Alexander et al. 2015; Pelclová et al. 2012).

22.3.1.3 Land Use Mix

Higher levels of land use mix have been consistently related to higher levels of active transport (Cerin et al. 2014; Ding et al. 2014b; Etman et al. 2014; Nathan et al. 2014; Nyunt et al. 2015; Shigematsu et al. 2009; Van Cauwenberg et al. 2012a; Van Holle et al. 2016). In terms of destination categories important for transportation walking, there is strong evidence to support access to shops and commercial services (Cerin et al. 2013b; Inoue et al. 2011; Nathan et al. 2014; Van Cauwenberg et al. 2012a), public transport (Cerin et al. 2013b, 2014; Ding et al. 2014b; Nathan et al. 2014), parks, open space, and recreational facilities (Barnett et al. 2016; Cerin et al. 2013a; Corseuil et al. 2011; Ding et al. 2014a; Shigematsu et al. 2009). In terms of specific destinations, Cerin et al. (2013b) found the prevalence of non-food retails and services, food/grocery stores and restaurants, the presence of a health clinic/service and place of worship, and the diversity in recreational destinations to be positively related to within-neighbourhood walking for transport. Such research into the importance of specific destinations is necessary to advise policymakers about how to develop walkable neighbourhoods most effectively.

For recreational PA, positive associations with access to parks and public open space (Hanibuchi et al. 2011; Salvador et al. 2009) and recreational facilities (Kim and Kosma 2013; Tsunoda et al. 2012) have been reported. Using longitudinal data from the Multi-Ethnic Study of Atherosclerosis, Ranchod et al. (2014) found that higher baseline values and three-year increases in recreational facility density resulted in less pronounced age-related declines in recreational PA. A review of qualitative studies on environment-PA relationships in a variety of countries revealed that older adults felt that there was a lack of nearby recreational facilities and limited transportation to them (Moran et al. 2014). They also commented that the facilities were often expensive to use, designed with younger people in mind, and that there was a need for supervised group activities designed for seniors. The preferred facilities for recreational PA appeared to be indoor gyms and pools.

22.3.2 Functional Features

22.3.2.1 Street Connectivity

Higher levels of street connectivity (i.e., the number of intersections in a given area) were related to higher levels of transportation walking among older adults in Hong Kong (Barnett et al. 2016; Cerin et al. 2014), Belgium (Van Holle et al. 2016), Brazil (Giehl et al. 2016), and Singapore (Nyunt et al. 2015). Moreover, although the results were less consistent (Hanibuchi et al. 2011; Nagel et al. 2008), some studies reported that higher levels of street connectivity were associated with higher levels of recreational walking.

22.3.2.2 Pedestrian and Bicycle Infrastructure

A review of qualitative studies exploring environment-PA relationships among older adults showed that pedestrian infrastructure emerged as an important theme in all 31 reviewed studies (Moran et al. 2014). Several sidewalk characteristics emerged as being relevant for older adults' PA, not only their presence and continuity but also sidewalk quality and maintenance, slopes and curbs, obstacles, and separation from other non-motorised transport (i.e., cyclists). Concerning sidewalk quality and maintenance, participants discussed issues such as sidewalk width, evenness of sidewalk surfaces, holes, and cracks. The importance of such a wide variety of detailed sidewalk characteristics may explain the inconsistent relationships observed between measures of pedestrian infrastructure and older adults' PA in quantitative observational studies (Van Cauwenberg et al. 2011). In a more-controlled, experimental study using photographs of a street in which nine street characteristics (e.g., sidewalk evenness, traffic volume, presence of trees) were manipulated, sidewalk evenness had by far the strongest influence on a street's appeal for transportation walking among Belgian older adults (Van Cauwenberg et al. 2016). In a study in Hong Kong, objectively assessed path quality (by means of auditing) moderated the relationships between the presence of a swimming pool, playground, and outdoor sports field and the odds of engaging in recreational PA other than walking (Cerin et al. 2013a). The presence of such facilities was only related to recreational PA other than walking if path quality was high. These findings suggest that recreational facilities may only be used by older adults for PA if the surrounding pedestrian infrastructure is of good quality.

A qualitative study in the UK showed that the presence of high-quality cycling paths was an important contributor to older adults' cycling experiences (Jones et al. 2016). Older cyclists preferred paths exclusively dedicated to cycling. They also highlighted the poor state of surfacing and how this made them feel uncomfortable and vulnerable. No quantitative study has previously examined the relationships between presence and quality of cycling infrastructure and older adults' cycling levels.

22.3.2.3 Benches

In a Swedish mixed-methods study, one third of the participating older adults reported a lack of benches as a barrier preventing them from walking within their neighbourhood, despite a strong desire to undertake this walking (Stahl et al. 2008). The participants complained that there were too few benches and that the distances between those that existed were too long. Participants also emphasised the importance of the comfort and convenience of benches. Among a sample of Belgian older adults, the presence of benches appeared to be especially important for those with functional limitations and fear of falling (Van Cauwenberg et al. 2016). In Hong Kong, the perceived presence of benches was indeed related to more transportation walking, especially among the oldest participants (aged over 75 years) (Barnett et al. 2016; Cerin et al. 2014).

22.3.3 Safety Features

Safety from traffic and crime are often considered to be particularly relevant for older adults' PA behaviours (Alfonzo 2005). However, the majority of quantitative studies in this area reported no significant relationships (Bracy et al. 2014; Nathan et al. 2014; Nyunt et al. 2015; Van Cauwenberg et al. 2011).

22.3.3.1 Traffic Safety

Perceptions of traffic-related safety can be influenced by traffic volume and speed and the presence of safe crossings. High levels of traffic volume and speeding cars are generally found to be barriers for PA in qualitative research (Moran et al. 2014; Stahl et al. 2008; Van Cauwenberg et al. 2012b). In a qualitative study focusing on the environmental factors influencing Belgian older adults' cycling for transport, traffic safety emerged as the most important concern (Van Cauwenberg et al. 2018). The most important factor influencing participants' feelings of traffic safety during cycling was the presence of cycling paths that were well-separated from motorised traffic. However, evidence from quantitative studies is less consistent. For example, higher levels of traffic volume have been reported to be related to lower levels of recreational PA among Hong Kong older adults (Cerin et al. 2013a, c). However, no relationships between traffic volume and recreational PA were observed in other studies based in Brazil and England (Salvador et al. 2009; Wu et al. 2016). Some studies have even reported the opposite, whereby higher levels of traffic volume were related to higher levels of transportation walking (Nathan et al. 2014) and recreational PA (Nagel et al. 2008). Such inconsistencies may be explained by older adults wanting to walk on streets with less traffic, but being forced to walk on streets with heavier traffic to reach daily destinations.

The presence of safe crossings is a frequently discussed topic by older adults during qualitative studies. Older adults prefer to have regular and clearly indicated crossings with short crossing distance. In case of signalled crossings, signal times should be adequate in length (Moran et al. 2014). Among US older adults, the objectively assessed (i.e., audited) presence of 'safe' crossings was positively related to transportation walking, but not to recreational walking (Cain et al. 2014). The perceived presence of crossings was not related to transportation and recreational walking and cycling among Belgian older adults (Van Cauwenberg et al. 2012a).

22.3.3.2 Safety from Crime

Qualitative studies have observed that some older adults felt unsafe being physically active in areas with vacant houses, overgrown lots, vandalism, and inadequate street lighting. The presence of people may increase or decrease feelings of safety when being physically active. Older adults felt safer when friendly, smiling, and familiar people, families with children, socially responsible residents, or people walking, biking, or jogging were present. In contrast, the presence of large crowds, criminality, intimidating groups of youths, beggars, immigrants, and homeless people fostered feelings of lack of safety (Moran et al. 2014).

The majority of quantitative studies reported no relationships between safety from crime and older adults' transportation and recreational PA (Bracy et al. 2014; Corseuil et al. 2011; Nathan et al. 2014; Nyunt et al. 2015; Van Cauwenberg et al. 2011). These non-significant relationships may be due to the assessment of perceived safety from crime without including the source of danger and emotional reactions attached to these perceptions (Foster and Giles-Corti 2008). A study using a more comprehensive measure of perceived safety from crime found higher levels of safety to be related to a higher likelihood of transportation and recreational walking and cycling among Belgian older adults (Van Cauwenberg et al. 2012a). In this study the presence of street lighting was also related to a higher likelihood of walking and cycling, especially among women. Providing evidence for the importance of surveillance ('eyes on the street'), Borst et al. (2009) reported that streets with blind walls (low surveillance) were used less for transportation walking by Dutch older adults. In line with this, the perceived presence of people in neighbourhood streets was related to higher levels of transportation walking and an increased likelihood of recreational walking among Hong Kong older adults (Barnett et al. 2016). This latter study also reported higher levels of perceived crime to be related to higher levels of transportation walking. Such a counterintuitive finding may be explained by higher levels of crime being inherent to areas with high levels of pedestrian activity (i.e., shopping areas). Furthermore, older adults from lower socio-economic backgrounds may be less able to afford motorised forms of transport and may inhabit areas with higher levels of crime (hence, they are forced to walk despite low levels of safety from crime).

22.3.4 Aesthetic Features

Coherent with the socio-ecological model's domain-specific reasoning, aesthetics (e.g., greenery, well-maintained gardens) appeared to be positively related to older adults' recreational walking but unrelated to transportation walking (Kolbe-Alexander et al. 2015; Nathan et al. 2014; Sugiyama and Ward Thompson 2008). Moreover, qualitative studies have reported that older adults prefer streets with well-maintained houses and gardens and including historical buildings and attractive streetscapes (e.g., statues, distinctive buildings, or architectural variation between houses) (Moran et al. 2014). This is supported by humans' general preference for vegetation and greenery (Van Den Berg et al. 2003) and the fact that they enjoy being physically active in areas with trees and water (Moran et al. 2014). However, there are potential side effects of greenery that should be considered. Specifically, leaves may cause sidewalks to become slippery, trees or their roots may be obstacles on the sidewalk, and unkempt greenery may narrow sidewalks (Van Cauwenberg et al. 2014, 2012b).

In some cities, air pollution may constitute a hazard for PA (Lu et al. 2015). In Hong Kong, the objectively assessed presence of noise and air pollution was found to be related to lower levels of recreational walking (Cerin et al. 2013a). Furthermore, the presence of a swimming pool, playground, and park was only related to engagement in recreational PA other than walking when noise and air pollution levels were low. This suggests that such facilities are only used by older adults for recreational PA when the surroundings are free from noise and air pollution.

22.4 Key Practical Implications

22.4.1 Implications for Policy and Practice

To promote transportation walking among older adults, neighbourhoods should provide: (1) easy access to local shops and services (possibly achieved by high residential density, land use mix, and street connectivity); (2) easy access to a high-quality public transit system; (3) continuous, even sidewalks that are well-separated from other road users (cars and cyclists); and (4) benches at regular distances to allow older adults to rest.

To promote recreational PA among older adults, neighbourhoods should provide: (1) recreational facilities adapted to the needs of older adults (e.g., supervised group activities); (2) parks and public open spaces; and (3) aesthetically pleasing and well-maintained streets with greenery.

When the above described guidelines are implemented, policymakers and researchers should collaborate to evaluate the effects of such environmental modifications on older adults' PA levels. Such evaluations will strengthen the knowledge-base and can be used to help shape future policy initiatives. It should be acknowledged as well that socio-ecological theory posits that multi-level interventions are needed to effectively increase older adults' PA levels (Sallis et al. 2006). This implies that environmental modifications should be complemented by strategies targeting individual's psychosocial attributes (e.g., attitudes and self-efficacy), social norms, social capital, and initiatives at the economic and policy level (e.g., reduced bus fares).

22.4.2 Recommendations for Future Research

Several issues remain unresolved. First, little is known about the optimal 'dose' of an environmental factor necessary to stimulate PA. Second, further studies using GPS-devices may yield insights into which areas of their older adults' environments are most strongly influencing their PA behaviours. Third, very little is known about which environmental factors matter most for which demographic subgroups. Fourth, few studies have examined interactions between environmental factors. Fifth, research outside North America, Europe, East Asia, and Oceania is necessary to confirm the generalisability of the current findings. Lastly, there is a need for longitudinal and experimental studies to infer causality.

22.5 Conclusion

There is a clear need to provide older citizens with neighbourhoods, streets, and public open spaces that stimulate active living. About 15 years of research into the environmental determinants of older adults' PA has provided us with some clear priorities to target during environmental interventions. Access to local shops, services, public transit, parks, public open spaces, and recreational facilities within walking distance along well-maintained and aesthetically pleasing streets with high-quality pedestrian infrastructure appear to be paramount for promoting PA among older adults. Policy initiatives aimed at providing such environments should be evaluated to strengthen the evidence base, which is currently mainly observational. Researchers across the world should be encouraged to strive for more detailed insights (e.g., dose-response relationships, interaction effects) to come up with cost-effective solutions to promote active living among older adults.

Suggested Further Reading

- Moran, M., Van Cauwenberg, J., Hercky-Linnewiel, R., Cerin, E., Deforche, B., & Plaut, P. (2014). Understanding the relationships between the physical environment and physical activity in older adults: A systematic

review of qualitative studies. *International Journal of Behavioural Nutrition and Physical Activity, 11*. Available on: http://ijbnpa.biomedcentral.com/articles/10.1186/1479-5868-11-79
- Cerin, E., Barnett, D., Nathan, A., Van Cauwenberg, J., & Barnett, A. (2017). The neighbourhood physical environment and active travel in older adults: A systematic review and meta-analysis. *International Journal of Behavioural Nutrition and Physical Activity, 14*. Available on: http://ijbnpa.biomedcentral.com/articles/10.1186/s12966-017-0471-5
- Website of the Active Living Research program with links to research papers, article summaries and measurement tools. http://activelivingresearch.org/

References

8 80 Cities. (2016). 8 1 Cities. Retrieved from http://www.880cities.org/

Alfonzo, M. A. (2005). To walk or not to walk? The hierarchy of walking needs. *Environment & Behavior, 37*(6), 808–836.

Barnett, A., Cerin, E., Zhang, C. J. P., Sit, C. H. P., Johnston, J. M., Cheung, M. M. C., & Lee, R. S. Y. (2016). Associations between the neighbourhood environment characteristics and physical activity in older adults with specific types of chronic conditions: The ALECS cross-sectional study. *International Journal of Behavioral Nutrition & Physical Activity, 13*. https://doi.org/10.1186/s12966-016-0377-7.

Berke, E. M., Koepsell, T. D., Moudon, A. V., Hoskins, R. E., & Larson, E. B. (2007). Association of the built environment with physical activity and obesity in older persons. *American Journal of Public Health, 97*(3), 486–492.

Borst, H. C., De Vries, S. I., Graham, J. M. A., Van Dongen, J. E. F., Bakker, I., & Miedema, H. M. E. (2009). Influence of environmental street characteristics on walking route choice of elderly people. *Journal of Environmental Psychology, 29*(4), 477–484. https://doi.org/10.1016/j.jenvp.2009.08.002.

Bracy, N. L., Millstein, R. A., Carlson, J. A., Conway, T. L., Sallis, J. F., Saelens, B. E., et al. (2014). Is the relationship between the built environment and physical activity moderated by perceptions of crime and safety? *International Journal of Behavioral Nutrition & Physical Activity, 11*. https://doi.org/10.1186/1479-5868-11-24.

Cain, K. L., Millstein, R. A., Sallis, J. F., Conway, T. L., Gavand, K. A., Frank, L. D., et al. (2014). Contribution of streetscape audits to explanation of physical activity in four age groups based on the microscale audit of pedestrian streetscapes (MAPS). *Social Science & Medicine, 116*, 82–92. https://doi.org/10.1016/j.socscimed.2014.06.042.

Cao, X. Y., Mokhtarian, P. L., & Handy, S. L. (2010). Neighborhood design and the accessibility of the elderly: An empirical analysis in Northern California. *International Journal of Sustainable Transportation, 4*(6), 347–371. https://doi.org/10.1080/15568310903145212.

Carlson, J. A., Sallis, J. F., Conway, T. L., Saelens, B. E., Frank, L. D., Kerr, J., et al. (2012). Interactions between psychosocial and built environment factors in explaining older adults' physical activity. *Preventive Medicine, 54*(1), 68–73. https://doi.org/10.1016/j.ypmed.2011.10.004.

Cerin, E., Conway, T. L., Saelens, B. E., Frank, L. D., & Sallis, J. F. (2009). Cross-validation of the factorial structure of the neighborhood environment walkability scale (NEWS) and its abbreviated form (NEWS-A). *International Journal of Behavioral Nutrition & Physical Activity, 6*, 32. https://doi.org/10.1186/1479-5868-6-32.

Cerin, E., Chan, K. W., Macfarlane, D. J., Lee, K. Y., & Lai, P. C. (2011). Objective assessment of walking environments in ultra-dense cities: Development and reliability of the environment in Asia scan tool-Hong Kong version (EAST-HK). *Health & Place, 17*(4), 937–945. https://doi.org/10.1016/j.healthplace.2011.04.005.

Cerin, E., Lee, K. Y., Barnett, A., Sit, C. H. P., Cheung, M. C., & Chan, W. M. (2013a). Objectively-measured neighborhood environments and leisure-time physical activity in Chinese urban elders. *Preventive Medicine, 56*(1), 86–89. https://doi.org/10.1016/j.ypmed.2012.10.024.

Cerin, E., Lee, K. Y., Barnett, A., Sit, C. H. P., Cheung, M. C., Chan, W. M., & Johnston, J. M. (2013b). Walking for transportation in Hong Kong Chinese urban elders: A cross-sectional study on what destinations matter and when. *International Journal of Behavioral Nutrition & Physical Activity, 10*, 78. https://doi.org/10.1186/1479-5868-10-78.

Cerin, E., Macfarlane, D. J., Sit, C. H. P., Ho, S. Y., Johnston, J. M., Chou, K. L., et al. (2013c). Effects of built environment on walking among Hong Kong older adults. *Hong Kong Medical Journal, 19*(Suppl 4), 39–41.

Cerin, E., Sit, C. H. P., Barnett, A., Cheung, M. C., & Chan, W. M. (2013d). Walking for recreation and perceptions of the neighborhood environment in older Chinese urban dwellers. *Journal of Urban Health, 90*(1), 56–66. https://doi.org/10.1007/s11524-012-9704-8.

Cerin, E., Sit, C. H. P., Barnett, A., Johnston, J. M., Cheung, M. C., & Chan, W. M. (2014). Ageing in an ultra-dense metropolis: Perceived neighbourhood characteristics and utilitarian walking in Hong Kong elders. *Public Health Nutrition, 17*(1), 225–232. https://doi.org/10.1017/s1368980012003862.

Corseuil, M. W., Schneider, I. J. C., Silva, D. A. S., Costa, F. F., Silva, K. S., Borges, L. J., & D'Orsi, E. (2011). Perception of environmental obstacles to commuting physical activity in Brazilian elderly. *Preventive Medicine, 53*(4–5), 289–292. https://doi.org/10.1016/j.ypmed.2011.07.016.

Davison, K. K., & Lawson, C. T. (2006). Do attributes in the physical environment influence children's physical activity? A review of the literature. *International Journal of Behavioral Nutrition & Physical Activity, 3.* https://doi.org/10.1186/1479-5868-3-19.

De Sa, E., & Ardern, C. I. (2014). Neighbourhood walkability, leisure-time and transport-related physical activity in a mixed urban-rural area. *PeerJ, 2,* e440. https://doi.org/10.7717/peerj.440.

Ding, D., & Gebel, K. (2012). Built environment, physical activity, and obesity: What have we learned from reviewing the literature? *Health & Place, 18*(1), 100–105. https://doi.org/10.1016/j.healthplace.2011.08.021.

Ding, D., Gebel, K., Phongsavan, P., Bauman, A. E., & Merom, D. (2014a). Driving: A road to unhealthy lifestyles and poor health outcomes. *PLoS One, 9*(6). https://doi.org/10.1371/journal.pone.0094602.

Ding, D., Sallis, J. F., Norman, G. J., Frank, L. D., Saelens, B. E., Kerr, J., et al. (2014b). Neighborhood environment and physical activity among older adults: Do the relationships differ by driving status? *Journal of Aging & Physical Activity, 22*(3), 421–431. https://doi.org/10.1123/japa.2012-0332.

Etman, A., Kamphuis, C. B. M., Prins, R. G., Burdorf, A., Pierik, F. H., & Van Lenthe, F. J. (2014). Characteristics of residential areas and transportational walking among frail and non-frail Dutch elderly: Does the size of the area matter? *International Journal of Health Geographics, 13.* https://doi.org/10.1186/1476-072x-13-7.

Forsyth, A., Oakes, J. M., Lee, B., & Schmitz, K. H. (2009). The built environment, walking, and physical activity: Is the environment more important to some people than others? *Transportation Research Part D, 14*(1), 42–49. https://doi.org/10.1016/j.trd.2008.10.003.

Foster, S., & Giles-Corti, B. (2008). The built environment, neighborhood crime and constrained physical activity: An exploration of inconsistent findings. *Preventive Medicine, 47*(3), 241–251. https://doi.org/10.1016/j.ypmed.2008.03.017.

Frank, L. D., Sallis, J. F., Saelens, B. E., Leary, L., Cain, K. L., Conway, T. L., & Hess, P. M. (2010). The development of a walkability index: Application to the neighborhood quality of life study. *British Journal of Sports Medicine, 44*(13), 924–933. https://doi.org/10.1136/bjsm.2009.058701.

Giehl, M. W. C., Hallal, P. C., Corseuil, C. W., Schneider, L. J. C., & D'Orsi, E. (2016). Built environment and walking behavior among Brazilian older adults: A population-based study. *Journal of Physical Activity & Health, 13*(6), 617–624. https://doi.org/10.1123/jpah.2015-0355.

Hanibuchi, T., Kawachi, I., Nakaya, T., Hirai, H., & Kondo, K. (2011). Neighborhood built environment and physical activity of Japanese older adults: Results from the Aichi Gerontological evaluation study (AGES). *BMC Public Health, 11.* https://doi.org/10.1186/1471-2458-11-657.

Inoue, S., Ohya, Y., Odagiri, Y., Takamiya, T., Kamada, M., Okada, S., et al. (2011). Perceived neighborhood environment and walking for specific purposes among elderly Japanese. *Journal of Epidemiology, 21*(6), 481–490. https://doi.org/10.2188/jea.JE20110044.

Iwarsson, S. (2005). A long-term perspective on person-environment fit and ADL dependence among older Swedish adults. *The Gerontologist, 45*(3), 327–336. https://doi.org/10.1093/geront/45.3.327.

Jones, T., Chatterjee, K., Spinney, J., Street, E., Van Reekum, C., Spencer, B., et al. (2016). *Cycle BOOM: Design for lifelong health and wellbeing*. Retrieved from Oxford Brookes University, Oxford. http://d1qmdf3vop2l07.cloudfront.net/quaint-manatee.cloudvent.net/compressed/5ab7ab985c867240c4f1883d77e0fbb1.pdf

Kerr, J., Emond, J. A., Badland, H., Reis, R. S., Sarmiento, O., Carlson, J. A., et al. (2016). Perceived neighborhood environmental attributes associated with walking and cycling for transport among adult residents of 17 cities in 12 countries: The IPEN study. *Environmental Health Perspectives, 124*(3), 290–298. https://doi.org/10.1289/ehp.1409466.

Kim, Y. H., & Kosma, M. (2013). Psychosocial and environmental correlates of physical activity among Korean older adults. *Research on Aging, 35*(6), 750–767. https://doi.org/10.1177/0164027512462412.

King, A. C., Sallis, J. F., Frank, L. D., Saelens, B. E., Cain, K. L., Conway, T. L., et al. (2011). Aging in neighborhoods differing in walkability and income: Associations with physical activity and obesity in older adults. *Social Science & Medicine, 73*(10), 1525–1533. https://doi.org/10.1016/j.socscimed.2011.08.032.

Kolbe-Alexander, T. L., Pacheco, K., Tomaz, S. A., Karpul, D., & Lambert, E. V. (2015). The relationship between the built environment and habitual levels of physical activity in South African older adults: A pilot study. *BMC Public Health, 15*, 518. https://doi.org/10.1186/s12889-015-1853-8.

Lawton, M. P., & Simon, B. (1968). The ecology of social relationships in housing for the elderly. *The Gerontologist, 8*(2), 108–115. https://doi.org/10.1093/geront/8.2.108.

Lu, J. J., Liang, L. C., Feng, Y., Li, R. N., & Liu, Y. (2015). Air pollution exposure and physical activity in China: Current knowledge, public health implications, and future research needs. *International Journal of Environmental Research & Public Health, 12*(11), 14887–14897. https://doi.org/10.3390/ijerph121114887.

Moran, M., Van Cauwenberg, J., Hercky-Linnewiel, R., Cerin, E., Deforche, B., & Plaut, P. (2014). Understanding the relationships between the physical environment and physical activity in older adults: A systematic review of qualitative studies. *International Journal of Behavioral Nutrition & Physical Activity, 11*. https://doi.org/10.1186/1479-5868-11-79.

Nagel, C. L., Carlson, N. E., Bosworth, M., & Michael, Y. L. (2008). The relation between neighborhood built environment and walking activity among older adults. *American Journal of Epidemiology, 168*(4), 461–468. https://doi.org/10.1093/aje/kwn158.

Nathan, A., Wood, L., & Giles-Corti, B. (2014). Perceptions of the built environment and associations with walking among retirement village residents. *Environment & Behavior, 46*(1), 46–69. https://doi.org/10.1177/0013916512450173.

Nyunt, M. S. Z., Shuvo, F. K., Eng, J. Y., Yap, K. B., Scherer, S., Hee, L. M., et al. (2015). Objective and subjective measures of neighborhood environment (NE): Relationships with transportation physical activity among older persons. *International Journal of Behavioral Nutrition & Physical Activity, 12*. https://doi.org/10.1186/s12966-015-0276-3.

Owen, N., Cerin, E., Leslie, E., Dutoit, L., Coffee, N., Frank, L. D., et al. (2007). Neighborhood walkability and the walking behavior of Australian adults. *American Journal of Preventive Medicine, 33*(5), 387–395. https://doi.org/10.1016/j.amepre.2007.07.025.

Pelclová, J., Frömel, K., Bláha, L., Zając-Gawlak, I., & Tlučáková, L. (2012). Neighborhood environment and walking for transport and recreation in central European older adults. *Acta Universitatis Palackianae Olomucensis Gymnica, 42*(4), 49–56.

Pikora, T., Giles-Corti, B., Bull, F., Jamrozik, K., & Donovan, R. (2003). Developing a framework for assessment of the environmental determinants of walking and cycling. *Social Science & Medicine, 56*(8), 1693–1703. https://doi.org/10.1016/s0277-9536(02)00163-6.

Ranchod, Y. K., Roux, A. V. D., Evenson, K. R., Sanchez, B. N., & Moore, K. (2014). Longitudinal associations between neighborhood recreational facilities and change in recreational physical activity in the multi-ethnic study of atherosclerosis, 2000–2007. *American Journal of Epidemiology, 179*(3), 335–343. https://doi.org/10.1093/aje/kwt263.

Roux, A. V. D. (2001). Investigating neighborhood and area effects on health. *American Journal of Public Health, 91*(11), 1783–1789.

Saelens, B. E., Sallis, J. F., Black, J. B., & Chen, D. (2003). Neighborhood-based differences in physical activity: An environment scale evaluation. *American Journal of Public Health, 93*(9), 1552–1558. https://doi.org/10.2105/ajph.93.9.1552.

Sallis, J. F., Cervero, R., Ascher, W., Henderson, K., Kraft, M., & Kerr, J. (2006). An ecological approach to creating active living communities. *Annual Review of Public Health, 27*(1), 297–322. https://doi.org/10.1146/annurev.publhealth.27.021405.102100.

Sallis, J. F., Saelens, B. E., Frank, L. D., Conway, T. L., Slymen, D. J., Cain, K. L., et al. (2009). Neighborhood built environment and income: Examining multiple health outcomes. *Social Science & Medicine, 68*(7), 1285–1293. https://doi.org/10.1016/j.socscimed.2009.01.017.

Salvador, E. P., Florindo, A. A., Reis, R. S., & Costa, E. F. (2009). Perception of the environment and leisure-time physical activity in the elderly. *Revista de Saúde Pública, 43*(6), 1–8.

Satariano, W. (2006). *Epidemiology of aging: An ecological approach*. Sudbury: Jones and Bartlett Publishers.

Shigematsu, R., Sallis, J. F., Conway, T. L., Saelens, B. E., Frank, L. D., Cain, K. L., et al. (2009). Age differences in the relation of perceived neighborhood environment to walking. *Medicine & Science in Sports & Exercise, 41*(2), 314–321. https://doi.org/10.1249/MSS.0b013e318185496c.

Spivock, M., Gauvin, L., Riva, M., & Brodeur, J. (2008). Promoting active living among people with physical disabilities: Evidence for neighborhood-level buoys. *American Journal of Preventive Medicine, 34*(4), 291–298.

Stahl, A., Carlsson, G., Hovbrandt, P., & Iwarsson, S. (2008). "Let's go for a walk!": Identification and prioritisation of accessibility and safety measures involving elderly people in a residential area. *European Journal of Ageing, 5*(3), 265–273. https://doi.org/10.1007/s10433-008-0091-7.

Stokols, D. (1996). Translating social ecological theory into guidelines for community health promotion. *American Journal of Health Promotion, 10*, 282–298.

Sugiyama, T., & Ward Thompson, C. (2008). Associations between characteristics of neighbourhood open space and older people's walking. *Urban Forestry & Urban Greening, 7*, 41–51.

Sundquist, K., Eriksson, U., Kawakami, N., Skog, L., Ohlsson, H., & Arvidsson, D. (2011). Neighborhood walkability, physical activity, and walking behavior: The Swedish neighborhood and physical activity (SNAP) study. *Social Science & Medicine, 72*(8), 1266–1273. https://doi.org/10.1016/j.socscimed.2011.03.004.

Transportation Research Board. (2005). Does the built environment influence physical activity? Examining the evidence. Retrieved from Washington, DC. http://onlinepubs.trb.org/onlinepubs/sr/sr282.pdf

Tsunoda, K., Tsuji, T., Kitano, N., Mitsuishi, Y., Yoon, J., Yoon, J., & Okura, T. (2012). Associations of physical activity with neighborhood environments and transportation modes in older Japanese adults. *Preventive Medicine, 55*(2), 113–118. https://doi.org/10.1016/j.ypmed.2012.05.013.

Van Cauwenberg, J., De Bourdeaudhuij, I., De Meester, F., Van Dyck, D., Salmon, J., Clarys, P., & Deforche, B. (2011). Relationship between the physical environment and physical activity in older adults: A systematic review. *Health & Place, 17*(2), 458–469. https://doi.org/10.1016/j.healthplace.2010.11.010.

Van Cauwenberg, J., Clarys, P., De Bourdeaudhuij, I., Van Holle, V., Verte, D., De Witte, N., et al. (2012a). Physical environmental factors related to walking and cycling in older adults: The Belgian aging studies. *BMC Public Health, 12*. https://doi.org/10.1186/1471-2458-12-142.

Van Cauwenberg, J., Van Holle, V., Simons, D., Deridder, R., Clarys, P., Goubert, L., et al. (2012b). Environmental factors influencing older adults' walking for transportation: A study using walk-along interviews. *International Journal of Behavioral Nutrition & Physical Activity, 9*. https://doi.org/10.1186/1479-5868-9-85.

Van Cauwenberg, J., Van Holle, V., De Bourdeaudhuij, I., Clarys, P., Nasar, J., Salmon, J., et al. (2014). Using manipulated photographs to identify features of streetscapes that may encourage older adults to walk for transport. *PLoS One, 9*(11). https://doi.org/10.1371/journal.pone.0112107.

Van Cauwenberg, J., De Bourdeaudhuij, I., Clarys, P., Nasar, J., Salmon, J., Goubert, L., & Deforche, B. (2016). Street characteristics preferred for transportation walking among older adults: A choice-based conjoint analysis with manipulated photographs. *International Journal of Behavioral Nutrition & Physical Activity, 13*. https://doi.org/10.1186/s12966-016-0331-8.

Van Cauwenberg, J., Clarys, P., De Bourdeaudhuij, I., Ghekiere, A., de Geus, B., Owen, N., & Deforche, B. (2018). Environmental influences on older adults' transportation cycling experiences: A study using bike-along interviews. *Landscape and Urban Planning, 169*, 37–46.

Van Den Berg, A. E., Koole, S. L., & Van Der Wulp, N. Y. (2003). Environmental preference and restoration: (How) are they related? *Journal of Environmental Psychology, 23*(2), 135–146. https://doi.org/10.1016/s0272-4944(02)00111-1.

Van Dyck, D., Cardon, G., Deforche, B., Sallis, J. F., Owen, N., & De Bourdeaudhuij, I. (2010). Neighborhood SES and walkability are related to physical activity behavior in Belgian adults. *Preventive Medicine, 50*, S74–S79. https://doi.org/10.1016/j.ypmed.2009.07.027.

Van Holle, V., Van Cauwenberg, J., Van Dyck, D., Deforche, B., Van De Weghe, N., & De Bourdeaudhuij, I. (2014). Relationship between neighborhood walkability and older adults' physical activity: Results from the Belgian environmental physical activity study in seniors (BEPAS seniors). *International Journal of Behavioral Nutrition & Physical Activity, 11*, 110. https://doi.org/10.1186/s12966-014-0110-3.

Van Holle, V., Van Cauwenberg, J., Gheysen, F., Van Dyck, D., Deforche, B., Van De Weghe, N., & De Bourdeaudhuij, I. (2016). The association between Belgian older adults' physical functioning and physical activity: What is the moderating role of the physical environment? *PLoS One, 11*(2), e0148398. https://doi.org/10.1371/journal.pone.0148398.

Weden, M. M., Carpiano, R. M., & Robert, S. A. (2008). Subjective and objective neighborhood characteristics and adult health. *Social Science & Medicine, 66*(6), 1256–1270. https://doi.org/10.1016/j.socscimed.2007.11.041.

Wen, M., Hawkley, L. C., & Cacioppo, J. T. (2006). Objective and perceived neighborhood environment, individual SES and psychosocial factors, and self-rated health: An analysis of older adults in Cook County, Illinois. *Social Science & Medicine, 63*(10), 2575–2590.

WHO. (2007). *Global age-friendly cities: A guide*. Geneva: WHO Press. http://apps.who.int/iris/bitstream/10665/43755/1/9789241547307_eng.pdf.

Wu, Y. T., Jones, N. R., Van Sluijs, E. M. F., Griffin, S. J., Wareham, N. J., & Jones, A. P. (2016). Perceived and objectively measured environmental correlates of domain specific physical activity in older English adults. *Journal of Aging & Physical Activity, 24*(4), 599–616. https://doi.org/10.1123/japa.2015-0241.

23

Indoor Environments and Promoting Physical Activity Among Older People

Maureen C. Ashe

23.1 Introduction

House, abode, building, dwelling, quarters, residence, home. Does where we live influence the amount of activity incorporated into our daily life routines? An important consideration given that many people (especially older adults) spend so much time inside (Matz et al. 2014). Age-friendly communities, "a place where older people are actively involved, valued, and supported with infrastructure and services that effectively accommodate their needs" (Alley et al. 2007, page 4), include a focus on housing to support older adults' daily life routines. Although there is a rapidly developing field looking at the role of physical activity (recreational and utilitarian) and the outdoor built environment (Eisenberg et al. 2017; Hanson et al. 2012; Saelens and Papadopoulos 2008), few studies consider the *indoor* environment as a potential intervention to support day-to-day activity patterns of older adults (Gitlin 2003; Joseph 2006; Marmot and Ucci 2015). But it is not always "build it and they will come" (or *move*, as is the case here). Engaging in regular physical activity is a confluence of different personal, environmental, and societal factors (Carlson et al. 2012; Sallis et al. 2006). Further, social interaction and destinations are essential elements to support physical activity, just as in the outdoor built environment (Chudyk et al. 2015; Hanson et al. 2012, 2013).

M. C. Ashe (✉)
Department of Family Practice, The University of British Columbia Centre for Hip Health & Mobility, Vancouver, BC, Canada

This chapter will examine physical activity in later life from the perspective of building design to support (or hinder) physical activity across the spectrum of mobility, from older adults who aim to "age in place" to older adults who already moved into more supportive housing, such as assisted living. The aim of this chapter is to summarize what is currently known on indoor environments and older adults' physical activity, identify gaps in theory and knowledge, and consider future policy implications for this important field of ageing.

23.1.1 Housing in Later Life

Housing for older adults can vary greatly depending on individual characteristics, needs and preferences, geography, cultural norms, social support, and available finances (Kinsella et al. 2002). Generally, women live longer than men, but also live with more chronic conditions (World Health Organization 2011). But recent data from the United States (US) suggest that while the life expectancy for men may be increasing, older women's disability compression is not occurring (Freedman et al. 2016). In general, for many countries, more older women live alone, while older men tend to live with families (Kinsella et al. 2002). Based on an international report of ten countries (Ferreira 2013), most older adults live independently within the community, and not in more supportive housing (e.g., communal or care facilities). However, this can vary. For example, in the UK 89% of older adults live independently, while in Brazil almost all of the older adult population (99%) live in the community, most often with family. In 2008, only 1.5% of older adults in China lived in nursing homes (Chu and Chi 2008), although the numbers are expected to increase (Chu and Chi 2008; Feng et al. 2012), especially as nearly one third of older Chinese adults may require some form of assistance (Feng et al. 2012). In Canada 7.9% of older adults live in supportive care, while the remaining 92% (4.5 million) reside in private dwellings (https://www12.statcan.gc.ca/census-recensement/2011/as-sa/98-312-x/98-312-x2011003_4-eng.cfm). There are 1.4 million older Americans living in long-term care facilities (Harris-Kojetin et al. 2016), but 85% (32.6 million) of the older American population (≥65 years) live in traditional housing settings (Freedman and Spillman 2014). These figures are to highlight that although there are many older adults who reside in supportive accommodation settings, the preponderance of older adults live "at home".

Given the projected growth in the number of older adults, the number and types of buildings that currently exist may not meet future demands. Although more supportive housing is available in high-income countries, there is greater demand across the globe given the ubiquitous increase in the number of older adults (Kinsella et al. 2002). Different needs arise in health and housing globally, and particularly for the baby boomers (people born between 1946 and 1964), who may be different (from previous generations) because of their access to resources, health (Martin et al. 2009; Rice et al. 2010), and perspectives on ageing.

As data suggest that older adults spend the majority of their day (89%) inside (Matz et al. 2014), the indoor environment has the potential to play a significant role in how we create our daily life routines. This is especially true for older adults who may have mobility limitations. Given the number of older adults living in private dwellings, this presents some challenges to retrofit or update the vast number (and diversity) of current buildings. The life space of supportive care buildings has the opportunity to impact on more people simultaneously, but making changes at scale can be prohibitive. Regardless of location (and challenges), there still exists microelement changes (e.g., adding benches, clear pathways, destinations) and behaviour change interventions to create active indoor spaces. Recognizing the projected global increase in ageing populations, there is an opportunity *now* to reflect upon building design to encourage more physical activity, thus in turn support the active ageing of present and future older adults around the world.

23.1.2 Spectrum of Physical Activity at Home

There are many opportunities for older adults to be active inside their homes, and other indoor spaces. For example, balance and strength training conducted at home is feasible to incorporate into daily life routines (Clemson et al. 2012; Fleig et al. 2016) and may also reduce the risk of falling (Clemson et al. 2012). Further, as per the results from a Cochrane Systematic Review, although centred-based physical activity programs may result in greater performance-based measures in the short term, over time, older adults had greater adherence to home-based exercises (Ashworth et al. 2005). Therefore, it is not surprising that population-level data from older Canadians highlight that home exercise was the second most commonly reported physical activity for people aged 65 years and older (Ashe et al. 2009). Given the potential benefits (and opportunities) to be active at home (both recreational and utilitarian activity), a shift in mindset may be in order. That is, should we create spaces and habits within the home to be a source of household activities, opportunities to engage in everyday balance and strength exercises, and/or a place to conduct more traditional "exercise" such as using a stationary bike, treadmill, stepper or cycle ergometer? Even without the perfect house design, clean open (safe) spaces along with behaviour change interventions can support older adults to remain active within their home environment.

23.2 Related Theories

Lawton and Nahemow's concept of the person-environment (competence-press) fit (Lawton and Nahemow 1979) describes how a person's capacity can be influenced by their physical surrounds: an imbalance between a person's capacity (e.g., loss of mobility) and environment demands (challenging home setup, stairs, etc.) can result in a necessary adaption to housing and/or relocation. For example, after a significant health event such as a hip fracture or stroke, stairs in the home may be an insurmountable barrier for independent-living. An older adult who lives on the second floor of an apartment building, without access to an elevator, who develops mobility challenges would need to relocate because of the barriers to leave their home (regardless of the apartment's accessibility). To some degree architectural determinism (Marmot 2002) is a related concept, as this theory posits that we adapt our behaviour to the physical surrounds. In another example, an older adult who lived for years in a small home but could no longer manage stairs, moved to a slightly larger apartment with access to corridors (and strategically-placed chairs and benches) and an elevator. In this scenario, the increase in living space and indoor corridor can "nudge" the older adult to include more physical activity into their daily life routine, and thus, activity by design.

23.3 Accommodation Mode and Physical Activity

Many older adults would like to *age in place*; however, this term may be more familiar to policymakers (Wiles et al. 2012). Ageing in place is "viewed as a positive approach to meeting the needs of the older person, supporting them to live independently, or with some assistance, for as long as possible. It implies that older people prefer to live in their own home, rather than in an institution or care centre." (Horner and Boldy 2008 page 356). This is aligned with the principles extolled by the WHO endorsed Age-Friendly movement. Housing is one of eight focal areas; other related foci include transportation, and outdoor spaces and buildings. From an Age-Friendly perspective, there should be enough secure and well-constructed housing stock (including rental accommodation), located in safe areas, with access to destinations and amenities (e.g., home maintenance, support services). The interior of the home should have features such as level surfaces, sufficiently wide hallways and areas to navigate within rooms and other spaces (http://www.who.int/ageing/age-friendly-world/en/).

Many countries advocate ageing in place for a number of reasons, including the ability to support independence, community engagement in familiar environments, and potential cost-reduction by avoiding institutionalization (Wiles et al. 2012). Wiles and colleagues put forth that ageing in place should consider both the home *and* the neighbourhood. In essence, ageing in place extends beyond the physical home and recognizes that the familiarity, social connections, and destinations within a neighbourhood may be just as important. The ideal scenario would be a home *and* neighbourhood that supports older adults' physical activity, social interactions, and destinations nearby to promote ageing in place. But some older adults may struggle to maintain a home (and yard) because of their preference for independence within familiar surrounds (neighbourhood destinations and social connections). What needs further investigation is to determine if moving to a different living space (i.e., more aligned with an older adults' abilities and preferences), but within the same neighbourhood would support ageing in place.

It is essential over the next decade to work collaboratively with health professionals, housing industry, technology sector, and other stakeholders to co-create active living environments guided by the voices of older adults, to develop accommodation options that can adapt to a person's changing physical, cognitive, and mental capabilities associated with ageing. An existing example of this is in the UK, called Care and Repair (http://careandrepair-england.org.uk/), which provide a number of services to support older people by modifying living spaces. Similarly, the Canadian Mortgage and Housing Corporation has funding programs to assist older adults with home renovations and offers education on how to adapt living spaces to encourage ageing in place (Canadian Mortgage and Housing Corporation). The movement to support the indoor built environment to encourage physical activity (and ageing in place) at a national/international level is beginning, but will require time and resources to evolve.

23.3.1 Assessing Indoor Spaces

What factors are important to encourage more activity in the home? What is the best way to determine if home renovations and/or new housing projects meet the need for age-friendly and/or ageing in place? There are instruments available to evaluate home setup, such as the Housing Enabler Tool, developed in Sweden in the 1990s (Iwarsson and Isacsson 1996) based on work published in the 1970s (Steinfeld 1979). The Home Enabler Tool has undergone psychometric testing (Helle et al. 2010; Iwarsson and Isacsson 1996), translation into other languages, and development of a shortened (screening) version (Carlsson et al. 2009). What sets the Home Enabler Tool apart from other environment assessment tools for older adults is its grounding in the person-environment fit theory. Operationally, the Home Enabler Tool consists of three steps: (i) determine the capacity of the person (either through questionnaire or performance-based tasks); (ii) assess key components of the indoor environment (e.g., stairs, doorways, turning circles, toilet heights, etc.) and outdoor areas in close proximity (entrance, backyards, balconies, etc.); and (iii) calculate a score based on the interaction of the person in their environment. As this is done for each person, it can be time consuming, thus the motivation for developing the valid, shorter screening version (Carlsson et al. 2009). The Home Enabler Tool also has the potential to facilitate a tailored plan, to identify places and routines that encourage more daily physical activity.

23.3.2 Houses, Apartments, Flats, Condos

To date, evidence is sparse on indoor environment to encourage physical activity in later life. There are some basic principles that may support more active living, including the adoption of accessibility, universal design, and age-friendly principles, including consideration of home size, location, entrances/doors, number of stories (stairs), social environment, the immediate outdoor spaces, and nearby destinations. These are discussed briefly below; however, as per the person-environment fit (and the principles of the Home Enabler Tool), there remains the interaction of older adults' ability/capacity/preferences and the home environment to encourage adoption and maintenance of physical activity within daily life routines.

There are relatively few studies that have looked specifically at features of the indoor environment and their impact on physical activity. In a Swedish study (Niva and Skar 2006) conducted in 2000, investigators looked at the activity patterns of five older adults after housing modifications (based on recognized needs). Specifically, participants identified features such as narrow entrances and thresholds and room design (e.g., challenges navigating bathroom and kitchen spaces) impaired their activity (and possibly increased their risk of falls). They also highlighted that stairs and entrance/exits were problematic to enter/leave the home. Following the home modifications, participants reported increased activity and reduced rest time (Niva and Skar 2006). However, this was a small project that used self-report measures, and therefore the study design makes it difficult to generalize the results to the wider community of older adults.

Cress and colleagues (Cress et al. 2011) investigated the effect of room size on physical activity (step counts). In this cross-sectional study, they compared daily step counts between community-dwelling older adults and adults living in residential care. Overall, the community-dwelling older adults had more than double the available floor space (179 m^2 vs 69 m^2). They also accumulated 2000 more steps per day indoors compared with older adults in residential care (5000 vs 3000 steps per day; $p = 0.001$), controlling for age (and excluding exercise). This study was hypothesis-generating around size of home and amount of physical activity: more data are required to ascertain the extent of home size on overall activity, especially given the context of the person-environment fit, and opportunities and preferences to be physically active.

Benzinger and colleagues incorporated the Home Enabler Tool and self-report measures of physical activity within a cross-sectional study of community-dwelling older adults. Of note, for 81 older adults [79 (76–83) years median (Q1–Q3)], there was a significant association between the measure of person-environment fit (using the Home Enabler Tool) and physical activity, but there were no significant associations between the number of identified barriers in the home (and close proximity) and physical activity. However, participants were doing well functionally as evidenced by a median (Q1–Q3) gait (walking) speed of 1.1 (0.9–1.2) m/s: a speed compatible with what is needed to cross many city streets (1.2 m/s) (Asher et al. 2012). Conversely, functional limitations were associated with physical activity. At first glance, these data suggest that older adults' ability (and not environmental barriers) were associated with physical activity. However, what remains unknown is the type and degree of obstruction that barriers created, and if participants adapted to the barriers within their home over time.

As older adults constitute a large group with distinct abilities and economic resources, there are environmental features appropriate for some, but may be a barrier for others. Using a qualitative design (focus groups and semi-structured interviews) (Brookfield et al. 2015), investigators explored the components of what helped or hindered activity within the home. Key features that emerged included the adoption of universal design, room size, and stairs: although room size and stairs resulted in diverse perceptions. For example, although stairs were a significant barrier for some (especially if designed poorly) they were viewed by others as an opportunity for being physically active. This study also reiterated the importance of room size and completion of everyday activities. While some participants noted that smaller areas present hazards (e.g., bumping into furniture or problems with using mobility aids) and restrict activity, a few participants highlighted small living quarters were more manageable to navigate their living space. That is, narrow passageways and proximity to sturdy structures (e.g., walls) and furniture provided additional support to reduce their perceptions of falling (Brookfield et al. 2015).

Some older adults may not be able to engage in prolonged exercise within their home (e.g., moderate to vigorous physical activity; MVPA), yet their housing may not preclude the ability to reduce sitting time and perform balance and strength activities. Studies, such as the Lifestyle-Integrated Functional Exercise (LiFE) program by Clemson and colleagues, use behavioural change theory and techniques to support older adults to use their *home as a gym* (Clemson et al. 2012). This large randomized controlled trial (n = 317 older adults aged 70 years+ with a history of falls) noted that integrating exercises within the home as part of daily routines resulted in a statistically significant reduction in the rate of falls compared with participants in a control group and those allocated to a structured exercise program. There may be other physical activity options for those older adults living in apartments/condominiums, for example, walking within interior corridors in the winter months and/or when weather is inclement, or the use of on-site gyms to engage in more strength and/or cardiovascular training. Beyond the bricks and mortar of a home, how furniture is arranged and/or the elimination of clutter can also encourage more physical activity and potentially reduce the risk of falls and injury. Below is an example of how one older adult encourages more activity into her day supported by the indoor environment and destinations in close proximity.

> Grace is 90 years old and lives independently in a condominium within a small urban setting. Her condo is located on the third floor of a multistory building which is wheelchair accessible and has two elevators. The living area is 1000 feet^2 with two bathrooms and spacious rooms and hallways. Grace has a small balcony where she has a container garden and within her building she has access to two long corridors, a common area and mailroom on the first floor. Grace is doing very well and, despite having some chronic conditions, has maintained a

high level of physical activity. She manages all household tasks including, cleaning, laundry and cooking. In the spring and summer she has a garden to encourage the use of the balcony. She also does her home program of balance and strength exercises that are incorporated into her daily routine. For instance, when she is washing the dishes, she holds onto the counter and completes mini squats and challenges her balance doing tandem and one-leg stance. Doing the tasks close to the sink provides additional hand support. Grace does her best to keep her home free of clutter and obstacles that can impede moving around the condo. On a daily basis Grace leaves her home and travels a short distance with a wheeled walker to the local grocery store (about 200m away) and other adjacent shops. On the days that she is not able to leave her home, she adds more physical activity within her building, such as walking up and down the halls on her floor, and checking her mailbox.

23.3.3 Assisted Living

Assisted living is a relatively new housing option that is based on a social model of care, and offers hospitality services plus personal assistance to support independence in a homelike environment (Sikorska-Simmons and Wright 2007). The US and Canada have emerged as leaders in assisted living; however, even between these two countries, definitions vary, and consequently so do the profile of the residents and on-site services. Another name for a similar type of accommodation is retirement homes (US, Canada) and/or retirement villages (e.g., in Australia and UK), although again, definitions vary by country and region.

In Canada, social and recreational opportunities are a hallmark of assisted living facilities in some provinces. Hanson and colleagues conducted a comprehensive review of social and recreational opportunities within 51 assisted living sites in two health authorities. Although they noted that most activities were social, there were still opportunities to blend physical activity within daily life and social routines (Hanson et al. 2014), such as walking to meals and/or social events. Participation in social and recreational opportunities supports ageing in place: Tighe and colleagues (2008) noted that older US adults who participated in physical activities remained in assisted living longer, even after adjusting to levels of cognition, health, and mobility. An example of physical activity and retirement villages is from Australia (Holt et al. 2016), where researchers audited 50 sites and interviewed 200 older adults. Of note, only half of the participants reported using physical activity resources within the facility, and barriers to walking outside included hills and safety. However, there were no significant associations between perceived neighbourhood barriers and physical activity. Destinations within close proximity to housing (combined with a supportive built environment) may facilitate regular physical activity and/or outdoor trips (Chudyk et al. 2015), but these features may not always be present. In a study conducted assessing the areas in close proximity to four assisted living sites in British Columbia, Canada (Chudyk et al. 2014), there were environmental features supportive of physical activity (safety, presence of sidewalks, etc.), but few areas surveyed (25%) had destinations within walking distance such as grocery stores, restaurants, and transit stops (Chudyk et al. 2014).

Assisted living environments can contribute to activity through walking programs (Lu 2010; Lu et al. 2011), within or around their sites. Features to consider are the length and width of hallways, appropriately placed furniture (benches and/or chairs) for breaks, wayfinding, and adequate lighting, which is a necessity for falls prevention (Lu 2010). In a recent study by Lu and colleagues (Lu et al. 2015), they investigated environmental features that impacted on older adults' walking patterns within assisted living. Researchers surveyed 18 assisted living sites in Texas to inquire about walking and related behaviours; they also conducted on-site evaluations of the built environment. In sum, they noted significant associations between the indoor environment and walking behaviour among the tenants. In particular, destinations within facilities encouraged activity: specifically walking to destinations such as meals, the mailbox, and/or the front entrance (Lu et al. 2015).

> It has been two years since Mateo fractured his hip and moved into the assisted living site. Although he was reluctant to move, he felt comforted knowing that there would be more resources available to him. Mateo moved to a facility that prioritized physical activity and social opportunities. For example, although his apartment was only 400 feet^2, he requested a unit located further away from the dining and social areas of the building. In this way, despite his mobility limitations, he takes (at least) three long walks daily with his walker inside the building and the nearby gardens. This has been made easier because the assisted living site has wide corridors, adequate lighting, and the occasional chair (or bench) along the way, so that if Mateo gets tired he can stop and rest. Mateo continues with his home exercise program that he was given after his hip fracture, and this is supplemented with the regular exercise programs within the facility. The building has also been constructed to have a few small areas where ramps and steps are present. These have been well thought out, and provide an opportunity for Mateo to safely practice going up and down stairs to build leg strength and challenge his balance. The assisted living site offers many social opportunities that simultaneously encourage physical activity, such as gardening, volunteering at the library, and reading to other older adults in the building.

As there is a coffee shop nearby, Mateo walks there weekly to meet with friends from his old neighbourhood.

The indoor built environment has the potential to play an important role in fostering an active lifestyle. However, even the best environment may need interventions to educate, prioritize, and strategize with older adult residents to adopt a more active lifestyle. Resnick and colleagues (Resnick et al. 2013, Resnick 2011) are leaders in the field of function-focused care for older adults who reside in supportive care. Based on this approach, staff were trained to recognize the capability of tenants/residents and encourage them to adopt more physical activities into their day. This is accomplished by older adults completing more of their activities of daily living (e.g., laundry, self-care) (Resnick et al. 2011): some of these tasks/responsibilities are almost entirely eliminated when entering into more supportive living arrangements. Thus, an ideal building design and function-focused care in combination may be the best option to maximize activity in daily life routines.

23.3.4 Technology, Housing, and Physical Activity

This chapter would be remiss without the mention of a recent development within the health, design, and technology spheres: smart homes—dwellings equipped with technology and sensors to monitor and assist occupants to maximize function and ultimately improve quality of life (Demiris and Hensel 2008). Although the concept (and technology) has been available for some time, there has been a recent increase in studies investigating the health outcomes related to smart home technology, and the acceptance of older adults to live in smart homes (Courtney et al. 2008; Demiris et al. 2008). To date, many studies report older adults' satisfaction with smart technology (especially if there is no need for them to directly interact with it). But, in a recent systematic review, researchers (Liu et al. 2016) noted that widespread readiness to implement smart homes remains low, and there are few high-level studies assessing the effectiveness of smart homes.

Personal monitoring has increased exponentially over the past few years, and thus, forward-looking technologies may be optimal to support older adults to better age in place. In addition to personal monitoring systems (for falls prevention, physical activity, and reducing prolonged sedentary behaviour), new homes may be adapted to address the person-environment fit. An example is related to counter tops; technology exists to raise and lower counter heights. This home feature would permit people of different heights to use the same space for activities of daily living, and/or it may be used if an older adult's mobility status changes (e.g., necessitating the need to sit more for meal preparation). Sensing technology can also support the automatic detection of lighting both during the day and at night. In an ideal world, future opportunities could include stairs that could be electronically reconfigured to account for an addition of a walking aid, for hip, knee or ankle impairment. At the press of a button, a full flight of stairs could become an escalator (or similar) that has adequate space to accommodate mobility and/or a caregiver. Some current activity monitors learn activity patterns and interpret the type undertaken (machine learning). Perhaps in future our homes can also learn to adapt to our changing needs over the life course. These are all possibilities, but it will take time to repurpose existing technologies into the home setting, resources to install and monitor the technology, and acceptance, instruction, and habit-building for older adults to use the new features. Ageing in place is possible, but it requires resources and the collective wisdom of many stakeholders (including older adults) and the adoption by the primary users.

23.4 Implications for Practice

Despite the fact that we spend so much time in our homes, we have limited knowledge of best evidence for indoor built environment and physical activity (active design) for older adults. Further, policy and practice for promoting physical activity with older people using indoor spaces to encourage active living is an evolving field. Although there are currently policies on physical activity and ageing, and separate policies on housing and ageing, few, if any, target the indoor environment as a possible physical activity intervention. For older adults, and especially those with limited mobility, there is a need to shift perspectives and embrace all activity types of physical activity to promote health and longevity. Initiatives such as age-friendly communities is an excellent global platform to begin the conversion to add more physical activity (recreational and utilitarian) into the routine and homes of the growing number of older adults. Related to housing (in general) and older adults, as per age-friendly communities, there is a need for affordable, accessible/age-friendly options in a variety of housing forms (homes, apartments/condos/communal dwelling) with access to destinations and services within close proximity. We require *activity by design* policies to promote physical activity across the lifespan and for a shift in community culture to support behaviour change (to reduce sedentary behaviour and encourage all physical activity). In particular, it is essential to integrate health into the design and building of future housing options across the life course, but especially in later life.

23.5 Conclusion

Regular physical activity contributes to active ageing, which in turn can lead to increased community mobility and quality of life. As we spend so much time indoors, it is incumbent on the research and health professional communities, housing industry, and policymakers to collectively work towards an evidence-informed foundation to maximize activity in the home (activity by design), especially for adults in later life. However, regardless of size or design of accommodation, behavioural strategies are needed to adopt more physical activity across the lifespan throughout everyday routines. Within the wider accommodation footprint, socialization, and destinations within, and around, buildings are key to encourage more activity. Given the advancements in understanding behaviour change and progressions in technology, it is imperative to move forward looking for feasible and acceptable solutions to maximize physical activity to support ageing well.

Suggested Further Reading

- Satariano, W. (2006). Aging, health, and the environment: An ecological model. *Epidemiology of aging: An ecological approach* (pp. 39–84). Toronto: Jones and Bartlett.
- Wahl, H. W., & Weisman, G. D. (2003). Environmental gerontology at the beginning of the new millennium: Reflections on its historical, empirical, and theoretical development. *The Gerontologist, 43*(5), 616–627.

References

Alley, D., Liebig, P., Pynoos, J., Banerjee, T., & Choi, I. H. (2007). Creating elder-friendly communities: Preparations for an aging society. *Journal of Gerontological Social Work, 49*(1–2), 1–18. https://doi.org/10.1300/J083v49n04_01.

Ashe, M., Miller, W. C., Eng, J. J., Noreau, L., Physical, A., & Chronic Conditions Research, T. (2009). Older adults, chronic disease and leisure-time physical activity. *Gerontology, 55*(1), 64–72. https://doi.org/10.1159/000141518.

Asher, L., Aresu, M., Falaschetti, E., & Mindell, J. (2012). Most older pedestrians are unable to cross the road in time: A cross-sectional study. *Age and Ageing, 41*(5), 690–694. https://doi.org/10.1093/ageing/afs076.

Ashworth, N. L., Chad, K. E., Harrison, E. L., Reeder, B. A., & Marshall, S. C. (2005). Home versus center based physical activity programs in older adults. *Cochrane Database of Systematic Reviews, 1*, CD004017. https://doi.org/10.1002/14651858.CD004017.pub2.

Brookfield, K., Fitzsimons, C., Scott, I., Mead, G., Starr, J., Thin, N., et al. (2015). The home as enabler of more active lifestyles among older people. *Building Research and Information, 43*(5), 616–630. https://doi.org/10.1080/09613218.2015.1045702.

Canadian Mortgage and Housing Corporation. *Aging in Place*. https://www.cmhc-schl.gc.ca/en/co/acho/index.cfm

Carlson, J. A., Sallis, J. F., Conway, T. L., Saelens, B. E., Frank, L. D., Kerr, J., et al. (2012). Interactions between psychosocial and built environment factors in explaining older adults' physical activity. *Preventive Medicine, 54*(1), 68–73. https://doi.org/10.1016/j.ypmed.2011.10.004.

Carlsson, G., Schilling, O., Slaug, B., Fange, A., Stahl, A., Nygren, C., & Iwarsson, S. (2009). Toward a screening tool for housing accessibility problems a reduced version of the housing enabler. *Journal of Applied Gerontology, 28*(1), 59–80. https://doi.org/10.1177/0733464808315293.

Chu, L. W., & Chi, I. (2008). Nursing homes in China. *Journal of the American Medical Directors Association, 9*(4), 237–243. https://doi.org/10.1016/j.jamda.2008.01.008.

Chudyk, A. M., Winters, M., Gorman, E., McKay, H. A., & Ashe, M. C. (2014). Agreement between virtual and in-the-field environmental audits of assisted living sites. *Journal of Aging and Physical Activity, 22*(3), 414–420. https://doi.org/10.1123/japa.2013-0047.

Chudyk, A. M., Winters, M., Moniruzzaman, M., Ashe, M. C., Gould, J. S., & McKay, H. (2015). Destinations matter: The association between where older adults live and their travel behavior. *Journal of Transport Health, 2*(1), 50–57. https://doi.org/10.1016/j.jth.2014.09.008.

Clemson, L., Fiatarone Singh, M. A., Bundy, A., Cumming, R. G., Manollaras, K., O'Loughlin, P., & Black, D. (2012). Integration of balance and strength training into daily life activity to reduce rate of falls in older people (the LiFE study): Randomised parallel trial. *BMJ, 345*, e4547. https://doi.org/10.1136/bmj.e4547.

Courtney, K. L., Demiris, G., Rantz, M., & Skubic, M. (2008). Needing smart home technologies: The perspectives of older adults in continuing care retirement communities. *Informatics in Primary Care, 16*(3), 195–201.

Cress, M. E., Orini, S., & Kinsler, L. (2011). Living environment and mobility of older adults. *Gerontology, 57*(3), 287–294. https://doi.org/10.1159/000322195.

Demiris, G., & Hensel, B. K. (2008). Technologies for an aging society: A systematic review of "smart home" applications. *Yearbook of Medical Informatics, 3*, 33–40.

Demiris, G., Hensel, B. K., Skubic, M., & Rantz, M. (2008). Senior residents' perceived need of and preferences for "smart home" sensor technologies. *International Journal of Technology Assessment in Health Care, 24*(1), 120–124. https://doi.org/10.1017/S0266462307080154.

Eisenberg, Y., Vanderbom, K. A., & Vasudevan, V. (2017). Does the built environment moderate the relationship between having a disability and lower levels of physical activity? A systematic review. *Preventive Medicine, 95S*, S75–S84. https://doi.org/10.1016/j.ypmed.2016.07.019.

Feng, Z., Liu, C., Guan, X., & Mor, V. (2012). China's rapidly aging population creates policy challenges in shaping a viable long-term care system. *Health Affairs, 31*(12), 2764–2773. https://doi.org/10.1377/hlthaff.2012.0535.

Ferreira, M. (2013). Housing for older people globally. What are best practices? *ILC Global Alliance Discussion Paper*. http://www.ilc-alliance.org/images/uploads/publication-pdfs/Housing_for_older_people_-_an_ILC_Global_Alliance_Discussion_Paper.pdf

Fleig, L., McAllister, M. M., Chen, P., Iverson, J., Milne, K., McKay, H. A., et al. (2016). Health behaviour change theory meets falls prevention: Feasibility of a habit-based balance and strength exercise intervention for older adults. *Psychology of Sport and Exercise, 22*, 114–122. https://doi.org/10.1016/j.psychsport.2015.07.002.

Freedman, V. A., & Spillman, B. C. (2014). The residential continuum from home to nursing home: Size, characteristics and unmet needs of older adults. *Journals of Gerontology Series B – Psychological Sciences and Social Sciences, 69*(Suppl 1), S42–S50. https://doi.org/10.1093/geronb/gbu120.

Freedman, V. A., Wolf, D. A., & Spillman, B. C. (2016). Disability-free life expectancy over 30 years: A growing female disadvantage in the US population. *American Journal of Public Health, 106*(6), 1079–1085. https://doi.org/10.2105/AJPH.2016.303089.

Gitlin, L. N. (2003). Conducting research on home environments: Lessons learned and new directions. *The Gerontologist, 43*(5), 628–637.

Hanson, H. M., Ashe, M. C., McKay, H. A., & Winters, M. (2012). Intersection between the built and social environments and older adults' mobility: An evidence review. *National Collaborating Centre for Environmental Health*. http://www.ncceh.ca/sites/default/files/Built_and_Social_Environments_Older_Adults_Nov_2012.pdf

Hanson, H. M., Schiller, C., Winters, M., Sims-Gould, J., Clarke, P., Curran, E., et al. (2013). Concept mapping applied to the intersection between older adults' outdoor walking and the built and social environments. *Preventive Medicine, 57*(6), 785–791. https://doi.org/10.1016/j.ypmed.2013.08.023.

Hanson, H. M., Hoppmann, C. A., Condon, K., Davis, J., Feldman, F., Friesen, M., et al. (2014). Characterizing social and recreational programming in assisted living. *Canadian Journal on Aging, 33*(3), 285–295. https://doi.org/10.1017/S0714980814000178.

Harris-Kojetin, L., Sengupta, M., Park-Lee, E., Valverde, R., Caffrey, C., Rome, V., & Lendon, J. (2016). Long-term care providers and services users in the United States: Data from the national study of long-term care providers, 2013–2014. *Vital Health Statistics, 3*(38), x–xii, 1–105.

Helle, T., Nygren, C., Slaug, B., Brandt, A., Pikkarainen, A., Hansen, A. G., et al. (2010). The Nordic Housing Enabler: Inter-rater reliability in cross-Nordic occupational therapy practice. *Scandinavian Journal of Occupational Therapy, 17*(4), 258–266. https://doi.org/10.3109/11038120903265014.

Holt, A., Lee, A. H., Jancey, J., Kerr, D., & Howat, P. (2016). Are retirement villages promoting active aging? *Journal of Aging and Physical Activity, 24*(3), 407–411. https://doi.org/10.1123/japa.2015-0194.

Horner, B., & Boldy, D. P. (2008). The benefit and burden of "ageing-in-place" in an aged care community. *Australian Health Review, 32*(2), 356–365.

Iwarsson, S., & Isacsson, A. (1996). Development of a novel instrument for occupational therapy of assessment of the physical environment in the home – A methodologic study on "The enabler". *Occupational Therapy Journal of Research, 16*(4), 227–244.

Joseph, A. (2006). *Health promotion by design in long-term care settings*. Report prepared for Laguna Honda Foundation on flagrant funded by the California Health Care Foundation. The Center for Health Design.

Kinsella, K., Velkoff, V. A., & Bureau, U. S. C. (2002). Living arrangements. *Aging Clinical and Experimental Research, 14*(6), 431–438.

Lawton, M. P., & Nahemow, L. (1979). Social areas and the Wellbeing of tenants in housing for the elderly. *Multivariate Behavior Research, 14*(4), 463–484. https://doi.org/10.1207/s15327906mbr1404_6.

Liu, L., Stroulia, E., Nikolaidis, I., Miguel-Cruz, A., & Rios Rincon, A. (2016). Smart homes and home health monitoring technologies for older adults: A systematic review. *International Journal of Medical Informatics, 91*, 44–59. https://doi.org/10.1016/j.ijmedinf.2016.04.007.

Lu, Z. (2010). Investigating walking environments in and around assisted living facilities: A facility visit study. *HERD, 3*(4), 58–74.

Lu, Z., Rodiek, S. D., Shepley, M. M., & Duffy, M. (2011). Influences of physical environment on corridor walking among assisted living residents: Findings from focus group discussions. *Journal of Applied Gerontology, 30*(4), 463–484. https://doi.org/10.1177/0733464810370325.

Lu, Z., Rodiek, S., Shepley, M. M., & Tassinary, L. G. (2015). Environmental influences on indoor walking behaviours of assisted living residents. *Building Research and Information, 43*(5), 602–615. https://doi.org/10.1080/09613218.2015.1049494.

Marmot, A. (2002). Architectural determinism. Does design change behaviour? *British Journal of General Practice, 52*(476), 252–253.

Marmot, A., & Ucci, M. (2015). Sitting less, moving more: The indoor built environment as a tool for change. *Building Research & Information, 43*(5), 561–565. https://doi.org/10.1080/09613218.2015.1069081.

Martin, L. G., Freedman, V. A., Schoeni, R. F., & Andreski, P. M. (2009). Health and functioning among baby boomers approaching 60. *Journals of Gerontology Series B – Psychological Sciences and Social Sciences, 64*(3), 369–377. https://doi.org/10.1093/geronb/gbn040.

Matz, C. J., Stieb, D. M., Davis, K., Egyed, M., Rose, A., Chou, B., & Brion, O. (2014). Effects of age, season, gender and urban-rural status on time-activity: Canadian Human Activity Pattern Survey 2 (CHAPS 2). *International Journal of Environmental Research for Public Health, 11*(2), 2108–2124. https://doi.org/10.3390/ijerph110202108.

Niva, B., & Skar, L. (2006). A pilot study of the activity patterns of five elderly persons after a housing adaptation. *Occupational Therapy International, 13*(1), 21–34.

Resnick, B., Galik, E., Gruber-Baldini, A., & Zimmerman, S. (2011). Testing the effect of function-focused care in assisted living. *Journal of the American Geriatrics Society, 59*(12), 2233–2240. https://doi.org/10.1111/j.1532-5415.2011.03699.x.

Resnick, B., Galik, E., & Boltz, M. (2013). Function focused care approaches: Literature review of progress and future possibilities. *Journal of the American Medical Directors Association, 14*(5), 313–318. https://doi.org/10.1016/j.jamda.2012.10.019.

Rice, N. E., Lang, I. A., Henley, W., & Melzer, D. (2010). Baby boomers nearing retirement: The healthiest generation? *Rejuvenation Research, 13*(1), 105–114. https://doi.org/10.1089/rej.2009.0896.

Saelens, B. E., & Papadopoulos, C. (2008). The importance of the built environment in older adults' physical activity: A review of the literature. *Washington State Journal of Public Health Practice, 1*, 13–21.

Sallis, J. F., Cervero, R. B., Ascher, W., Henderson, K. A., Kraft, M. K., & Kerr, J. (2006). An ecological approach to creating active living communities. *Annual Review of Public Health, 27*, 297–322. https://doi.org/10.1146/annurev.publhealth.27.021405.102100.

Sikorska-Simmons, E., & Wright, J. D. (2007). Determinants of resident autonomy in assisted living facilities: A review of the literature. *Care Management Journals, 8*(4), 187–193.

Steinfeld, E. (1979). *Access to the built environment: A review of literature.* The Office: For sale by the Supt. of Docs., US Govt. Print. Off.

Tighe, S. K., Leoutsakos, J. M. S., Carlson, M. C., Onyike, C. U., Samus, Q., Baker, A., et al. (2008). The association between activity participation and time to discharge in the assisted living setting. *International Journal of Geriatric Psychiatry, 23*(6), 586–591. https://doi.org/10.1002/gps.1940.

Wiles, J. L., Leibing, A., Guberman, N., Reeve, J., & Allen, R. E. (2012). The meaning of "aging in place" to older people. *The Gerontologist, 52*(3), 357–366. https://doi.org/10.1093/geront/gnr098.

World Health Organization. (2011). *Global health and aging.* Geneva: World Health Organization.

24

Restorative Environments and Promoting Physical Activity Among Older People

Jenny Roe and Alice Roe

24.1 Introduction

This chapter offers an overview of what is known about restorative environments (REs) for older adults (65+). First, it describes what constitutes an RE and considers these attributes in relation to the needs of older people. Next, it considers the processes of psychological restoration and how this intersects with physical activity. Then it sets out what is known about REs, first, for healthy older adults and, second, for those experiencing cognitive impairment and dementia by RE setting (e.g. the home, the neighborhood, and street context). Finally, it suggests some new inquiries for future research and policy implications.

24.2 Restorative Environments: Theoretical Context

The relationship between older people's mobility and the built environment (BE) is largely explored via the physical opportunities or constraints that the BE offers for mobility, that is, the *functional* affordances of the environment

---

J. Roe (✉)
School of Architecture, University of Virginia, Charlottesville, VA, USA

A. Roe
Age UK, Tavis House, London, UK

and what's 'do-able' in the setting. We argue that ambience and the mood of a place, together with curiosity and complexity in the environment, are important dimensions of the BE that motivate older people to explore and investigate their everyday environments. We explore this psychological dimension of setting via the concept of REs.

Psychological restoration has been defined as the process of renewing a psychological, physiological, or social resource that has become depleted (Hartig 2007). An RE is therefore any environment that promotes recovery from a depleted resource such as cognitive fatigue, stress, or low mood. Two theories have dominated the literature on REs for the last four decades, each dealing with different forms of resource depletion: the first deals with cognitive depletion, the second with affective depletion, which in turn, triggers a physiological response.

Cognitive Recovery Under the first model, Attention Restoration Theory (ART) (Kaplan and Kaplan 1989), it is posited that an RE needs to offer a combination of four attributes:

(1) The opportunity to escape from everyday stressors (defined as 'being away'): this restorative capability might be accomplished by experiencing a new environment for the first time—but it can also be experienced by perceiving an old environment in a new way (Kaplan 1995). This latter experience has not much been explored in the literature but is very pertinent to older people who may have become overfamiliar with their everyday settings or simply are unable to easily access further away 'new' destinations such as a national park or city. In addition, 'being with'—rather than 'being away'—may be more pertinent to the social needs of older people.
(2) Offer expansive spaces and contexts that allow us to find a 'whole other world' (defined as 'extent') with sufficient scope to engage the mind: *It must provide enough to see, experience, and think about so that it takes up a substantial portion of the available room in one's head* (Kaplan 1995, p. 173). Places that evoke memories, stories, and histories provide this, and this attribute of REs may therefore be particularly pertinent to older people.
(3) Facilitate activities that are 'compatible' with our intrinsic goals and motivations, known as 'person-environment fit' (Kaplan 1995). Compatibility is thought to be particularly important to restorative experiences in older people (Scopelliti and Giuliani 2005). Recently, it has been suggested that

if a setting is to be restorative, the environmental cues need to be compatible with our personalities, that is, if we are extroverted, we will seek out REs that offer social stimuli; if introverted, we will seek out REs that offer stillness and quiet (Newman 2016). We also suggest compatibility has greater leaning in the RE framework from the perspective of an older person.

(4) Provide stimuli that are 'fascinating' such as the 'soft' stimuli of natural settings: light patterns of trees, plants in bloom, and sunsets all offer highly restorative environments. These cues have sufficient enough interest to hold our attention effortlessly but not so much to as to exclude room for reflection. By contrast, urban environments that are rich in 'hard' fascination grab the attention dramatically, leaving no room for reflective thought and requiring directed attention to overcome the stimulation. This attribute is particularly important to integrate into residential environments for older people, many of whom live in under-stimulated environments, lacking a range of sensory stimulations.

In summary, ART posits that the cues in the natural environment support 'involuntary' or 'indirect attention' and enable our 'voluntary' or 'directed' attention capacities to recover and restore from cognitive fatigue, stress, and low mood (Kaplan and Kaplan 1989; Kaplan 1995). We suggest there is a need to re-evaluate the attributes of the model from the perspective of older people and that certain attributes—such as compatibility—have greater weighting in this model.

Stress Reduction The second model, stress reduction theory (SRT) focuses on stress depletion under a psycho-physiological theoretical model (Ulrich 1983; Ulrich et al. 1991). The *preferenda* (cues) of REs activate our parasympathetic nervous system in ways that reduce stress and autonomic arousal owing to our innate evolutionary connection to the natural world. There is growing evidence to show effects of REs on stress reduction, using biomarkers such as skin conductance, heart rate variability, and cortisol, the stress hormone (Gladwell et al. 2012; Park et al. 2007; Roe et al. 2013; van den Berg and Custers 2011).

Typically, RE research has explored well-being outcomes using a natural versus human-made urban environment dichotomy, or what is referred to as a *grey* versus *green* difference (Wright and Lund 2000; White et al. 2010). This dichotomous approach is now being challenged: urban environments which offer a calm place—such as a bookstore, library, or art gallery—can equally restore us (Newman and Brucks 2016). We explore this body of emerging research, and its relevance to older people, below.

24.3 The Benefits of Restorative Environments in Older Age

The specific context of REs for older people has been poorly examined with much of the research focusing on students or the general population, or in specific environments, such as residential care homes. There is also a lack of longitudinal studies exploring REs and their benefits and how they might change with age. We posit REs are a *multifaceted* health resource for older adults, providing a range of physical, mental, and social well-being benefits:

Mobility and Well-being Benefits of Restorative Environments Mobility has an important role to play in the quality of life of older people, facilitating independence, social interactions, and neighbourhood ties. Whilst the relationship between exercise and mental well-being in older people is well evidenced (Catalan-Matamoros et al. 2016), mobility research is almost exclusively focused on the *functional* affordances of the RE that impede or enable mobility in older people such as steps, curbs, and uneven pavements (Brookfield et al. 2017). However, well-being is context dependent and contemporary mobility planning has so far failed to account for the *distinctive* experience of older people's daily travel (Nordbakke and Schwanen 2014) or how mood of place intersects with physical activity. REs improve our mood (Roe 2008); this, in turn, is associated with improved decision-making (Isen and Means 1983); improved working memory (Brose et al. 2014); increased curiosity and the ability to engage in novel, exploratory thoughts and actions (Fredrickson 2004); and greater likelihood to exercise (Carels et al. 2007). In turn, our environmental context can positively change our mood whilst navigating the city (Aspinall et al. 2013). Mood of place, therefore, is particularly important for older people as they navigate urban environments. By exploring mood outcomes of our city streets in older people, recent research has significantly advanced the mobility agenda from a focus on the environmental attributes that restrict mobility towards a focus on wellness and the emotional experiences of different urban settings (Neale et al. 2017). Using mobile electroencephalography, or *mobile EEG*, this research has shown that older people experience varying moods, measured as levels of 'excitement', 'engagement', and 'frustration', in different urban environments whilst walking. Excitement—an indicator of arousal and increased alertness—was higher in urban busy streets than in urban parks; by comparison, levels of engagement—an indicator of immersion or interest—were higher in the park setting. The findings are consistent with RE theory suggesting a restorative effect of urban green space, which in turn, may drive motivations to visit and be more active in such settings.

Cognitive Health Benefits of Restorative Environments The evidence base has tended to focus on attention recovery from contact with REs; but increasingly, RE research is turning to study cognitive processes that include self-control, self-regulation, rumination, executive functioning, and goal planning. We argue REs are particularly important for older adults, often facing complex and consequential decisions, in relation to future financial planning, healthcare, and living. In turn, older people need to sustain healthy behaviours and exert self-regulation to maintain health and fitness in older age. But attention declines in older age, in turn associated with poorer decision-making. Older people may become more forgetful and experience lapses in memory. Self-regulation tends to become increasingly more difficult in older age (Gerstoff and Ram 2009): a factor associated with increased risk of chronic health problems such as obesity (Fan and Jin 2014) and poor motivation to maintain healthy lifestyles in old age. REs incorporating nature can support many aspects of cognitive health, including brooding (or rumination) (Bratman et al. 2015), short-term memory (Bratman et al. 2015), and task recall (Fägerstam and Blom 2012), but to date, this research has been carried out exclusively in younger adults and has yet to be demonstrated in older people. REs could support cognitive health in older people to a far greater extent than we are yet aware of.

Social Aspects of Restorative Environments Social interaction plays an important and place-specific role in restorative experiences of older people. Scopelliti and Giuliani (2005) found social interactions increased perceived restorative experiences in urban built settings in older people; this concords with Staats and Hartig (2004) who showed that social interaction increases the restorative potential of an urban environment. In addition, Kewon et al. (1998) showed that greater use of green space among older adults from an inner-city neighbourhood in the United States corresponded with stronger social ties and sense of community. However, the social aspects of REs in older people are generally poorly understood; we would argue that 'being with'—as well as 'being away'—are important attributes of an RE for older people with significant potential health benefits. Social isolation is not only detrimental to mental well-being, it has also been significantly associated with increased mortality in older people (Steptoe et al. 2013). It is therefore vital—in a population where many are experiencing loneliness and social isolation—that we better understand the significance of social processes within restorative experiences and the distinction between organised social contact with 'significant others' (i.e. partner, friend, relatives) and impromptu social contact with those unknown to us.

24.4 Specific Restorative Environments and Their Mobility and Well-being Benefits in Older People

Next, we consider the benefits of specific REs, first for healthy older adults and then for older people experiencing specific cognitive decline, focusing on REs within the wider community context (see Chap. 23 for discussion on the home environment). REs explored below include private and communal gardens; access to parks and local green space; outdoor gyms/intergenerational settings; water settings (referred to in the literature as 'blue space'); and community/cultural facilities such as libraries, art galleries, and museums.

24.5 Healthy Older People

24.5.1 The Home Living Environment

The everyday residential context in which older people spend so much of their time arguably offers the most important context for restoration and leisure activity. The functional attributes of the home that enable or impede mobility in older people (e.g. steps, layout of space, the location and form of facilities, fixtures, and fittings) are well researched (see Chap. 25). However, sensory stimulation in the living environment triggers curiosity and, in turn, our motivation to move around and explore. Important characteristics that stimulate fascination and trigger restoration include architectural variation (Lindal and Hartig 2013), but it is not known how such attributes contribute to well-being—and mobility—in older populations. The need for visual delight and aesthetic stimulation—both indoors and out—are additional factors to consider. There is a need for more research on the home—particularly in relation to sensory stimulation and the relationship to psychosocial and mobility benefits in older people living independently and those living in residential care homes.

24.5.2 Gardens: Private and Communal

Private or communal gardens offer a direct restorative benefit for older people through contact with nature, whether actively or passively encountered (e.g. by a view). Gardens, and gardening, support a wide range of physical, cognitive, and psychosocial benefits in older people, including reductions in stress, improvements in mood, depression, anxiety, prevention of dementia, and cognitive decline (Buck 2016); improved physical activity/activeness; and increases in life satisfaction, quality of life, and sense of community and belonging (see Soga et al. for general review 2016; Wright and Wadsworth 2014; Wang and MacMillan 2013 for reviews in older people). Van den Berg and Custers (2011) found that gardening, in particular, promoted restoration in older adults, relieving stress, as measured by cortisol, and promoted affective restoration.

Gardening also promotes physical strength and coordination. There are surprisingly few studies of gardening as a form of physical activity in older people, despite its popularity (Buck 2016). Nicklett et al.'s (2014) review summarises what is known but most of the studies are limited to small sample sizes and focus on container or indoor gardening. There are few consistent findings across the studies. There is emerging evidence to show gardening can help in falls prevention: Chen and Janke (2012) explored the health outcomes between non-gardeners and gardeners in a US study of older adults and showed that gardeners were healthier overall, had fewer chronic health problems, fewer functional limitations, and better balance and gait, resulting in fewer falls. Heliker et al. (2001) found that gardening was instrumental in increasing a sense of psychological well-being in racially and culturally diverse groups in the United States and that it increased a sense of spirituality and connection to nature.

Gardens also carry special meanings for older individuals (Gross and Lane 2007) providing, for example, a connection to past memories, a sense of achievement (Milligan et al. 2004), and other outcomes akin to meditative practice (Wright and Wadsworth 2014). Gardening increases connection to future generations: it is a 'bridge-building' activity for enhancing intergenerational cooperation in community settings (Wright and Wadsworth 2014), a dimension further considered below. Pettigrew and Roberts (2008), in a small-scale qualitative study, found gardening to be one of the activities that can ameliorate loneliness in older age—something we increasingly understand to be as damaging to health for older people as behaviours such as smoking (Holt-Lunstad et al. 2010).

However, it is important to consider that the care of a garden can become incredibly burdensome for older people and a cause for psychological stress (Fänge and Ivanoff 2009). Where garden upkeep becomes difficult—or the residential context does not provide access to a garden—communal gardening (e.g. allotments) can offer a more suitable alternative setting, offering similar scope for promoting mental well-being, physical activity, and engaging socially and across generations. A better understanding of the potential burden of a garden is needed, together with support to facilitate gardening in older people.

24.6 The Local Neighbourhood

The wider neighbourhood environment—and the outdoor attributes that support active living in elders—is well evidenced, particularly in relation to the benefits of green space in the immediate neighbourhood setting. For instance, the UK's Inclusive Design for Getting Outdoors (I'DGO) research programme (http://www.idgo.ac.uk/) found that older people who live in environments where it is easy and enjoyable to go outdoors are more likely to be physically active and satisfied with life and twice as likely to achieve recommended levels of healthy walking. Later, we explore these neighbourhood settings in more depth.

24.6.1 Parks, Gardens, and Local Green Space

Parks, urban woodlands, and botanical gardens provide an important context for active living in older people, alongside opportunities for psychological restoration and social contact. There are significant positive effects of green space in the neighbourhood among older people for physical activity (see Broekhuizen et al. 2013 for a systematic review); perceived health (de Vries et al. 2003) and mental health (Wu et al. 2015); and social contact and community belonging (Kweon et al. 1998). Higher park density (Parra et al. 2010) and distance to a park (Nagel et al. 2008) are two dimensions associated with active park use in older people. This relationship, however, will vary by physical capability and the social support available to facilitate park access, particularly for those who are less mobile.

The perceived quality of a park and the facilities available also impact frequency of visiting and mobility outcomes in older people. Sugiyama and Ward Thompson (2008) found an association between the quality of neighbourhood open space and increased walking in older people in the UK. Alongside trees and greenery, specific park attributes that motivate older people to be active outdoors include the presence of seating and facilities such as toilets (Aspinall et al. 2010).

Further, the health benefits of green spaces among older people may be more significant than in younger populations (Astell-Burt et al. 2014; de Vries et al. 2003), and findings are more consistent in this age group (Broekhuizen et al. 2013). This is possibly due to older people's greater dependence on the local neighbourhood; however, as identified above, there is a need to understand patterns between the 'older' old and the 'younger' old. Surprisingly, we found no evidence of the effect of urban botanical gardens on well-being or mobility in older people. Considering older people's frequent visitation patterns, we suggest botanical gardens may hold a special purpose for activity and mental well-being in older people.

24.6.2 The Urban Street

The street design attributes that promoting walkability in older people are well evidenced (see Chap. 25). However, there is a need to understand more than just the *functional* properties of the street that promote mobility. An older person's emotional connection to the street will also affect their motivation to move and explore. The street aesthetic—and variation in the building façade (e.g. form, proportion, materials and colour)—together with the prospect of social interactions (impromptu or otherwise) are all characteristics that will motivate older people to be more mobile. Whilst a lack of visual complexity in street-level facades is known to foster boredom and reduced attentional capacity in the general population (Ellard 2017), older people may be at greater risk from lack of stimuli in the street setting, but as yet this is not proven.

Fleig et al. (2016) highlights that how older people *perceive* the built environment is important for physical activity, largely because these environmental perceptions are positively linked to older adults' confidence in walking. This concords with evidence from Brookfield et al. (2017), showing how perceptions of the street—and the meanings and possibilities older adults derive from the environmental context—shape their mobility choices. In summary, the affective quality of a street—its level of calm or busyness—together with opportunities for aesthetic and social stimulation are all attributes that impact on mobility and well-being in older people.

24.6.3 Outdoor Gyms and Multigenerational Playgrounds

In recent years, outdoor gyms designed especially for older adults (also called 'geriatric parks' or 'senior playgrounds') have increased in popularity, especially in Europe, the United States, and Asia (Chow 2013). Given that older adults are often observed as remaining sedentary during park visits (Kaczynski et al. 2011), these spaces provide local and low-cost opportunities for older adults to remain physically active and to socialise. To date, evidence on the use and impact of outdoor gyms among older adults is limited. Nonetheless, initial studies suggest that outdoor fitness equipment can have a positive impact on physical activity (Cohen et al. 2012), as well as psychological health and social integration among older adults. Playground users report 'feeling happier' and empowered after using the gym (i.e. when they managed to overcome a difficult piece of equipment) (Chow 2013; Pahtaja et al. 2006). Moreover, these playgrounds offer an environment for many older adults to socialise while exercising.

Following on from the success of playgrounds for older people, multigenerational playgrounds are gaining popularity, designed for use by people of all ages (e.g. in Finland and the United States). While there is no research on intergenerational outdoor play, it is thought that intergenerational indoor settings may affect physical, mental, and social well-being among older adults, through promoting intellectual activity, social networks, and physical activity (Sakurai et al. 2015). By extension, we posit the same may apply for playgrounds. Finlay et al. (2015) found that the mix of multigenerational activity with public green and blue spaces was a significant factor in older adults' improved social well-being and enjoyment of them; this research adds an important and under-researched multigenerational element to literature linking REs to the formation of social networks, explored earlier in this chapter. In summary, we suggest there is much scope to explore the possible physical, cognitive, emotional, and social benefits of multigenerational play in nature.

24.6.4 Water Settings

Older adults have distinctly therapeutic relationships with water settings (referred to in the field as 'blue space') (Finlay et al. 2015). 'Blue space' includes inland bodies of water—such as lakes, rivers and canals—natural or engineered spaces (including water fountains in urban settings), as well as coasts and oceans. Interactions with blue spaces offer a range of physical, mental, and social health benefits, much akin to green space. But blue space also offers additional benefits: it provides alternative opportunities for physical activity to walking, for example, swimming or canoeing (Finlay et al. 2015); it offers greater multisensory enjoyment, including the sounds of moving water, tranquil surroundings (e.g. calm, still waters for mental restoration), visual contact with wildlife (e.g. fish, dragon flies) and opportunities in warmer weather to physically experience the water (e.g. dipping one's fingers or feet in the water). The psychological benefits of access to blue space for older people constitute a symbolic connection with the self, evoking memories of people, events, and eliciting a reminder of the positive feelings experienced; the memory of a blue space, it is argued, is uplifting (Coleman and Kearns 2014).

Incorporating easy access for older people to blue spaces—from urban fountains to a river boardwalk or ocean-side pathway—offers much potential for both mobility and psychological well-being. However, issues of safety, accessibility, and personal perceptions of the risks of water settings need to be understood better by age and could impact on well-being outcomes.

24.6.5 Adventurous Restorative Environments Further Afield

Older people need opportunities to experience challenge in the environment; challenge is linked to well-being and offers a means of discovering inner strengths and resources (Patmore 2006). Adventure—and its accompanying sense of thrill—is important for well-being; the psychological process accompanying challenge has been conceptualised as 'flow' by Csikszentmihalyi (1990). Flow is an optimal form of experience achieved when a challenge is matched with the level of skill someone brings to it and promotes strong positive affect, absorption, and a sense of timelessness. This type of experience is often obtained by taking part in leisure activities that challenge us in some way. It is therefore important to keep these opportunities alive in older age.

This includes providing recreational opportunities in wilder natural settings further away from home. In Italy, further afield countryside and mountains were a preferred RE in healthy older adults (Scopelliti and Giuliani 2005). But we found no evidence of the value of adventure experiences in wilder nature on mobility and well-being in older people. Perhaps owing to accessibility difficulties, these types of environments are less well explored among older adults.

24.6.6 The City

Some urban settings—particularly downtown districts offering visual intrigue and complexity—have restorative potential. In older people, urban historic districts and museums can offer potential restorative experiences (Scopelliti and Giuliani 2005) and, in turn, increased opportunities for mobility. Others have identified the restorative potential of urban settings (Fornara and Troffa 2009), art galleries (Clow and Fredhoi 2006), cafes (Staats et al. 2016), bookstores and libraries (Newman and Brucks 2016) among younger populations; however, we found no evidence for positive effects in older people specifically. Urban farmers' markets offer older people a wide range of health opportunities including: healthy food options, visual stimuli that changes seasonally,

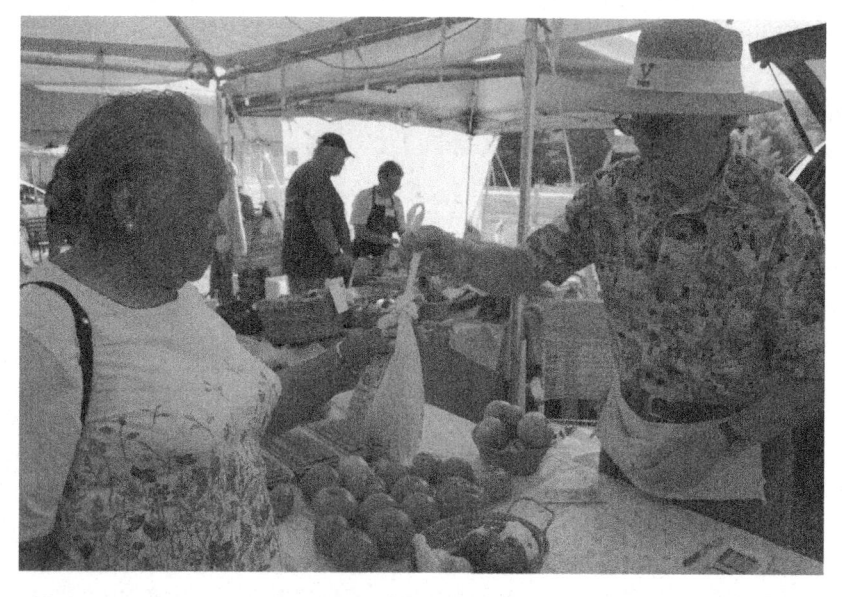

Fig. 24.1 Urban farmers' markets offer older people a wealth of health opportunities. (Source: The image is © JABA (Jefferson Area Board for Aging))

increased social connection to the local community, and increased mobility (Fig. 24.1). However, farmers' markets need to be inclusive, for example, by offering discounted produce for low-income seniors. As yet, the farmers' market as a potential RE for health benefits in older people is unexplored.

24.7 Older Adults with Dementia

As with healthy older adults, evidence suggests that access to REs among older adults experiencing cognitive impairment and dementia can improve well-being and physical health. Contact with nature among those living with dementia can lead to improvements in emotional state (i.e. reduced stress, agitation), physical health, verbal expression, memory and attention, awareness (i.e. multi-sensory engagement), sense of well-being, and social interaction (Clarke et al. 2013). To date, much of the research on REs and older adults with dementia has focused on residential care homes and access to gardens. Evidence suggests that the availability of gardens or outdoor areas in residential homes offers a range of physical and emotional benefits, including serving as alternatives to pharmacological interventions for management of behavioural symptoms (see Whear et al. 2014 for review of the evidence). Studies suggest significant improvements to levels of agitation after visiting a garden (Edwards et al. 2013); improvements to physical activity, sleep, and cognition (Lee and Kim 2008); and positive emotional outcomes (Whear et al. 2014). For individuals with dementia, gardening was found to be effective for encouraging activity participation and improving affect (D'Andrea et al. 2007; Gigliotti et al. 2004; Gurski 2004). The potential of therapeutic gardens and gardening as a source of stimulation may be particularly important for adults with dementia. Access to activities involving plants and gardening can spark memories of earlier pleasurable experiences and keep individuals with dementia actively involved in their lives (Edwards et al. 2013).

In contrast to private gardens and residential care homes, public spaces and the mental and physical effects on those living with dementia are much less well researched. With a majority of adults with dementia living independently (Mapes et al. 2016), the potential restorative benefits of public parks and gardens is an important area of research. In a qualitative study of older adults living with dementia in England (Mapes et al. 2016), urban parks and public gardens emerged as the most popular places to visit, in comparison with more 'natural' settings such as the countryside, coast, or woods. Ease of access to outdoor spaces is a driving factor of use, as well as 'managed' environments with facilities (e.g. paths, signs). This study also found that blue space is particularly popular for people with dementia (45% of respondents mentioned water): participants spoke strongly about lakes being an environment which promoted relaxation. This finding reflects literature about the benefits of blue space among the general older adult population (see above) and suggests a possible research avenue into exploring the benefits among those with dementia, including quantifying this evidence. Evidence suggests that participating in activities is a strong motivating factor for engaging with the natural environment (Mapes et al. 2016). Activities include informal walking, wildlife watching (especially bird watching), and social activities such as guided walks, community gardening, and farming.

Despite the perceived benefits of natural environments among older adults with dementia, there are significant and multiple barriers to access. Problems with mobility, tiredness, and disorientation can have a significant impact on the ability of people living with dementia to enjoy outdoor spaces, as well as additional health conditions or physical disabilities. We suggest that understanding and improving these barriers to access are an important area of research, and the possible health and cost benefits from such interventions are potentially huge.

24.8 Practical Implications

(1) *Improving access to and provision of REs:* design practice should pay more attention to the provision of sensory stimuli and visual complexity in the BE for older people (e.g. colour, architectural detail, natural stimuli). Visual diversity not only improves mental engagement with and alertness to one's environment but also encourages mobility and the motivation to move around and explore. In turn, social and recreational policy needs to improve both access to, and provision of, REs (inherently rich in curiosity and fascination), for example, libraries, farmers' markets, historic urban districts, museums, cafes, bookstores, botanical gardens, and parks. These REs also offer an important context for impromptu social interactions; indeed, for older people, these interactions may be their only opportunity for direct human contact over the course of a day. In addition, REs—owing to their collective restorative value—potentially nurture a wider 'civic consciousness' that can improve social capital in a community by raising mood and mindfulness, and perhaps even awareness of older people's needs.

(2) *Facilitating meaningful engagement with REs:* older people may need help engaging more mindfully with their everyday settings, for example, by

becoming more mindful of nature in a nearby green space and/or seeing their world through fresh eyes, say through the eyes of a child via inter-generational interactions outdoors or indoors. Social and recreational policy that fosters deeper connections to place should be encouraged via the provision of inter-generational opportunities (e.g. in residential care contexts) as well as fostering the use of technological tools, including mobile phone apps, that can raise awareness of the BE and its features.

(3) *Equitable access to REs:* poorer people living in poorer quality neighbourhoods have less access to the REs flagged above, for instance, they have less access to green space, and the quality is also poorer. Improving access to these settings is a health equity issue (Allen and Balfour 2014). In addition to improving access, policy and practice needs to better understand how to cater the provision of REs to diverse needs (e.g. by gender, ethnicity, cognitive difficulty, etc.) and how local culture—and its complexities— mediates in restorative processes.

24.9 Conclusions

REs offer a wealth of psychological well-being benefits to older people, including improved cognitive, emotional, and social well-being. Travelling to and from RE destinations and interacting with and moving through REs generates additional mobility benefits. Our findings suggest a need to understand the benefits for older people across a wider diversity of REs since the literature to date has focused almost entirely on the benefits of natural settings. More attention should be paid to the residential context, immediate street environs, and popular leisure places for older people, including museums and botanical gardens. We posit that the environmental attributes in the RE model (i.e. being away, soft fascination, extent, and compatibility) will vary according to age and need, and that, for older people, important attributes of REs are compatibility, social context, and a need for greater connection with the everyday setting (rather than *being away*). We also suggest memory recall is an important potential contributor to the restorative experience in older people. We believe that visual complexity and sensory stimuli in REs may be particularly important for generating well-being and mobility in older people, for example, by fostering better alertness that may assist in better decision-making—and reduced risk of falls—when navigating city streets. We conclude that an RE research framework—of the nature described above—provides a valuable framework by which to consider social and emotional well-being in older people and their interaction with physical activity.

Suggested Further Reading

- Collado, S., Staats, H., Corraliza, J., & Hartig, T. (2017). Restorative environments and health. In I. G. Fleury-Bahi, E. Pol, & O. Navarro (Eds.), *Handbook of environmental psychology and quality of life research* (pp. 127–148). Heidelberg: Springer.
- Roe, J. (forthcoming). *A new health urbanism*. In T. Banerjee & A. Loukaitou-Sideris (Eds.), *Urban design companion: A sequel*. London: Routledge.
- Staats, H. (2012). Restorative environments. In S. Clayton (Ed.), *The Oxford handbook of environmental and conservation psychology* (pp. 445–458). Oxford: Oxford University Press.

References

Allen, J., & Balfour, R. (2014, October). Natural solutions for tackling health inequalities, UCL Institute of Health Equity. Available online: https://www.gov.uk/government/news/natural-solutions-for-tackling-health-inequalities-conference-report. Accessed 8 Sept 2017.

Aspinall, P. A., Thompson, C. W., Alves, S., Sugiyama, T., Brice, R., & Vickers, A. (2010). Preference and relative importance for environmental attributes of neighbourhood open space in older people. *Environment and Planning B, 37*, 1022–1039.

Aspinall, P. A., Mavros, P., Coyne, R., & Roe, J. (2013). Urban brain: Analyzing outdoor physical activity with mobile EEG. *British Journal of Sports Medicine*. 06.03.2013. http://bjsm.bmj.com/content/49/4/272.

Astell-Burt, T., Mitchell, R., & Hartig, T. (2014). The association between green space and mental health varies across the lifecourse. A longitudinal study. *Journal of Epidemiology and Community Health, 68*, 578–583.

Bratman, G. N., Daily, G. C., Levy, B. J., & Gross, J. J. (2015). The benefits of nature experience: Improved affect and cognition. *Landscape and Urban Planning, 138*, 41–50.

Broekhuizen, K., De Vries, S., & Pierik, F. (2013). *Healthy aging in a green living environment: A systematic review of the literature*. Leiden: TNO.

Brookfield, K., Thompson, C. W., & Scott, I. (2017). The uncommon impact of common environmental details on walking in older adults. *International Journal of Environmental Research and Public Health, 14*(2), 190.

Brose, A., Lövdén, M., & Schmiedek, F. (2014). Daily fluctuations in positive affect positively co-vary with working memory performance. *Emotion, 14*, 1–6.

Buck, D. (2016). *Gardens and health: Implications for policy and practice*. London: The King's Fund.

Carels, R. A., Coit, C., Young, K., & Berger, B. (2007). Exercise makes you feel good, but does feeling good make you exercise?: An examination of obese dieters. *Journal of Sport & Exercise Psychology, 29*, 706–722.

Catalan-Matamoros, D., Gomez-Conesa, A., Stubbs, B., & Vancampfort, D. (2016). Exercise improves depressive symptoms in older adults: An umbrella review of systematic reviews and meta-analyses. *Psychiatry Research, 244*(2016), 202–209.

Chen, T.-Y., & Janke, M. C. (2012). Gardening as a potential activity to reduce falls in older adults. *Journal of Aging and Physical Activity, 20*(1), 15–31.

Chow, H. (2013). Outdoor fitness equipment in parks: A qualitative study from older adults' perceptions. *BMC Public Health, 13*, 1216.

Clarke, P., Mapes, N., Burt, J., & Preston, S. (2013). *Greening Dementia: A literature review of the benefits and barriers facing individuals living with dementia in accessing the natural environment and local greenspace*. Natural England Commissioned Reports, No. 137(5).

Clow, A., & Fredhoi, C. (2006). Normalisation of salivary cortisol levels and self-report stress by a brief lunchtime visit to an art gallery by London City workers. *Journal of Holistic Healthcare, 3*(2), 29–32.

Cohen, D. A., Marsh, T., Williamson, S., Golinelli, D., & McKenzie, T. L. (2012). Impact and cost-effectiveness of family fitness zones: A natural experiment in urban public parks. *Health & Place, 13*(1), 39–45.

Coleman, T., & Kearns, R. (2014). The role of blue spaces in experiencing place, aging and wellbeing: Insights from Waiheke Island, New Zealand. *Health & Place, 35*, 206–217.

Csikszentmihalyi, M. (1990). *Flow: The psychology of optimal experience*. New York: Harper & Row.

D'Andrea, S. J., Batavia, M., & Sasson, N. (2007). Effect of horticultural therapy on preventing the decline of mental abilities of patients with Alzheimer's type dementia. *Journal of Therapeutic Horticulture, 18*, 9–17.

De Vries, S., Verheij, R. A., Groenewegen, P. P., & Spreeuwenberg, P. (2003). Natural environments – Healthy environments? An exploratory analysis of the relationship between greenspace and health. *Environment and Planning A, 35*, 1717–1731.

Edwards, C. A., McDonnell, C., & Merl, H. (2013). An evaluation of a therapeutic garden's influence on the quality of life of aged care residents with dementia. *Dementia, 12*(4), 494–510.

Ellard, C. (2017). A new agenda for urban psychology: Out of the laboratory and onto the street. *Journal of Urban Design and Mental Health, 2*, 3.

Fägerstam, E., & Blom, J. (2012). Learning biology and mathematics outdoors: Effects and attitudes in a Swedish high school context. *Journal of Adventure Education & Outdoor Learning, 13*(1), 56–75.

Fan, M., & Jin, Y. (2014). Obesity and self-control: Food consumption, physical activity and weight-loss intention. *Applied Economic Perspectives and Policy, 36*(1), 125–145.

Fänge, A., & Ivanoff, S. D. (2009). The home is the hub of health in very old age: Findings from the ENABLE-AGE project. *Archives of Gerontology and Geriatrics, 48*(3), 340–345.

Finlay, J., Franke, T., McKay, H., & Sims-Gould, J. (2015). Therapeutic landscapes and wellbeing in later life: Impacts of blue and green spaces for older adults. *Health & Place, 34*, 97–106.

Fleig, L., Ashe, M. C., Voss, C., Therrien, S., Sims-Gould, J., McKay, H. A., & Winters, M. (2016). Environmental and psychosocial correlates of objectively measured physical activity among older adults. *Health Psychology, 35*(12), 1364–1372.

Fornara, F., & Troffa, R. (2009). Restorative experiences and perceived affective qualities in different built and natural urban places. In H. T. Yildiz & Y. I. Guney (Eds.), *Revitalising built environments: Requalifying old places for new uses. Proceedings of the IAPS-CSBE & Housing Networks International Symposium* (pp. 1–10). Istanbul: Istanbul Technical University.

Fredrickson, B. L. (2004). The broaden-and-build theory of positive emotions. *Philosophical Transactions of The Royal Society, London, 359*, 1367–1377.

Gerstoff, D., & Ram, N. (2009). Limitations on the importance of self-regulation in old age. *Human Development, 52*(1), 38–43.

Gigliotti, C., Jarrott, S., & Yorgason, J. (2004). Harvesting health: Effects of three types of horticultural therapy activities for persons with dementia. *Dementia, 3*(2), 161–180.

Gladwell, V. F., Brown, D. K., Barton, J. L., Tarvainen, M. P., Kuoppa, P., Pretty, J., Suddaby, J. M., & Sandercock, G. R. (2012). The effect of views of nature on autonomic control. *European Journal of Applied Psychology, 112*(9), 3379–3386.

Gross, H., & Lane, N. (2007). Landscapes of the lifespan: Exploring accounts of own gardens and gardening. *Journal of Environmental Psychology, 27*, 225–241.

Gurski, C. (2004). Horticultural therapy for institutionalized older adults and persons with Alzheimer's disease and other dementias: A study and practice. *Journal of Therapeutic Horticulture, 15*, 25–31.

Hartig, T. (2007). Three steps to understanding restorative environments as health resources. In C. W. Thompson & P. Travlou (Eds.), *Open spaces, people space* (pp. 163–180). Abingdon: Taylor and Francis.

Heliker, D., Chadwick, A., & O'Connell, T. (2001). The meaning of gardening and the effects on perceived well being of a gardening project on diverse populations of elders. *Activities, Adaptation & Aging, 24*(3), 35–56.

Holt-Lunstad, J., Smith, T. B., & Bradley Layton, J. (2010). Social relationships and mortality risk: A meta-analytic review. *PLoS Medicine, 7*(7), e1000316.

Isen, A. M., & Means, B. (1983). The influence of positive affect on decision-making strategy. *Social Cognition, 2*(1), 18–31.

Kaczynski, A. T., Stanis, S. A. W., Hastmann, T. J., & Besenyi, G. M. (2011). Variations in observed park physical activity intensity level by gender, race, and age: Individual and joint effects. *Journal of Physical Activity and Health, 13*, 151–160.

Kaplan, S. (1995). The restorative benefits of nature: Toward an integrative framework. *Journal of Environmental Psychology, 15*, 169–182.

Kaplan, R., & Kaplan, S. (1989). *The experience of nature: A psychological perspective.* New York: Cambridge University Press.

Kewon, B., Sullivan, W., & Riley, A. (1998). Green common spaces and the social integration of inner city older adults. *Environment and Behavior, 30*(6), 832–858.

Lee, Y., & Kim, S. (2008). Effects of indoor gardening on sleep, agitation, and cognition in dementia patients – A pilot study. *International Journal of Geriatric Psychiatry, 23*, 485–489.

Lindal, P. J., & Hartig, T. (2013). Architectural variation, building height, and the restorative quality or urban residential streetscapes. *Journal of Environmental Psychology, 33*, 26–36.

Mapes, N., Milton, S., Nicholls, V., & Williamson, T. (2016). *Is it nice outside? – Consulting people living with dementia and carers about engaging with the natural environment.* Natural England Commissioned Reports, No. 211.

Milligan, C., Gatrell, A., & Bingley, A. (2004). 'Cultivating health': Therapeutic landscapes and older people in northern England. *Social Science & Medicine, 58*(9), 1781–1793.

Nagel, C. L., Carlson, N. E., Bosworth, M., & Michael, Y. L. (2008). The relation between neighborhood built environment and walking activity among older adults. *American Journal of Epidemiology, 168*(4), 461–468.

Neale, C., Aspinall, P. A., Roe, J., et al. (2017). The ageing urban brain: Analysing outdoor physical activity using the Emotiv Affectiv suite in older people. *Journal of Urban Health, 94*(6), 869–880. https://link.springer.com/article/10.1007/s11524-017-0191-9.

Newman, K. P., & Brucks, M. (2016). When are natural and urban environments restorative? The impact of environmental compatibility on self-control restoration. *Journal of Consumer Psychology, 26*(4), 535–541. https://doi.org/10.1016/j.jcps.2016.02.005

Nicklett, E. J., Anderson, A., & Yen, I. H. (2014). Gardening activities and physical health among older adults: A review of the evidence. *Journal of Applied Gerontology, 35*(6), 678–690.

Nordbakke, S., & Schwanen, T. (2014). Well-being and mobility: A theoretical framework and literature review focusing on older people. *Mobilities, 9*(1), 104–129.

Pahtaja, P., Hämäläinen, H., & Tero, L. (2006). *Exercising senior citizens' balance and motor coordination, Rovaniemi Polytechnic (RAMK).* School of Sports and Leisure MOTO+ project.

Park, B. J., Tsunetsugu, Y., Kasetani, T., Hirano, H., Kagawa, T., Sato, M., & Miyazaki, Y. (2007). Physiological effects of Shinrin-yoku (taking in the atmosphere of the forest) using salivary cortisol and cerebral activity as indicators. *Journal of Physiological Anthropology, 26*, 123–128.

Parra, D. C., Gomez, L. F., Fleischer, N. L., & David Pinzon, J. (2010). Built environment characteristics and perceived active park use among older adults: Results from a multilevel study in Bogotá. *Health & Place, 16*(6), 1174–1181.

Patmore, A. (2006). *The truth about stress*. London: Atlantic Books.

Pettigrew, S., & Roberts, M. (2008). Addressing loneliness in later life. *Aging Mental Health, 12*(3), 302–309.

Roe, J. (2008). *The restorative power of natural and built environments*. Doctoral dissertation. Edinburgh: School of Built Environment, Heriot-Watt University. Retrieved from http://www.ros.hw.ac.uk/bitstream/handle/10399/2250/RoeJ_0908_sbe.pdf

Roe, J., Thompson, C. W., Aspinall, P. A., Brewer, M. J., Duff, E., Miller, D., Mitchell, R., & Clow, A. (2013). Green space and stress: Evidence from cortisol measures in deprived urban communities. *International Journal of Environmental Research and Public Health, 10*(9), 4086–4103.

Sakurai, R., Yasunaga, M., Murayama, Y., Ohba, H., Kumiko, N., Suzuki, H., Sakuma, N., Nishi, M., Hayato, U., Shinkai, S., Rebok, G. W., & Fujiwara, Y. (2015). Long-term effects of an intergenerational program on functional capacity in older adults: Results from a seven-year follow-up of the REPRINTS study. *Archives of Gerontology and Geriatrics, 64*, 13–20.

Scopelliti, M., & Giuliani, M. V. (2005). Restorative environments in later life. An approach to well-being from the perspective of environmental psychology. *Journal of Housing for the Elderly, 19*, 205–222.

Soga, M., Gaston, K. J., & Yamaura, Y. (2016). Gardening is beneficial for health: A meta-analysis. *Preventive Medicine Reports, 5*, 92–99.

Staats, H., & Hartig, T. (2004). Alone or with a friend: A social context for psychological restoration and environmental preferences. *Journal of Environmental Psychology, 24*(2), 199–211.

Staats, H., Jahncke, H., Herzog, T. R., & Hartig, T. (2016). Urban options for psychological restoration: Common strategies in everyday situations. *PLoS One, 11*(1), e0146213.

Steptoe, A., Shankar, A., Demakakos, P., & Wardle, J. (2013). Social isolation, loneliness, and all-cause mortality in older men and women. *PNAS, 110*(15), 5797–5801.

Sugiyama, T., & Thompson, C. W. (2008). Associations between characteristics of neighbourhood open space and older people's walking. *Urban Forestry & Urban Greening, 7*, 41–51.

Ulrich, R. S. (1983). Aesthetic and affective responses to natural environment. In I. Altman & J. F. Wohlwill (Eds.), *Behavior and the natural environment* (pp. 85–125). New York: Springer.

Ulrich, R. S., Simons, R. F., Losito, B. D., Fiorito, E., Miles, M. A., & Zelson, M. (1991). Stress recovery during exposure to natural and urban environments. *Journal of Environmental Psychology, 11*, 201–230.

Van den Berg, A. E., & Custers, M. H. (2011). Gardening promotes neuroendocrine and affective restoration from stress. *Journal of Health Psychology, 16*(1), 3–11.

Wang, D., & MacMillan, T. (2013). The benefits of gardening for older adults: A systematic review of the literature. *Activities, Adaptation & Aging, 37*(2), 153.

Whear, R., Thompson Coon, J., Bethel, A., Abbott, R., Stein, K., & Garside, R. (2014). What is the impact of using outdoor spaces such as gardens on the physical and mental well-being of those with dementia? A systematic review of quantitative and qualitative evidence. *The Journal of Post-Acute and Long-Term Care Medicine, 15*(10), 697–705.

White, M., Smith, A., Humphryes, K., Pahl, S., Snelling, D., & Depledge, M. (2010). Blue space: The importance of water for preference, affect, and restorativeness ratings of natural and built scenes. *Journal of Environmental Psychology, 30*, 482–493.

Wright, S. D., & Lund, D. A. (2000). Gray and green? Stewardship and sustainability in an aging society. *Journal of Aging Studies, 14*(3), 229–249.

Wright, S. D., & Wadsworth, A. M. (2014). Gray and green revisited: A multidisciplinary perspective of gardens, gardening, and the aging process. *Journal of Aging Research, 2014*, 283682.

Wu, Y., Prina, A. M., Jones, A., Matthews, F. E., & Brayne, C. (2015). Older people, the natural environment and common mental disorders: Cross-sectional results from the cognitive function and ageing study. *BMJ Open, 5*(9), e007936.

25

Transportation and Promoting Physical Activity Among Older People

Charles Musselwhite

25.1 Introduction

Maintaining mobility in later life is important for maintaining health and well-being. It enables older people to stay in close contact with family and friends and reduces loneliness. It keeps people connected to neighbourhoods, reducing isolation through affording access to services, shops and facilities, and allows people to engage in sports and leisure (WHO 1999). Walking and cycling ('active travel') as part of a daily routine can promote moderate physical activity, improving overall health and well-being (WHO 1999; Saelens et al. 2003).

In the wealthy Western world, people live in a hypermobile society where people must traverse further distances than ever before to stay connected to family and friends and to be able to access work, services, shops and hospitals. Consequently, this is most conveniently met through the use of cars. This is especially true for people who may have mobility difficulties due to age that make walking, cycling and using a bus more problematic and is especially true in rural areas poorly served by public transport and with dispersed services and shops (Parkhurst et al. 2014). Unsurprisingly, there has been an unprecedented growth in the use of private mechanised mobility among the older population in most wealthy countries, most notably a huge increase in driver licences held among older people and also the number of miles driven.

C. Musselwhite (✉)
Centre for Innovative Ageing, Swansea University, Swansea, UK

© The Author(s) 2018
S. R. Nyman et al. (eds.), *The Palgrave Handbook of Ageing and Physical Activity Promotion*, https://doi.org/10.1007/978-3-319-71291-8_25

25.2 Active Travel: Walking and Cycling

There are direct benefits of continuing active travel in later life. Regular walking or cycling has been found to reduce cardiovascular disease by around 30% and reduce all-cause mortality by 20% (Hamer and Chida 2008), through reducing the risk of coronary heart disease, stroke, cancer, obesity and type 2 diabetes (NICE 2013). It also keeps the musculoskeletal system healthy and is good for mental health (NICE 2013).

Many older people's physiological or cognitive changes can restrict their personal mobility. This is amplified for those who have to give up driving (Musselwhite and Shergold 2013). A lack of personal mobility can be a significant contributing factor to societal exclusion, for example, reducing accessibility to shops and services and limiting chances for social or cultural activity and exchange (Preston and Raje 2007). Unsurprisingly, older people who are restricted in getting out and about are far more likely to report being lonely and depressed (Fonda et al. 2001; Ling and Mannion 1995; Ziegler and Schwanen 2011) and have reduced quality of life (Schlag et al. 1996).

25.2.1 Amount of Walking and Cycling Among Older People

In many Western cultures, there is an increase in driving, especially among the older age groups. As an example, in 1975, in Great Britain, only 15% of people aged over 70 held a driving licence. This has increased to 62% in 2013 (DfT 2015a). This increase is more profound in females. In 1975, only 4% of females over 70 held a driving licence and now almost half do (DfT 2014, 2015a).

Number of miles driven per person per year falls from 70 years onwards (e.g. 1,905 miles/person per year against an average across all ages of 3,235 miles/person per year in Britain) but has increased compared to previous generations. For example, since 1995, Britain has seen an 8% reduction in the number of miles driven across all age groups. Yet for those aged 60–69, number of miles driven per person per year has increased by 37%, for the over 70s the figure is a 77% increase (DfT 2014, 2015a).

In many countries the increase in driving is also coupled with a decrease in use of active modes of transport. For example, the average distance walked per person per year has fallen over the last 20 years. In Great Britain this is by about 9% since 1995/97; Germany and France have seen very similar decline in walking as Britain. The United States has not seen a decline but has a far lower rate of walking at around 11% of all trips made across all ages. This rate is lower the older the resident in the United States, with only 9% of all trips made by 65+ year olds. Conversely, in developing countries older people are much more likely to walk long distances, especially those from lower socio-economic backgrounds (Prohaska et al. 2012).

There are different patterns in the Netherlands and in Denmark. Although a similar percentage of walking trips are made per person as in Britain, this has remained steady over the past 30 years (compared to a huge decline in Britain) (see Pucher and Buehler 2012). Over one-quarter of trips made are on foot in the Netherlands and almost one-fifth of all trips in Denmark. This does not differ by age much; in the Netherlands 23% of all trips made are on foot for those aged 60–69 and also for those aged 70–84 years. In Denmark, 15% of all trips made by 60–69-year olds and 70–84-year olds are made on foot. There has not been a significant change in walking among older people in Netherlands and Denmark that is seen elsewhere. Quality infrastructure, planning for walking and cycling and cultural norms are generally seen as reasons for this (Pucher and Buehler 2012).

For older people, cycling accounts for fewer miles and trips per person across all European countries, especially for those aged 70 and over. Distance cycled per person per year in England was 15 miles for those over the age of 70, 52 miles for 60–69-year olds and 53 miles across all age groups. Number of miles cycled per person per year has increased over the past 13 years for 60–69-year olds but not so for the 70+ age group (DfT 2014, 2015a). Despite a low amount of cycling in the 60+ age groups, it is worth noting that over one-quarter of British 60–69-year olds own a bicycle (27%) and 17% report having ridden a bicycle during the last year (Jones et al. 2016). In the United Kingdom, older people who own and use a bicycle are more likely to be wealthy, White and male (Jones et al. 2016). In addition, older people living in rural areas cycle three times as far as those in urban areas (Jones et al. 2016).

In summary, the amount of cycling in the UK among the older (and indeed the younger) population are low compared to other northern European countries. For example, cycling accounts for 23% of trips made by older people in the Netherlands, 15% in Denmark and 9% in Germany against less than 1% in the UK (Pucher and Buehler 2012; DfT 2014, 2015a).

25.2.2 Walking and Road User Safety

In the UK, people over the age of 70 make up 11.8% of the population (ONS 2015) and account for around 8% of pedestrian activity (DfT 2015a, b).

Yet, older people also account for 42.8% of all pedestrian fatalities: 191 deaths from 446 across all age groups in total (DfT 2015a, b). That means almost half the pedestrians killed on roads come from just over 11% of the population. Countries that have more stringent licence renewal process for older drivers can face an increase in the number of road traffic-related injuries and deaths with older people, as people switch from the car to being a pedestrian (Mitchell 2013).

A look at police data, collected at the scene of road collisions in Britain, shows that failure to judge vehicle speed is a significant factor in older people's road collisions as pedestrians (DfT 2015b). This correlates with data in Australia (Job 1998), France (Domnes, et al. 2014), the Netherlands (Dijkstra and Bos 1997) and several other countries (See PROMISING 2001). Generally, older pedestrians look less at traffic and accept significantly smaller gaps in traffic when crossing the road than younger pedestrians. Looking at the barriers to walking for older people may help reveal where safety improvements can occur.

25.3 Key Barriers to Being a Pedestrian in Later Life

Barriers to walking as seen through the eyes of older people have been identified in a number of projects from various places across the world (Alves et al. 2008; Dunbar et al. 2004; Newton and Ormerod 2008, 2012; Newton et al. 2010; Stahl et al. 2008; Sugiyama and Ward-Thompson 2007, 2008; Wennberg 2009). They can be summarised as follows:

- *Poorly maintained pavements.* Maintenance of pedestrian areas is crucial, not just for aesthetics but also for safety and concerns for falling, again as evidenced by older people themselves. Research for the Inclusive Design for Going Outdoors (IDGO) project in the United Kingdom, for example, using Go-Along interviews, where the older person leads the researcher on a walking route and describes enablers and barriers, has found how frequently cracked or poorly maintained pavements hamper walking, creating difficulties walking and balancing on tactile pavements (Newton and Ormerod 2012) and the importance of using appropriate non-slip materials to use that are easily replaceable when necessary (Newton and Ormerod 2008). Poor surfaces, caused by fallen leaves, rain, ice or snow, for example, can also be a barrier. There is a tendency amongst councils to clear roads of ice

and snow but not always pavements and this becomes a real barrier and hazard for older people's active mobility in winter months across Europe and North America (Wennberg 2009).
- *Continuous ability to walk.* To enable walking, older people need a distinct area dedicated to walking, where a pathway, pavement (or sidewalk) is preferred and the wider and more away from the intrusion of vehicles the better. There are also concerns over sharing the space with cyclists and also where there are other pedestrians in large numbers. In addition, to foster continuous walking, there needs to be space to stop and dwell along with appropriately located and safe and accessible public conveniences and seating (Newton et al. 2010).
- *Poor crossing facilities.* Inability to cross the road has been cited as a crucial factor that reduces older people's confidence with getting out and about and can mean older people make large detours to avoid crossing dangerous roads, make fewer trips or even stay at home (Lord et al. 2010; Zijlstra et al. 2007). Time spent travelling tends to be viewed by authorities as wasted time, a cost to the individuals and society. As such, transport policy and strategy is often geared around the need to reduce travel time. An example of this is evident when transport modes compete, where the emphasis is placed on reducing the travel time of vehicles on business while increasing the travel time for those not on business. Hence, crossing points tend to be put in largely where vehicles might be hampered by large volumes of pedestrians crossing. In the UK, the most common form of crossing is the Pelican crossing. This consists of a traffic-lighted crossing point, with green (go) and red (stop) phases for drivers and pedestrians. The Department for Transport in the UK typically suggest the time for the green phase for pedestrians should be set at a walking speed of between 1 and 1.22 metres per second (or around 4 feet per second). Suggesting walking speeds of around 1.2 metres per second for signalised pedestrian crossings is found almost universally around the world. Research suggests older people do not walk anywhere near this speed. Musselwhite (2015), using three case study areas in the UK, found 88% of people aged over 65 did not walk at this speed. This increased to 94% of older females over the age of 65. Previous research has found similar results, suggesting older people's average speeds are between 0.7 and 0.9 metres per second. This concurs with previous research which has found similar issues with crossing times for older people (e.g. Asher et al. 2012, Newton and Ormerod 2008).
- *Poor or no lighting.* Poorly lit streets especially in poor weather or at night have a negative effect on older people using the street, especially as older

people are more likely to have difficulty with luminance. It can also reduce confidence through concerns about safety (Shumway-Cook et al. 2003).
- *Noise.* High levels of noise, especially from heavy traffic, can be especially distressing to older people who are more likely to suffer from hearing problems (Balfour and Kaplan 2002; Burholt et al. 2016).
- *Legibility.* Spaces must be legible for the user, in that they must demonstrate to the user what can happen in the space and be broken up into separate areas for different types of activity clearly marked. Formal signage is not always necessary, as the space itself can afford to others what activity is expected in the area. Spaces that are too open and wide can be viewed negatively as they are difficult to navigate and lack legibility, even if they are totally pedestrianised (Atkin 2010). Conversely, small spaces meaning older people have restricted passing space can be an issue, especially if the older person cannot turn their body quickly which can be an issue in later life (Musselwhite 2015).
- *Pollution.* Smog is a deterrent for older people to go out walking, especially in developing nations. Cities in India are particularly a no-go area for older people at certain times of high pollution. Wealthier nations can also suffer similar problems; Japanese cities and at times European cities can be at risk for older people (Deguen and Zmirou-Navier 2010).
- *Natural elements.* The climate can affect older people's walking (Burholt et al. 2016). High or very low temperatures can stop people walking, as can weather variability or extreme weather conditions, for example, wind, snow, ice or rain especially. This can be mitigated through shelter, especially natural green vegetation cover (e.g. Williams et al. 2012). Topography is also an issue, especially, hills can be a barrier to walking for older people.
- *Land use.* Having services within walking distance from home has been linked to increased walking (Strath et al. 2012). In addition, access to nature, especially green fields, trees and sounds of nature, is also related to more walking among older people (Burholt et al. 2016; Gauvin et al. 2012; Strath et al. 2012).

25.4 Improving Street Design at a Strategic, Policy and Practitioner Level

To design a street network, there needs to be a full understanding of the needs, wishes and desires of the users, including understanding of issues and problems. Transport planning in all countries has for too long overrelied on statistics, models and technical manuals and guidelines at the expense of beauty, harmony, interiority and animals, and this has inevitably led to the development of bland, vehicle-centric roads and streets with little understanding of humanness or humanity (King 1991). There has also been an overreliance on collecting vehicular data at the expense of pedestrian or cyclist behaviour adding to an imbalance of representation when designing streets. Traffic calming measures, physical changes in the road layout made to slow down vehicles such as speed humps, build outs or chicanes, have a bad name for themselves because they have traditionally been implemented using poor materials or are not in keeping with the area. They may make the area look problematic, since they can indicate an area with speeding vehicles. There may be better ways of using traffic calming, perhaps by using more natural materials: utilising cattle grids, hedges or overhanging trees as gateways; or psychological calming—the use of narrowing (e.g. by trees or hedges); or altering perceptual cues (e.g. using road markings to create the impression of narrower roads or to eradicate road markings altogether) have had some success, for example (for reviews see Elliott et al. 2003 and Kennedy et al. 2005).

Building on work by Alves et al. (2008), Sugiyama and Ward-Thompson (2007, 2008) and Musselwhite (2014), and taking the principles of good design, it is possible to design streets around recognised objectives of urban design as set out by Centre for Architechture and the Built Enviornment (CABE) (2011) (see Table 25.1):

(a) *Safe and accessible space*

- *Ease of movement*: Movement should be enhanced for all users, giving space for users to pass each other. There should be places to stop and dwell such as provision of benches. There should be focal points to commune at including fountains, works of art, sculptures, memorials and greenery.

(b) *Legible place*

- *Legibility*: The area should be designed in a way that is easy to understand and interpret, not just with signage but with other visual and tactile cues as well to help determine legitimacy in activity and determine use. Legibility does not always have to be constant; people can adapt as with new designs, for example, older people are able to adapt to changes in the urban environment that allow vehicles and pedestrians to use the same space; they were fine using shared space (Hammond and Musselwhite 2013). This case study was at Widemarsh Street,

Table 25.1 Designing streets for older people based on CABE (2011) principles (Musselwhite 2014)

(1) *Safe and accessible space*—feel you are safe there Sharing space—feel you have room to move, space to dwell for safe interactions with other users	*Ease of movement*	Movement should be enhanced for all users, along with permission to stop and dwell at benches and places to lean and creating focal points to commune at including fountains, works of art, sculptures, memorials or trees, gardens and other greenery
(2) *Legible place*—Psychological attachment and legitimacy—feel you should be there	*Legibility*	Area should be designed in a way that is easy to understand and interpret, not just with signage but with other visual and tactile cues as well to help determine legitimacy in activity and determine use
	Adaptability	The place should be built to adapt to changes in the needs of users, policy and legislation over time
	Diversity and choice	Allowing area to be used by a large variety of individuals and uses, with minimum exclusion
(3) *Distinctive and aesthetically pleasing*—somewhere you want to go and spend time—feel you want to be there	*Character*	Streets should have character and reflect local identify, history and culture. Utilising local art and architecture can help enhance distinct and unique character and identity
	Continuity and enclosure	Where public and private spaces are easily distinguished
	Quality public realm	Good-quality materials easily maintained and replaced

Hereford, in the UK, an area of low traffic volume, and more research is needed where high volumes of traffic may be found.

- *Adaptability*: The place should be built to adapt to changes in the needs of users, policy and legislation over time. There will be a higher percentage of older people using the built environment and a need to reflect that in design, for example.
- *Diversity and choice*: Allowing area to be used by a large variety of individuals and uses, with minimum exclusion. Space heterogeneity is to be encouraged where possible.

(c) *Distinctive and aesthetically pleasing space*

- *Character*: The streets should have character and reflect local identify, history and culture. Utilising local art and architecture can help enhance distinct and unique character and identity. Older people, especially those living with cognitive decline or dementia, connect well to elements of a past that they know and recognise (Mitchell and Burton 2006; Musselwhite 2014). In the built environment, connectivity occurs therefore through distinct buildings, road layouts and names of streets and buildings. Consideration must be given to understanding people's connections to place in order to help people navigate and feel confident with the space
- *Continuity and enclosure*: Continuity of public space helps older people define their role within that place. A sense of purpose can be afforded from the layout of space—is it somewhere they can sit and dwell? Is it a corridor to another place? Can it be gleaned from the layouts provided? Increasing privatisation of public space is a threat to older people. Private space is often heavily managed and designed for particular commercial reasons, for example, as a managed corridor to encourage certain groups of people into shops, offices or housing. Hence they tend to lack public amenities of other areas and can restrict behaviours of older people that may exclude them from using that space, for example, a lack of benches and lack of public conveniences which may be deemed by the landowner as unnecessarily costly or indeed a direct threat to further use of the space nearby (Musselwhite 2014). For example, not providing public benches near cafes, coffee shops, restaurants and bars in the hope of encouraging people who need to sit to purchase goods.
- *Quality public realm*: uneven or cracked pavements are a large contributor to falls in later life. Research from the UK suggests around half of falls occur outdoors, many of which are attributed to uneven or damaged pavements (Age UK 2012; Nyman et al. 2013). Having a fall can have a large detrimental effect on older people's confidence to go out, increasing isolation and reducing independence. There needs to be careful consideration for materials used, Newton and Ormerod (2008) provide excellent guidance based on discussions and trials with older people in the UK. They found older people prefer tarmac as a surface, largely for its smoothness, as long as it is not slippery. Paving slabs are seen as aesthetically pleasing in the environment, but must be laid and maintained properly and all be a similar height without cracks. Cobbles

were seen as very aesthetically pleasing and in keeping with historical perspective of many cities, towns and villages in Europe, in particular, but were conversely seen as very difficult to walk on in later life. Gravel was almost uniformly rejected on aesthetics and ease of walking. Maintenance and repair is vital and older people are encouraged to be active in reporting problems to the relevant authorities and be much more involved in the design of materials used (Age UK 2012). All councils need to ensure that pavement repairs are carried out promptly and that people are encouraged to report problem areas.

25.5 Barriers to Cycling

As stated earlier, there are few older people cycling in the UK, but there is evidence for demand; 42% of older people would cycle more if barriers to cycling were removed or support given to overcome them (UK Department for Transport 2011). The barriers include both built environment factors and personal and cultural factors.

The main reason that puts older people off cycling in the UK is the perception that the roads are dominated by large numbers of fast-moving motorised vehicles and as such are seen as very dangerous (Pooley et al. 2013). It is not surprising that the highest level of cycling among older people, in Europe at least, is in countries Denmark and the Netherlands, for example, with greater dedicated cycling infrastructure to allow cycling to occur off road away from busy traffic. Research by Jones et al. (2016) with 95 experienced older cyclists in 4 UK cities involving velo observations and video elicitation interviews identified the following key barriers in addition to high traffic levels:

- *Dismounting:* Having to dismount and get back on the bike, as often happens at dangerous or difficult-to-negotiate junctions, is seen negatively, not least for the physical difficulty of getting on and off a bike is increased in later life.
- *Sharing space*: Uncertainty and anxiety among users where cyclists have to share paths with pedestrians with particular concern for unpredictable pedestrian activity. There are particular concerns about dogs and children as they are viewed as even more unpredictable.
- *Poor surfaces*: Lack of upkeep of surfaces and deliberate changes in surfaces such as speed cushions and rumble strips cause discomfort and increase vulnerability.

- *Uncertainty*: Lack of understanding what is expected of them as a cyclist is key issue for older cyclists, for example, start/stop cycle lanes and lanes moving across traffic.

These kinds of barriers could reduce cycling for some older people. In others, it meant they compensated by breaking the rules, for example, not using dangerous cycle lanes or by using pavements especially at junctions. Performing such illegal behaviours made older people feel very uncomfortable (Jones et al. 2016).

There are also personal and cultural factors at play. There are concerns over personal levels of fitness required for cycling that older people don't feel they possess (Davies et al. 1997), especially in countries where there is little cycling across all age groups and cycling across the life course is fragmented (Jones et al. 2016). The difference in cultures and cycling rates among older people is also based on cultural norms; how normal is it to see older people on their bikes, for example, differs between Denmark, where it is much more normal and expected, and the UK, where it is an exception (Pucher and Beuhler 2008, 2012).

25.5.1 Improving Cycling for Older People

The overwhelming desire, perhaps not surprisingly, is for better quality cycle provision that is safe and comfortable to use. The following suggestions are adapted from Jones et al. (2016):

- *Dedicated lanes for cycling*: Separation and segregation of cycle routes away from traffic are necessary.
- *Ensuring momentum of cycling is maintained*: This is very pertinent for older people, some of whom have less physical ability to keep getting on and off their bike.
- *Legibility*: Urban spaces will also need to be designed so that it is clear where cyclists are 'meant to be', that is, they should be clearly signposted and legible on the ground being consistent in surface quality, colour and design. Spaces for cycling should be free of potholes, clear of debris and smooth.
- *Training*: Helping older people re-engage with cycling is needed in later life. Dedicated support for older people to help their confidence in riding has had some success, but there are relatively few examples of it around the UK.

- *E-bikes*: Electronic bikes or E-bikes are bicycles that can be used normally but also have a small engine which can be used to aid propulsion. The potential for E-bikes to overcome some of the concerns about the physically demanding aspects of cycling for older people is huge—a mixture of pedal power supplemented by power-assisted engine is ideal for physically demanding hills or when fatigue sets in. E-bikes are, however, heavy and expensive to use at present but they are improving and hence could be part of the future for active mobility for older people.

25.6 Using Public Transport and Walking

It is worth noting that use of buses has been correlated with increased walking. Older people's use of buses increases, especially with the advent of free or concessionary bus fares as introduced in the UK under the Transport Act of 2000 and introduced from 2002. In later life, miles travelled on buses increase for the over 70s (529 miles/person per year for over 70s compared to 331 miles/person per year across all ages (DfT 2014, 2015a)). Bus use is higher among females, as it is across the life course and this extends into older age, although with the advent of the free bus pass, this has begun to even up among the genders, with more males using the bus than previous generations. The percentage of eligible older people taking up bus pass is 76% female and 79% male, 73% up from 61% and 50% in 2005 (year before free bus travel was introduced) but not as high as the peak in 2012 at 78%. Humphrey and Scott (2012) found that ownership of a free bus pass is higher (around 80–82%) among those with lower income (less than £15,000). This group are also more likely to use the bus once a week than those on higher incomes who use it less frequently.

There is compelling evidence that use of the bus system increases with 'free' travel for older people (Mackett 2013a, b). The most commonly reported activity older people cite as their destination across all these surveys is shopping, followed by social and leisure, day trips, visiting friends then medical, meaning people are socially connected and hence reduce isolation (Mackett 2013b). Mackett (2013b) also notes how such journeys support volunteering and caring work older people undertake which would otherwise not take place. Dargay et al. (2010) modelled bus use against what would have happened if no free bus pass had been introduced and suggested the number of bus stages (groups of bus stops) travelled through by older people increased by 45.4% in rural areas and 26.5% in urban areas. The journeys made are not just more numerous but also often longer in duration and distance (Dargay et al. 2010). Additionally, Andrews (2011) found 74% of his respondents stated that the free bus pass improved their quality of life and general well-being.

Webb et al. (2011) used logistic regression analyses on three waves of data (2004, 2006 and 2008) from the English Longitudinal Study of Ageing. They found becoming eligible for a free bus pass is associated with increased use of public transport and older people who used more public transport between 2004 and 2008 had a reduced chance of being obese. They conclude that the introduction of free bus travel for older residents is associated with increased public transport use and may have a protective effect against obesity.

25.7 Implications for Policy and Practice

To improve walking and cycling, a change in culture and governance is needed, as well as changes to the walking and cycling environment and infrastructure:

25.7.1 Changing Cultures

As a research community, we have a job to spread the word as to how important being active is in later life and how being active can form part of ordinary everyday walking and cycling. Too often, activity in later life is viewed as something additional to the norm, but with walking and cycling it can be built into everyday activity. Health practitioners need to be able to emphasise the value of active travel to their patients, potentially being able to prescribe exercise into the lives of older people especially in relation to everyday activity.

People who are more active in later life tend to be people who have always been active and have been much more multi-modal throughout their life. However, current generations of older people are more wedded to their car than ever before. More work is needed to address behaviour change with regard to encouraging older people out of their vehicles and into more active travel. Support groups can help overcome some of the social and physical barriers (Jones et al. 2016) but more is needed to integrate and embed changes into everyday life.

25.7.2 Changing Governance

Overall, walking and cycling for older people must be given greater priority among decision-makers. Multiple stakeholders often control public space and have different interests. A comprehensive strategy bringing together the different elements of the street, in terms of usability for older people, is needed. The Welsh Government's Active Travel (Wales) Act 2013 places a requirement on Local Authorities in Wales, for example, to improve facilities and routes for walkers and cyclists, to enable everyday journeys to be made by walking and cycling. Age is not mentioned in the Act, but there is room for it to be a central focus (Musselwhite 2016). Provision of shops and services at a local neighbourhood level within walking distance of residential areas results in more older people walking. An Active Travel Act can help feed into master planning to encourage local services and shops to be among residential areas (Musselwhite 2016).

25.7.3 Changing Environments

Improvements need to be made so that the environment is safe, accessible and desirable for older people. At the microscopic level, quality paving is needed that is maintained well, is non-slip and free from ice and snow. Spaces for walking and cycling need to be placed, where possible, on dedicated infrastructure as far away from vehicles as is possible. Crossings need to be made more accessible, not least with giving older people more time to cross safely. Key walking routes need to ensure benches and toilets are provided at regular intervals. Where natural barriers exist, for example, heat and sunshine, providing a green canopy can mitigate the negative affect and allow people to walk or cycle. Areas must also be attractive and neighbourhood aesthetics are important in encouraging older people to be active pedestrians or cyclists in their local area.

25.8 Conclusions

There are low numbers of walkers and especially cyclists in later life. Too often walking is seen as something only for leisure purposes whereas it needs to be better integrated into everyday lives of older people and accompany more functional trips to shops and to access services and see family and friends.

The barriers and enablers are similar for both walking and cycling. Having a dedicated space for walking and for cycling seems imperative where possible. Keeping active travel away from speeding traffic is vital. Where this can't be done, creating clear and legible rules and spaces for walking and cycling is needed. Reducing speeds of vehicles where sharing occurs is also vital; speeding traffic is not only intrusive and reduces people walking and cycling but it is overtly dangerous too. Where crossings are put in, there must be more time allowed for older people to complete the crossing before vehicles take over the carriageway again. Creating legible space for both walking and cycling is needed. Too often, space is ambiguous making it hard for older people to ascertain their legitimacy as an active road user.

Changes in culture are also required for both walking and cycling. Older people need to feel like psychologically legitimate road users as walkers or cyclists and not seen as unusual or dangerous. Walking needs to be viewed as a legitimate activity for older people, something that can happen away from just for leisure purposes and something that can be done at any time and any place. Such cultural shifts will take time to happen and need to be evident across the life course in order to make change in later life.

In creating age-friendly communities, there is a need to address mobility. Too often mobility is forgotten about when thinking about how communities engage and connect. Active travel needs to be central to fostering supportive communities and infrastructure in later life.

Suggested Further Reading

- Mitchell, L., & Burton, E. (2006). Neighbourhoods for life: Designing dementia-friendly outdoor environments. *Quality in Ageing and Older Adults, 7*(1), 26–33.
- Newton, R., Ormerod, M., Burton, E., Mitchell, L., & Ward-Thompson, C. (2010). Increasing independence for older people through good street design. *Journal of Integrated Care, 18*(3), 24–29.
- Sinnett, D., Williams, K., Chatterjee, K., & Cavill, N. (2011). *Making the case for investment in the walking environment: A review of the evidence* (Technical Report). London: Living Streets. Available from: http://eprints.uwe.ac.uk/15502

References

AGE UK. (2012). *Pride of place. How councillors can improve neighbourhoods for older people*. London: AGE UK Campaign.

Alves, S., Aspinall, P., Ward Thompson, C., Sugiyama, T., Brice, R., & Vickers, A. (2008). Preferences of older people for environmental attributes of local parks: The use of choice-based conjoint analysis. *Facilities, 26*(11/12), 433–453.

Andrews, G. (2011). *Just the ticket? Exploring the contribution of free bus fares policy to quality of later life*. A thesis submitted in partial fulfilment of the requirements of the University of the West of England, Bristol, for the degree of Doctor of Philosophy.

Asher, L., Aresu, M., Falaschetti, E. A., & Mindell, J. (2012). Most older pedestrians are unable to cross the road in time: A cross-sectional study. *Age and Ageing, 41*, 690–694.

Atkin, R. (2010). *Sight line. Designing better streets for people with low vision*. London: Helen Hamlyn Centre/Centre, Royal College of Art.

Balfour, J. L., & Kaplan, G. A. (2002). Neighborhood environment and loss of physical function in older adults: Evidence from the Alameda County study. *American Journal of Epidemiology, 155*, 507–515.

Burholt, V., Roberts, M. S., & Musselwhite, C. B. A. (2016). Older People's external residential assessment tool (OPERAT): A complementary participatory and metric approach to the development of an observational environmental measure. *BMC Public Health, 16*, 1022.

CABE. (2011). Seven principles of good design. http://webarchive.nationalarchives.gov.uk/20110118095356/http:/www.cabe.org.uk/councillors/principles. Last accessed 1 June 2017.

Dargay, J., Last, A., & Goodwin, P. (2010). *Concessionary travel: The research papers* (A report to the Department for Transport). Leeds: Institute for Transport Studies, University of Leeds.

Davies, D. G., Halliday, M. E., Mayes, M., & Pocock, R. L. (1997). *Attitudes to cycling: A qualitative study and conceptual framework*. Crowthorne: Transport Research Laboratory.

Deguen, S., & Zmirou-Navier, D. (2010). Social inequalities resulting from health risks related to ambient air quality—A European review. *European Journal of Public Health, 20*, 27–35.

Department for Transport (DfT). (2011). Climate change and transport choices segmentation – Underlying data. http://webarchive.nationalarchives.gov.uk/20121105134522/http://assets.dft.gov.uk/publications/climate-change-transport-choices/climate-change-transport-choices-segment-variables.csv. Last accessed 1 June 2017.

Department for Transport (DfT). (2014). *Transport statistics great Britain: (2013)*. London: DfT. Available at: www.gov.uk/government/uploads/system/uploads/attachment_data/file/264679/tsgb-2013.pdf. Accessed 1 June 2017.

Department for Transport (DfT). (2015a). National travel survey. Available at: https://www.gov.uk/government/collections/national-travel-survey-statistics. Last accessed 1 June 2017.

Department for Transport (DfT). (2015b). Facts on pedestrian casualties. Available at: https://www.gov.uk/government/uploads/system/uploads/attachment_data/file/448036/pedestrian-casualties-2013-data.pdf. Last accessed 1 June 2017.

Dijkstra, A., & Bos, J. M. J. (1997). *ACEA – Dutch contribution: Road safety effects of small infrastructural measures with emphasis on pedestrians*. Leidschendam: SWOV.

Domnes, A., Cavallo, V., Baptiste Dubuisson, J., Tournier, I., & Vienne, F. (2014). Crossing a two-way street: Comparison of young and old pedestrians. *Journal of Safety Research, 50*, 27–34.

Dunbar, G., Holland, C. A., & Maylor, E. A. (2004). *Older pedestrians: A critical review of the literature road safety research report no. 37*. London: Department for Transport.

Elliott, M. A., McColl, V. A., & Kennedy, J. V. (2003). *Road design measures to reduce drivers' speed via "psychological" processes: A literature review* (TRL Report TRL564). Crowthorne: TRL Limited.

Fonda, S. J., Wallace, R. B., & Herzog, A. R. (2001). Changes in driving patterns and worsening depressive symptoms among older adults. *Journal of Gerontology: Social Sciences, 56B*(6), S343–S351.

Gauvin, L., Richard, L., Kestens, Y., Shatenstein, B., Daniel, M., Moore, S. D., Mercille, G., & Payette, H. (2012). Living in a well-serviced urban area is associated with maintenance of frequent walking among seniors in the VoisiNuAge study. *The Journals of Gerontology. Series B, Psychological Sciences and Social Sciences, 67*, 76–88.

Hamer, M., & Chida, Y. (2008). Walking and primary prevention: A meta-analysis of prospective cohort studies. *British Journal of Sports Medicine, 42*(4), 238–243.

Hammond, V., & Musselwhite, C. B. A. (2013). The attitudes, perceptions and concerns of pedestrians and vulnerable road users to shared space: A case study from the UK. *Journal Of Urban Design, 18*(1), 78–97.

Humphrey, A., & Scott, A. (2012). *Older people's use of concessionary bus travel*. Report by NatCen Social Research for Age UK. Available from: http://www.ageuk.org.uk/documents/en-gb/for-professionals/research/concessionary_bus_travel_2012.pdf?dtrk=true. Accessed 10 Apr 2017.

Job, R. F. (1998). Pedestrians at traffic light controlled intersections: Crossing behaviour of the elderly and non-elderly. *Proceedings of the conference on pedestrian safety*, 29 and 30 June, Melbourne, 40–4.

Jones, T., Chatterjee, K., Spinney, J., Street, E., Van Reekum, C., Spencer, B., Jones, H., Leyland, L. A., Mann, C., Williams, S., & Beale, N. (2016). *cycle BOOM. Design *for lifelong health and wellbeing. Summary of key findings and recommendations.* Oxford, UK: Oxford Brookes University.

Kennedy, J. V., Gorell, R., Crinson, L., Wheeler, A., & Elliott, M. A. (2005). *Psychological traffic calming* (TRL Report TRL641). Crowthorne: Transport Research Laboratory.

King, G. (1991). *No particular place to go.* Report for transport 2000: Transport and environment in Wales, Llandrindod Wells.

Ling, D. J., & Mannion, R. (1995). *Enhanced mobility and quality of life of older people: Assessment of economic and social benefits of dial-a- ride services.* Proceedings of the seventh international conference on Transport and Mobility for Older and Disabled People, Vol. 1. London: Department for the Environment Transport and the Regions (DETR).

Lord, S. E., Weatherall, M., & Rochester, L. (2010). Community ambulation in older adults: Which internal characteristics are important? *Archives of Physical Medicine and Rehabilitation, 91*(3), 378–383.

Mackett, R. (2013a). The impact of concessionary bus travel on the wellbeing of older and disabled people. *Transportation Research Record, 2352,* 114–119.

Mackett, R. (2013b). The benefits of a policy of free bus travel for older people. *Proceedings of the 13th world conference on transport research,* Rio de Janeiro, 15–18 July.

Mitchell, C. G. B. (2013). The licensing and safety of older drivers in Britain. *Accident Analysis and Prevention, 50,* 732–741.

Mitchell, L., & Burton, E. (2006). Neighbourhoods for life: Designing dementia-friendly outdoor environments. *Quality in Ageing and Older Adults, 7*(1), 26–33.

Musselwhite, C. (2014). Designing public space for older people. *Generations Review, 24*(3), 25–27.

Musselwhite, C. (2016). Vision for an age friendly transport system in Wales. *EnvisAGE, Age Cymru, 11,* 14–23.

Musselwhite, C. B. A. (2015). Further examinations of mobility in later life and improving health and wellbeing. *Journal of Transport & Health, 2*(2), 99–100.

Musselwhite, C. B. A., & Shergold, I. (2013). Examining the process of driving cessation in later life. *European Journal of Ageing, 10*(2), 89–100.

Newton, R., & Ormerod, M. (2008). The design of streets with older people in mind: Design guide – Materials of footways and footpaths. I'DGO inclusive design for getting outdoors. Available at: http://www.idgo.ac.uk/design_guidance/factsheets/materials_footways_footpaths.htm. Last accessed 1 June 2017.

Newton, R. A., & Ormerod, M. G. (2012). The design of streets with older people in mind: Tactile paving. I'DGO. Inclusive design for getting outdoors. Available at: www.idgo.ac.uk/design_guidance/streets.htm. Accessed 1 June 2017.

Newton, R. A., Ormerod, M. G., Burton, E., Mitchell, L., & Ward-Thompson, C. (2010). Increasing independence for older people through good street design. *Journal of Integrated Care, 18*(3), 24–29.

NICE. (2013). Walking and cycling: Local measures to promote walking and cycling as forms of travel or recreation NICE public health guidance 41. Available at: https://www.nice.org.uk/guidance/ph41. Last accessed 8 Jan 2017.

Nyman, S., Ballinger, C., Phillips, J., & Newton, R. (2013). Characteristics of outdoor falls among older people: A qualitative study. *BMC Geriatrics, 13*(1), 125.

Office for National Statistics (ONS). (2015). Annual mid-year population estimates for the UK. Available at: https://www.ons.gov.uk/peoplepopulationandcommunity/populationandmigration/populationestimates/bulletins/annualmidyearpopulationestimates/latest. Last accessed 10 Apr 2017.

Parkhurst, G., Galvin, K., Musselwhite, C., Phillips, J., Shergold, I., & Todres, L. (2014). Beyond transport: Understanding the role of mobilities in connecting rural elders in civic society. In C. Hennesey, R. Means, & V. Burholt (Eds.), *Countryside connections: Older people, community and place in rural Britain* (pp. 125–175). Bristol: Policy Press.

Pooley, C., Jones, T., Tight, M., Horton, D., Scheldeman, G., Mullen, C., Jopson, A., & Strano, E. (2013). *Promoting walking and cycling: New perspectives on sustainable travel*. Bristol: Policy Press.

Preston, J. M., & Raje, F. (2007). Accessibility, mobility and transport-related social exclusion. *Journal of Transport Geography, 15*(3), 151–160.

Prohaska, T., Anderson, L., & Binstock, R. (Eds.). (2012). *Public health for an aging society*. Baltimore: The Johns Hopkins University Press.

PROMISING. (2001). *Measures for pedestrian safety and mobility: A cross Europe study*. Leidschendam: SWOV Institute for Road Safety Research.

Pucher, J., & Buehler, R. (2008). Making cycling irresistible: Lessons from The Netherlands, Denmark and Germany. *Transport Reviews, 28*(4), 495–528.

Pucher, J., & Buehler, R. (2012). *City cycling*. Cambridge, MA: MIT Press. isbn:9780262517812.

Saelens, B. E., Sallis, J. F., Black, J. B., & Chen, D. (2003). Neighborhood-based differences in physical activity: An environment scale evaluation. *American Journal of Public Health, 93*(9), 1552–1558.

Schlag, B., Schwenkhagen, U., & Trankle, U. (1996). Transportation for the elderly: Towards a user- friendly combination of private and public transport. *IATSS Research, 20*(1), 75–82.

Shumway-Cook, A., Patla, A., Stewart, A., Ferrucci, L., Ciol, M. A., & Guralnik, J. M. (2003). Environmental components of mobility disability in community-living older persons. *Journal of the American Geriatrics Society, 51*, 393–398.

Ståhl, A., Carlsson, G., Hovbrandt, P., & Iwarsson, S. (2008). "Let's go for a walk!": Identification and prioritisation of accessibility and safety measures involving elderly people in a residential area. *European Journal of Ageing, 5*, 265–273.

Strath, S. J., Greenwald, M. J., Isaacs, R., Hart, T. L., Lenz, E. K., Dondzila, C. J., & Swartz, A. M. (2012). Measured and perceived environmental characteristics are related to accelerometer defined physical activity in older adults. *International Journal of Behavioral Nutrition and Physical Activity, 9*, 40.

Sugiyama, T., & Ward Thompson, C. (2007). Outdoor environments, activity and well-being of older people: Conceptualising environmental support. *Environment and Planning A, 39*(8), 1943–1960.

Sugiyama, T., & Ward Thompson, C. (2008). Associations between characteristics of NBH open space and older people's walking. *Urban Forestry and Urban Greening, 7*(1), 41–51.

Webb, E., Netuveli, G., & Millett, C. (2011). Free bus passes, use of public transport and obesity among older people in England. *Journal of Epidemiology and Community Health, 66*(2), 176–180.

Wennberg, H. (2009). *Walking in old age: A year-round perspective on accessibility in the outdoor environment and effects of measures taken*. Doctoral thesis. Institutionen för Teknik och samhälle, Trafik och väg. Available at: http://www.fot.se/documents/Wennberg_-_Walking_in_old_age_KAPPAN_-_2009.pdf. Last accessed 6 Apr 2017.

WHO (World Health Organisation). (1999). *Charter on transport, environment and health, European Series* (Vol. 89). Geneva: WHO Regional Publications.

Williams, K., Gupta, R., Smith, I., Joynt, J., Hopkins, D., Bramley, G., Payne, C., Gregg, M., Hambleton, R., Bates-Brkljac, N., Dunse, N., & Musselwhite, C. (2012). *Suburban neighbourhood adaptation for a changing climate (SNACC)* (Final Report). University of the West of England, Oxford Brookes University and Heriot-Watt University.

Ziegler, F., & Schwanen, T. (2011). I like to go out to be energised by different people: An exploratory analysis of mobility and wellbeing in later life. *Ageing and Society, 31*(5), 758–781.

Zijlstra, G. A., van Haastregt, J. C., van Eijk, J. T., van Rossum, E., Stalenhoef, P. A., & Kempen, G. I. (2007). Prevalence and correlates of fear of falling, and associated avoidance of activity in the general population of community living older people. *Age and Ageing, 36*(3), 304–309.

Section 6

Sociological Factors and Physical Activity Among Older People

Khim Horton

Following on from Section 5 that focuses on the environmental science perspective on physical activity (PA) among older people, this section takes a sociological stance to enable the reader to develop a deeper and broader understanding of the sociological factors that facilitate or hinder the promotion of physical activity among older people. More specifically, the reader will appreciate the value and relevance of key sociological theories and concepts to their professional development and practice from the evidence in the discussion of the following chapters.

As outlined in Chap. 1, the model of the determinants of active ageing (WHO 2002) and Dahlgren and Whitehead's (1991) main determinants of health both have identified not only individual-level factors but also wider levels of influence that are at work in promoting or hindering physical activity. From an individual perspective, one's experiences are influenced by social structures that support them; these structures are multilayered, ranging from family, community, government, as well as international. Their influences may change over time. Hence, in Chap. 26 Palmer and her colleagues argue that the ability to be physically active is conditional on a physical, cultural, and phenomenological understanding of the body. Through an outline of the sociological understandings of the ageing body and locating PA within this, the authors examine the processes that lead to the development of one's disposition to be physically active over time. Drawing on empirical data from

K. Horton (✉)
School of Health Sciences, University of London, London

three studies, they encapsulate the complexities of the meaning of ageing that men and women associate PA with. The typologies of PA responding to physical ageing as well as the cultural understanding of PA are highlighted. They emphasise that negotiating PA through our ageing body in that 'becoming, being, and remaining physically active' as we age is not that straightforward.

In Chap. 27, Evans and his co-authors contend that how older people ascribe meaning to experiences of being active are influenced by the subjective, lived aspects of old age. In their critical consideration of Atchley's theory of continuity, the authors highlight the lack of clarity in the interactions of various factors on the individual's sense of self. They further stress that 'older people's sense of self can be interdependent on how others define them, and how they define others', explaining that such relationships (situating 'I' identities within the 'We' and 'They' group) are not static as they change over time and space. By contrasting various sociological perspectives, Evans and his co-authors offer an alternative approach by drawing on the principles of figurational sociological framework. Their consideration of this framework highlights the social change processes and how older people might (re)negotiate their changing social position. The discussion in this chapter promotes the empowerment of older people as active agents within PA and health promotion.

Another key focus in this section is gender and social class. In Chap. 28, Tamar Semerjian examines critically the complex relationship between gender, social class, and PA in later life. Whilst such relationships are further influenced by cultural expectations and gender ideologies as well as media portrayal of older people's engagement in PA, less is known from a sociological perspective, for example, how PA among men and women and its impact may differ culturally. Semerjian advocates a move to consider issues beyond simply 'gender'. The complex relationship of social class or socio-economic status (SES) and PA demands a more sociocultural examination of the intersections, amongst other factors, of class, gender, and ethnicity. Semerjian's review of the evidence highlights that intervention studies are often targeted at low-income communities. Her chapter also explores the impact of dog ownership on sedentary behaviours, and Semerjian argues that more work needs to be undertaken to determine how social class interacts with the physical environments in the creation of spaces that increase or decrease the likelihood of PA.

In the light of the ongoing social and demographic changes in Great Britain, there is a greater need to understand ethnicity in terms of research, policy, and practice. Hence, in Chap. 29, Victor focuses on PA and ethnic minority elders in Great Britain. Measuring PA can be challenging; older people both under-report the target levels of PA and over-estimate their own activity levels. Where ethnic minority groups are concerned, in studies on PA, there is a significant omission to consider ethnicity. Victor highlights the tendency of research to focus on specific issues among individual minority populations. As evidence in the UK suggests that ethnic minorities tend to have poorer health profiles than the majority of the population in the same age, there is a pressing need to disentangle the different factors that may help our understanding and response to the low levels of PA among older people from minority groups.

In the final chapter of this section, Rose and Fisher examine the role of government policies in shaping and developing PA initiatives to promote PA and highlight the limited translational evidence into policy and practice, within specific context of Australia, Canada, and the United States. Their critical review of national- and community-level initiatives across these countries offers a valuable insight into the barriers and facilitators to engaging in PA among older people. This chapter also outlines the types of intervention strategies that work and the extent to which they are both cost-effective and cost-efficient. Examples of successful evidence-based health promotion strategies illustrate the value of evidence as the core of any population-based initiatives (both at community and national levels) in promoting PA. Rose and Fisher also identified policy evaluation frameworks that can help strengthen strategies in PA promotion.

This section underlines the importance of understanding the sociological factors that influence older people and PA. Without this appreciation, it will be challenging for policymakers and health professionals to address the pressing global issue of obesity in the long run whilst attempting to enhance quality of life in later life.

26

Physical Activity and the Ageing Body

Victoria J. Palmer, Emmanuelle Tulle, and James Bowness

26.1 Introduction

Exploring understandings and experiences of physical activity (PA) in ageing requires engagement with the ageing body and in particular how it has been constructed, how this has informed how older people themselves are embodied and ultimately how they can envisage their future.

Rapid transformations in norms of aged embodiment reflecting societal changes and shifts in understandings about biological ageing appear to have positioned PA as a way of managing what had previously been assumed to be inescapable processes of deterioration. The implications of the turn to PA for the cultural value attributed to ageing, in particular, visible physical ageing (functional limitations and ill-health), and the cultural position of older persons are worth exploring. If we are to accept that PA is an effective weapon against ageing decrements, we need to consider the feasibility of encouraging people to become physically active, especially as they become older and have to contend with the fleshy, lived body (Turner 2008).

Our argument is that there is nothing straightforward about becoming, being and remaining physically active as we get older. The challenges that we

---

V. J. Palmer (✉)
Institute of Health and Wellbeing, College of Social Science, University of Glasgow, Glasgow, UK

E. Tulle • J. Bowness
Department of Social Sciences, Media and Journalism, Glasgow Caledonian University, Glasgow, UK

might have to overcome are physical, cultural, structural and historical. Using empirical evidence from three research projects which explore ageing and PA (understood broadly), we show that whilst our body is the condition for our existence, its fleshiness has to be reckoned with. Our experience of physical ageing is mediated by cultural norms and discourses which give us the frame to imagine what is 'thinkable' (Castoriadis 1975) and feasible. Then, we will highlight the processes which led to the development of a disposition to be physically active over time and how this can be facilitated or hindered by cultures and structures, putting the body in tension between conflicting effects. Lastly, we will point to the ambiguous meanings of PA in relation to prevailing attitudes towards ageing. But first we turn to a brief presentation of recent theoretical and conceptual developments in understandings of bodily ageing.

26.1.1 Reinventing the Ageing Body

In the last 25 years, bodily ageing has been the subject of much theoretical development and empirical investigation in the social sciences, a trend that has been described as the turn to the body (Cregan 2006). Until then, the dominant perception of the body was as a material thing with its own laws dictating its functioning and the course of its development over time. This apprehension of bodies owes much to Cartesian dualism, a philosophical stance derived from the writings and insights of René Descartes. Descartes (1966) envisaged a separation of the mind from the body, arguing that our minds as the bearers of our power of reasoning were what made us distinctive as humans. The early social sciences largely reflected this Cartesian approach, giving primacy to the social and agency, whilst leaving the body to the biological sciences.

The recent discovery of the body as a legitimate target of sociological enquiry reflected the realisation that whilst the body is the condition for our participation in the world, it is not just a biological thing: our bodily experiences are themselves socially and culturally mediated. As such, there have emerged several ways of theorising ageing bodies in the social sciences and in sociology: positions informed by social constructionism, phenomenological developments and neo-structuralist insights which combine the fleshiness of the body with its structural position. Of necessity what follows is a brief outline of the developments that have taken place and in the process some subtleties will be missed (see Tulle 2015).

Social construction approaches focus on historical, discursive, ideological and structural *conditions* in which bodies are brought to visibility and on the strategies available to achieve particular social aims. We can use the conceptual apparatus of Michel Foucault (cf. Katz 1997) to bring to light the ways in which, since the nineteenth century, old age and old bodies have been understood and constructed by biomedicine. A new discourse emerged which gave priority to biological processes over other aspects of ageing, and problematised them into 'a crisis of thought' and, crucially, into sets of 'universal dilemmas' (Katz 2000, p. 137, 138): aged bodies were problematic bodies and their functioning came to be seen as both deviant and normal. Experts also constituted themselves by literally mapping these bodies, naming the conditions of old age and setting up an apparatus of intervention designed to name and control individuals (Katz 1996). In return, individuals who come under the purview of this apparatus would subject themselves to these techniques of control. Thus, aged embodiment means allowing regimes of truth to dictate the naming of one's body as old and problematic. Thus, to say that biologically compromised bodies are socially constructed is to say that they are given meaning and brought to visibility by particular systems of classification and, in some historical circumstances, this will make them the targets of intervention. For instance, the adoption of the term 'frailty' (Grenier 2007) is a social process with cultural implications because it tells us what normal functioning is.

The social constructionist approach is valuable because it captures the historical and social contingencies of bodily ageing. It also enables us to see that bodies are the object of regulation, pointing to the role that we play as social actors in 'performing' old age. However, the lived, fleshy experience of embodiment is not in evidence here.

Thus, scholars have sought to uncover rich insights into how people experience their ageing using a *phenomenological* approach. Informed by the work of Merleau-Ponty (1945) and his premise that during our everyday sensate engagement with the world (being-in-the-world), we lay down habits which become *meaningful* automatisms, the manifestations of practical mastery. This process renders our actions pre-reflective. In other words, over time, we develop ways of living with and in our bodies, and these inform the decisions that we make. Thus, agency is always embodied. This takes place in intersection with the demands, values and norms which exist in the social world during our lifetime. Physical ageing can disrupt the close relationship which we develop with our bodies. How we respond to this disruption is contingent on the social world and its values.

We have already seen that we live in a society which provides the context in which ageing and, in particular, bodily ageing are understood and managed. Then we saw that the physical body and how it is experienced must be taken into account. Now we need to consider how in our negotiations of wider societal norms, we come to embody our social location, that is, how class, gender, ethnicity and also age are inscribed in what we do and of relevance here, in how we age and respond to it. Bourdieu (1984) suggests we develop an embodied awareness of our social location, or habitus, during socialisation. We discover and rehearse what position we occupy by managing different forms of capital (economic, social, cultural and also physical) (Bourdieu 1977). This is manifested in the range of dispositions and aspirations that we build over time. What we aspire to do with our bodies, or what we think might not be feasible, reflects our habitus. Thus, how we work with our bodies reproduces the class and gender hierarchy which prevails as we move through life.

In order to understand better how aged embodiment intersects with social location, we turn to a consideration of PA as a practice which brings together social and phenomenological factors.

26.1.2 PA and Ageing

Since the 1990s, PA has become inextricably linked with health, particularly for older people. Many of the health benefits associated with older people's PA are associated with reducing the risk of, or delaying the onset of, 'the chronic diseases of ageing' (Paterson et al. 2007, p. S92). Being active in later life is seen to postpone the onset of morbidity and ultimately prolong life (Paterson et al. 2007). More specifically, participating in PA has been linked to reversing age-related deterioration of the cardiovascular system, reduce the rate and delay onset of sarcopenia (age-related loss of muscle mass) and maintain bone strength (Taylor et al. 2004). As a result, older people who are active are expected to have a greater number of years of functional independence, as well as an increased health-related quality of life (Paterson et al. 2007). Older people are, however, viewed as being at the greatest risk of morbidity and mortality as a result of prolonged inactivity (Brown et al. 2012).

This narrative places the ageing body as in decline. By situating it in discourses of disease, decline and dysfunction, the ageing body becomes 'risky' and thus a site for intervention, to be trained and improved. As such, the sport and exercise sciences position PA as a tool for resisting ageing, reflecting the medicalisation of PA, as well as the medicalisation of the ageing body itself (Gilleard and Higgs 2000; Nye 2003; Tulle 2008a). There have been many attempts within the sport exercise and life sciences to increase older people's PA levels. Interventions to increase PA participation among older people have used various designs and approaches which are largely developed using theories of motivation and behaviour change with roots in social psychology. However, these have produced varied results. In particular, it appears that interventions are successful for the duration of the intervention, but long-term success is more difficult to achieve (Chase 2013; Hobbs et al. 2013). One particular critique of such attempts to increase PA is that they are focussed on the individual and overlook the wider social and cultural context in which PA occurs.[1]

There is therefore a need to understand how PA in later life is shaped by wider social and cultural expectations of old age and ageing. Despite a recent shift towards 'active ageing', historical analysis reveals that PA participation was not viewed as appropriate for older people, particularly women (Vertinsky 1995). Moreover, older adulthood is often viewed as a time to 'take it easy' and for rest (Kirk 1997 in Grant 2008). Despite definitions of ageing constantly evolving and moving away from these traditional ideas of ageing, many older people's beliefs about ageing, PA and the body are still rooted in these cultural norms (Grant 2002). Thus, older people face a paradox, whereby, on one hand, health promotion experts are informing them to be more active, but on the other, traditional societal views are telling them to slow down and rest. In addition, they are faced with negotiating PA within class and gender relations.

For older people who have been physically active throughout the life course, maintaining PA also becomes entangled in their experiences of ageing. While many of these older people do not primarily participate in PA for health or to prolong life (Tulle 2008b), they acknowledge its health benefits. Moreover, they are driven by a fear of losing physical capital (Dionigi 2010) reinforcing dominant discourses of ageing as a period of decline. For older people who are beginning or returning to PA, health may feature more prominently. However, it is worth noting that an awareness of the health benefits of PA alone is not enough to elicit participation. Grant (2008) notes that there is a misalignment between knowing the benefits of PA and engaging in PA in later life. Similarly, Dionigi et al. (2011) found that while (inactive) older people acknowledged that PA was good for their health, they rejected that it was an essential part of ageing well, demonstrating a resistance to the active ageing discourse. For those who do engage with PA in later life, negotiating and maintaining PA is complex. Grant (2008) found that very few older people were able to maintain PA regularly. She notes that modifying one's life with PA was viewed as daunting and particularly difficult to maintain if the activity was unfamiliar or if the individual did not view PA as meaningful. Tulle and Dorrer (2012), however, found that older people were able to successfully negotiate PA and embed physically active practice into their everyday lives but within strict limits set by themselves and their own understandings of their capabilities.

26.2 Methodological Considerations

We have outlined the key philosophical and sociological perspectives that have enabled us to capture bodies as embodiment. By embodiment we mean not only the actual experiences that people forge with their bodies over time but also the social and cultural circumstances which provide the spaces and discourses in which our bodies are shaped and managed. We have also reviewed what is known about PA in later life. What emerges clearly is that we cannot do justice to older people's attitudes towards PA without capturing what it feels like to put one's body in movement. In order to do this, we need to use appropriate methods. We contend that life history interviews fulfil this purpose.

Life history interviewing has been used across a variety of social sciences (Atkinson 2002) to understand how individuals make sense of their own experience across the life course (Josselson and Lieblich 1995). This form of interview places the interviewer as guide whilst the interviewee orally weaves through their lived experience. The sociological uses of the life history interview allow the reconciliation of the individual with the social, providing the lived experience of the interviewee. This approach allows us to look to common themes across individuals which suggest a link between a specific topic/subject and multiple individuals, and casting out further to the social, cultural and historical environment in which lives are led, decisions made and experiences interpreted.

The following discussion combines empirical data from three studies which all had elements of life-history interviewing inherent in their design. All three studies (see Table 26.1) dealt with the place of PA in later life. It is worth noting that some of the master athletes are chronologically still fairly young and may not be thought of as 'older people'. However, they are deemed too old to take part in mainstream sport and are therefore forced to contend with physiological ageing.

Using life history interviews allowed for the elaboration of life events which challenged engagement with PA. We will present three major themes which emerged across the three datasets, encapsulating the complex meanings ageing men and women associate with PA: 1. typologies of PA, 2. responding to physical ageing and 3. cultural understandings of PA.

Table 26.1 Characteristics of three studies presented in this chapter

	Study 1 Master runners	Study 2 Highland gamers	Study 3 Active grandparents
Description of participants	Competitive masters runners	Competitors in masters highland games	Grandparents in three generational family, self-defined as active
No. participants	21	19	5[a]
Age	48–86	40–75	59–79
Males	14	13	2
Females	7	6	3

[a]Grandparents were interviewed as part of a larger project exploring physical activity in families (Palmer 2015)

26.3 Typologies of PA

As already identified, participation in PA is the product of social structures and an individual's biography. PA can be thought of as fluid in that the meanings attributed to the PA that we do can mutate as societies change and individual lives develop over time. Dionigi (2015) previously created a typology of how older individuals became physically active: 'rekindlers'—those who return to PA as older people, 'continuers'—those who are continuously engaged in PA throughout the life course and 'late bloomers'—adults who become active later in life. This helps us to understand PA participation in relation to older people's biographical history. However, it does not tell us of the complex meanings which PA assumes. The structures of class and gender, amongst others, augment and shape the logic of practice of PA, inflecting why and how individuals engage with PA. Extending Dionigi's (2015) model, we suggest three modalities of engaging with PA which we have conceptualised as functional, sporting and performative. These begin to tell us how individuals negotiate being physically active and how PA is situated in their life-worlds.

Functional PA relates to uses of the body which fulfil an instrumental role in the lives of individuals. Everyday chores may require use of the body, which may not be consciously understood or recognised as PA, but are physically demanding. For older people, examples may include walking grandchildren to school or collecting weekly groceries. This type of PA is woven into the everyday lives of men and women, and as they negotiate relationships, roles and responsibilities within their lives, their PA may change. Thus, meanings of PA often morph into new conceptions. For example, a 'continuer' in study 3, Elaine, aged 62, talking about walking, notes: 'walking gets me from A to

B as well as keeping well reasonably fit'. In this case, we see the functional nature of walking for transport, however, this serves a dual purpose of maintaining fitness. Elaine subsequently discusses how she tries to maintain fitness levels in order to fulfil her familial role as a grandparent:

> I like to be able to keep myself fit so that I can still keep up with [my grandchildren] like you know[…]Don't want to be lagging behind them [laughs] sitting in the park saying no I can't play football I'm too old [laughs].

This demonstrates that while Elaine's lifelong participation in PA is walking from A to B, her experience has more recently been shaped by a desire to maintain fitness in order to fulfil obligations as a grandparent. Thus, the disposition to use walking as a method of transport is translated into being able to play with her grandchildren, highlighting how an initial disposition can be maintained over time with meanings of PA developing coterminously.

The second, perhaps most ubiquitous, form of PA is sport. Sport occupies a multitude of fields, each with specific customs and values. Each sport has its own logic of practice inflected by class and gender. Bourdieu (1978) suggested that class habitus was intricately linked with sporting choices, with the use of the body finding different spaces of legitimacy between classes.

Many masters athletes begin a sporting career after an absence from activity often after leaving formal education. In Dionigi's (2015) typology, these individuals are 'rekindlers'. Many of the Highland Games athletes fit this description. One example comes from Jack, aged 47, who describes the social context in which he returned to competitive sport:

> I was a Division III college shotputter, and won a couple of conference titles and a state championship. I threw until I was roughly 26, competing in various meets around the east. […] When I turned 40, a recently graduated thrower from my Alma matter contacted me and asked me why I stopped throwing and if I would be interested in throwing again. I was recently divorced, and without a whole lot of entertainment funds, so I took him up on his offer, and we started to train hammer throw together.

Jack's recent divorce was instrumental in rekindling his PA. His initial disposition to take part in throwing events in college translated first to masters-level track and field and later to the Highland Games, an event which requires similar physical capital. In this vein, an initial disposition allowed for a subtle change in the mode of PA.

For those who engage in sporting activities for prolonged periods, a process of identification with the field occurs. New forms of identity may also be created as the by-product of PA. In this sense, PA becomes *performative* of identity. Forms of PA may allow for the performance of traditional masculinity, in sports such as weightlifting or rugby, with other sporting fields allowing for the performance of national identity. Routes to these performative physical activities are also structured by class and gender. This example, from 'continuer' Tina, aged 52, highlights her route into the Highland Games, a space where Scottish identity can be performed:

> That was a really great story. There was a Scottish festival near our hometown and my husband had read about it or heard about it on the radio and said hey I want to go out there. We had the whole family, at that point our daughter was 2 and our son was 5. So we got them in the stroller and headed out there to the park and we got there before it even started, he starts talking to a few of the athletes and he comes back and says 'I'm going to do this today'. Do what today?

Tina's husband (and later her) participation in sport is closely tied up with the development of an affinity with Scottish culture as displayed in Highland Games. In addition, the performance of identity involves the material body. In another example, Colin, started his athletic career as a cyclist but switched to long-distance running. He articulates his transformation from cyclist to runner:

> So this is when I thought I am going to learn to become a runner. But it took me two years before I called myself a runner, you know, two years before I could honestly say the pains have gone and I was running properly.

Kate, aged 50, is a 'late bloomer'; she started running in her mid-30s. Her family roles were such that she could only continue expressing her growing disposition to PA by using very creative means and with her husband's tacit support:

> I just use my work [as a part-time aerobics instructor] as part of my training. My family life is a lot easier now […] and I don't have to be here for meal times and that sort of thing. When they were younger it was more awkward because when I first started running they were still at junior school […] the school holidays were a problem for me because my husband is in the car trade so July was his busy month and he worked seven days a week. So I used to have a mile measured outside the house and I used to go out and run this mile 20 times? (laughter).

All of these examples highlight how structures such as gender and family circumstances can influence older people's engagement with PA throughout the life course. By extending Dionigi's (2015) typology, we can begin to grasp the complexity of becoming and remaining active over time. For those who continue or rekindle, dispositions which were previously held are either maintained or reignited. But for those who have not shown a disposition previously, starting PA in mid-adulthood or older adulthood, such as the people featured here, is a fragile undertaking. Regardless of existing dispositions, disposable income, time and permission are necessary to facilitate activity. For some, PA may require creative capacities, as demonstrated by Kate or support structures, as in the case of Tina. However, these are not available to all. In addition, these already fragile careers are made more insecure by ageing. As we age, our relationship to our bodies becomes increasingly appropriated by biomedicine. Whether this would facilitate and legitimise the development of PA careers must be examined.

26.4 Responding to PA

While the older people who participated in our research were able to engage in physically active pursuits, they did so while negotiating their own 'real' experiences of physical ageing, albeit in different ways. What we can see in all cases are examples of the medicalisation of PA and ageing, with ageing bodies viewed as sites to be managed and trained. As such, being healthy is associated with self-assessment, self-regulation and self-care reflecting public health promotion policies that, in the face of an ageing population and the erosion of the welfare state, promote self-responsibility for health (Ballard and Elston 2005). This operates in two interrelated modalities: firstly, PA is reconstructed as medical prescription, and secondly, the body is understood within a risk framework.

26.4.1 PA as Prescription

Throughout the developed world, PA has become a prescription to address the decrements of old age and maintain health. This appears to be accepted by older people themselves for whom health is at the centre of their PA understandings and practices. However, their view of health and PA is reactive, rather than preventative, thus it is lived experience of poor health, rather than *perceived* threat of poor health, that prompts engagement with PA, as illustrated by Donald, aged 68:

> … there is a kind of eh…I was going to say desire but maybe it realisation's maybe a better word that I need to do something or the body's just going to give up on me, so eh yip[…]Exercise or start pushing up the daisies [laughs].

Donald had been prescribed PA for cardiovascular health issues. For him and others with similar experiences in study 3, the initial prescription was short term and included an exercise programme as well as a series of lectures about the dangers of an 'unhealthy lifestyle'. This reflects a shift in the responsibility of health from the medical professional to the individual, by assuming that having knowledge of health-related practices individuals will make informed choices and follow a PA programme over the long term (Lhussier and Carr 2008).

However, the presence of health issues also makes PA participation more difficult. Older people discussed how health can restrict PA in many ways. Often participants reported that they were in pain, ranging from general aches and pains to specific conditions such as arthritis. Thus, experiences of health and PA present a site of moral conflict, where on the one hand, older people accept the need to be PA for health, but their experiences of their bodies do not allow them to do so. Being active means having to engage with risk.

26.4.2 Risky Bodies

In order to take responsibility for one's health, individuals need an awareness of what's at stake. We find that PA in later life is situated within a discourse of risk. In the public health context, epidemiological evidence is used to identify high-risk groups and introduce preventative measures for 'risky individuals' (Rose 2000). Often older people are identified as an 'at-risk population'. Older individuals are expected to be able to identify themselves as 'at risk' and engage 'in the ethical work necessary to decrease their probability of disease or health problems' (Dallaire et al. 2012, p. 327).

However, for older people, some types of PA are considered to be damaging to their ageing bodies. A good example of this relates to the Highland Games. Robert, aged 49, demonstrates how ageing is discussed in relation to injury and risk:

> Certainly, my age has a lot to do with my injuries. When I was younger playing American Football, I only ever suffered one injury which was a deep thigh bruise during a game. It knocked me out for just one practice. I have been invincible for most of my life. I'd heal from injury in just a day or two. Not so much anymore.

Thus, in master athletes, we see a different form of management of the body. In these examples, older people carefully harness physical capital in order to *continue* to compete and even improve upon previous performances. In contrast to PA as prescription, the expert knowledge is not sought in medical discourse, especially in situations where medical professionals have discouraged participation in 'risky' sports and suggested more age-appropriate activities. A good illustration of this is James who was still a regular runner at age 65. In his 50s, he sought help from his physician for knee pain: 'the doctor told me to go and play bowls. I said "I don't want to play bowls, I want to run"'. This process of discouragement can affect athletes at even younger ages:

> I'd been complaining about symptoms for four years but my doctor would just say you're just getting old, three different doctors you're just getting old, this is what I do for fun, I go out with military forces guys but for fun I throw telephone poles and stuff, I am not accepting the answer I'm just getting old. (Chris, aged 47)

As such, athletes can become sceptical of the medical profession. If they want to continue being active, they have to assume the role of expert in the management of their own bodies or turn to other, more sympathetic, sources of expertise, for example, coaches, chiropractors and osteopaths:

> it almost becomes a pain/body management game, if you can imagine, I have an extra vertebrae in my lower spin and it tends to keep my hip out of balance, so I've done all sorts of things learning how to manage that, because yesterday when I left the field it felt like it was jammed, if there is a chiropractor on the field that's wonderful because they can fix me right up, but if not, then I've got to do it myself. And so I've spent a great deal of time last night and this morning trying to stretch it, and dislocate it and impinge it and just all of those things which you have to do, I'm feeling pretty good this morning, but it's a tricky business. (Tina, aged 52)

This presents a paradox where, on one hand, PA is seen as a solution to or treatment of 'ageing' and the management of 'risky ageing bodies'. On the other hand, the belief that some forms of physical engagement are too risky remains strong, which could curtail physical activity in the very late years. The examples above demonstrate the persistence of the decline narrative—as articulated by experts and older people—of old age.

26.5 Cultural Understandings of PA in Later Life

So far, we have described the factors which facilitate or hinder how older people encounter PA. This enabled us to highlight the fragility of a PA career and the increasing but ambiguous role played by the medical model to give meaning to PA in old age. Now, we want to show that this is part of a pervasive cultural framework, what in ageing studies (Gullette 2004) has been referred to as the decline narrative—where ageing is perceived primarily as a biological process of inevitable decline.

The following exchange between the author and a long-distance runner (Colin aged 52) is instructive:

ET: […] However your times have been going down a bit in the last few years? […] why is that?

Colin: I don't know, I just presume, I mean I don't know anything about the body but I just think *it is maybe the cells in the body turning off, slowing down* [our emphasis], they don't recover the same. I talk to other colleagues… runners who are equals, they do the same training, run as hard, mentally apply themselves to it, yet some are half a minute down.

When pressed to explain why he runs marginally more slowly than before, he finds an explanation in the decline of bodily systems, here using a cellular explanation. This is consistent with the recent science of ageing (Tulle 2008a; Hunter et al. 2004). This calls for a response in terms of managing physiological changes and in personal terms. Colin and his 'colleagues' persist with their training regime, while the loss of speed is observed and felt. This calls into question people's identification with old age.

One response to this consists of dissociating *feel* age from *physical* age (Öberg and Tornstam 1999). Here, Harry, aged 65, like 19 of the 21 master runners who took part in study 1, rejects an aged identity and prioritises how he *feels* to account for himself:

ET: Now then, are you old?

Harry: What do you mean exactly? Do I think I am old? I am getting on I suppose is what I would say, no-one ever likes to say they are old do they? No I wouldn't say 'I am old'. No. It is all comparative of course against other people but I don't *feel* [Informant's emphasis] old I suppose. Of course when I was younger I would say middle-aged is halfway to the grave so if you lived to 72 then when you are 32 you are middle-aged but of course middle-age starts later, the older you get, doesn't it?

Harry avoids identifying himself as *old* by going through several stages: 1. he claims not to understand the question. 2. he reappropriates it by answering from his subjective point of view, eschewing the question as referring to an objective state of being old. 3. he shifts from being to feeling. 4. he locates the issue to wider social and cultural processes, comparing himself to others, and his position in the life course then and now. It could be argued that by claiming not to feel old, people resist the decline narrative. But others might not see it like this, and older people end up having to manage their own bodies as well as other people's expectations of appropriate and therefore normative ageing. In other words, being old has to be reckoned with.

Elaine, aged 62, as a walker describes how others view her as follows:

> I think sometimes they [friends] think I'm a wee bit [gestures] daft or something always rushing about and say 'slow down slow down' but if I slow down I'll never get there so I've got to keep going [laughs].

She expresses her desire to keep going, stressing that if she slowed down, she will be 'finished'. Thus, she articulates her desire to continue being active into her 'old' age:

> I'd still like to be able to get my at least a walk everyday like you know *even when I'm…old* [our emphasis] [laughs] I'm not old yet [laughs].

We find that older people who exercise regularly can hold apparently conflicting balls in the air: they clearly accepted ageing as decline, located deep in the body whilst refusing to accept old age as a desirable constituent of their identity, despite the incontrovertible evidence that they have aged. They also had to contend with pressure from others to accept the inevitable in line with the decline narrative and associated cultural norms. Women appeared to be particularly sensitive to what others might think although if they were injured, men also had to deal with doctors' own expectations of appropriate behaviour and risk-taking.

26.6 Conclusion

The purpose of this chapter was to explore how experiences of PA in later life are shaped by orientations to, lived experiences of and social constructions of the ageing body. We demonstrate that becoming, being and remaining active in later life is not easy. Understanding PA in later life must appreciate the structural, cultural and phenomenological contexts of its participants.

As we have seen in our three data sources, specific rules and customs contextualise PA. Whether this is the performance of national identity in the Highland Games or the undertaking of familial responsibilities, PA is never a-cultural or a-historical. Therefore, we argue that regardless of 'how' or 'why' older people engage in PA, it is difficult, particularly for older people who are faced with a (re)negotiation of their ageing bodies and what it means to get older. Our findings echo Dionigi's (2015) pathways to masters sport: we realise that being active in later life is owed largely to available structural resources. However, PA in later life is also largely pinned on the materiality of our bodies. In this sense, we should comprehend what the body has been through and what previous injuries or illnesses imprint upon the body. We must also consider forces which shape sensate experience and create a unique feeling of PA in later life. For example, this may come in the form of an injury which occurred decades previously and now causes pain during activity. Thus, it is the combination of sensate experience and cultural context which provides the framework for meanings of PA in later life.

Responding to and managing the ageing body intersects with narratives of medicalisation which place PA as a weapon for combatting the 'inevitable' declines associated with ageing. Older people who faced health issues were expected to start a PA programme, but perceptions of their own bodies' capabilities were not taken into account by professionals. In contrast, master athletes' PA was viewed as 'risky', that is, understood within the same discursive space which dictates that vigorous PA is incompatible with ageing bodies. Receiving no support from medical experts, they became experts in managing their bodies in order to harness physical capital and continue to play sport. This sort of tenacity could be interpreted as a challenge to the traditional medical model, but we argue that this is more complex. As Dionigi (2015) previously noted, these master athletes could be seen as embodying the 'active ageing agenda', which itself assumes that there are 'good' and 'bad' ways to grow old (Pike 2011).

Thus, physically active older people must negotiate cultural expectations of appropriate uses of the ageing body. It could be argued that 'active ageing' discourses have shifted these cultural norms and legitimised PA practices in later life. However, as we have highlighted, the discourse of ageing prevails, reinforced, ironically, by the medicalisation of PA. Moreover, these cultural aspects of ageing are deeply embedded in older people's experiences of ageing. Lastly, the materiality of the body is inflected strongly by the physical and health capital we accumulate from our class, gender and ethnic background. Therefore, older people who wish to be active in later life must negotiate what appears to be a series of moral, cultural and phenomenological conflicts.

26.7 Implications for Practice

Putting the ageing body into movement is complex. It is vital that policymakers and practitioners take into account that PA is an embodied practice. Thus, there is a need to create environments which view ageing bodies as 'being-in-the-world'. This means that ageing bodies and PA should not be viewed through the exclusive prism of health. Instead, physically active practices should be considered as ways through which older people can enjoy and gain pleasure through the use of their bodies.

It is also vital that in promoting PA to older people, we do not create moral binds such as those presented by the medicalisation of ageing and PA as this has the potential to isolate those who choose not to, or feel that they cannot, be physically active. We therefore encourage policymakers and practitioners to recognise that there are multiple modalities of physical engagement in later life. Older people should be supported to engage in a wide variety of opportunities to remain in-the-world and manage physical decrements not exclusively to minimise the 'burden of ageing' but to enhance happiness.

Suggested Further Reading

- Tulle, E. (2008). *Ageing, the body and social change: Running in later life.* Basingstoke: Palgrave.
- Tulle, E., & Phoenix, C. (Eds). (2015). *Physical activity and sport in later life: Critical perspectives.* London: Palgrave.

Note

1. There has been a recent shift in the development of interventions that are underpinned by the socio-ecological model of health, exploring the individual's relationship with environmental, social and cultural factors. However, these still place the individual at the centre, and in PA research, multi-level interventions have tended to focus on the physical environment rather than social or cultural factors.

References

Atkinson, R. (2002). The life story interview. In J. Gubrium & J. Holstein (Eds.), *Handbook of interview research: Context and method* (pp. 121–140). Thousand Oaks: Sage.

Ballard, K., & Elston, M. A. (2005). Medicalisation: A multi-dimensional concept. *Social Theory & Health, 3*(3), 228–241.

Bourdieu, P. (1977). *Outline of a theory of practice.* Cambridge: Cambridge University Press.

Bourdieu, P. (1978). Sport and social class. *Social Science Information, 17*(6), 819–840.

Bourdieu, P. (1984). *Distinction: A social critique of the judgement of taste.* Cambridge: Harvard University Press.

Brown, W. J., McLaughlin, D., Leung, J., McCaul, K. A., Flicker, L., Almeida, O. P., & Dobson, A. J. (2012). Physical activity and all-cause mortality in older women and men. *British Journal of Sports Medicine, 46*(9), 664–668. https://doi.org/10.1136/bjsports-2011-090529.

Castoriadis, C. (1975). *L'Institution Imaginaire De La Société.* Paris: Seuil.

Chase, J.-A. D. (2013). Physical activity interventions among older adults: A literature review. *Research and Theory for Nursing Practice, 27*(1), 53–80. https://doi.org/10.1891/1541-6577.27.1.53.

Cregan, K. (2006). *The sociology of the body: Mapping the abstraction of embodiment.* London: Sage.

Dallaire, C., Gibbs, L., Lemyre, L., & Krewski, D. (2012). The gap between knowing and doing: How Canadians understand physical activity as a health promotion strategy. *Sociology of Sport Journal, 29*(3), 325–347.

Descartes, R. (1966). *Discours De La Méthode.* Paris: Garnier-Flammarion.

Dionigi, R. A. (2010). Masters sport as a strategy for managing the aging process. In J. Baker, S. Horton, & P. Wier (Eds.), *The masters athlete: Understanding the role of sport and exercise in optimizing aging* (pp. 137–155). London: Routledge.

Dionigi, R. A. (2015). Pathways to masters sport: Sharing stories from sport 'continuers', 'rekindlers' and 'late bloomers'. In E. Tulle & C. Phoenix (Eds.), *Physical activity and sport in later life* (pp. 54–68). London: Palgrave.

Dionigi, R. A., Horton, S., & Bellamy, J. (2011). Meanings of aging among older Canadian women of varying physical activity levels. *Leisure Sciences, 33*(5), 402–419. https://doi.org/10.1080/01490400.2011.606779.

Gilleard, C., & Higgs, P. (2000). *Cultures of ageing self, citizen and the body.* Harlow: Pearson Education.

Grant, B. C. (2002). Physical activity: Not a popular leisure choice in later life. *Loisir Et Société/Society and Leisure, 25*(2), 285–302. https://doi.org/10.1080/07053436.2002.10707590.

Grant, B. C. (2008). An insider's view on physical activity in later life. *Psychology of Sport and Exercise, 9*(6), 817–829. https://doi.org/10.1016/j.psychsport.2008.01.003.

Grenier, A. (2007). Constructions of frailty in the English language, care practice and the lived experience. *Ageing & Society, 27*(03), 425–445.

Gullette, M. M. (2004). *Aged by culture.* Chicago: University of Chicago Press.

Hobbs, N., Godfrey, A., Lara, J., Errington, L., Meyer, T. D., Rochester, L., & Sniehotta, F. F. (2013). Are behavioral interventions effective in increasing physical activity at 12 to 36 months in adults aged 55 to 70 years? A systematic review and meta-analysis. *BMC Medicine, 11*(1), 1.

Hunter, G. R., McCarthy, J. P., & Bamman, M. M. (2004). Effects of resistance training on older adults. *Sports Medicine, 34*(5), 329–348.

Josselson, R., & Lieblich, A. (1995). *Interpreting experience* (Vol. 3). London: Sage.

Katz, S. (1996). *Disciplining old age: The formation of gerontological knowledge*. Charlottesville: University Press of Virginia.

Katz, S. (1997). Foucault and gerontological knowledge: The making of the aged body. In C. O'Farrell (Ed.), *Foucault: The legacy* (pp. 728–735). Kelvin Grove: Queensland University of Technology.

Katz, S. (2000). Busy bodies: Activity, aging and the management of everyday life. *Journal of Aging Studies, 14*(2), 135–152.

Lhussier, M., & Carr, S. M. (2008). Health-related lifestyle advice: Critical insights. *Critical Public Health, 18*(3), 299–309.

Merleau-Ponty, M. (1945). *Phénomenologie De La Perception*. Paris: Tel Gallimard.

Nye, R. A. (2003). The evolution of the concept of medicalization in the late twentieth century. *Journal of the History of the Behavioral Sciences, 39*(2), 115–129. https://doi.org/10.1002/jhbs.10108.

Öberg, P., & Tornstam, L. (1999). Body images of men and women of different ages. *Ageing and Society, 19*(5), 629–644.

Palmer, V. J. (2015). *The negotiation of physical activity in three generational families*. Unpublished Doctoral Thesis, Glasgow Caledonian University.

Paterson, D. H., Jones, G. R., & Rice, C. L. (2007). Ageing and physical activity: Evidence to develop exercise recommendations for older adults. *Canadian Journal of Public Health, 98*(suppl. 2), S69–S108.

Pike, E. C. J. (2011). The *active aging* agenda, old folk devils and a new moral panic. *Sociology of Sport Journal, 32*(2), 209–225.

Rose, N. (2000). Government and control. *British Journal of Criminology, 40*(2), 321–339.

Taylor, A. H., Cable, N. T., Faulkner, G., Hillsdon, M., Narici, M., & Van, D. B. (2004). Physical activity and older adults: A review of health benefits and the effectiveness of interventions. *Journal of Sports Sciences, 22*(8), 703–725. https://doi.org/10.1080/02640410410001712421.

Tulle, E. (2008a). Acting your age? Sports science and the ageing body. *Journal of Aging Studies, 22*(4), 340–347. https://doi.org/10.1016/j.jaging.2008.05.005.

Tulle, E. (2008b). *Ageing, the body and social change: Running in later life*. Basingstoke: Palgrave.

Tulle, E. (2015). Theoretical perspectives on ageing and embodiment. In J. Twigg & W. Martin (Eds.), *The Routledge handbook of cultural gerontology* (pp. 125–132). London: Routledge.

Tulle, E., & Dorrer, N. (2012). Back from the brink: Ageing, exercise and health in a small gym. *Ageing & Society, 32*(7), 1106–1127.

Turner, B. S. (2008). *Body and society: Explorations in social theory* (3rd ed.). London: Sage.

Vertinsky, P. A. (1995). Stereotypes of aging women and exercise: A historical perspective. *Journal of Aging and Physical Activity, 3*(3), 223–237.

27

Physical Activity Across the Life Course: Socio-Cultural Approaches

Adam B. Evans, Anne Nistrup, and Jacquelyn Allen-Collinson

27.1 Introduction

There is increasing awareness of the importance of older people's subjective experiences of physical activity (PA) in shaping their participation (Phoenix and Grant 2009). Predominantly taking socio-cultural or socio-psychological approaches, this chapter highlights how older people's participation in PA is closely linked to their beliefs about what PA is, the perceived benefits of participation and how it is experienced throughout the life course (Tulle 2008b; Phoenix and Smith 2011; Evans and Crust 2015). This chapter is important in seeking to empower older people, as well as to challenge several commonly held assumptions in PA promotion. These include the tendency to: (i) view PA as a means to attenuate multiple (negative) age-related physiological and psychological changes (Taylor et al. 2004), (ii) suggest older people require expert support, advice and guidance about the mode, amount and intensity of activity that is 'appropriate' for them (Tulle 2008a), and (iii) treat older people as passive recipients within PA programmes (e.g. Evans and Crust 2015).

A. B. Evans (✉) • A. Nistrup
Department of Nutrition, Exercise and Sport, Faculty of Science, University of Copenhagen, København, Denmark

J. Allen-Collinson
Human Performance Centre, School of Sport & Exercise Science, University of Lincoln, Lincoln, Lincolnshire, UK

In contrast, several socio-cultural approaches focus upon empowering older people to make activity choices, to be active stakeholders, or agents in PA programmes and promote empathy amongst exercise and health practitioners about what it actually means to be an active older person in largely ageist societies (Phoenix and Smith 2011; Tulle and Phoenix 2015). Here, the term 'human agency' is often used within sociological approaches as a synonym for voluntary individual action, as opposed to those actions which are more determined by social structures such as class, gender, race/ethnicity, and socio-cultural constructions of 'age.' Such socio-cultural approaches also attempt to theorise the manner in which experiences of the past can inform present attitudes and older people's changing conception of self by taking a longitudinal approach (e.g., Atchley 1999; Elias 2001; Vincent 2005; Evans and Sleap 2014). One conceptual challenge is to overcome the tendency to 'retreat to the present' when examining older people's experiences of PA. Studies suggest reflections on past experiences can be juxtaposed against the present (Evans and Crust 2015), and both the experiential and biological experiences of ageing are heterogeneous and set within broader socio-cultural constructions of age. Such approaches can have important implications for PA promotion, such as encouraging exercise and health practitioners to look beyond the present-day 'older adult' to perceive the person with a lifetime's experiences. In short, older people were not always 'old,' and their experiences and memories of PA are not limited to a time when they considered themselves 'old.' In this chapter, we begin by outlining the key principles of Atchley's continuity theory, before highlighting the additional potential offered by socio-cultural approaches to the continuity of the self in PA promotion. In so doing, we focus upon the figurational approach to understanding ageing, before offering concluding comments on the implications of these approaches for PA promotion.

27.2 The Key Principles of Continuity Theory

In his 'continuity theory' (1989), Atchley examines how older people' activities, behaviours and attitudes develop towards, during and after the time of retirement. Classified as a feedback system theory (similar to the work of Buckley 1967 & Bailey 1990), continuity theory holds that an initial pattern of behaviour and sense of self are influenced by previous life experiences, which in turn are used to evaluate and revise the process of making behavioural choices (Atchley 1989, 1998). Such feedback system theories assume that people need mental frameworks to organise and interpret their life experiences (Atchley 1999). Initially based upon a longitudinal study in which more than 1000 older people were followed through a period of 20 years in middle age (from 50 years), continuity theory has been used as a conceptual framework to examine how individuals maintain life satisfaction or adapt to changing circumstances in old age (Atchley 1992; Finchum and Weber 2000; Agahi et al. 2006; Von Bonsdorff et al. 2009). According to continuity theorists, the theory demonstrates how a large proportion of older people will continue their patterns of thinking, activities, and social lives despite changes in health, functioning, and social circumstances (e.g., Wan and Odell 1983; Atchley 1999). Hence, events such as retirement offer opportunities for individuals to maintain earlier lifestyle patterns, previous levels of self-esteem, and to support long-standing values internally (e.g., in terms of personality structure) or externally (e.g., in seeking to maintain familiar surroundings) (Richardson and Kilty 1991).

Furthermore, continuity theory has a specific focus on adult development as a strategy for maintaining existing internal or external factors relating to a person's sense of self through continuity and adaptation. Thus, Atchley defines *continuity* as:

> A character evolving over a lifetime of action and learning and struggle and joy and heartbreak. The character remains recognizable in most cases, but evolution is also obvious. Continuity of values and beliefs, lifestyles, and relationships constitutes a solid base from which to greet changes in circumstances, both positive and negative. (Atchley 2006: 20–21).

Additionally, continuity can be subdivided into *internal continuity* where ideas of self, coping strategies, values, attitudes, and beliefs are maintained as consistent frameworks (Atchley 1999) and *external continuity* including 'social roles, activities, living arrangements and relationships with others' (Atchley 1999: 10). Continuity is distinguished from discontinuity when basic patterns are upheld, although the precise details of the nature of such patterns remain less clear (Atchley 1999). Hence, the principal of continuity has been used to predict the behaviour of older people based on the presumption that people are motivated to continue to use adaptive strategies developed throughout adulthood to diagnose situations, chart future courses and adapt to change (Parker 1995; Atchley 1999). Consequently for Atchley, the self is continuous and independent from disruption in health status and circumstances of life, although continuity and adaptation to change can still coexist. Moreover, both continuity and adaptation to change are not necessarily positive. For example, they can include continuity or adaptation to potentially negative self-conceptualisations such as low self-esteem and abusive relationships (Atchley 1999). Atchley (1999) therefore describes adaptive capacity largely as the extent to which a person is able to maintain morale in the face of discontinuity. Nevertheless, Atchley's empirical study highlights how declining morale was rarely seen amongst those who maintained their basic behaviour patterns. Thus, being able to adapt, even if imperfectly, is associated by Atchley with a greater likelihood of preserving morale (Atchley 1992). Indeed, despite the fact that Atchley acknowledges the 'downward slope' of physical ageing and recognises how the individual can experience disability or signs of pathological ageing, Atchley considers that: '…most individuals cope with these changes and continue on to lead a fully normal life. Only a small proportion must learn to cope with significant, negative changes brought about by ageing' and '..only in cases of extreme disability does ageing result in an experience of more discontinuity than continuity' (Atchley 1992: 12). Hence, according to the continuity approach, those coping with role loss and associated behavioural changes are still likely to try to preserve pre-existing behavioural patterns, even in a reduced way.

This notion is problematic, however, because continuity theory can appear to underplay the transition to retirement as disruption, changes of activity patterns, or similar events evoking a loss or change in role and identity (Richardson and Kilty 1991). Rather, it suggests that older people tend to use continuity to adapt to changing circumstances as the individual sees them, to become more of what they have always been (Atchley 1992; Agahi et al. 2006). Indeed, although the theory focuses on psychological, physiological, social, and behavioural patterns of ageing, the precise interaction of these factors on a person's sense of self is not always clear. Instead, the individual is largely situated independently, and although society is mentioned, the interaction of social norms and individual choice is not clarified. Instead, the emphasis is placed upon how continuity and adaptation to ageing are dependent upon a person's access to 'resources' (Richardson and Kilty 1991). By putting emphasis on how the life experiences of the individual influence behavioural choices, continuity theory therefore suggests that, in conjunction with the availability of resources, individuals can age in directions of their own choosing (Atchley 1999).

Consequently, Atchley (1999: 6) proposes that individuals are free to decide life paths themselves, no matter 'how strong society's effort to influence personal constructs.' In this regard, Atchley considers continuity theory to be constructivist, in that individuals construe personal knowledge, ideas of self and relationship to others based on their individual experiences. Moreover, placing ultimate responsibility on the individual to stay healthy and age in a certain way has drawn criticism because it fails to recognise the intensely disruptive effects that such events as retirement can have (Covey 1981; Palmore et al. 1984) and does not always explain individual variability in life choices, particularly if those choices lead to unhealthy behaviour (Agahi et al. 2006). Atchley (1999: 7), however, stresses that the theory does not suggest strategies to successful ageing but instead predicts how most people: '…will try continuity as their first adaptive strategy' during periods of change. It is therefore unclear whether Atchley's theory allows for the changeability of personal identity over the life course. By placing the individual at the centre, the theory potentially underplays the social, cultural, and contextual influences upon an individual's subjective sense of self and how these factors can cause individuals to experience ageing in a way that is co-produced and contested by other subjects according to socio-cultural power dynamics.

27.3 Contrasting Sociological Perspectives: Social Constructionism and Symbolic Interactionism

In contrast to Atchley's focus on the individual and on notions of 'correct' ageing, we now consider alternative approaches, to give a flavour of how other sociological, theoretical, and conceptual frameworks have examined ageing and the life course. There is a wealth of perspectives that offer such alternatives, and here we focus first on social constructionism as an umbrella term for a range of theories. Whilst Atchley (1999) considers his theory to be 'constructivist' or constructionist, in that social actors construct their personal knowledge, ideas of self, and relationship to others, other sociological traditions are more radical in their approach to the notion of 'social construction.' Whilst accepting that birth and death are biological givens, social constructionist perspectives highlight the emergent, processual, and negotiated character of people's journeys through the life course, the impact of socio-cultural and social-structural forces upon individuals, and social relationships. Rather than taking an individualistic, atomistic approach to people's perspectives on ageing and 'healthy ageing,' social constructionism investigates the ways in which meanings are constructed by *social groups*, for example, in relation to conceptualisations of time, the ageing process, and what is deemed 'old' in different contexts.

Social constructionism, rather than constituting a singular theoretical framework, represents a multi-stranded body of work, a mosaic of theoretical and methodological perspectives (Gubrium and Holstein 2008). Adopting some of the social-phenomenological insights of Alfred Schütz, along with those of the sociological tradition of symbolic interactionism, Berger and Luckmann (1991) were some of the earliest proponents of the social constructionist approach in the 1960s. In their groundbreaking work, *The Social Construction of Reality*, drawing on phenomenological principles of 'bracketing' or 'standing aside from' (Allen-Collinson 2011), Berger and Luckmann (1991) exhorted sociologists fundamentally to question taken-for-granted assumptions about the 'realities' of everyday life and to explore and examine how such realities came to be accepted as facts and embedded in common-sense knowledge. They were thus interested in processes of knowledge production and how people come to 'know things' about the everyday world. This includes challenging taken-for-granted assumptions about the realities of ageing, how people should age 'correctly,' and notions of what is and is not possible for older people to do in terms of PA and other health-related behaviours. Berger and Luckmann (1991) argued that the meanings surrounding objects and processes were not given or inherent but rather were constructed in social interaction. The impact of society, social groups, and social others is thus seen as hugely influential on the individual and her/his attitudes and behaviours vis-à-vis ageing, as highlighted by a specific tradition within social constructionism: symbolic interactionism.

In relation to ageing processes and the life course, for example, Clair et al. (1993) draw on Blumer's (1961) classic symbolic interactionist work on meaning and meaning-making processes. Using Blumer's (1961) three tenets, Clair et al. (1993) argue that: (i) age, ageing, and the life course have multiple meanings for social actors; (ii) these meanings are constructed in everyday social interaction; (iii) these meanings are subject to modification in the light of changing social and societal definitions of situations. For symbolic interactionists, the self is very much a *social* and relational self, formed, reformed, and 'tried out' in ongoing interactional encounters. Importantly, too, Goffman (1958) emphasises that social actors actively engage in a 'presentation of self' to an audience. A key component of that presentation, along with, for example, gender, ethnicity, and familial role, is age. Individuals thus draw on generally agreed (but not deterministic) normative 'scripts' for how people of certain ages should act within the relevant socio-cultural (and historical) context. They then receive acceptance (or rejection) of that presentation by others in the interactional context. For example, if a woman in her 80s takes up distance running, this might be construed as diverging somewhat from general, everyday meanings and norms surrounding age-appropriate behaviour and presentation of self. Commensurate with Blumer's (1961) formulation, however, if the running woman lives in a family or community of physically active older people, their 'definition of the situation' might well frame her involvement in distance running as 'natural' and perfectly acceptable, rather than exceptional or risky. From a symbolic interactionist perspective, therefore, it makes no sense to seek to understand older people (including their PA behaviours) in isolation, without understanding and acknowledging the social context in which they are embedded, and the social relationships that influence their identities and behaviours.

Social constructionist and other sociological approaches to ageing therefore offer significant promise to promoters of PA to older people, because they recognise the significance of socio-cultural influences on the construction of self across the life course. They also highlight how the heterogeneity of older people's perceptions of self can shape their experiences of being active in both positive and negative ways. Hence, we focus upon one such theoretical framework, figurational or process sociology (Elias and Dunning 1986), which offers promise in health promotion and the study of ageing and older people's experiences of PA. The key points of this theory relating to the interaction of power dynamics and agents' sense of self will be outlined in brief, before the implications for PA and health promotion of this approach are highlighted.

27.4 The Figurational Approach to Ageing and the Life Course: Continuity of Self as a Social Phenomenon

The figurational approach centres upon the sociological work of Norbert Elias. Elias' primary objective was to challenge what he called 'false dichotomies' in sociological thought, including 'artificial' divisions between individual and society, object and subject, macro- and micro-scales of analysis, and synchronic (or present-oriented) and diachronic (or longitudinal) explanations of social phenomena (Elias and Schröter 1991; Jarvie and Maguire 1994). Hence, this approach has specific relevance to the conceptualisation of the older 'self.'

In order to achieve this, Elias calls for a reorientation in our conceptualisation of individuals (or 'social agents') and structures. For Elias, the notion that 'society' (or structures) exists independently of individuals is flawed. Instead, society is a reflection of the individuals who constitute it; no 'society' exists without individuals, whilst no individual exists in a vacuum. Thus, the division of individual and society represents a recent, socially constructed, *Homo clausus* (or enclosed human) representation of humanity. This artificial division of 'individual' and 'society' results in a view of humans as individual units who exist within externally existing structures, rather than as beings interconnected in webs of interdependent relationships which constitute structures. The result is a shift to 'psychologisation' (Horrocks and Johnson 2014) and 'lifestyle drift' (Popay, Whitehead and Hunter 2010), that is, the tendency to view people as units to be treated in isolation and the consequent reduction of complex social problems to solutions based upon lifestyle choices. In overcoming this artificial division, Elias suggests that studying people in plural is central because agents cannot 'know' their sense of self in isolation from others. For example, to understand what it 'means' to be 'old,' one must also define what it means to be 'younger.' The two terms are relational. The adoption of such a *homines aperti* (or open human being) terminology that situates individuals *within* societies is therefore necessary, which replaces reference to either 'individuals' and/or 'societies' as mutually exclusive categories with the use of 'I,' 'he,' and 'she' identities that are simultaneously situated within networks of 'we' and 'they' relationships. These networks are referred to as figurations.

This is potentially an important shift in orientation for those in PA promotion. By situating 'I' identities within networks of 'we' and 'they' groups, together with recognising the mutual impact such relationships can evoke, a wider focus is required than those which target or 'treat' individuals in isolation. Instead, the interaction of individuals in contouring experiences and meanings becomes central. Here, the 'self' is co-produced, and the continuity of self, therefore, is contested. What's more, power balances within figurational networks can be mapped because they represent an unplanned social order made up of a multiplicity of 'I' identities connected through interdependency chains. These chains form webs of relationships that run throughout a society in such a manner that individual agents are largely unaware of their full extent (Evans et al. 2016). For example, in the production of a magazine, reciprocal relationships exist between writer, printer, editor, consumer, and web designer even though many of these individuals might never meet. Yet, a social order with a specific configuration of power balances exists in such a context, which both influences social action and mutually defines norms, roles, and identities of all within the figuration.

Relationships are not static; both I-identities and figurations of I-We and They groups change over time and space. This also has implications for an agent's continuity of self. For example, in a study of older people's experiences of PA in cardiac rehabilitation, participants' self-perceptions were based upon constant comparison with other 'similar' bodies in the same context (Evans and Crust 2015). Such comparisons were based upon participants' description of the process of rebuilding trust in their bodies related to several coexisting, competing, and ephemeral 'I' identities, including a sense of self originating in earlier 'healthier' life stages, a dangerous and 'uncivilised' embodied self immediately prior to and during treatment, and perceptions of self relating to participants' actual and potential embodied capacity in the present and future. These internal conceptualisations of self were interdependent with each other, with exercise and health professionals' assessments of participants' bodies, and with participants' perceptions of other participants' bodies in the rehabilitation figuration. For this group of older people, therefore, rehabilitation was simultaneously an individual and a social experience, understood through participants' present, past, and possible future senses of self in relation to other bodies within the rehabilitation figuration.

Thus, the reciprocity of relationships in figurations means that both PA and health promoters and their participants are interdependently involved in producing, reproducing, and challenging the norms and behaviours of PA and ageing figurations. Here, non-intentional interconnections prevail over intentional acts, and intentional acts have at their root non-intentional interconnections (Jarvie and Maguire 1994). Indeed, the short-term, intended actions of all agents, or 'I-s' within a figuration, interact with the actions of others so that they create more enduring unintended consequences. Such dynamics seemingly give 'society' its own 'game sense,' maintaining the illusion that independent structures exist (Elias and Schröter 1991; Jarvie and Maguire 1994). Elias uses the game of chess to illustrate this point. Each player makes moves based upon both their pre-conceived plan and in reaction to the moves of the other so that after several moves the game takes on a form that neither player intended nor can fully control (Jarvie and Maguire 1994). Instead, the 'game dynamic' produced is an unintended consequence of both players' actions. Similarly, the dynamic nature of wider figurations remains beyond the control of any individual-I or we-group and is instead a direct product of the aggregation of their actions.

Hence, in contrast to the continuity theory approach, social order does not exist independently as an influence on human actions; instead, it is *constituted* and *shaped* by human actions. The extent to which individual actions influence figurations is a product of the *relative* power or influence I-we groups have. This creates hierarchies amongst we- and they-groups, or between 'established' and 'outsider' groups, according to changes in the relative intensity and duration of bonds of association within and between social agents in specific contexts (Elias and Scotson 1994). Such groups have certain characteristics. For example, established groups tend to have stronger we-group bonds of association than outsider groups, for whom a shared identity can be more superficial or recent. Moreover, established and outsider groups define one another interdependently. For example, members of established groups have a tendency to perceive outsiders as dangerous, status violators or scapegoats, and characterise them in terms of the 'minority of the worst.' Furthermore, outsider groups often accept the established group's characterisation of them as 'natural' (Elias and Scotson 1994).

Thus, an older adult can begin to rationalise and uncritically accept their marginal status in exercise figurations. Previously strong bonds of association can become weaker as older people become more marginalised in fields such as employment, whereas many health-related relationships can see power balances shift away from older people towards health professionals (Elias 2001; Evans and Sleap 2012). For instance, health professionals may design PA interventions based upon a specific idea of which activities are 'appropriate' for the maintenance of older bodies (Tulle 2008a, b; Evans and Sleap 2012; Tulle and Phoenix 2015). Often, the widely accepted 'frailty' of older bodies is used as a rationale for tailoring provision (Evans and Sleap 2012, 2013; Tulle and Dorrer 2012), which is then internalised by older people as 'natural,' thereby inducing them to unintentionally reproduce their own marginalisation through the choices they make (Tulle 2008a). Increasingly, therefore, body-age and health status, rather than perceptions of embodied self, defines the experiences of being a physically active older body and of differentiating its exercising capacity from 'normal' (younger) bodies. This, at a time when scientific knowledge about the (negative) changes associated with advanced age has increased, can reproduce an ageist rationality in sport and exercise science discourses that emphasise older peoples' declining or inferior physical capacity and the need for expert supervision (Elias 2001; Tulle 2008a), which can then be internalised by older people as 'only natural' (Evans and Crust 2015).

In contrast, PA provision can foster the development of newer bonds of association where positive meanings associated with PA and ageing can be created, particularly where others perceive and value these meanings. For example, older people can value PA programmes to which they have exclusive access and feel a sense of commonality with other participants. Perceptually, this reduces the risk of their ageing bodies being placed under (potentially negative) scrutiny by other, younger groups (Evans and Sleap 2012). Such programmes also offer the potential to develop new, enabling, and supportive bonds of association, even in some cases empowering older people to resist biomedical discourses of decline, and begin to retake control of their activity choices (Allen-Collinson and Hockey 2011; Phoenix and Smith 2011;

Tulle and Dorrer 2012; Evans and Crust 2015). Moreover, the interdependent nature of power in the figurational approach draws attention to how older people are neither passive nor powerless in terms of (re)negotiating their changing social position. Relationships are not something that 'happen to' older people; they are reciprocal. Therefore, instead of considering 'isolation' or 'inactivity' amongst older people as individual lifestyle problems, it is important to recognise older people's roles in actively re-negotiating their position within figurations of health and PA (Evans and Sleap 2012; Pavey et al. 2013). In short, alterations in older people's relationship networks can offer opportunities as well as challenges.

Indeed, health promoters must be aware that hierarchies still exist amongst participants within such programmes and services. Hence, participants can begin to define themselves according to established or outsider group identities even within a programme, potentially (re)creating social hierarchies (Wheatley 2005; Evans and Crust 2015). Such within-programme relationship networks can be both enabling and constraining to older people's choices, often simultaneously. For example, the provision of PA exclusively for older people, such as an 'over-65' swimming session, can enable inactive or sedentary old adults to be physically active alongside others with perceived commonalities, at the same time as 'othering' participants in relation to other (younger) groups by highlighting age-related differences (Evans and Sleap 2012). Such exclusion can consequently constrain participants' opportunities to be active and potentially reinforce stereotypes about the age appropriateness of the activity (e.g., low intensity, low 'impact,' professionally supervised) (Evans and Sleap 2012, 2013). Furthermore, the meanings attached to PA are contested, and, PA takes on different meanings according to who is participating. For older people, moreover, these meanings are set against a backdrop of ageist ideologies grounded in wider social processes (Mennell 1989). A brief outline of how these factors can influence an individual's continuity of self therefore follows.

27.4.1 Situating Older People's Sense of Self Within the Social Construction of Age: Some Figurational Points for Consideration

Old age is not experienced in an isolated way; the meanings associated with it are co-produced. Many sociological approaches to old age and the ageing process challenge the tendency to consider them 'objective' facts. Instead, both are regarded as social constructs, albeit grounded in heterogeneous biological changes. For example, in 'Time: An essay,' Elias (1992) describes how physical time and social time have become differentiated, and the increasing emphasis on the former has led to the dominance of physical sciences in defining what time—and the ageing process—is. When associated with ageing processes, however, the assumption that time is objective and runs independently of human agency is problematic because it tends to reduce all lives to a linear, uniform trajectory (Elias and Jephcott 1992). Where such assumptions prevail, ageing becomes viewed as 'natural' and ordered and is therefore often represented in numerical quantities such as chronological age (Phoenix and Grant 2009; Tulle and Phoenix 2015). Whilst undoubtedly the rise in this knowledge has reduced uncertainty about physical ageing and led to considerable development in how older people's health is managed, it has also unintentionally contributed to the marginalisation of older people. A detailed description of these processes is beyond the scope of the present chapter, although a brief outline of the key points is perhaps valuable.

In the figurational approach, understanding long-term processes of social change (or 'Civilising Processes') are central. These include the development of a gradual, unplanned refinement of social standards and a lowering of the threshold of repugnance to previously acceptable behaviours. This in turn led to a shift of several previously public acts into the private sphere, such as reproduction, medical treatment, the care of the self, and death (Elias 2001). Whilst in the Middle Ages people died surrounded by their dependants, family, and friends, today Elias (2001) argues they often die in isolation, behind closed doors, often under the care of medical practitioners. As Elias (2001: 23) expounds, 'Never before in the history of humanity have the dying been removed so hygienically behind the scenes of social life.' Ageing and death have become 'repressed' both as processes and as memories, and clinical care has simultaneously become individualised and controlled by healthcare professionals (Elias 2001). Bodies are objectified, treatments emphasise the need for maintenance of functionality, and care for part processes that allow a person's body to go on functioning 'correctly' tends to supersede care for the emotional or social human being.

Neglect for the empowerment of older people as *homines aperti* can be common (Elias 2001). Awareness of this problem can draw attention to the way in which specific meanings associated with exercise and health can 'other' older people. Such meanings are relational and bound within a more general ageist culture within the 'exercise body-beautiful complex' (Maguire and Mansfield 1998). This culture often promotes the production and maintenance of a specific, 'civilised,' slim, toned, youthful, and attractive idealised body as a central object of cultivation that is unobtainable for many older people (Maguire and Mansfield 1998; Shilling 2003). Some older people may have sought to cultivate such embodied techniques themselves at some point in their lives and may still do so!

Such socio-cultural norms become internalised by agents beneath the level of conscious decision-making and therefore influence their sense of self. As in many sociological frameworks, Elias emphasised the interdependence of 'external,' relational processes and 'internal' bio-psychological processes in how people learn and negotiate dominant socio-cultural norms. These norms then influence behaviour, which is considered both a product of individual choice and social regulation (Jarvie and Maguire 1994). Thus, in part due to the emphasis of the ageing-as-decline narrative, it can become 'common sense' that an older person participates in less intense PA than a younger person. In the figurational approach, this internalisation of social regulation produces the habitus, which influences—but does not determine—behaviour (Jarvie and Maguire 1994). Put simply, the habitus reflects the social regulation of many of the 'taken-for-granted' attitudes people hold about PA, exercise, health, and other fields.

Furthermore, meanings associated with PA also change over time, so that within the habitus of older participants, different meanings can coexist. For example, discourses of hygiene, management of water hazards, and learning to swim can coexist with present-day perceptions of swimming, regardless of participation recentness (Evans and Sleap 2014). Often, such recollections are grounded in participants' embodied experiences during youth. Here, more visceral experiences can be recounted, suggesting these were 'magnified moments' within participants' recollections that most influenced present perceptions (Hochschild 1998). Thus, youthful experiences of cold, unhygienic swimming 'baths' gave rise to perceptions of the pool environment as dirty and swimming as cold and uncomfortable (Evans and Sleap 2014).

The problem is that within an ageist culture, the ageing body can become a mask to which others give meaning, rather than reflecting who an older person considers themselves to be (Featherstone and Hepworth 2005). What's more, many of the ideals of the exercise body-beautiful complex are unobtainable to the older adult, where the jeopardy of health risk associated with advanced age is perceived to be concurrent with a loss of productivity and physical capital, and the open display of the ageing body in public spaces has become less acceptable. That said, when promoted to emphasise the positive aspects of old age, PA offers considerable scope for the empowerment of older people. Where choice and active engagement from older people are fostered in terms of *both* participation and programme design and delivery, the potential to challenge ageist stereotypes which reproduce ideas of older adults' dependency on other would seem to exist.

The figurational approach also provides a framework where the sociocultural construction of meanings associated with sport, leisure, and PA can be supported through the 'Quest for Excitement.' Rather than uncritically viewing sport, leisure, and PA as synonymous with 'freedom' and 'choice,' activities are instead viewed as products of specific historical contexts which are more accessible for some groups than others. Moreover, Elias and Dunning (1986) highlight how leisure, sport, and PA actually produce emotions via arousal of pleasurable forms of excitement, depending upon the nature of the activity. Several factors influence this process, including the degree to which the emotions flow freely, the degree of controlled decontrolling of the emotions that is evident, the degree to which excitement imitates 'real'-life situations, the degree to which de-routinisation occurs (i.e., the higher the level of unpredictability), and the degree to which the activity seems to counteract stress tensions. Activities can therefore be placed on a continuum running from purely sociable pastimes including leisure 'work,' via activities involving only motility, up to 'mimetic' (or sports) activities. Frequently, because of an emphasis on the benefits of PA to fitness and health, the emotional and affective possibilities of PA can be overlooked (Tulle 2008a; Allen-Collinson et al. 2011; Tulle and Phoenix 2015).

27.5 Implications for Physical Activity Promotion

Based upon the above discussion, we can make several points relating to practice in PA and health promotion. First, professionals must aim to empower older people by making them active stakeholders in PA programmes. We can do this by offering choice, making PA relevant to older people' needs and preferences as defined by themselves, and by emphasising older peoples' potential to create, innovate, and have fulfilling experiences of PA in and of itself. Rather than promoting PA as a means simply to attenuate decline or to just 'keep going,' emphasising the emotional and sociable potential of PA in accordance with participants' preferences together with its undoubted health benefits can have a significant positive impact.

We must also avoid the 'retreat to the present' in how we think about older people by looking beyond the 'mask' of the older body, to see the person beneath. This person has lived a life, experienced success and failure, and may have relationships with family and friends stretching back decades. Her/his understanding of what PA is began to be produced at a time when the meanings associated with PA and health were very different from those of today.

Talking about these experiences can be vital in understanding a person's attitudes to being active/inactive.

Third, we need to critique the simplistic *Homo clausus* model of understanding older people's sense of self. A sense of self is not singular, or purely individualised, but is instead co-produced, socially mediated, and is interdependent with the meanings others attribute to a person, as well as that person's understandings of, and reaction to, those meanings. Hence, we need to avoid treating individuals as isolated units to be 'corrected.' Indeed, the importance of avoiding simple solutions to complex social problems, particularly those which focus upon individual behaviour, is an important observation. The tendency towards lifestyle drift and focusing narrowly on changing the individual in PA promotion can overlook the sometimes restrictive social contexts within which individuals are situated both in the present and throughout their life course. PA programmes must avoid the tendency to equate morals with lifestyle choices and victim blaming where healthy behaviours are not adopted. They must also pay attention to the ways in which social inequalities can be reproduced, even widened, by the propagation of health messages and how hierarchies can be produced within groups of older people.

Finally, rather than viewing ageing as 'objective' fact, it is important to acknowledge how heterogeneous physiological and psychological processes at the individual level are understood at the societal level. Ageing is never experienced in quite the same way by any two individuals. Consequently, instead of viewing old age simply as a period only of decline, isolation, and withdrawal, we must instead see it as a time of creative potential, a time when new relationships can be forged, and when the positives of age, such as wisdom and experience, can be promoted. In such a way, we can ensure that we as health professionals take greater account of older people's sense of self and ways of being.

27.6 Conclusions

The current chapter has outlined several approaches to understanding older people's temporally changing sense of self in relation to PA promotion. Beginning with continuity theory, we summarised how older people's previous attitudes towards their concept of self and the activities that they choose to participate in can be inherently linked to previous phases of the life course. Such approaches are undoubtedly valuable in terms of considering the interaction between attitudes developed earlier in life and perceptions of self and activity habits during older age. However, we also argue that it is important to consider socio-cultural contexts within which ageing takes place and how these, together with the people who inhabit them, can contribute to the *co-production* of a sense of self. This is also necessary in understanding how individuals understand the meanings associated with the contexts in which PA takes place, together with the socio-cultural meanings attached to PA and PA settings, historically and in the present. These meanings are produced, reproduced, and contested over time. In short, there is a clear need to understand and counteract the wider socio-cultural factors that 'other' older people experience if we are effectively to tailor PA programmes to their needs (Tulle and Phoenix 2015). To this end, symbolic interactionist and the figurational theoretical frameworks are possible approaches that offer insight for health promoters.

Suggested Reading

- Elias, N. (2001). *The loneliness of the dying.* New York: Continuum International Publishing Group.
- Featherstone, M., & Wernick, A. (1995). *Images of ageing: Cultural representations of later life.* London: Routledge.
- Tulle, E., & Phoenix, C. (2015). *Physical activity and sport in later life: Critical perspectives.* London: Palgrave Macmillan.

References

Agahi, N., Ahacic, K., & Parker, M. G. (2006). Continuity of leisure participation from middle age to old age. *The Journals of Gerontology Series B: Psychological Sciences and Social Sciences, 61*(6), S340–S346.

Allen-Collinson, J. (2011). Intention and epochē in tension: Autophenomenography, bracketing and a novel approach to researching sporting embodiment. *Qualitative Research in Sport, Exercise and Health, 3*(1), 48–62.

Allen-Collinson, J., & Hockey, J. (2011). Feeling the way: Notes toward a haptic phenomenology of distance running and scuba diving. *International Review for the Sociology of Sport, 46*(3), 330–345.

Allen-Collinson, J., Curry, N., Leledaki, A., & Clark, M. (2011). 'Mentro Allan'/'Venture Out' evaluation: Lived experiences of physical activity in outdoor environments. Report to Sport Wales.

Atchley, R. C. (1989). A continuity theory of normal aging. *The Gerontologist, 29*(2), 183–190.

Atchley, R. C. (1992). What do social theories of aging offer counselors? *The Counseling Psychologist, 20*(2), 336–340.

Atchley, R. C. (1998). Activity adaptations to the development of functional limitations and results for subjective well-being in later adulthood: A qualitative analysis of longitudinal panel data over a 16-year period. *Journal of Aging Studies, 12*(1), 19–38.

Atchley, R. C. (1999). *Continuity and adaptation in aging*. Baltimore: The John Hopkins University Press.

Atchley, R. C. (2006). Continuity, spiritual growth, and coping in later adulthood. *Journal of Religion, Spirituality & Aging, 18*(2–3), 19–29.

Bailey, K. D. (1990). *Social entropy theory*. Albany: State University of New York Press.

Berger, P. L., & Luckmann, T. (1991). *The social construction of reality: A treatise in the sociology of knowledge (penguin social sciences)*. Garden City: Doubleday.

Blumer, H. (1961). *Symbolic interactionism: Perspective and method* (1st ed.). Upper Saddle River: Prentice Hall.

Buckley, W. (1967). *Sociology and modern systems theory*. Englewood Cliffs: Prentice Hall.

Clair, J. M., Karp, D. A., & Yoels, W. C. (1993). *Experiencing the life cycle: A social psychology of aging*. Springfield: CC Thomas.

Covey, H. C. (1981). A reconceptualization of continuity theory: Some preliminary thoughts. *The Gerontologist, 21*(6), 628–633.

Elias, N. (2001). *The loneliness of the dying*. New York: Continuum International Publishing Group.

Elias, N., & Dunning, E. (1986). *Quest for excitement: Sport and leisure in the civilizing process*. Oxford/New York: Basil Blackwell.

Elias, N., & Jephcott, E. (1992). *Time: An essay*. Oxford: Blackwell.

Elias, N., & Schröter, M. (1991). *The society of individuals*. New York: Continuum International Publishing Group.

Elias, N., & Scotson, J. L. (1994). *The established and the outsiders: A sociological enquiry into community problems* (Vol. 32). London: Sage.

Evans, A. B., & Crust, L. (2015). 'Some of these people aren't as fit as us …': Experiencing the ageing, physically active body in cardiac rehabilitation. *Qualitative Research in Sport, Exercise and Health, 7*(1), 13–36. https://doi.org/10.1080/2159676x.2014.908945.

Evans, A. B., & Sleap, M. (2012). "You feel like people are looking at you and laughing": Older people' perceptions of aquatic physical activity. *Journal of Aging Studies, 23*(4), 515–526.

Evans, A. B., & Sleap, M. (2013). "Swim for health": Program evaluation of a multi-agency aquatic activity intervention in the United Kingdom. *International Journal of Aquatic Research and Education, 7*(1), 24–38.

Evans, A. B., & Sleap, M. (2014). 'Older people' lifelong embodied experiences of leisure time aquatic physical activity in the United Kingdom. *Leisure Studies*, 1–19. https://doi.org/10.1080/02614367.2014.923492.

Evans, A. B., Carter, A., Middleton, G., & Bishop, D. C. (2016). Personal goals, group performance and 'social' networks: Participants' negotiation of virtual and embodied relationships in the 'workplace challenge' physical activity programme. *Qualitative Research in Sport, Exercise and Health, 8*(2), 301–318. https://doi.org/10.1080/2159676X.2016.1154096.

Featherstone, M., & Hepworth, M. (2005). *Images of ageing: Cultural representations of later life*. Cambridge: Cambridge University Press.

Finchum, T., & Weber, J. A. (2000). Applying continuity theory to older adult friendships. *Journal of Aging and Identity, 5*(3), 159–168.

Goffman, E. (1958). *The presentation of self in everyday life*. London: Penguin Books.

Gubrium, J. F., & Holstein, J. A. (2008). *Handbook of constructionist research*. New York: Guilford Press.

Hochschild, A. R. (1998). The sociology of emotion as a way of seeing. In *Emotions in social life: Critical themes and contemporary issues* (pp. 3–15). London: Routledge.

Horrocks, C., & Johnson, S. (2014). A socially situated approach to inform ways to improve health and wellbeing. *Sociology of Health & Illness, 36*(2), 75–186.

Jarvie, G., & Maguire, J. A. (1994). *Sport and leisure in social thought*. London: Taylor & Francis.

Maguire, J., & Mansfield, L. (1998). "No-body's perfect": Women, aerobics, and the body beautiful. *Sociology of Sport Journal, 15*(2), 109–137.

Mennell, S. (1989). *Norbert Elias: Civilization and the human self-image*. Oxford: Basil Blackwell.

Palmore, E. B., Fillenbaum, G. G., & George, L. K. (1984). Consequences of retirement. *Journal of Gerontology, 39*(1), 109–116.

Parker, R. G. (1995). Reminiscence: A continuity theory framework. *The Gerontologist, 35*(4), 515–525.

Pavey, A., Allen-Collinson, J., & Pavey, T. (2013). The lived experience of diagnosis delivery in motor neurone disease: A sociological-phenomenological study. *Sociological Research Online, 18*(2), 11.

Phoenix, C., & Grant, B. (2009). Expanding the agenda for research on the physically active aging body. *Journal of Aging and Physical Activity, 17*(3), 362–379. Retrieved from http://www.ncbi.nlm.nih.gov/pubmed/19799105

Phoenix, C., & Smith, B. (2011). Telling a (good?) counterstory of aging: Natural bodybuilding meets the narrative of decline. *The Journals of Gerontology Series B: Psychological Sciences and Social Sciences, 66*((5), 628–639.

Popay, J., Whitehead, M., & Hunter, D. J. (2010). Injustice is killing people on a large scale—But what is to be done about it? *Journal of Public Health, 32*(2), 148–149.

Richardson, V., & Kilty, K. M. (1991). Adjustment to retirement: Continuity vs. discontinuity. *The International Journal of Aging and Human Development, 33*(2), 151–169.

Shilling, C. (2003). *The body and social theory*. London: Sage.

Taylor, A., Cable, N., Faulkner, G., Hillsdon, M., Narici, M., & Van Der Bij, A. (2004). Physical activity and older people: A review of health benefits and the effectiveness of interventions. *Journal of Sports Sciences, 22*(8), 703–725.

Tulle, E. (2008a). Acting your age? Sports science and the ageing body. *Journal of Aging Studies, 22*(4), 340–347.

Tulle, E. (2008b). The ageing body and the ontology of ageing: Athletic competence in later life. *Body & Society, 14*(3), 1–19.

Tulle, E., & Dorrer, N. (2012). Back from the brink: Ageing, exercise and health in a small gym. *Ageing and Society, 32*(7), 1106–1127.

Tulle, E., & Phoenix, C. (2015). *Physical activity and sport in later life: Critical perspectives*. London: Palgrave Macmillan.

Vincent, J. A. (2005). Understanding generations: Political economy and culture in an ageing society. *The British Journal of Sociology, 56*(4), 579–599.

Von Bonsdorff, M. E., Shultz, K. S., Leskinen, E., & Tansky, J. (2009). The choice between retirement and bridge employment: A continuity theory and life course perspective. *The International Journal of Aging and Human Development, 69*(2), 79–100.

Wan, T. T., & Odell, B. G. (1983). Major role losses and social participation of older males. *Research on Aging, 5*(2), 173–196.

Wheatley, E. E. (2005). Discipline and resistance: Order and disorder in a cardiac rehabilitation clinic. *Qualitative Health Research, 15*(4), 438–459. https://doi.org/10.1177/1049732304273044.

28

The Role of Gender and Social Class in Physical Activity in Later Life

Tamar Z. Semerjian

28.1 Introduction

The benefits of physical activity for older people have been well established in the research literature (as outlined in Chap. 2) but less discussion has occurred about how gender and social class impact participation in physical activity in later life. Perhaps older people are not seen as exciting, or dynamic, or perhaps as some have contended, feminists (Jermyn 2016) and other social theorists are anxious about their own impending ageing (Tulle and Krekula 2013). Broadly speaking, it is clear that older men engage in more physical activity than older women (mirroring trends seen across the lifespan and starting at an early age) and have higher levels of physical performance, and that those enjoying higher socioeconomic conditions are more likely to engage in leisure time physical activities (Bauman et al. 2012; Hansen et al. 2014; Lee and Levy 2011; Lee 2005; Trost et al. 2002). These relationships, however, quickly become complicated. Whilst men may engage in more physical activity, they are more likely to do so alone and engage in self-guided activities such as walking and weight training, but women are more likely to seek out structured programmes (Tischer et al. 2011). Engagement in these structured programmes is influenced by the ability to afford them, with women from higher economic groups participating in swimming, water aerobics, and tennis at higher levels than women from lower economic groups (Lee and Levy 2011). Environmental factors are also influential in determining the likelihood of an

---

T. Z. Semerjian (✉)
Department of Kinesiology, San José State University, San Jose, CA, USA

© The Author(s) 2018
S. R. Nyman et al. (eds.), *The Palgrave Handbook of Ageing and Physical Activity Promotion*, https://doi.org/10.1007/978-3-319-71291-8_28

individual to exercise (Trost et al. 2002), thus considerations of neighbourhoods become important.

The lack of literature in the area of social class and gender as social constructs highlights the lack of attention given to ageing by sociologists of sport and the lack of attention given to social constructs by those who study ageing and physical activity.

28.2 Gender

Sport and physical activity are increasingly being marketed to older people as a way to experience "healthy ageing". Some argue that this marketing is not as gendered for older people as it is for younger people, such that whilst sport and exercise are typically marked as masculine activities, for older people, women are welcome too (Higgs and Gilleard 2015; Tischer et al. 2011). Despite this assertion that exercise is becoming increasingly acceptable for older women, much of the research to date points to lower levels of physical activity among older women as compared to older men.

Many studies that consider gender within the context of exercise and physical activity are demographic or epidemiological studies that focus on participation rates. One such study, conducted in Turkey, found that for men there were no differences in physical activity between younger (60–69 years) and older (70–80) age groups; however younger women were more active than older women. Men also demonstrated higher levels of physical activity than women among the population studied (Çırak et al. 2015).

Hankonen et al. (2010) were interested in identifying if there were gender differences in psychosocial variables which then would predict behaviour in a lifestyle-change intervention study. They found that men had more social support for physical activity than did women, however the intervention, which provided social support from lifestyle counselling nurses who encouraged participants to develop an action plan for lifestyle changes, seemed to be more effective for the women. After three months of the intervention, the women in the study were more likely to have developed plans to exercise. Self-efficacy, the confidence that the individual can execute a behaviour successfully (Bandura 1977), was an important factor for both older men and women in predicting exercise behaviour.

A comprehensive epidemiological study considering community-dwelling Canadians found an association with gender and socioeconomic status (SES) linked to frequency of physical activity (Kaplan et al. 2001). Specifically males, and those with higher SES, were more likely to be physically active than women and those with lower levels of education. The authors note that there were significant regional variations in activity levels among older people. These findings highlight that more ethnographic methodologies that consider multiple variables are important for understanding the relationships between SES and physical activity.

To better understand the barriers and facilitators of exercise for low-income individuals, Clark (1999) conducted focus groups with White and African-American men and women, aged 55–70. In the study, they had a great deal of difficulty recruiting White men. Studies involving exercise intervention often have low numbers of male participants, and Clark commented that despite active recruitment of White males, they were more likely to decline participation, and among those who had agreed to participate, many did not attend the focus groups. Clark found that the African-American women who participated in the focus group identified very few physical activities that they engaged in, the primary one being walking. The distances they walked were quite short, as compared to the other groups interviewed. African-American men reported a more robust list of physical activities they engaged in and tended to walk further distances than the other groups. These walks were conscious exercise behaviours the men reported engaging in and not necessarily a reflection of lack of transportation or environmental conditions. All groups identified walking as their preferred physical activity. Notably, women were more likely to report that they wanted a leader and supportive group, whilst men seemed to prefer more independent exercise experiences. This is consistent with anecdotal reports of the relative underrepresentation of men at senior centres and group exercise classes. There has not been a systematic analysis of why this phenomenon occurs, and few studies have explored differential use of senior centres by men and women with the exception of Bøen (2012) who provides some preliminary demographic data regarding senior centre users. Often the primary attendees of these classes are women. There would be value in future research lines to query whether men tend to feel more comfortable being autonomous in exercise activities, do not enjoy the social aspects of group exercise settings, or if there is some other deterrent.

Tischer et al. (2011) reference a "diminishing or blurring gender gap" (p. 86) in regard to differential sport participation among older people in Germany. In their review of literature considering sport participation across the lifespan, Tischer et al. note ambiguous findings. While the earlier studies they reviewed found higher rates of participation in sport among men, more recent studies have found higher rates of sport participation among women over the age of 50, while others did not find significant differences based on gender. They point out that socialisation has a significant impact on these participation rates. Among the oldest age groups (80+), women's sport participation rates are indeed lower, but this is largely a cohort effect and a reflection of a generation of women who had minimal access to physical education and sport experiences. However, as sport has slowly become more acceptable for girls and women, there appear to be higher participation rates. They note that the strongest increase in sport participation among women occurred in the age groups of 45–54 and 55–64. This may indicate that as women who were socialised to see sport as a gender-appropriate activity age, we will see more and more women engaging in sport throughout the lifespan and into their later years.

In contrast to the research which seems to over-represent women's experiences in exercise, Sparkes (2015) provides an autoethnography of his experiences lifting weights at a gym in England, inhabiting what he describes as his ageing body. Autoethnography is a research method involving intense personal reflection and analysis of experiences of the researcher. These experiences are often used to draw broader conclusions about sociocultural epistemologies. At 59, Sparkes' age becomes increasingly visible, and whilst he is seen as stronger than many in the gym, he finds himself questioning his masculinity as others highlight his advanced age as compared to the others exercising in the space. Sparkes' experience highlights that ageing is subjective, embodied, and gendered. Within the context of the gym, youth is idealised, and in the narrative he presents his body fails him. A trainer in the gym tells him, "You're looking pretty good. You're doing ok-for your age" (p. 142). The compliment, however, is seen more as a reflection of his age, and haunts him later, looking at his body, and seeing only decline. This narrative reminded me of a story related by a member of my cycling club. He twice now has told me the story of a conversation he had with several female triathletes he encountered during a road bike ride. At the end of their exchange, the women told him he was "Fast for a guy his age". Like Sparkes, his interpretation of the remark was highly negative and I suspect perceived to be a threat to his masculinity. It is not coincidental perhaps that both of these comments were made by younger women, to older men. Men who had both been highly competitive athletes, who still take pride in their physique and work hard to maintain their strength and endurance. But rather than these moments boosting their pride, they are received as a jab. The entanglement of masculinity with embodiment is critical to consider when theorising about gender and exercise as we age, and yet Sparkes is one of very few theorists to consider this in a critically cultural and theoretical way. More of these types of analyses and narratives are necessary to better understand how men and women make sense of their physicality and exercise experiences over the lifespan.

In a study conducted in Scotland, Tulle and Dorrer (2012) interviewed exercisers and instructors at a gym that had programmes targeted towards older people with chronic conditions. Although they do not specifically discuss gender differences in perceptions of ageing and physical activity, it is clear that such perceptions of how older bodies should work, the dissonance between how older people felt psychologically and how their bodies behaved physically, point to the importance of perceptions. Gender ideologies strongly shape our sense of how we should move and what are appropriate activities to engage in. Ideologies related to both gender and ageing will thus influence the choices older people make as to what types of physical activity to engage in and how they will feel when they engage in these activities. Tulle and Dorrer highlight quotes from two women in their study regarding sweating during exercise. Both women state that they never sweat in the past but in their exercise class they often sweat, and they perceive this as an indicator that they are working hard and it appears to give them a sense of accomplishment. Sweating may not have been seen as appropriate for these women, 73 and 83 years of age at the time of the interview, when they were younger. Within the context of an exercise class, designed for older people, they embrace the physical experience and feel a sense of satisfaction. In the exercise classes that I have taught, I have often had older women comment when they sweat. They seem to find it both surprising and satisfying, as though sweating whilst exercising is something novel. These types of anecdotes may be indicative of the differences in the ways that men and women experience their gender identities, bodies, and therefore, exercise.

Gender as a variable is often included in research regarding ageing but is less often considered from a sociological perspective. Although there may be differences in physical activity among men and women, there is much less attention to how these differences emerge culturally and their differential impact on men and women. The research available to date indicates that older men participate in physical activity at higher levels than women (Çırak et al. 2015; Clark 1999; Kaplan et al. 2001), but they are less likely to engage in group exercise activities, preferring to exercise alone. Perhaps as a result of this preference, men are rarely included in intervention studies (e.g. Toto et al. 2012 present a study where the intervention group is 100% women despite being open to both genders). Women are overrepresented in intervention studies, focus groups studies, in fact, nearly all studies that require voluntary participation (e.g. Clark 1999; Manson et al. 2013; Plow et al. 2011; Toto et al. 2012). The differential levels of participation in sport and physical activity in later life are likely a result of a lifetime of socialisation, whereby men have been encouraged to be physically active and see sport and exercise as their rightful domain, whilst women have been taught that physicality is not consistent with gender ideologies of femininity and were either actively discouraged from sport participation or denied opportunities to participate (O'Brien Cousins 1997). What will happen to these disparities as future generations reach old age? Girls and women are participating in sport and exercise at higher rates than in the past. Additionally, the pressures on women to age gracefully and the anti-ageing movement will also contribute to not only encouragement but an imperative to stay active, fit, and attractive into later life (Brown and Knight 2015; Jermyn 2016).

Future research pertaining to gender and physical activity in later life also needs to consider issues beyond simply "gender" as it is often conceptualised. In the field of ageing studies, there has been increased attention to lesbian, gay, bisexual, transgender, queer, and intersex (LBGTQI) communities but nothing comparable within the study of sport or exercise. This dearth of attention to the LGBTQI population within sport and exercise among older people reflects the general lack of attention to these communities. As gender roles and ideologies are strongly related to the level and type of sport engagement, it is likely that LGBTQI older people will have unique relationships to sport and physical activity settings. Their access to welcoming physical activity environments may be a barrier to their sport participation. It is difficult to conjecture what the unique issues facing the LGBTQI community might be but not hard to imagine that there may be many barriers to participation that are not currently being addressed within community-based exercise programmes (anxiety about facing homophobia from peers or instructors, discomfort in physical activity settings resulting from negative experiences during their youth, apprehension about non-conforming gender identities when entering a locker room, and lack of recognition by instructors or gate-keepers that there are LGBTQI older persons).

28.3 Social Class

Just as gender is related to physical activity, so too is social class. Among low-income older people, one study found that 78% were inactive (Plow et al. 2011). Social class, or socioeconomic status (SES), are generally conceptualised as being related to income and education. Access to more material wealth makes it likely that seniors will have more options to attend exercise classes, drive to places where they can exercise outdoors, and have access to healthcare providers who encourage physical activity. However, the relationship between class and physical activity is complex and requires a more sociocultural examination that considers intersections of class, gender, ethnicity, and many other factors to more fully understand these relationships, and thereby to propose interventions that are relevant and effective within unique communities.

Barnett et al. (2012) found that socioeconomic status was associated with physical activity, with those enjoying higher SES engaging in more physical activity whilst those occupying lower SES brackets engaged in less physical activity. They reviewed research which examined changes in physical activity during the transition to retirement and paid particular attention to how SES impacted physical activity during this transition. In reviewing 19 articles meeting their selection criteria, the authors found that results from the studies reviewed indicated that after transition to retirement, there was an increase in exercise and leisure-time physical activity. This differed, however, based on SES. Individuals retiring from manual occupations tended to reduce their physical activity after retirement, whilst those in "high-grade" occupations increased the amount of physical activity they engaged in. Increases in physical activity post-retirement were more pronounced for men than women in most of the studies reviewed.

Rautio et al. (2005) considered the physical capacity of individuals over the age of 75 years in Finland and conducted 5- and 10-year follow-ups to determine if functional capacity and changes in these capacities over time were related to SES. These authors considered education and income separately in their analyses and found that income was more strongly associated with physical capacity than education. Chronic conditions, as well as behaviours such as smoking and physical activity, were controlled for in the analyses. Higher education and income were related to greater maximal walking speed, hand grip strength, and maximal vital capacity. Overall, income was more strongly related to physical capacity than education level. Whilst previous research had shown that individuals in lower SES groups demonstrated more significant levels of decline in physical capacity over time than those in higher SES groups (Deeg et al. 1992; Hemingway et al. 1997), Rautio et al. (2005) found that the rate of declines were similar across the SES groups. The authors suggest that differences between these groups may be a result of disparities in access to material wealth, as education had less of an impact than income. They highlight a materialist theory explanation, stating that while education may be a factor in SES, in this study health was more related to income than education. Thus, as individuals have less access to material wealth, they are less likely to have access to preventative healthcare, opportunities for physical activity in safe environments, and more likely to engage in harmful health behaviours such as smoking or excessive alcohol consumption.

Citing differential participation rates along lines of social class, Hammerback et al. (2012) implemented the Physical Activity for a Lifetime of Success (PALS) programme in Seattle, Washington. The goal of the programme was to increase physical activity among sedentary older people through a telephone-support intervention. Volunteers were recruited and trained to use motivational interviewing to encourage participants to increase their physical activity levels. The intervention was successful in terms of increasing physical activity of older people who participated, but recruiting sufficient numbers of volunteers and participants proved a significant challenge. The programme ended early, with the researchers determining that the intervention was too costly to maintain and did not have the impact desired. The PALS programme is evidence-based, but this study highlights that within certain communities, in this case, a low-income ethnically diverse community, evidence-based programmes may not work effectively. Peer-led programmes such as PALS are designed to be lower cost, but the recruitment of volunteers within these communities is often quite challenging. Identifying programmes that are viable, and sustainable, and meet the needs of diverse communities is critical if the interventions are to be effective and sustainable.

Intervention studies are often aimed at low-income communities, due to lower participation rates in physical activities in these communities and citing lack of access as a barrier to participation (Dye et al. 2012; Manson et al. 2013; Toto et al. 2012). These studies consistently demonstrate that exercise interventions are effective at increasing physical activity levels, functional fitness, strength, and a variety of important variables which increase the likelihood to exercise, including self-efficacy.

Several research groups have worked to better understand the relationship between environment and physical activity as it relates to socioeconomic and safety factors (Bracy et al. 2014; Carlson et al. 2012; Van Holle et al. 2014). The findings of these studies portray a complex view of how built environments, perceptions of crime and traffic safety, and other variables relate to physical activities.

Carlson et al. (2012) considered how older people's gender, ethnicity, and SES moderated their perception of safety within their neighbourhood and physical activity, in two cities in the USA. Interestingly, the results revealed that perceptions of traffic and pedestrian safety were associated with higher levels of moderate to vigorous physical activity (MVPA) among highly educated and high-income older people but that these perceptions of safety did not have an impact on MVPA among those of lower SES. Similar results were found in the association between pedestrian and traffic safety and walking for transportation and walking for leisure. The researchers also found that traffic safety was positively related to walking for transportation for women, but not for men, and that traffic safety was positively related to walking for leisure for men, but not for women. The authors highlight that sociodemographic variables clearly impacted how individuals perceived and responded (through physical activity) to neighbourhood safety variables, however, the results of their study do not create a coherent story. There appears to be greater complexity to these relationships than was captured in this study. They suggest that it may be that for more affluent groups, perceptions of safety have a greater influence on physical activity because "a small difference in safety may be influential for affluent/advantaged people who live in mostly safe areas, whereas a small difference in people who already feel unsafe may not be as perceptible and thus may be less influential on physical activity" (Carlson et al. 2012, p. 1561).

Van Holle et al. (2014) conducted a study similar to that of Carlson et al. (2012) in Belgium, the Belgian Environment and Physical Activity Study in Seniors (BEPAS Seniors). Their results indicated a positive relationship between walkability (often related to the proximity of shopping, access to necessary services, safety, in terms of crime and the ability to navigate through traffic safely, attractiveness of area, and walkways that are wide, safe, and well-maintained) and MVPA in residents of low-income neighbourhoods but no relationship for those in high-income neighbourhoods. They also found that individuals in high-income areas engaged in more low to light levels of physical activity compared to those in low-income areas. These findings are in contrast to those of Carlson et al., and the authors point out that their North American setting is quite unique. They also explain that walkability impacts high- and low-income neighbourhood residents differently, in that those in low-income neighbourhoods are influenced more by the walkability of their surroundings because they spend more time in their neighbourhoods, whilst higher-income neighbourhood residents may have more mobility options and can go to other neighbourhoods for exercise and leisure needs.

In a further analysis of the BEPAS Seniors (Van Holle et al. 2014) study, Van Cauwenberg et al. (2016) highlighted additional findings. In this study, the authors considered the relationship between a number of health outcomes, walkability, and how these factors varied in differing income neighbourhoods. In low-income neighbourhoods, walkability was associated with lower BMI and lower waist circumference. These associations were moderated by an increase in walking for transport. Thus, individuals in lower-income neighbourhoods, within higher walkability, were more likely to walk for transportation, which appears to have led to better health outcomes. These relationships were not evident from those in higher-income neighbourhood.

The authors point out that this is in contrast to the work of King and her colleagues (Bracy et al. 2014; Carlson et al. 2012; King et al. 2011; White et al. 2016) where increased safety and walkability were related to more walking in higher, but not lower, income neighbourhoods, or were not related to income at all.

White et al. (2016) investigated the impact of dog ownership on sedentary behaviours. They found that individuals who owned a dog had lower levels of sedentary behaviour, but this relationship had the greatest benefit for the most educated individuals in the sample. Interestingly, the most educated individuals in this sample also experienced the highest levels of sedentary behaviour, and thus dog ownership seemed to have a greater impact in this group. Individuals who were drivers, however, also had lower rates of sedentary behaviours as compared to those who did not have access to a car or could no longer operate one. The authors suggest that those with cars may engage in less walking for transportation but have more access to social and physical activities, reducing sedentary time. Presumably access to a car may be associated with income level. This study, like the others reviewed here indicates that SES factors influence physical activity in ways that are complex and multifaceted.

As pointed out by Van Holle et al. (2014), there are significant variations across countries. Whilst many of the studies discussed have been conducted within the USA, the USA is quite unique in its reliance on personal automobiles as the primary mode of transportation. In contrast, much of Europe and the UK have communities designed for better walkability and access to shops and community services. This will have a significant impact on physical activity associated with walking. Thus studies across various types of urban and rural environments are warranted, and policy recommendations will likely be quite different in varying locals.

Ageing expectations vary among those of low and high SES and appear to be associated with physical activity (Dogra et al. 2015). Among low SES individuals over the age of 60, ageing expectations were strongly associated with mental health, physical activity, and self-rated health. Individuals with positive expectations of ageing engage in higher levels of physical activities than those with poorer expectations of ageing. These expectations may mediate relationships between income, health, and physical activity.

In one of the few studies to consider SES using qualitative methodologies and incorporating a strong theoretical framework, Gray et al. (2016) conducted focus groups with low- and high-SES older people in Northern Ireland. They incorporated self-determination theory (Deci and Ryan 1985) and self-efficacy theory (Bandura 1977). The groups were predominantly female, aged

50 and older, with a mean age of 70.3 years. Across both low and high SES groups, anticipated health benefits, enjoyment of physical activity, opportunities to socialise, and social support to exercise were strong motivators for physical activity participation. Among the high SES group, continuation of activities from their youth, being among other older people participating in sport leading to higher levels of confidence, rehabilitation from health conditions, and influences from the media were also noted as motivation for participation in sport and physical activity. These motives were not apparently shared by the lower SES group. Interestingly, cost, access, and transportation, commonly cited barriers to physical activity participation among older people, were salient across both groups. The lower SES group experienced chronic health conditions, neighbourhood safety, walkability, weather, and lack of knowledge of physical activity guidelines as unique barriers. The only unique barrier salient to the high SES group was time, whereby participants stated that they had other obligations that kept them from exercising.

Several of the studies reviewed here look at social class and gender in tandem. Given the emphasis of these studies, it is perhaps surprising that many of them, particularly intervention and qualitative studies, had very low rates of male participants (often less than 70%) (Gray et al. 2016; Hankonen et al. 2010; Manson et al. 2013; Toto et al. 2012). These researchers are to be applauded for considering both aspects of gender and social class together; however, it appears that the results of these studies may be more reflective of the experiences of women than men, and that interventions are more likely to be attractive and effective for women. Further exploration of what types of interventions are effective for men across the SES spectrum are warranted. A final consideration that is warranted of intervention studies, is that whilst they are often quite effective, there are rarely long-term plans for the sustainability of the programme. Once funding ends, or the study concludes, these interventions typically end. Although researchers often state that the intervention is low cost, in increasingly fiscally strained times, even a low-cost programme may be beyond the capacity of community centres. Programmes that require expert staff or equipment may not be practical in areas serving low-income communities.

In conclusion, much more work needs to be done to determine how social class interacts with physical environments in the creation of spaces that increase or decrease the likelihood of physical activity. Most studies to date rely on epidemiological and quantitative perspectives. More qualitative studies that include both interviews and ethnographic work, where researchers themselves spend time in diverse neighbourhoods, may provide more insights into what factors facilitate physical activity, and what leads to either a reliance on motor transportation or isolation among older people in these communities. Jones et al. (2015) demonstrated that in the USA, there was great variation in the availability of parks and recreation facilities. Overall, there was a higher prevalence of parks in lower-income areas but fewer recreation facilities. In general, access to parks and recreation facilities is associated with higher physical activity levels in lower-income areas in the USA, as higher-income residents are able to gain access to recreation facilities in which to exercise outside of their immediate neighbourhoods. This study, however, highlights the complexities of these relationships. Parks may provide opportunities for physical activity for older people, but they can also be a site for crime and drug activities in certain areas as well. Thus simply having a park does not mean that seniors will feel safe engaging in walking or other activities therein.

28.4 Media

Broadly speaking, images of older people in the media, and particularly in advertising, are lacking. Previous research has consistently found that older people are underrepresented and that images of older women are significantly underrepresented as compared to older men (Zhang et al. 2006). Although the images of older people are generally positive (Robinson 1998), they are few, and do not represent an accurate depiction of older people.

Chen (2015) conducted a comparative analysis of representations of older people in television advertising in the UK and Taiwan. Chen found that whilst older people were more prominently portrayed in television advertisements in Taiwan, they were depicted in less active physical environments, such as the home or medical settings. UK advertisements were more likely to portray older people outdoors and engaging in enjoyable activities.

Media images of older people engaging in physical activity are quite rare, and there has been virtually no media analysis of depictions of older people within sporting or physical activity contexts. A recent advertisement provides an example of how Western cultures may sensationalise older people's engagement in physical activity. During the television airing of the Rio 2016 Olympics, Nike produced an advertisement featuring the "Iron Nun", an 86-year-old nun named Sister Madonna Buder, who has participated in 45 Iron distance triathlons. The title of the advertisement is "Unlimited Youth". The advertisement starts with her in prayer in a church or chapel:

Narrator: Sister Madonna Buder goes out for a morning run. (Image of Buder running) Good for you sister. (Image of

	Buder open water swimming) She's still active at her age, that's…great? (Image of Buder biking on hilly terrain) Whoa. Maybe a little too active? Nap time Sister?
Madonna Buder:	I don't think so.
Narrator:	The Sister doesn't think so.
Narrator:	(Image of Buder at start of Ironman triathlon) Wait, what? Ironman? Oh no, no, no, no, no. This is a bad idea Sister. A real bad idea.
A younger male competitor:	Relax! She's the Iron Nun!
Narrator:	But she won't make it, this is an Ironman!
Madonna Buder:	The first 45 didn't kill me.
Narrator:	You've done 45 of these? Okay! Do your thing Sister. Do your thing.
Picture on Screen:	UNLIMITED YOUTH

The notion that one can be active through the lifespan is important when considering the plethora of benefits of physical activity at all ages. The valorisation of "youth", however, belies any valuing of ageing and suggests that individuals like Sister Madonna Buder are forever young, not ageing and powerful. These images may be intended to be inspirational, but they can also be so unrealistic and unattainable for the average individual that they are demotivating. They play into the anti-ageing narrative, critiqued by Tulle and her colleagues (Tulle 2008; Tulle and Krekula 2013; Vincent et al. 2008) and highlight the sportification of ageing as well. Now we can be eternally youthful through exercise. Sparkes (2015) highlights how inspirational elements can be counterproductive, because eventually our bodies do experience differences in our abilities, and thus this ideal of "Unlimited Youth" sets us up to fail.

28.5 Implications for Practice

Interventions to increase access to, and a belief in the value of, physical activity among older women and those in lower social-class groups seem warranted based on the research reviewed. That said, it is quite clear that interventions must be tailored to the unique needs of communities. Women, men, and communities stratified by income levels are not the same across countries or regions. The research, particularly related to walkability, highlights that communities are quite idiosyncratic, and interventions that will increase physical activity among those who are the least likely to participate must address the unique needs of each community and populations within those communities. Additionally, whilst women may have lower levels of participation in physical activity, they have much higher levels of engagement in research and interventions. Determining the best way to target interventions to men may be important if we are to address their healthcare needs as well. The implementation of evidence-based exercise programmes which are culturally sensitive and address the needs of diverse older people may be the key to increasing physical activity among all genders and social classes.

28.6 Conclusion

The relationship between gender, social class, and physical activity has been examined but largely in epidemiological and demographic studies. The findings of this research indicate that older women who are in higher social-class groups may have more freedom to exercise and have more autonomy than working class women. The pressures to support the family, cook, and provide caregiving may encroach on working-class women's ability to exercise and engage in self-care activities. This is also further impacted by cultural expectations, thus ethnicity, class, and gender will all intersect to impact how, when, and if women have the ability to exercise. For men, being physically capable is consistent with gender ideologies, and men have more social support to be physically active (Hankonen et al. 2010). The implications of social class on physical activity are complex, and whilst generally those from higher-social class groups enjoy better health and engage in more physical activity, a variety of factors, including the safety and walkability of the neighbourhoods they live in, access to transportation, and access to exercise facilities and parks, influence the physical activities older people engage in. Media has a strong influence on our perceptions of others as well as ourselves. The limited images of older people in the media limits our notions of what ageing can and should look like.

Suggested Reading
- Gilleard, C. J., & Higgs, P. (2000). *Cultures of ageing: Self, citizen and the body*. London: Prentice Hall.
- Gilleard, C., & Higgs, P. (2013). *Ageing, corporeality and embodiment*. London: Anthem Press.
- Tulle, E., & Phoenix, C. (Eds.). (2015). *Physical activity in sport in later life*. Basingstoke: Palgrave Macmillan.

References

Bandura, A. (1977). Self-efficacy: Toward a unifying theory of behavioral change. *Psychological Review, 84*, 191–215.

Barnett, I., van Sluijs, E. M. F., & Ogilvie, D. (2012). Physical activity and transitioning to retirement: A systematic review. *American Journal of Preventive Medicine, 43*, 329–336.

Bauman, A. E., Reis, R. S., Sallis, J. F., Wells, J. C., Loos, R. J. F., & Martin, B. W. (2012). Correlates of physical activity: Why are some people physically active and others are not? *The Lancet, 380*, 258–271.

Bøen, H. (2012). Characteristics of senior centre users – And the impact of a group programme on social support and late-life depression. *Norsk Epidemiologi, 22*(2), 261–269.

Bracy, N. L., Millstein, R. A., Carlson, J. A., Conway, T. L., Sallis, J. F., Saelens, B. E., et al. (2014). Is the relationship between the built environment and physical activity moderated by perceptions of crime and safety? *International Journal of Behavioral Nutrition & Physical Activity, 11*(1), 24. https://doi.org/10.1186/1479-5868-11-24.

Brown, A., & Knight, T. (2015). Shifts in media images of women appearance and social status from 1960 to 2010: A content analysis of beauty advertisements in two Australian magazines. *Journal of Aging Studies, 35*, 74–83.

Carlson, J. A., Sallis, J. F., Conway, T. L., Saelens, B. E., Frank, L. D., Kerr, J., et al. (2012). Interactions between psychosocial and built environment factors in explaining older adults' physical activity. *Preventive Medicine: An International Journal Devoted to Practice and Theory, 54*(1), 68–73. https://doi.org/10.1016/j.ypmed.2011.10.004.

Chen, C. (2015). Advertising representations of older people in the United Kingdom and Taiwan: A comparative analysis. *The International Journal of Aging, 80*, 140–183.

Çırak, Y., Yılmaz Yelvar, G. D., Parlak Demir, Y., Dalkılınç, M., Mustafa, K., & Tağıl, S. M. (2015). Age-and sex-related differences in physical fitness and physical activity levels of the physically independent community-dwelling older adults. *Turkish Journal of Geriatrics, 18*, 273–279.

Clark, D. O. (1999). Identifying psychological, physiological, and environmental barriers and facilitators to exercise among older low income adults. *Journal of Clinical Geropsychology, 5*(1), 51–62. https://doi.org/10.1023/A:1022942913555.

Deci, E. L., & Ryan, R. M. (1985). *Intrinsic motivation and self-determination in human behavior.* New York: Plenum.

Deeg, D. J. H., Haga, H., Yasumura, S., Suzuki, T., Shichita, K., & Shibata, H. (1992). Predictors of a 10-year change in physical, cognitive and social function in Japanese elderly. *Archives of Gerontology and Geriatrics, 15*, 163–179.

Dogra, S., Al-Sahab, B., Manson, J., & Tamim, H. (2015). Aging expectations are associated with physical activity and health among older adults of low socioeconomic status. *Journal of Aging & Physical Activity, 23*, 180–186.

Dye, C. J., Williams, J. E., Kemper, K. A., McGuire, F. A., & Aybar-Damali, B. (2012). Impacting mediators of change for physical activity among elderly food stamp recipients. *Educational Gerontology, 38*, 788–798. https://doi.org/10.1080/03601277.2011.645444.

Gray, P. M., Murphy, M. H., Gallagher, A. M., & Simpson, E. E. A. (2016). Motives and barriers to physical activity among older adults of different socioeconomic status. *Journal of Aging & Physical Activity, 24*, 419–429.

Hammerback, K., Felias-Christensen, G., & Phelan, E. A. (2012). Evaluation of a telephone-based physical activity promotion program for disadvantaged older adults. *Preventing Chronic Disease, 9*, E62–E62.

Hankonen, N., Absetz, P., Ghisletta, P., Renner, B., & Uutela, A. (2010). Gender differences in social cognitive determinants of exercise adoption. *Psychology and Health, 25*, 55–69. https://doi.org/10.1080/08870440902736972.

Hansen, Å. M., Andersen, L. L., Skotte, J., Christensen, U., Mortensen, O. S., Molbo, D., et al. (2014). Social class differences in physical functions in middle-aged men and women. *Journal of Aging & Health, 26*(1), 88–105. https://doi.org/10.1177/0898264313508188.

Hemingway, H., Stafford, M., Stansfeld, S., Shipley, M., & Marmot, M. (1997). Is the SF-36 a valid measure of change in populations heath? Results from the Whitehall II study. *British Medical Journal, 315*, 1273–1279.

Higgs, P., & Gilleard, C. (2015). Fitness and consumerism in later life. In E. Tulle & C. Phoenix (Eds.), *Physical activity in sport in later life* (pp. 32–42). Basingstoke: Palgrave Macmillan.

Jermyn, D. (2016). Pretty past it? Interrogating the post-feminist makeover of ageing, style and fashion. *Feminist Media Studies, 16*, 573–589.

Jones, S. A., Moore, L. V., Moore, K., Zagorski, M., Brines, S. J., Diez Roux, A. V., et al. (2015). Disparities in physical activity resource availability in six US regions. *Preventive Medicine, 78*, 17–22. https://doi.org/10.1016/j.ypmed.2015.05.028.

Kaplan, M. S., Newsom, J. T., McFarland, B. H., & Lu, L. (2001). Demographic and psychosocial correlates of physical activity in late life. *American Journal of Preventive Medicine, 21*(4), 306–312. https://doi.org/10.1016/S0749-3797(01)00364-6.

King, A. C., Sallis, J. F., Frank, L. D., Saelens, B. E., Cain, K., Conway, T. L., Chapman, J. E., Ahn, D. K., & Kerr, J. (2011). Aging in neighborhoods differing in walkability and income: Associations with physical activity and obesity in older adults. *Social Science & Medicine, 73*, 1525–1533.

Lee, Y. (2005). Gender differences in physical activity and walking among older adults. *Journal of Women & Aging, 17*, 55–70. https://doi.org/10.1300/J074v17n01_05.

Lee, Y., & Levy, S. S. (2011). Gender and income associations in physical activity and blood pressure among older adults. *Journal of Physical Activity & Health, 8*(1), 1–9.

Manson, J., Ritvo, P., Ardern, C., Weir, P., Baker, J., Jamnik, V., et al. (2013). Tai chi's effects on health-related fitness of low-income older adults. *Canadian Journal on Aging, 32*(3), 270–277. https://doi.org/10.1017/S0714980813000305.

O'Brien Cousins, S. (1997). Elderly tomboys? Sources of self-efficacy for physical activity in late life. *Journal of Aging & Physical Activity, 5*, 229–243.

Plow, M. A., Allen, S. M., & Resnik, L. (2011). Correlates of physical activity among low-income older adults. *Journal of Applied Gerontology, 30*(5), 629–642. https://doi.org/10.1177/0733464810375685.

Rautio, N., Heikkinen, E., & Ebrahim, S. (2005). Socioeconomic position and its relationship to physical capacity among elderly people living in Jyväskylä, Finland: Five- and ten-year follow-up studies. *Social Science & Medicine, 60*, 2405–2416. https://doi.org/10.1016/j.socsimed.2004.11.029.

Robinson, T. E. (1998). *Portraying older people in advertising*. New York: Garland.

Sparkes, A. C. (2015). Ageing and embodied masculinities in physical activity settings: From flesh to theory and back again. In E. Tulle & C. Phoenix (Eds.), *Physical activity in sport in later life* (pp. 137–148). Basingstoke: Palgrave Macmillan.

Tischer, U., Hartmann-Tews, I., & Combrink, C. (2011). Sport participation of the elderly-the role of gender, age, and social class. *European Reviews of Aging & Physical Activity, 8*(2), 83–91.

Toto, P. E., Raina, K. D., Holm, M. B., Schlenk, E. A., Rubinstein, E. N., & Rogers, J. C. (2012). Outcomes of a multicomponent physical activity program for sedentary, community-dwelling older adults. *Journal of Aging & Physical Activity, 20*(3), 363–378.

Trost, S. G., Owen, N., Bauman, A. E., Sallis, J. F., & Brown, W. (2002). Correlates of adults' participation in physical activity: Review and update. *Medicine & Science in Sports & Exercise, 34*(12), 1996–2001. https://doi.org/10.1097/00005768-200212000-00020.

Tulle, E. (2008). Acting your age? Sports science and the aging body. *Journal of Aging Studies, 22*, 340–347. https://doi.org/10.1016/j.jaging.2008.05.005.

Tulle, E., & Dorrer, N. (2012). Back from the brink: Ageing, exercise and health in a small gym. *Ageing & Society, 32*(7), 1106–1127. https://doi.org/10.1017/S0144686X11000742.

Tulle, E., & Krekula, C. (2013). Ageing embodiment and the search for social change. *International Journal of Ageing & Later Life, 8*(1), 7–10.

Van Cauwenberg, J., Van Holle, V., De Bourdeaudhuij, I., Van Dyck, D., & Deforche, B. (2016). Neighborhood walkability and health outcomes among older adults: The mediating role of physical activity. *Health & Place, 37*, 16–25. https://doi.org/10.1016/j.healthplace.2015.11.003.

Van Holle, V., Van Cauwenberg, J., Van Dyck, D., Deforche, B., Van de Weghe, N., & De Bourdeaudhuij, I. (2014). Relationship between neighborhood walkability and older adults' physical activity: Results from the Belgian environmental physical activity study in seniors (BEPAS seniors). *International Journal of Behavioral Nutrition & Physical Activity, 11*, 1–18. https://doi.org/10.1186/s12966-014-0110-3.

Vincent, J. A., Tulle, E., & Bond, J. (2008). The anti-ageing enterprise: Science, knowledge, expertise, rhetoric and values. *Journal of Aging Studies, 22*(4), 291–294. https://doi.org/10.1016/j.jaging.2008.05.001.

White, M. N., King, A. C., Sallis, J. F., Frank, L. D., Saelens, B. E., Conway, T. L., et al. (2016). Caregiving, transport-related, and demographic correlates of sedentary behavior in older adults: The senior neighborhood quality of life study. *Journal of Aging and Health, 28*(5), 812–833. https://doi.org/10.1177/0898264315611668.

Zhang, Y. B., Harwood, J., Williams, A., Ylänne-McEwen, V., Wadleigh, P. M., & Thimm, C. (2006). The portrayal of older adults in advertising: A cross-national review. *Journal of Language & Social Psychology, 25*, 264–282.

29

Physical Activity Amongst Ethnic Minority Elders: The Experience of Great Britain

Christina Victor

29.1 Introduction

Cassel (2002, p. 2334) observed that physical activity offers the 'the best treatment for aging' given the well-established benefits of physical activity for health and well-being across the life course. Within a public health context there is a clear trend evident for exercise and physical activity interventions to be adopted within Europe, North America and Austrasia, as methods of improving the health of the general population. In addition, guidelines for desirable levels of physical activity have been articulated for the general populations in a range of countries including Australia, Ireland and America. The first general guidance on desirable levels of physical activity for adults seems to be the set of guidance issued by the American College of Sports Medicine (ACSM) in 1975 and the 1978 position statement (see Chodzko-Zajko et al. 2009; Troiano 2016). Since these initial statements there has been a refining of the activity guidance in response to the developing evidence base. Guidelines have moved away from an 'athletic' focus on vigorous activity as the benefits of population-based moderate intensity exercise targeted at specific populations have been identified (Troiano 2016). At the same time, there has been a developing awareness that guidance on physical activity needs to be tailored to meet the specific requirements of different population subgroups, most

---

C. Victor (✉)
College of Health and Life Sciences, Department of Clinical Sciences,
Brunel University London, Uxbridge, UK

© The Author(s) 2018
S. R. Nyman et al. (eds.), *The Palgrave Handbook of Ageing and Physical Activity Promotion*, https://doi.org/10.1007/978-3-319-71291-8_29

notably children and older adults. The American guidelines on physical activity published in 2008 included a section specific to older adults (Chodzko-Zajko et al. 2009) whilst in the UK the 2011 guidelines for physical activity for the UK older adults (aged 65+) were published for the UK (Chief Medical Officers 2011) as part of the overall guidance. This included both guidance upon appropriate duration and intensity of activity as well as specific advice for those at risk of falls which emphasised strength and balance training and is now standard in both national and international guidelines (WHO 2010). This inclusion of older adults as a distinct group for whom such guidance is offered represents a 'paradigm shift' in terms of the remit of such guidelines. This has developed in response to the developing body of evidence about the benefits of physical activity for older adults in terms of promoting general well-being as well as promoting health (McPhee et al. 2016; Tulle and Dorrer 2012). However, as we consider later in this chapter, older people are not a heterogeneous group. However, this differentiation in terms of age, gender or ethnicity and other factors such as income or geographical location rarely features in guidelines promoting physical activity in later life. We may speculate that the next stage of guideline developments may take more nuanced and tailored approaches for specific subgroups of older people defined by care needs (the frail, those with dementia or residents of long-term care) or by socio-demographic factors such as gender or ethnicity.

29.2 How Physically Active Are Older People?

As noted elsewhere in this book there are a range of different ways of measuring and reporting physical activity levels which range from the use of standardised questionnaires such as the International Physical Activity Questionnaire or objective measures such as pedometers or accelerometers (see Chap. 31). Regardless of the method of collecting activity data, one of the most common forms of reporting is in terms of the percentages of older people achieving physical activity guidelines. Given the complexity of the different ways that physical activity data can be recorded, this is a (relatively) straightforward reporting mechanism that is easily understood by older people, practitioners and policymakers and can be used to compare differences across and within populations and over time. Typical of this approach is the 2012 Health Survey for England (HSE). This classifies self-reported physical activity into four bands linked to the current UK physical activity guidance: (a) those who meet the recommendation of 150 minutes a week; (b) those with some activity in the range of 60–149 minutes per week; (c) those with low levels of activity in the 30–59 minutes of activity per week; and (d) the inactive (less than 30 minutes of activity per week).

There is a clear age-related decrease in the achievement of physical activity targets which is not unique to the UK. In 2012, 58% of males aged 65–74 reported that they achieved the recommended activity level compared with 43% aged 75–84 and 11% of those aged 85+ (Anokye et al. 2013). There are also differences in terms of gender with females consistently reporting lower levels of physical activity. Again in 2012, 52% of females aged 65–74 achieved the physical activity target; 21% of those aged 75–84 and 8% for those aged 85+. When we look at the opposite end of the distribution and look at those in the low, HSE data demonstrate a clear step change in levels of physical activity for those aged 75+. Almost two-thirds, 60%, of this age group are in the inactive category as are 90% of those aged 85+.

However, there are concerns as to the reliability and validity of questionnaire and self-report methods of physical activity assessment (see Chap. 31). Consistently accelerometry-based studies of physical activity indicate that these levels of self-reported activity over-report activity although the degree of difference depends somewhat on the 'cut points' used (Harris et al. 2009a; Shiroma et al. 2015; Scholes et al. 2014). Data from the 2008 HSE demonstrate that 5% of men aged 65+ achieve the activity target and none of the women, with 75% of both groups defined as 'low activity'. However, whilst self-report data may 'over-estimate' levels of activity and the proportions meeting specified guidelines, the general patterns observed are supported by objective data. Thus, self-report data are useful in establishing and characterising the least and most active groups of older adults and can serve a useful public health/policy evaluation function.

Given that these data are derived from a survey in England, how representative are these findings for adults living in other parts of the world? Sun et al. (2013) reported a systematic review of the proportion of older adults meeting physical activity guidance across a range of mostly developed countries. Given the different surveys, samples, populations, methods of measuring physical activity and guidelines, drawing a detailed conclusion is challenging. However, for those aged 65+ resident in Europe, Australia and North American, approximately 20–30% of adults achieved physical activity guidelines using self-report measures. When physical activity guidance was measured objectively, then the proportions meeting the guidance ranged from 0 to 10%. Older adults both under-reported the target levels of physical activity and over-estimated their own levels of activity resulting in a clear perceptual gap between their understanding of desired activity levels and their own levels of activity.

Physical activity, regardless of the method of measurement, consistently showed an age-related decrease and gender difference (men report more activity than women).

Are levels of physical activity for older adults increasing over time in response to both the increased prominence of the guidelines advocating physical activity for older people and the changing nature of the older population? Over the 15 years, the 1997–2012 Health Survey for England data have reported an increase in the 65–74 years age group meeting the primary physical activity target of 150 minutes per week of moderate-to-vigorous activity. For men, this increased from 12% in 1997 to 26% in 2012 with women's self-reported physical activity increasing from 8% to 22%. However there has been little change for males and females aged 75+ over this period (males 7% vs 11% and females 5–8%). Internationally, Sun et al. (2013) suggest that physical activity levels for older adults in America and Australia are also increasing for those aged 65+ and that this is largely accounted for by those aged 65–74. This may reflect a cohort or generational change as the 'baby boomer' group enters old age or a period effect of increased physical activity across the population more generally. It will be interesting to observe if this increase is maintained as this cohort ages. However, it remains the case that most older adults do not achieve current physical activity guidelines.

29.3 What Factors Are Associated with Physical Activity in Later Life?

It is clear that a proportion of older people remain physically active. As noted elsewhere in this book, there are older people who participate in a range of sporting activities (see Chap. 33) and who participate in national or international events such as the World Masters Swimming Championships or the four yearly World Masters Games (Dionigi et al. 2013). Given that most older people are not physically active, what factors support older people to remain physically active? Answering this question is problematic in that the focus of research is usually upon barriers to physical activity rather than facilitators or enablers. This is problematic and limiting in that we cannot presume that facilitators are the inverse of barriers. In addition, developing a definitive list of 'risk factors' that are consistently associated with physical (in)activity is challenging because of: (a) the variability and diversity across studies in the potential barriers/facilitators included such as socio-demographic characteristics, material and/or social resources, health status, personality or environmental factors; (b) their method of operationalisation and measurement; and (c) variability in populations studied in terms of age, sample size and sample types (national, local or focus upon specific populations in terms of disease states or types of residence).

Both quantitative and qualitative approaches have been used to determine what factors promote/inhibit physical activity in later life in both descriptive studies or reporting outcomes from a range of trials and interventions. Using the HSE 2008 data, Chaudhury and Shelton (2010) identified three key factors associated with low levels of physical activity for those aged 60–69: not being in employment (retirement has consistently been linked with a decrease in activity—see Barnett et al. 2012a); obesity; and the presence of a long-term illness. Harris et al. (2009b), using accelerometry data for people aged 65+, found that age; health factors (general health; disability; diabetes; body mass index); and psychological factors (exercise self-efficacy and perceived exercise control) were associated with physical activity. A systematic view of exercise post-retirement (Barnett et al. 2012b) reported 24 studies, of which 19 were quantitative and 10 were undertaken in the United States. Factors associated with activity uptake/maintenance were social factors (including giving structure to the day post-retirement and offering opportunities to build new social networks) and health benefits whilst the barriers focussed upon existing health problems, costs, caring responsibilities, psychological factors and social expectations (the inappropriateness of exercise for older people). Koeneman et al. (2011) reviewed factors promoting the uptake of physical activity/exercise by older adults (aged 55+) since 1990 and confirmed previously identified 'risk factors', namely, age, body mass index, exercise self-efficacy and social support but were much more cautious as to the robustness of these relationships because of the methodological weaknesses of the 30 studies reviewed. However, these quantitative studies tell us which groups are 'at risk' of being physically (in)active, but they do not tell us why. We explore insights into barriers and facilitators to physical activity from qualitative studies later in this chapter (Kosteli et al. 2016; Olanrewaju et al. 2016).

29.4 Understanding Diversity and Physical Activity

Typically studies looking at factors associated with physical activity among older adults focus their analysis on three key sets of factors: characteristics of the individual, the social network and physical environments. In terms of individual characteristics, the emphasis has been upon resources (social, material and health), personality/psychological resources and socio-demographic factors. With regard to the socio-demographic profile, three key axes of social differentiation, age, gender and socio-economic position, dominate our evidence base. The review by Olanrewaju et al. (2016) notes the importance of these factors in behaviour change for older people from a health inequalities perspective. Although within most developed countries ethnicity is an important and consistent facet of health inequalities, studies rarely consider ethnicity as a factor in understanding physical activity in later life. This is a significant omission but is largely explained by the comparative recency of the 'ageing' of the minority groups who migrated to Europe in the post-war period. Like many other Western societies, Britain is undergoing important social and demographic changes, most notably the 'ageing' of our black and ethnic minority populations. Within this broad demographic trend, we see emerging into 'old age' groups the minority communities who moved to Britain in the decades from 1950 to 1980 (approximately) from the Caribbean and South Asia (notably India, Pakistan and Bangladesh). Similar trends are evident in mainland Europe, but the nature of the migrant groups is rather different, being drawn from Turkey, North Africa and Southern Europe.

Within the British context, ethnicity is a concept that is based upon self-identification, usually from a list of predefined categories, and is a multidimensional concept that embraces a range of features including the country of birth, skin colour, language(s) spoken, nationality, culture and religion. Importantly ethnicity is linked with identity, either individual or group based, and embraces some or all of shared origins, background, culture, traditions, language and religion. As such it is distinct from ideas of race (Todd et al. 2007). At the 2011 national census, 12.5% of those aged 65+ self-defined themselves as 'non-white', compared with 6.5% in 1991. Overall, 18% of the white British population are aged 65+ compared with 14% for the African Caribbean group; 8% for Indians; and 4% each for both the Pakistani and Bangladeshi populations. Precise predictions about the relative size of the older population in any population are always subject to uncertainty. However, it is clear that future decades will see an increasing diversity in terms of ethnicity amongst the older population in Britain (Centre for policy on Ageing 2010).

A key feature of the population of minority elders in Britain, as compared with some other European countries, such as France, Germany or the Netherlands, is that they are from a range of distinct ethnic groups rather than a single group such as the case of Turkish 'guest workers' in Germany. Thus, there is an emergent research agenda examining the experiences of ageing amongst older people from minority communities and the similarities and differences across and between groups as well as drawing comparisons with the majority community. This agenda does not, however, always acknowledge that the majority of older people from minority communities in Europe are first-generation migrants. The status of these groups as predominantly unskilled, low-paid post-war labour migrants who worked in predominantly may well influence their experience of ageing and later life. It is a matter of considerable interest to consider how the ageing experience of first-generation migrants may differ from the next generations of minority elders who will largely be born in Europe or from their peers who did not migrate (see Victor 2015).

The ageing of our minority communities is an important but relatively neglected issue in terms of research, policy and practice. Specifically, research focussing upon the ageing experience of older black and ethnic minority adults, sometimes referred to as 'ethnogerontology' (Koehn et al. 2013; Torres 2015), is a relatively new field of research within the UK (Phillipson 2015; Zubair and Norris 2015). While there has been some focus upon those elders originally from the Caribbean and South Asia or other migrant groups, the Chinese population, especially, remain largely obscured from the public gaze, are relatively neglected by research and are much less visible in social policy terms. Whilst the specific minority groups may vary in other countries the pattern of less and more visible ethnic minority groups is almost always present. Within Britain, our largest ethnic group—the Irish—is almost invisible in gerontological research. Research with older people from ethnic minority groups within Britain has focussed upon specific issues amongst individual minority populations within locations (e.g. social support systems of older South Asians in the south of England (Victor et al. 2012)). Studies opting for a comparative approach across the key minority groups or adopting a national perspective are rarer but include a focus upon quality of life (see Bajekal et al. 2004) and loneliness/social exclusion (Victor et al. 2012). Again, similar observations apply to most developed countries where older people from minority and/or migrant groups are now growing older.

Data from the 2011 census indicate 55% of the white population of Britain aged 65+ report that they have a long-term limiting illness, a measure of chronic health problems (i.e. one that limits daily activities and which has lasted for at least 12 months). This compares with 56% for the Caribbean population, 60% for the Indians, 70% for Pakistani elders and 75% for the Bangladeshi group (Bécares 2013). This profile reflects a range of other long-term conditions such as diabetes and cardio-vascular diseases where minority elders demonstrate higher levels of ill health than the majority community. There is also a broad consistency in the hierarchy of health demonstrating what Karlsen and Nazroo (2010) termed the 'double jeopardy' of being both aged and from a minority group. However, there is clearly considerable scope for studies that examine these 'top-line' health data in more depth by looking at gender and socio-economic variations within and between different minority communities and across different countries and do not focus on ethnicity in isolation.

We must be cautious in ascribing these health differentials purely to ethnicity without considering the importance of socio-economic factors and other health determinants in explaining these health inequalities (Evandrou et al. 2016). There is also an interesting but largely neglected debate about drawing comparisons with older people in the country of origin of older minority elders. Do the high levels of morbidity observed for minority groups who are migrants represent the continuation of the pattern from their country of origin? Victor (2015) has started to explore this issue by comparing levels of loneliness for Indian elders (aged 50+) in England and Wales and their peers in India using similar questions. Levels of loneliness were identical at 9% for both populations which also mirrors that for the general adult population of that age.

29.5 How Physically Active Are Minority Elders?

Evandrou et al. (2016) observe that the pattern of health inequalities demonstrated by minority elders in Britain has largely remained unchanged since the 1990s and suggests that public health policy and practice should focus upon improving the health of these groups. As noted earlier, physical activity is an important component of interventions to promote the health of the population. How active are older people from minority groups? Our evidence base is limited because general surveys of adults such as Health Survey for England include comparatively small numbers of minority elders and, as such, often combine data for a single black and minority ethnic group (BME). This increases the power of the data for statistical analysis. However, it obscures differences between ethnic groups which may well be of considerable importance in policy and practice terms.

In a systematic review of sport, physical recreation and BME groups in Britain, Long et al. (2009) confirm a consensus of evidence that BME groups participate less compared to the wider population with the differential at around 20%. Asian (Indian, Pakistani, Bangladeshi and Chinese) males and females in Britain were much less likely to achieve the target activity guidelines, with Bangladeshi men and women being especially vulnerable (Williams et al.

2010). This echoes the systematic review of Fischbacher, Hunt and Alexander (2004) who reported that activity levels of South Asian adults (under the age of 60) were 50–75% of the white population: a result confirmed by Williams et al. (2011a, b) for the 18–55 age group who reported that 1% of Bangladeshi women aged 18–55 achieved the physical activity guidelines. Bhatnagar et al. (2015; 2016) looked at physical activity for South Asian groups aged 55+ in Britain and concluded that the vast majority did not meet guidelines. The hierarchy of physical activity was lowest for the Bangladeshi group and the Pakistani and Indian groups with all groups below the white British norm. However, the gender difference is consistent with women reporting lower rates than men but reproducing the pattern noted above. Bangladeshi women reported 1 episode of physical activity lasting 30 minutes in a 4-week period compared with 2 for Pakistani and Indian women and 6 for the white population. Bhatnagar et al. (2015) also suggested that second-generation South Asian populations showed increased levels of physical activity but the gap with the general population had not been closed.

Our evidence base about physical activity amongst minority elders in the UK is limited as we lack a clear and unambiguous data describing levels of physical activity amongst minority elders. In particular, there is an emphasis upon studies with the three major South Asian communities to the exclusion of our elders with African Caribbean backgrounds. This illustrates a key gap in the UK literature in that studies often focus upon one minority group. However, using the above estimates, it is plausible that levels of physical activity among minority elders could be 20–80% less than the majority community. Consequently, the proportion achieving key physical activity targets is probably in the range of 5–15% (based upon self-reports) and 0–10% using objective recording methods such as accelerometry. These estimates are roughly commensurate with the data reported by Long et al. (2009) where, for the population aged 65+, self-reported activity meeting the 150-minute guidelines was about 15% for the white population and 5% for a combined black and Asian group. These crude overall estimates do not take into account variations within and across groups so it is highly plausible that some groups may report levels of physical activity significantly below these estimates.

Qualitative research offers some insights into levels and types of physical activity among our minority elders. Victor (2014) undertook a secondary analysis of 109 transcripts of interviews from a study of the daily life of older people (aged 50+) from Pakistani and Bangladeshi backgrounds (Victor et al. 2012). Twenty-three participants talked about physical activity or exercise specifically. Our remaining participants did mention physical activity or exercise in the course of the interviews. We can interpret this as reflecting exercise/activity as a routine that was habituated into their daily lives to the degree that it was not mentioned. More plausibly in the light of the quantitative evidence it is highly probable that the lack of mention of physical activity was because it did not feature in their daily lives. Four individuals (three of whom were men) discussed why they could not exercise with work being the major explanatory factor, either because they did not have time or their work (as taxi drivers) does not provide opportunities for physical activity: a point made by participants in the study reported by Jepson et al. (2012). Six participants (two women) described how they had been advised by a medical professional to take (more) exercise but had not been able to do this despite the support of their families. For both of these two 'not active' groups the explanations are not dissimilar to the general population.

We had 12 (11%) participants who reported being active, equally divided between men and women. Although we do not know the duration, intensity or form of activities engaged in, this proportion would seem consistent with epidemiological estimates noted earlier. Four forms of activity/exercise were reported: exercise classes, going to the gym, swimming and walking with the latter the most commonly reported. Health benefits and the opportunity for social engagement and enhanced well-being were given as the reasons for being active: again, very similar narratives that would be articulated for the general population.

29.6 Explanations for Physical (In)activity

Quantitative studies do not enable us to understand why some older people are physically active and others are not. However, we can consider the types of factors that are linked with physical (in)activity. Victor (2014) proposes that there are five key explanatory domains when considering physical activity and older adults: personal (values and beliefs, expectations of ageing and psychological factors), resources (social, health and material), family (values, norms and expectations of older adulthood), environmental factors (urban, rural, facilities, access) and wider society (culture, media, global (health) economy/science). These broadly link to the 20 different barriers identified by Koshoedo et al. (2015) in their review of barriers to physical activity among minority groups which they classed into four broad themes of: (a) perceived personal barriers; (b) socio-economic barriers; (c) cultural barriers; and (d) environmental barriers. In examining these factors, it is important to consider which of these are general to all minority groups and which are more group generic and which reflect the deprived nature of the minority communities rather than ethnicity per se. Disentangling these different elements remains a challenge for researchers seeking to understand and respond to the low levels of physical activity demonstrated by minority elders and how these explanations may vary across and within groups.

Horne and Tierney (2012) undertook a synthesis of 11 qualitative studies of physical activity in relation to pre-existing conditions (e.g. Coronary heart disease) amongst older South Asian adults, of which six were undertaken in the UK. These studies highlight the importance of cultural norms about ageing and physical activity acting as significant barriers to engagement in theraputic exercise-based activities. However cultural norms about ageing were not discussed with regard to physical activity more broadly. More recently, Horne (2013) undertook a qualitative comparative study of white and South Asian older adults and identified that common to both groups was the fear that physical activity could exacerbate existing conditions (see also Horne et al. 2012). Interpersonal barriers were also important to both groups in terms of time, motivation and peer support. This study also identified barriers specific to South Asian groups in terms of language and religious and cultural practices. This latter point, especially in terms of the design and delivery of physical activity interventions and classes, was important, focussing predominantly on the lack of female-only sessions and/or facilities. Gender and expectations of gender roles in close-knit communities are clearly important in promoting and supporting physical activity for women. Victor (2014) reported how expectations about what 'people would think about them' restricted women's participation in walking, who they walked with or where they walked. It is not clear if these expectations are internally or externally generated (or some combination of the two).

Jepson et al. (2012) reported how their Asian participants talked about the importance of role models in prompting physical activity, support from community leaders and having minority group members leading classes/courses and involvement in the development of interventions/physical activity programmes. Babakus and Thompson (2012) reported the potential of faith groups and religious leaders as 'change agents' in supporting enhanced physical activity. These authors see a role for faith groups and leaders in addressing fatalistic ideas about health, addressing lack of knowledge about the benefits of activity that seems to be characteristic of the South Asian populations and changing perceptions that old age or later life that older people should 'slow down' rather than remaining active. Such developments may be beneficial as current evidence of effectiveness for interventions promoting physical activity for South Asian populations is, at best, modest (Chapman et al. 2013).

29.7 Implications for Practice

A number of key implications for policy and practice arise from this discussion.

Firstly, policymakers and practitioners require a more multidimensional approach to the concept of ethnicity which also engages with generation, gender, age and socio-economic status. Ethnicity is one facet of an individual's identity but is not the sole driver of physical activity or other health-related behaviours. To understand and change behaviour, we need to also include other important drivers such as those noted above.

Secondly, for South Asian populations in particular, we need to move beyond simple culturally based explanations for physical activity levels that focus only on gender. These are clearly important but so are religious and fatalistic ideas about health and expectations about 'appropriate ways' to grow old. We will not change ideas and engagement in physical activity and other preventive health behaviours without embracing and engaging with these broader sets of cultural values.

Thirdly, we need to appreciate the heterogeneity of our communities of minority elders and recognise the diversity when developing policies and interventions to promote physical activity. Less attention seems to have been paid to the African Caribbean population in terms of quantitative or qualitative studies of barriers and facilitators to physical activity and consequently any issues about physical activity engagement/disengagement that are specific to this population.

Furthermore, we need to appreciate the importance of 'hidden minorities' such as—in the British context—the Chinese or our Irish or Traveller populations who rarely feature in debates about ageing or physical activity. Allied to this is that the next generation of minority elders will not be migrants but British born—how will that influence their ideas and expectations around ageing and physical activity? Policy and practice needs to be 'future proof' and to anticipate changing behavioural patterns.

29.8 Conclusion

Harper and Levin (2005) argue that in the UK, ethnic minorities have poorer health profiles than the majority population of the same age. One way of promoting the health of any given population is via physical activity. This suggests that the need to promote physical activity for older people from these communities is a public health imperative. However, it is also a very significant challenge as we lack a detailed prevalence survey of objectively measured physical activity for the range of key communities which comprise the population of BME elders in Britain. It is important to recognise the diversity of these populations and how this may promote/inhibit participation in physical activity. The deprived nature of these populations is an important point of note and we need to consider the degree to which low levels of physical activity reflect socio-economic disadvantage and differentiate this from ethnicity. Furthermore, there is a need to determine if the risk factors for activity behaviour in previous studies apply to British BME populations. There is a pressing research agenda focussing on activity behaviour that differentiates the BME population and which does not treat the BME population as a homogenous category and examines key issues of gender and age. It is important to remember that ethnicity is one dimension of an individual's identity and we need to link this in our research with other dimensions of social position such as gender and socio-economic position. We also need to remember that the cohort experience of our current population of BME elders as first-generation migrants may well not apply to the next cohorts of elders from these populations. Our evidence base with regard to physical activity amongst minority elders is however weak and we lack clear and unambiguous data describing the levels of physical activity and sedentaryness amongst minority elders and identifying barriers and facilitators that influence these. However, it is also important to note that there is also evidence of similarities as well as differences in terms of barriers to physical activity. There seems to be a consensus emerging that a significant barrier to physical activity across all groups is a concern about exacerbating existing conditions by being physically active. There is clearly an important information-giving agenda to be developed in terms of how activity can be safely combined with a range of long-term conditions. Research evaluating the importance of factors in promoting physical activity in later life has rarely engaged with the broader gerontological empirical and conceptual work examining 'active and/or successful ageing'. We suggest that, potentially, we may have more success in promoting physical activity in later life if we embed this within a broader ecological framework of promoting 'active ageing' and which recognises the importance of the social and physical environment, health resources, intra-personal factors (identity, empowerment, autonomy, self-efficacy) and socio-demographic factors and age-related transitions (as outlined in Chap. 1). Within this framework ethnicity is embraced as one of a range of interrelated factors rather than being exceptionalised and treated as both unique and detached from the other elements of an individual's identity.

Suggested Further Reading

- Tayrose, G. A., Beutel, B. G., Cardone, D. A., & Sherman, O. H. (2015). The masters athlete: A review of current exercise and treatment recommendations. *Sports Health, 7*(3), 270–276. https://doi.org/10.1177/1941738114548999.
- An interview with Fauja Singh-the oldest London Marathon runner: http://www.bbc.co.uk/programmes/p00wzn5j
- Age UK: Fit as a Fiddle: Engaging faith and BME communities in physical activity. http://www.ageuk.org.uk/Documents/EN-B/FaithGood%20Practice%20GuideWEB.pdf?dtrk=true

References

Anokye, N. K., Pokhrel, S., Buxton, M., & Fox-Rushby, J. (2013). Physical activity in England: Who is meeting the recommended level of participation through sports and exercise? *The European Journal of Public Health, 23*(3), 458–464.

Babakus, W. S., & Thompson, J. L. (2012). Physical activity among South Asian women: A systematic, mixed-methods review. *International Journal of Behavioural Nutrition and Physical Activity, 9*(1), 150.

Bajekal, M., Blane, D., Grewal, I., Karlsen, S., & Nazroo, J. (2004). Ethnic differences in influences on quality of life at older ages: A quantitative analysis. *Ageing and Society, 24*(5), 709–728.

Barnett, I., van Sluijs, E. M., & Ogilvie, D. (2012a). Physical activity and transitioning to retirement: A systematic review. *American Journal of Preventive Medicine, 43*(3), 329–336.

Barnett, I., Guell, C., & Ogilvie, D. (2012b). The experience of physical activity and the transition to retirement: A systematic review and integrative synthesis of qualitative and quantitative evidence. *International Journal of Behavioural Nutrition and Physical Activity, 9*, 97.

Bécares, L. (2013). *Which ethnic groups have the poorest health? Ethnic health inequalities 1991 to 2011. Centre on dynamics of ethnicity (CoDE)briefing*. Manchester: Manchester University. Available at: http://www.ethnicity.ac.uk/medialibrary/briefingsupdated/which-ethnic-groups-have-the-poorest-health.pdf

Bhatnagar, P., Shaw, A., & Foster, C. (2015). Generational differences in the physical activity of UK South Asians: A systematic review. *The International Journal of Behavioral Nutrition and Physical Activity, 12*, 96.

Bhatnagar, P., Townsend, N., Shaw, A., & Foster, C. (2016). The physical activity profiles of South Asian ethnic groups in England. *Journal of Epidemiology and Community Health, 70*(6), 602–608.

Cassel, C. K. (2002). Use it or lose it: Activity may be the best treatment for aging. *Journal of the American Medical Association, 288*(18), 2333–2335.

Centre for Policy Studies on Ageing (CPA). (2010). The future ageing of ethnic minority populations England and Wales. Available at http://www.cpa.org.uk/policy/briefings/ageing_ethnic_minority_population.pdf. Downloaded.

Chapman, J., Qureshi, N., & Kai, J. (2013). Effectiveness of physical activity and dietary interventions in South Asian populations: A systematic review. *British Journal of General Practice, 63*(607), 104–114.

Chaudhury, M., & Shelton, N. (2010). Physical activity among 60–69-year-olds in England: Knowledge, perception, behaviour and risk factors. *Ageing and Society, 30*(8), 1343–1355.

Chief Medical Officers of England, Wales, Scotland & Northern Ireland. (2011). Start active, stay active. http://www.dh.gov.uk/en/Publicationsandstatistics/Publications/PublicationsPolicyAndGuidance/DH_128209

Chodzko-Zajko, W. J., Proctor, D., & Fiatarone Singh, M. (2009). American College of Sports Medicine position stand. Exercise and physical activity for older adults. *Medicine and Science in Sports and Exercise, 41*(7), 1510–1530.

Dionigi, R., Horton, S., & Baker, J. (2013). How do older masters athletes account for their performance preservation? A qualitative analysis. *Ageing & Society, 33*(2), 297–319.

Evandrou, M., Falkingham, J., Feng, Z., & Vlachantoni, A. (2016). Ethnic inequalities in limiting health and self-reported health in later life revisited. *Journal of Epidemiology and Community Health, 70*, 633–662.

Fischbacher, C. M., Hunt, S., & Alexander, L. (2004). How physically active are South Asians in the United Kingdom? A literature review. *Journal of Public Health, 26*, 250–258.

Harper, S., & Levin, S. (2005). Family care, independent living and ethnicity. *Social Policy and Society, 4*(2), 157–169.

Harris, T. J., Owen, C. G., Victor, C. R., Adams, R., Ekelund, U., & Cook, D. G. (2009a). A comparison of questionnaire, accelerometer, and pedometer: Measures in older people. *Medicine and Science in Sports and Exercise, 41*(7), 1392–1402.

Harris, T. J., Owen, C. G., Victor, C. R., Adams, R., & Cook, D. G. (2009b). What factors are associated with physical activity in older people, assessed objectively by accelerometry? *British Journal of Sports Medicine, 43*(6), 442–450.

Horne, M. (2013). Perceived barriers to initiating and maintaining physical activity among South Asian and white British adults in their 60s living in the United Kingdom: A qualitative study. *Ethnicity & Health, 18*(6), 626–645.

Horne, M., & Tierney, S. (2012). What are the barriers and facilitators to exercise and physical activity uptake and adherence among South Asian older adults: A systematic review of qualitative studies. *Preventive Medicine*. https://doi.org/10.1016/j.ypmed.2012.07.016.

Horne, M., Skelton, D. A., Speed, S., & Todd, C. (2012). Attitudes and beliefs to the uptake and maintenance of physical activity among community-dwelling South Asians aged 60–70 years: A qualitative study. *Public Health, 126*, 417–423.

Jepson, R., Harris, F. M., Bowes, A., Robertson, R., Avan, G., & Sheikh, A. (2012). Physical activity in South Asians: An in-depth qualitative study to explore motivations and facilitators. *PLoS One, 7*(10), e45333.

Karlsen, S., & Nazroo, J. (2010). Religious and ethnic differences in health: Evidence from the health surveys for England 1999 and 2004. *Health and Ethnicity, 15*(6), 122–132.

Koehn, S., Neysmith, S., Kobayashi, K., & Khamisa, H. (2013). Revealing the shape of knowledge using an intersectionality lens: Results of a scoping review on the health and health care of ethnocultural minority older adults. *Ageing & Society, 33*(3), 437–464.

Koeneman, M., Koeneman, M. A., Verheijden, M. W., Chinapaw, M. J., & Hopman-Rock, M. (2011). Determinants of physical activity and exercise in healthy older adults: A systematic review. *International Journal of Behavioral Nutrition and Physical Activity, 8*, 142.

Koshoedo, S., Paul-Ebhohimhen, V. A., & Jepson, R. G. (2015). Understanding the complex interplay of barriers to physical activity amongst black and minority ethnic groups in the United Kingdom: A qualitative synthesis using meta-ethnography. *BMC Public Health, 15*(1), 643.

Kosteli, M.-C., Williams, S. E., & Cumming, J. (2016). Investigating the psychosocial determinants of physical activity in older adults: A qualitative approach. *Psychology & Health, 31*(6), 730–749. https://doi.org/10.1080/08870446.2016.1143943.

Long, J, Hylton, K., Spracklen, K., Ratna, A., & Bailey, S. (2009). *Systematic review of the literature on black minority and ethnic communities in sport and physical recreation*. UK Sports Councils

McPhee, J. S., French, D. P., Jackson, D., Nazroo, J., Pendleton, N., & Degens, H. (2016). Physical activity in older age: Perspectives for healthy ageing and frailty. *Biogerontology, 17*, 567–580.

Olanrewaju, O., Kelly, S., Cowan, A., Brayne, C., & Lafortune, L. (2016). Physical activity in community dwelling older people: A systematic review of reviews of interventions and context. *PLoS One, 11*(12), e0168614.

Phillipson, C. (2015). Placing ethnicity at the centre of studies of later life: Theoretical perspectives and empirical challenges. *Ageing & Society, 35*(5), 917–934.

Scholes, S., Coombs, N., Pedisic, Z., Mindell, J. S., Bauman, A., & Rowlands, A. V. (2014). Age- and sex-specific criterion validity of the health survey for England physical activity and sedentary behavior assessment questionnaire as compared with accelerometry. *American Journal of Epidemiology, 179*(12), 1493–1502.

Shiroma, E. J., Cook, N. R., Manson, J. E., Buring, J. E., Rimm, E. B., & Lee, I.-M. (2015). Comparison of self-reported and accelerometer-assessed physical activity in older women. *PLoS One, 10*(12), e0145950.

Sun, F., Norman, I. J., & While, N. (2013). Physical activity in older people: A systematic review. *BMC Public Health, 213*, 1.

Todd, C., Ballinger, C., & Whitehead, S. (2007). Reviews of socio-demographic factors related to falls and environmental interventions to prevent falls amongst older people living in the community. Available at http://www.who.int/ageing/projects/3.Environmental%20and%20socioeconomic%20risk%20factors%20on%20falls.pdf

Torres, S. (2015). Expanding the gerontological imagination on ethnicity: Conceptual and theoretical perspectives. *Ageing & Society, 35*(5), 935–997.

Troiano, P. (2016). https://health.gov/paguidelines/second-edition/meetings/1/History-of-Physical-Activity-Recommendations-and-Guidelines-for-Americans.pdf. Accessed 1 May 17.

Tulle, E., & Dorrer, N. (2012). Back from the brink: Ageing, exercise and health in a small gym. *Ageing & Society, 32*(7), 1106–1127.

Victor, C. R. (2014). Understanding physical activity in the daily lives of Bangladeshi and Pakistani elders in Great Britain. *ISRN Geriatrics, 2014*, 529428.

Victor, C. R. (2015). The wellbeing of ageing Indian migrants in England and Wales. *International Journal of Contemporary Sociology, 52*(1), 77–92.

Victor, C. R., Martin, W., & Zubair, M. (2012). Families and caring in South Asian communities: Results of a pilot study. *European Journal of Social Work*. https://doi.org/10.1080/13691457.2011.573913.

Williams, E. D., Stamatakis, E., Chandola, T., & Hamer, M. (2010). Assessment of physical activity levels in South Asians in the UK: Findings from the health survey for England. *Journal of Epidemiology and Community Health, 65*, 517–521.

Williams, E. D., Stamatakis, E., Chandola, T., & Hamer, M. (2011a). Assessment of physical activity levels in South Asians in the UK: Findings from the health survey for England. *Journal of Epidemiology and Community Health, 65*, 517–521.

Williams, E. D., Stamatakis, E., Chandola, T., & Hamer, M. (2011b). Physical activity behaviour and coronary heart disease mortality among South Asian people in the UK: An observational longitudinal study. *Heart, 97*(8), 655–659.

World Health Organization. (2010). *Global recommendations on physical activity for health*. Geneva: World Health Organization.

Zubair, M., & Norris, M. (2015). Perspectives on ageing, later life and ethnicity: Ageing research in ethnic minority contexts. *Ageing and Society, 35*(5), 897–916.

30

The Role of Government Policy in Promoting Physical Activity

Debra J. Rose and Koren L. Fisher

30.1 Introduction

A number of countries have published recommended guidelines for physical activity (PA) for their constituents and embarked upon the development of national PA initiatives and policies (Department of Health 2011; Department of Health Australia 2014a; U.S. Department of Health and Human Services 2008). The World Health Organisation (WHO 2010) also published and disseminated global recommendations on PA for health. Since the passage of both global and national PA recommendations, the question remains whether or not population levels of PA have been appreciably and positively influenced. In 2016, The Lancet published its second series addressing PA and the progress being made to reduce the high level of physical inactivity and sedentary behaviour globally. The continuing failure to harness the power of PA in the prevention of non-communicable diseases, including dementia, is highlighted in a series of four papers addressing the ongoing global pandemic of physical inactivity (Andersen et al. 2016). While high-income countries bear a larger proportion of the economic burden associated with physical inactivity, low- and

D. J. Rose (✉)
Kinesiology Department, Center for Successful Aging and Fall Prevention Center of Excellence, California State University, Fullerton, CA, USA

K. L. Fisher
Center for Successful Aging and Department of Kinesiology, California State University, Fullerton, CA, USA

middle-income countries experience a larger proportion of the disease burden (Ding et al. 2016). Perhaps the most disturbing finding emerging from this series of papers is that while many countries have now developed national PA plans and policies, PA levels, particularly among the older adult segment of the population, are not increasing worldwide.

30.2 Translating Evidence into Policy

Reliable scientific evidence should be at the core of any population-based efforts to promote increased PA. Indeed, effective policymaking is predicated on the integration of "good" science that can help policymakers at many levels better understand the extent of the problem, the types of intervention strategies that actually work, and the degree to which they are both cost-efficient and cost-effective. Thus, both the efficacy and the effectiveness of PA interventions must be considered in the development of PA policy and guidelines (Reis et al. 2016; Weed 2016). Efficacy refers to the performance of an intervention under controlled conditions, whereas effectiveness considers its performance in "real-world" contexts (see Table 30.1; Singhal et al. 2014; Weed 2016). This distinction is often poorly described and understood, with many assuming efficacy data to be effectiveness data when, in fact, highly efficacious interventions may be less than effective when implemented in real-world contexts and on a broader scale (Singhal et al. 2014; Weed 2016). Reis et al. (2016) argue that despite an abundance of translational trials where efficacious PA interventions are implemented in a variety of real-world settings, these interventions often fail to be fully scaled up to the point of being embedded within a system that would make them more likely to be maintained and sustained over the long term.

PA policy and guideline development has, so far, prioritised the use of systematic reviews based on randomised clinical controlled trials (RCT) to grade the quality of the scientific evidence to determine policy recommendations (British Heart Foundation National Centre 2012; Brown et al. 2012; Paterson et al. 2007; Physical Activity Guidelines Advisory Committee 2008; Tremblay et al. 2011). Unfortunately, translational research studies are rarely included in systematic reviews, and thus, are not often considered in the policy development process (Reis et al. 2016). Recently, the Appraisal of Guidelines, Research, and Evaluation II (AGREE II) Instrument, the international gold standard for the assessment of practice guidelines in medicine, has been applied to the development of PA guidelines (Brouwers et al. 2010; Tremblay et al. 2011).

Table 30.1 Key considerations for evaluating evidence for physical activity interventions

Intervention trial	Study designs
Efficacy	
Examines benefits and harms under highly controlled conditions	Randomised controlled trial (RCT) designs
Well-defined, homogenous populations with strict inclusion and exclusion criteria	Standard care or waitlisted control group
Limited generalizability of results	
Interventions delivered in highly standardised manner	
Resource intensive	
Publication bias may lead to the reporting of only positive outcomes	
Analysis considerations	
Intention-to-treat approach	
Effectiveness	
Examines intervention in "everyday" settings	RCT designs with less rigorous control group (usual care, fewer restrictions)
More heterogeneous populations with limited exclusion criteria	Quasi-experimental approaches
Less rigorous control group (usual care; wait-listed)	
Greater proportion of non-compliant participants	
Greater prevalence of comorbid conditions	
Greater generalizability of results	
Standardize interventions to the extent possible	
May have limitations in study resources to maximize participant recruitment and adherence	
Analysis considerations	
Intention-to-treat approach; higher rates of missing data	

The AGREE II instrument provides a means to assess the methodological rigor and transparency in guideline development, including the process used to gather and synthesise the evidence (Brouwers et al. 2010).

Interestingly, in our review of policies and initiatives established in three developed countries (Australia, Canada, and the United States), the most significant policy initiative used to establish PA as a national public health priority has been the release of national PA guidelines for their respective populations. These guidelines include detailed recommendations on the amount, type, and frequency of PA that should be performed on a weekly basis as well as the intensity at which it should be performed based on systematic reviews of the "science" surrounding PA. In all cases, the guidelines advocate 150 minutes of moderate-intensity PA per week, with some qualifications related to vigorous-intensity activity, along with muscle-strengthening activities on two or more days per week (U.S. Department of Health and Human Services 2008; Canadian Society for Exercise Physiology 2011; Department of Health, Physical Activity, Health Improvement and Protection 2011; Department of Health Australia 2014a, b). These guidelines are aligned with (and in the case of the United States, likely informed by) the World Health Organisation (WHO 2010) global recommendations on PA for health. The recommendations for older adults mirror those for younger adults, with some caveats—the primary differences being in the emphasis placed on vigorous PA, balance and flexibility activities, and on the accommodation of different functional levels within the guidelines. As outlined in other chapters in this Handbook, the guidelines released by the UK government are the only ones that explicitly recognise the heterogeneity of the older adult population and outline specific accommodations, as appropriate, for older adults of differing levels of function (Department of Health, Physical Activity, Health Improvement and Protection 2011).

The American, Canadian, and Australian guidelines explicitly identify the general public as an intended direct audience; however, despite the release and widespread dissemination of these guidelines through the mass media, the percentage of adults, and older adults in particular, currently meeting the recommended levels of PA remains very low in each of the three countries (Garriguet and Colley 2014; Harris et al. 2013; Tucker et al. 2011). The question then becomes whether 150 minutes represents a realistic behavioural target, particularly for older adults, as suggested by Latimer-Cheung et al. (2013) and Weed (2016) in their recent analysis of PA guidelines as public health interventions.

In all countries, review papers or technical reports outlining the underlying evidence base and the methodology used to synthesise the research evidence and produce the guidelines are publicly available (Brown et al. 2012; Paterson et al. 2007; Physical Activity Guidelines Advisory Committee 2008; Tremblay et al. 2011). Recently, the extent to which current PA guidelines are actually based on available evidence has been called into question, with Weed (2016) noting that none of the supporting documents cite evidence for effectiveness or potential effectiveness of the PA guidelines as a public health intervention. Rather, it has been argued that the current recommendations are based on un-evidenced assumptions about what the public will value and judgements about what represents a "substantial health benefit". Weed (2016) further states that if the efficacy evidence is objectively considered, a recommendation of 90 minutes of moderate-intensity PA per week would be more appropriate and offers the conclusion that, as a public health intervention, PA guidelines do not meet the standards of evidence or ethics that governments themselves have established (Weed 2016). This criticism is particularly relevant to older adults, for whom the recommendations may not be realistic or attainable and where the lack of an obvious lower limit to the dose-response relationship between PA and health benefits has important implications for the comparable effectiveness of different PA recommendations (Weed 2016). It is because of these concerns, many of which are discussed in the scientific review papers accompanying the guidelines, that certain recommendations regarding PA for older adults have been scaled back or eliminated (Latimer-Cheung et al. 2013). Further evidence is needed regarding the longer-term functional outcomes of PA interventions for older adults and to determine the relative importance and benefit of each component in multicomponent PA programmes before more specific guidelines are warranted (Tremblay et al. 2011; Brown et al. 2012; Department of Health, Physical Activity, Health Improvement and Protection 2011).

The development of effective PA policies, whether at a national or community level, requires multi-sectoral partnerships that go beyond healthcare and are informed by evidence-based best practices (Bellew et al. 2008; Choi 2005; Craig 2011). Common characteristics of successful PA policies have been identified over the years as nations and communities have shared their experiences and practices globally. Nine criteria describing the necessary characteristics for effective PA policy development and successful policy outcomes have been proposed and are outlined in Table 30.2.

Table 30.2 "HARDWIRED" criteria for successful physical activity policy

1. **H**ighly consultative (between policymakers and stakeholders) in development to ensure broad-based stakeholder agreement
2. **A**ctive through multi-strategic, multi-level, partnerships
3. **R**esourced adequately
4. **D**eveloped in stand-alone and synergistic policy modes
5. **W**idely communicated
6. **I**ndependently evaluated
7. **R**ole-clarified and performance delineated
8. **E**vidence-informed and evidence-generating
9. **D**efined national guidelines for health-enhancing physical activity

Adapted from Bellew et al. (2008)

30.3 National- and Community-Based Initiatives in the United States

Following the release of the Physical Activity Guidelines for Adults (PAGA) in 2008, the National Physical Activity Plan (NPAP) was developed in 2010 with the aim of supporting efforts to achieve other national health goals, such as Healthy People 2020. This plan, subsequently revised in 2016, outlines a comprehensive set of policies, initiatives, and programmes designed to increase the PA levels of all Americans and across all sectors of US society. It established seven overarching priorities. These include the development of a comprehensive PA surveillance system, policies for adoption at state, regional and community levels, a national PA campaign, and increased funding for promotion of the PA strategies outlined in the NPAP. Several working sectors are identified in the revised plan with strategies and tactics outlined for each sector. A particular strength of the NPAP is the development of a detailed logic plan by the Physical Activity Policy Research Network that is being used to guide the ongoing evaluation over the next several years. The accomplishments and lessons learnt from the initial implementation of the NPAP were cited by Evenson and Satinsky (2014) in a review paper that included findings from in-depth interviews with leads of six of the sectors. Among the positive experiences identified were opportunities for additional inter-organisational collaboration that extended beyond the NPAP, a growing camaraderie across organisations involved in each of the sectors, the opportunity to learn what other previously unknown organisations were doing related to PA, and thereby avoid redundancy of efforts and pride in the amount of work that had actually already been accomplished towards achieving many of the NPAP goals. The qualitative interviews also revealed a number of challenges such as a lack of funding beyond that provided by participating organisations, insufficient time available, the need for better marketing and promotion of the plan, as well as greater organisational support.

One other notable national initiative that preceded the NPAP in the United States and specifically targeted middle-aged and older Americans is the *National Blueprint: Increasing Physical Activity Among Adults Age 50 and Older*. Based on input from more than 60 individuals representing 46 organisations with multi-disciplinary and multi-agency expertise (Armstrong et al. 2001), the overarching goal was to develop a coordinated national strategy for promoting PA among older adults. Another goal of the *National Blueprint* was to identify some of the societal barriers to PA among older adults and to outline specific strategies for overcoming these barriers. The blueprint identified barriers in the areas of research application, home and community programmes, workplace settings, medical systems, public policy and advocacy, and marketing and communications.

To evaluate the effectiveness of the *National Blueprint,* Park et al. (2010) interviewed both senior administration and junior staff members from several organisations that developed the document. The interviewees reported how the blueprint has influenced their own organisational missions and strategies by including goals about PA. Interviewees also highlighted how administrative and staff behaviour has changed to become more in line with the blueprint as well as changes in organisational behaviour, beliefs, attitudes, and performance.

A more recent initiative that addresses some of the strategies highlighted by the *National Blueprint* is the *Go4Life* mass media initiative led by the National Institute on Aging (http://go4life.nia.nih.gov/). *Go4Life* focuses on increasing the PA of older adults in their daily life. Unfortunately, due to the relatively short time that the *Go4life* initiative has been operating, its reach and overall effectiveness has yet to be determined.

30.3.1 Community-Based Initiatives

At the community level within the United States, several initiatives have specifically focused on promoting PA among the 50-plus segment of the population. The most successful of those conducted thus far is the Active for Life (AFL) initiative, funded by the Robert Wood Johnson Foundation between 2003 and 2007. In response to the need for researchers to move beyond efficacy-based studies conducted in controlled research settings, the AFL initiative was the first to examine the translation of two evidence-based PA programmes (Active Choices and Active Living Everyday) into community settings by quite diverse community-based organisations. The first of the two programmes, *Active Choices*, was developed by researchers at Stanford University (Castro and King 2002) and is comprised of a six-month telephone-counselling programme that begins with an initial face-to-face meeting while Active Living Everyday is a small group-based PA programme (Dunn et al. 1997, 1999; Wilcox 2016). Process and outcome evaluations for both programmes demonstrated significant increases in PA that were almost identical in magnitude to the increases observed in the RCT setting (Wilcox et al. 2008).

Key factors that contributed to the successful translation of these two evidence-based programmes were outlined in a large-scale process evaluation conducted in nine lead community-based organisations between 2003 and 2007 (Griffin et al. 2010). Central to the success of the effectiveness trials conducted for both programmes was the fact that the evaluation process was framed and implemented as an interactive process. Open communication between the sites, programme developers, the national programme office, and the programme evaluation team facilitated the maintenance of high fidelity to the essential elements that were clearly identified following completion of the original RCT. While each site was able to "fit" the programme to their unique participant characteristics and settings by modifying certain programme elements (e.g. combining session content to make it more culturally and age appropriate, completing homework assignments within class sessions to assist participants with lower educational levels, increasing size of group), those elements considered to be essential to maintaining programme fidelity were not modified before the potential benefits or costs of making any changes were evaluated (see Griffin et al. 2010). The authors also concluded that allowing individual sites to tailor the programme to the diverse backgrounds of their clients and organisational environment also helped them to enhance their own identity and attract a specific client base. Finally, conducting a qualitative evaluation, in addition to gathering quantitative data, allowed for the adaptation and localisation of the programmes while still maintaining high fidelity of essential programme elements. With ongoing support from the US Administration on Aging, the Active Living Everyday programme now operates in 37 states nationwide, while the Active Choices programme operates in 13 states, including Canada and Australia.

Additional examples of successful community-level programmes aimed at improving PA levels among older adults include Fit and Strong, a PA/behaviour change programme that targets older adults with osteoarthritis of the lower extremities (Hughes et al. 2004, 2006, 2010) and EnhanceFitness (Wallace et al. 1998). Originally developed and tested at the Center for Research on Health and Aging at the University of Illinois at Chicago, Fit and Strong programmes are offered at five sites across Chicago, all of which are accessible to the targeted population, which now includes more minorities (e.g. ethnic, low socio-economic status), as well as three sites in North Carolina and one in West Virginia. The reach of this community-based programme is expected to increase as a result of beginning a collaborative relationship with the National Arthritis Foundation that currently provides other PA programmes in communities throughout the United States. Finally, EnhanceFitness is a low-cost, evidence-based group PA programme developed specifically for older adults. The programme was developed and tested by the University of Washington Health Promotion Research Center in 1994, in partnership with Senior

Services and Group Health Cooperative. Programme participation has increased significantly since its humble beginnings as a small pilot project operating in four senior centres to a nationally disseminated programme that now serves over 25,000 older adults throughout the United States. Widespread implementation of this multicomponent exercise programme has been facilitated by the completion and publication of several effectiveness trials (Ackermann et al. 2008; Belza et al. 2006), the development of a complete programme package that includes instructor training, programme manuals, data collection forms, and the development of an interactive website with marketing materials, programme updates, and instructor resources (www.projectenhance.org). Moreover, the ongoing evaluation and dissemination of the programme (via the University of Washington Health Promotion Research Center) continues to be funded and/or supported by federal entities such as the Centers for Disease Control and Prevention, National Council on Aging, and the US Administration on Aging.

30.4 National- and Community-Based Physical Activity Initiatives in Canada

Canada has a long history of policy initiatives addressing PA and active living at both the federal and provincial/territorial (FPT) levels (Craig 2011; Spence et al. 2015). ParticipAction is one of the most well-known Canadian PA initiatives. Originally launched in 1971 by the federal government, ParticipAction was one of the longest-running social marketing campaigns to promote PA in the world, eventually becoming a model for future social and behavioural change initiatives (Edwards 2004). Its success in creating a PA movement with relatively small amounts of seed funding led to unrealistic expectations in terms of ongoing media support and population reach as the Canadian media landscape rapidly expanded in the 1990s, eventually reducing its ability to be seen as a leading organisation, and ultimately resulting in its closure in 2001 (Edwards 2004). In 2007, with the restoration of federal funding, ParticipAction was relaunched as a national communications strategy to address issues of physical inactivity and increased rates of childhood obesity. It now positions itself as a "thought leader", partnering in PA research and participating in national issue-based working groups in addition to developing new and modern social marketing campaigns (ParticipAction 2016). However, the extent to which ParticipAction actually affects PA behaviour remains unclear and critics question the degree to which ParticipAction can advocate for PA policy change when it is so reliant on federal funding (Gordon 2011).

After funding for PA policy initiatives peaked in the 1980s, the changing political climate in the 1990s led to a devolution in Canadian PA policy, demonstrated by national PA infrastructure changes and the reallocation of resources, including the defunding of ParticipAction (Craig 2011). Currently, the policy role of the federal government is limited to supporting the PA guidelines and national PA surveillance strategies; however, most Canadian provinces and territories have developed their own stand-alone PA policy agendas (Craig 2011). A multilevel, multi-sectoral approach to PA policy such as this allows for the development and implementation of strategies to address local or regional needs within a common framework; however, shifts in governmental priorities and periods of fiscal restraint have demonstrated that this approach is insufficient if its implementation is not adequately resourced (Craig 2011; Spence et al. 2015). Recent assessments have determined that the current PA policy environment is inadequate to increase PA at the population level, leading to calls for a long-term, sustained, and high-level commitment on the part of the federal government (Craig 2011; Spence et al. 2015).

The PA sector in Canada recently put forth an action plan, Active Canada 20/20 (2012), as a call to action and national plan to engage decision-makers, non-government, and public sectors and foster continued, consistent, and collaborative efforts among stakeholders at every level (Spence et al. 2015). While not a national PA policy per se, Active Canada 20/20 provides a clear vision and change agenda and has received support from sport and recreation ministers at the federal, provincial, and territorial levels of government. To this end, public consultations to inform the development of a national PA framework were announced in late 2016, with completion of the framework expected in mid-2017 (Conference Board of Canada 2016). If this PA framework is to lead to proactive and effective initiatives, it will require consistent leadership from federal and provincial-territorial governments to ensure coordinated efforts, ongoing and sustainable resourcing, and rigorous and meaningful evaluations of impact on the national secular trends in physical inactivity (Spence et al. 2015; Weed 2016).

30.4.1 Community-Level Provincial-Territorial Physical Activity Policies

Provincial-territorial PA policies vary in specific strategic approaches; however, most share common goals to encourage increased PA participation and to create more supportive environments for PA (Craig 2011). Provincial strategies are typically the result of highly consultative development approaches and make use of strategic, multi-sector partnerships in their implementation (Craig 2011). The majority of provincial-territorial strategies focus on whole population change with three provinces outlining specific policy objectives pertaining to older adults. In each instance, the policy objectives focus on improving awareness of and access to PA programmes for older adults and creating more supportive environments for older adults to engage in PA by removing barriers to participation (Craig 2011; MacArthur Group 2004; Sante et Services Sociaux Quebec 2005; Ministry of Health 2015).

In motion is an example of a successful evidence-based grassroots health promotion strategy that has been successfully scaled up to the provincial level. Launched in 2000 in the city of Saskatoon, Saskatchewan, *in motion* began as a partnership between the municipal government, the regional health authority, the University of Saskatchewan, and ParticipAction. The *in motion* model utilised a community-capacity building approach that emphasised four key components: (1) building non-traditional partnerships to encourage multi-sectoral collaboration and community capacity for PA promotion, (2) building community awareness, (3) targeting community-based strategies for key population groups, including older adults, and (4) measuring success through evaluation and programme reviews (In Motion 2005). One key to the success of the founding initiative was the particular focus on the social-marketing aspect of the initiative, including significant investment in the branding of the initiative (In Motion 2005; Saskatchewan *in motion* 2014). Engaging public awareness campaigns (television and radio commercials; public billboards and signage) with coordinated branding, including a recognisable logo, were developed and agreements regarding brand use were included when the initiative was subsequently adopted elsewhere.

The *in motion* model has been adopted by at least seven other cities across Canada with significant investments from provincial governments and other partners. It has also been scaled up to the provincial level in both Saskatchewan (2003, Saskatchewan *in motion*) and Manitoba, where it was adopted by the provincial government as their overall PA strategy (2005, Manitoba *in motion*).

A particular strength of the *in motion* initiative is that it is characterised by multi-level and multi-sectoral partnership working to build capacity to accomplish goals that would otherwise be out of reach if pursued in isolation (In Motion 2005). One example is the community-university research partnerships that have typically been responsible for evaluating the *in motion* initiative. In both Saskatchewan and Manitoba, population-based data are collected on awareness, PA participation, and PA facilitators and barriers (In Motion 2005; Health, Leisure and Human Performance Research Institute 2005).

The research agenda was initially funded through federal research grants and, in addition to the population-based survey, also included a parallel research programme to examine PA determinants, interventions, and outcomes in each of six target populations, including older adults (Lindstrom et al. 2004; Chad et al. 2005; Reeder et al. 2008; Temple et al. 2008). Nonetheless, like most community-based initiatives, publicly available programme evaluations of the *in motion* initiative itself are limited to annual or bi-annual assessments of initiative awareness and PA participation rates as well as periodic reports developed for initiative partners or funders (In Motion 2005; Health, Leisure and Human Performance Research Institute 2005).

30.5 National- and Community-Based Physical Activity Initiatives and Policies in Australia

In response to the alarming rise in physical inactivity and its associated economic cost ($13.8 billion in 2008), the National Heart Foundation of Australia released a major planning document in 2009 that outlined an ambitious plan to address physical inactivity among Australians. A revised and expanded document was subsequently published in 2014 (National Heart Foundation of Australia 2014). A total of 13 action areas were identified and strategies for immediate intervention were identified. Action areas included the built environment, workplaces, healthcare, transportation and urban planning, sedentary behaviour, sport and active recreation, and addressed different age groups, disadvantaged populations, and minorities (i.e. Aboriginal and Torres Strait Islander peoples). Action area 10 of the Heart Foundation's *Blueprint for an Active Australia* specifically addresses intervention strategies aimed at older adults. Brown and van Uffelen (2014), the authors of this section, provided four recommendations for immediate action that included the following: implementing policies that support older people living physically active lives; planning, developing, and retrofitting environments to provide older adults with more opportunities to participate in PA (e.g. provide safe and aesthetically appealing walking paths in aged-care settings, site retirement communities in areas with connected streets, and close proximity to shopping and services); implementing social and community interventions that support older Australians living more active lives (e.g. design age-friendly health clubs and recreation centres, implementing age-appropriate and evidence-based PA programmes in the community and home, training health professionals to assist older adults develop personalized activity goals); and helping older adults to understand the health benefits of living a more physically active life (e.g. mass media campaigns, education and awareness programmes). The final action area described in the *Blueprint* is devoted to research and programme evaluation, a critical and necessary piece of the document for guiding, monitoring, and ultimately evaluating the effectiveness of the many multi-level interventions described in each of the action areas.

30.5.1 Community-Based Initiatives

One excellent example of a grassroots community-based initiative that has achieved national penetration in Australia is the *Just Walk It* (JWI) programme that began in the state of Queensland in 1995. Not only does walking represent a low-cost method of reaching a large proportion of the population, it is an activity that has been shown to transcend potential cultural and socioeconomic barriers (Jones and Owen 1999; Belza et al. 2006). The goal of the JWI programme is to increase regular engagement in PA by promoting walking as an activity. As a result of empowering community members to address their own health needs and building partnerships between communities and government agencies, this volunteer-led programme has grown from 35 walking groups with an average of six members per group to 900-plus walking groups with over 12,500 members and hundreds of volunteer leaders. The initial success of the programme has garnered the attention of the National Heart Foundation that now operates the free community-based programme in most states and territories within Australia. The Heart Foundation provides the training and support of Area Coordinators who administer, support, and promote the programme. It also provides professional development opportunities, support materials, merchandise, printed resources, and promotional tools at minimal cost to the Area Coordinators. Although the JWI programme targets all ages, the programme has attracted a high percentage of adults over 50 years. An evaluation involving a sample of registrants ($N = 601$) provided further evidence of the programme's efficacy in promoting regular engagement in PA, particularly in men, middle-aged participants, and those members who reported being inactive or insufficiently active at the time they enrolled in the walking programme 12 months earlier (Foreman et al. 2012). In a recent evaluation of whether the *JWI* framework is an effective and sustainable model for engaging the participation of community-based organisations in implementing the walking programme, Foreman et al. (2017) identified six key factors to successfully implementing *JWI*. They included (1) interagency collaboration, (2) strategic programme planning, (3) targeting local organisations with strong community links and experience of implementing programmes, (4) frequent and ongoing support from coordinators implementing the programme, (5) community ownership of the programme and (6) promotion and support from a National Organisation such as the Heart Foundation.

30.6 Practical Implications

This review, albeit limited in scope, of PA policies and initiatives in three developed countries clearly suggests that the development of effective PA strategies, whether at a national or community level, requires multi-sectoral partnerships that go beyond healthcare and are well informed by evidence-based best practices (Bellew et al. 2008; Craig 2011). As noted by Weed (2016), current policy processes have been less than optimal, leading to the development of less than optimal policies, with unintended consequences and potential harms for population health.

There is a recognised need for a stronger and *independently evaluated* evidence base, particularly as it pertains to older adults and the dose-response effect of PA on various fitness and health outcomes as well as the effectiveness and efficacy of current PA guidelines. To that end, policymakers are beginning to apply stronger evaluative criteria, such as AGREE II and the Nesta Standards of Evidence to both policy development and policy outcomes (Tremblay et al. 2010; Latimer-Cheung et al. 2013; Public Health England 2014). These policy evaluation frameworks examine the policy process across multiple indicators that include: stakeholder and public consultation, sustainable allocation of resources, the establishment of stand-alone and synergistic policies, independent evaluation of all stages of the policy process, and the clear delineation of roles and responsibilities, among other criteria. Making use of these frameworks, beginning at the earliest stages of the PA policy process, will allow for the development of stronger and truly evidence-based PA strategies, the evaluation of which will provide rigorous and much-needed effectiveness and efficacy data to inform future PA policy initiatives.

Grassroots community-based PA initiatives and programmes can also have a positive impact on the health and well-being of individuals—both participants and leaders—as well as the larger community through the development of social capital (i.e. trust, reciprocity, networking, social norms). Encouraging ownership of programmes by community members while developing cooperative partnerships between local businesses, city councils, government, and non-government organisations appear to be key ingredients of successful and sustainable grassroots efforts.

30.7 Conclusions

If we are to achieve the World Health Organization (WHO) target of a 10% reduction in physical inactivity by 2025, policymakers must adopt a much more serious approach to the promotion of PA across the lifespan (WHO 2014). This can only be accomplished by building capacity through adequate and sustained funding to implement national policies aimed at reducing sedentary behaviour and increasing PA levels among its constituents, irrespective of age. It is time for all nations to take immediate action to eliminate the global pandemic of physical inactivity by scaling up effective policy and practice for PA promotion worldwide (Reis et al. 2016). If, indeed, PA is the "best buy" in public health as argued by Morris in 1994, why are so many countries still devoting so little time and money to making it a reality?

Suggested Further Reading

- Pate R., & Buchner, D. (2014). *Implementing physical activity strategies*. Champaign: Human Kinetics.
- Piggin, J., Mansfield, L., & Weed, M. (2017). *The Routledge handbook of physical activity policy and practice*. https://books.google.com/books/about/Routledge_Handbook_of_Physical_Activity.html?id=u8D5sgEACAAJ
- Weed, M. (2016). Evidence for physical activity guidelines as a public health intervention: Efficacy, effectiveness, and harm – A critical policy sciences approach. *Health Psychology and Behavioral Medicine, 4*, 56–69. https://doi.org/10.1080/21642850.2016.1159517.

References

Ackermann, R. T., Williams, B., Nguyen, H. Q., Berke, E. M., Maciejewski, M. L., & LoGerfo, J. P. (2008). Healthcare cost differences with participation in a community-based group physical activity benefit for medicare managed care health plan members. *The. Journal of the American Geriatrics Society, 56*, 1459–1465.

Active Canada 20/20. (2012). Active Canada 20/20: A physical activity strategy & change agenda for Canada. Creating a culture of an active nation. Retrieved from https://docs.google.com/viewer?a=v&pid=sites&srcid=YWN0aXZlY2FuYWRh MjAyMC5jYXxwYWdlMXxneDozNjEyNjViMjNkZmIwYTA

Andersen, L. B., Mota, J., & Di Pietro, L. (2016). The global pandemic of physical inactivity. *Lancet, 388*, 1256.

Armstrong, S., Sloan, S., Turner, M., & Chodzko-Zajko, W. J. (2001). National blueprint for increasing physical activity among adults 50 and older. *Journal of Aging and Physical Activity, 9S*, S5–S13.

Bellew, B., Schoeppe, S., Bull, F. C., & Bauman, A. (2008). The rise and fall of Australian physical activity policy 1996–2006: A national review framed in an international context. *Australia and New Zealand Health Policy, 5*, 18.

Belza, B., Shumway-Cook, A., Phelan, E. A., Williams, B., Snyder, S. J., & LoGerfo, J. P. (2006). The effects of a community-based exercise program on function and health in older adults: The EnhanceFitness program. *Journal of Applied Gerontology, 25*, 291–306. https://doi.org/10.1177/0733464806290934

British Heart Foundation National Centre. (2012). Physical activity statistics. Retrieved from https://bhf.org.uk/research/statistics

Brouwers, M. C., Kho, M. E., Browman, G. P., Burgers, J. S., Cluzeau, F., Feder, G., et al. (2010). AGREE II: Advancing guideline development, reporting and evaluation in health care. *Canadian Medical Association Journal, 182*(18), E839–E842.

Brown, W. J., & van Uffelen, J. G. Z. (2014). Action area 10: Older people. In *Blueprint for an active Australia* (2nd ed.). Melbourne: National Heart Foundation of Australia.

Brown, W. J., Bauman, A. E., Bull, F. C., & Burton, N. W. (2012). *Development of evidence-based physical activity recommendations for adults*. Canberra: Department of Health.

Canadian Society for Exercise Physiology. (2011). *Canada's physical activity guidelines*. Ottawa: Author.

Castro, C. M., & King, A. C. (2002). Telephone assisted counseling for physical activity. *Exercise and Sport Sciences Reviews, 30*, 64–68.

Chad, K. E., Reeder, B. A., Harrison, E. L., Ashworth, N. L., Sheppard, M. S., Schultz, S. L., et al. (2005). Profile of physical activity levels in community dwelling older adults. *Medicine & Science in Sports & Exercise, 37*(10), 1174–1184.

Choi, B. C. K. (2005). Twelve essentials of science-based policy. *Preventing Chronic Disease* (serial online). Available from http://www.cdc.gov/pcd/issues/2005/oct/05_0005.htm

Conference Board of Canada. (2016). Federal, provincial, and territorial governments seeking input to inform a framework for physical activity [Press Release]. Retrieved from http://www.conferenceboard.ca/press/newsrelease/16-10-20/federal_provincial_and_territorial_governments_seeking_input_to_inform_a_framework_for_physical_activity.aspx

Craig, C. L. (2011). Evolution and devolution of national physical activity policy in Canada. *Journal of Physical Activity and Health, 8*, 1044–1056.

Department of Health Australia. (2014a). *Australia's physical activity and sedentary behavior guidelines*. Canberra: Author.

Department of Health Australia. (2014b). Physical activity recommendations for older Australians (65 years and older). Retrieved from http://www.health.gov.au/internet/main/publishing.nsf/content/health-pubhlth-strateg-phys-act-guidelines

Department of Health, Physical Activity, Health Improvement and Protection. (2011). *Start active, stay active: A report on physical activity for health from the four home countries' Chief Medical Officers*. Retrieved from http://www.paha.org.uk/Resource/start-active-stay-active-a-report-on-physical-activity-from-the-four-home-countries-chief-medical-officers

Ding, D., Lawson, K. D., Kolbe-Alexander, T. L., Lancet Physical Activity Series 2 Executive Committee, et al. (2016). The economic burden of physical activity: A global analysis of major non-communicable diseases. *Lancet, 388*, 1311–1324. https://doi.org/10.1016/S0140-6736(16)30728-0

Dunn, A. L., Marcus, B. H., Kampert, J. B., Garcia, M. E., Kohl, H. L., & Blair, S. N. (1997). Reduction in cardiovascular disease risk factors: 6-month results from project active. *Preventive Medicine, 26*, 883–892. https://doi.org/10.1006/pmed.1997.0218

Dunn, A. L., Marcus, B. H., Kampert, J. B., Garcia, M. E., Kohl, H. W., & Blair, S. N. (1999). Comparison of lifestyle and structured interventions to increase physical activity and cardiorespiratory fitness: A randomized trial. *Journal of the American Medical Association, 281*, 327–334.

Edwards, P. (2004). No country mouse. Thirty years of effective marketing and health communications. *Canadian Journal of Public Health, 95*(Suppl), S6–S13.

Evenson, K. R., & Satinsky, S. B. (2014). Sector activities and lessons learned around initial implementation of the United States National Physical Activity Plan. *Journal of Physical Activity and Health, 11*, 1120–1128. https://doi.org/10.1123/jpah.2012-0424

Foreman, R., van Uffelen, J. G., & Brown, W. J. (2012). Twelve month impact of the Just Walk It program on physical activity levels. *Health Promotion Journal of Australia, 23*, 101–107.

Foreman, R., Brookes, L., Abernethy, P., Brown, W., & Stoneham, M. (2017, January 8–12). *Assessing the sustainability of the "Just Walk It" program model: Is it effective and will it enhance program success?* Transportation Research Board 96th annual meeting, Washington, DC.

Garriguet, D., & Colley, R. C. (2014). A comparison of self-reported leisure-time physical activity and measured moderate-to-vigorous physical activity in adolescents and adults. *Health Reports, 25*(7), 3–11.

Gordon, A. (2011). ParticipAction's back with a message for parents, but will it work? *The Toronto Star*. Retrieved from https://www.thestar.com/life/health_wellness/2011/01/21/participactions_back_with_a_message_for_parents_but_will_it_work.html

Griffin, S. F., Wilcox, S., Ory, M. G., Lattimore, D., Leviton, L., Castro, C., Carpenter, R. A., & Rheaume, C. (2010). Results from the active for life process evaluation: Program delivery fidelity and adaptations. *Health Education Research, 25*(2), 325–342. https://doi.org/10.1093/her/cyp017.

Harris, C. D., Watson, K. B., Carlson, S. A., Fulton, J. E., Dorn, J. M., & Elam-Evans, L. (2013). Adult participation in aerobic and muscle strengthening physical activities – United States, 2011. *Morbidity and Mortality Weekly Report, 62*,

326–330. Retrieved from http://www.cdc.gov/mmwr/preview/mmwrhtml/mm6217a2.htm

Health, Leisure and Human Performance Research Institute. (2005). *In motion survey*. Winnipeg: University of Manitoba.

Hughes, S. L., Seymour, R. B., Campbell, R., Pollak, N., Huber, G., & Sharma, L. (2004). Impact of the fit and strong! Intervention on older adults with osteoarthritis. *The Gerontologist, 44*, 217–228.

Hughes, S. L., Seymour, R. B., Campbell, R. T., Huber, G., Pollak, N., Sharma, L., & Desai, P. (2006). Long term impact of fit and strong! On older adults with osteoarthritis. *The Gerontologist, 46*, 801–814.

Hughes, S. L., Seymour, R. B., Desai, P., Campbell, R. T., Huber, G., & Chang, H. J. (2010). Fit and strong!: Bolstering maintenance of physical activity among older adults with lower-extremity osteoarthritis. *American Journal of Health Behavior, 34*(6), 750–763.

In Motion. (2005). *Saskatoon in motion: Five years in the making. 2000–2005*. Saskatoon: Saskatoon Regional Health Authority.

Jones, J. A., & Owen, N. (1999). Neighbourhood walk: A local community-based program to promote physical activity among older adults. *Health Promotion Journal of Australia, 8*, 145–147.

Latimer-Cheung, A. E., Rhodes, R. E., Kho, M. E., Tomasone, J. R., Gainforth, H. L., Kowalski, K., Nasuti, G., et al. (2013). Evidence-informed recommendations for constructing and disseminating messages supplementing the new Canadian physical activity guidelines. *BMC Public Health, 13*, 419.

Lindstrom, B., Chad, K., Ashworth, N., Dunphy, B., Harrison, E., Reeder, B., et al. (2004). Effectiveness of recruitment strategies for a physical activity intervention in older adults with chronic diseases. *Journal of Physical Activity & Health, 1*, 259–269.

MacArthur Group Inc. (2004). Physical activity strategy for Prince Edward Island 2004–2009. Retrieved from http://www.gov.pe.ca/photos/original/doh_actstrat.pdf

Ministry of Health. (2015). *Active people, active places: British Columbia physical activity strategy*. Victoria: Province of British Columbia.

Morris, J. (1994). Exercise in the prevention of coronary heart disease. Today's best buy in public health. *Medicine & Science in Sports & Exercise, 26*, 807–814.

National Heart Foundation of Australia. (2014). *Blueprint for an active Australia* (2nd ed.). Melbourne: National Heart Foundation of Australia.

Park, C.-H., Chodzko-Zajko, W., Ory, M. G., Gleason-Senor, J., Bazzarre, T. L., & Mockenhaupt, R. (2010). The impact of a national strategy to increase physical activity among older adults on national organizations. *Journal of Aging and Physical Activity, 18*, 425–438.

ParticipAction. (2016). *Moving with the times: Impact report*. Toronto: ParticipAction.

Paterson, D. H., Jones, G. R., & Rice, C. (2007). Ageing and physical activity: Evidence to develop exercise recommendations for older adults. *Applied Physiology, Nutrition, and Metabolism, 32*, S69–S108.

Physical Activity Guidelines Advisory Committee. (2008). *Physical activity guidelines advisory committee report.* Washington, DC: Department of Health and Human Services.

Public Health England. (2014). *Everybody active, every day. An evidence-based approach to physical activity.* London: Public Health England (PHE). Publications Gateway Number: 2014319.

Reeder, B. A., Chad, K. E., Harrison, E. L., Ashworth, N. L., Sheppard, M. S., Fisher, K. L., et al. (2008). Saskatoon in motion: Class-versus home-based exercise intervention for older adults with chronic health conditions. *Journal of Physical Activity & Health, 5,* 74–87.

Reis, R. S., Salvo, D., Ogilvie, D., Lambert, E. V., Goenka, S., Brownson, R. C., & Lancet Physical Activity Series 2 Executive Committee. (2016). Scaling up physical activity interventions worldwide: Stepping up to larger and smarter approaches to get people moving. *The Lancet, 388,* 1337–1348. https://doi.org/10.1016/S0140-6736(16)30728-0

Sante et Services sociaux Quebec. (2005). Summary of the Kino-Quebec program: 2005–2008 action priorities. Retrieved from http://www.santecom.qc.ca/bibliothequevirtuelle/hyperion/2550452631_s.pdf

Saskatchewan in motion. (2014). *Grass roots physical activity movement takes shape: Saskatchewan in motion – Our first ten years.* Retrieved from http://www.saskatchewaninmotion.ca/public/files/10_Year_Story_Web.pdf

Singhal, A. G., Higgins, P. D. R., & Waljee, A. K. (2014). A primer on effectiveness and efficacy trials. *Clinical and Translational Gastroenterology, 5,* e45.

Spence, J. C., Faulkner, G., Bradstreet, C. C., Duggan, M., & Tremblay, M. S. (2015). Active Canada 20/20: A physical activity plan for Canada. *Canadian Journal of Public Health, 106*(8), e470–e473.

Temple, B., Janzen, B. L., Chad, K., Bell, G., Reeder, B., & Martin, L. (2008). The health benefits of a physical activity program for older adults in congregate housing. *Canadian Journal of Public Health, 99*(1), 36–40.

Tremblay, M. S., Kho, M. E., Tricco, A. C., & Duggan, M. (2010). Process description and evaluation of Canadian physical activity guidelines development. *International Journal of Behavioral Nutrition and Physical Activity, 7,* 42.

Tremblay, M. S., Warburton, D. E. R., Janssen, I., Paterson, D. H., Latimer, A. E., Rhodes, R. E., et al. (2011). New Canadian physical activity guidelines. *Applied Physiology, Nutrition, and Metabolism, 36,* 36–46.

Tucker, J. M., Welk, G. J., & Beyler, N. K. (2011). Adults: Compliance with the physical activity guidelines for Americans. *American Journal of Preventive Medicine, 40,* 454–461. https://doi.org/10.1016/j.amepre.2010.12.016

U.S. Department of Health and Human Services. (2008). 2008 physical activity guidelines for Americans. Retrieved from http://www.health.gov/paguidelines/

Wallace, J., Buchner, D., Grothaus, L., Leveille, S., LaCroix, A., & Wagner, E. (1998). Implementation and effectiveness of a community-based health promotion program for older adults. *Journal of Gerontology: Medical Sciences, 53a,* M301–M306.

Weed, M. (2016). Evidence for physical activity guidelines as a public health intervention: Efficacy, effectiveness, and harm – A critical policy sciences approach. *Health Psychology and Behavioral Medicine, 4*, 56–69. https://doi.org/10.1080/21642850.2016.1159517

Wilcox, S. (2016). Behavioral interventions and physical activity in older adults: Gains and gaps. *Kinesiology Review, 5*, 57–64.

Wilcox, S., Dowda, M., Leviton, L. C., Bartlett-Prescott, J., Bazzarre, T., Campbell-Voytal, K., et al. (2008). Active for life: Final results from the translation of two physical activity programs. *American Journal of Preventive Medicine, 35*, 62–351.

World Health Organisation. (2010). *Global status report on non-communicable diseases*. Geneva: World Health Organisation.

World Health Organization. (2014). *World Health Statistics 2014*. Geneva: World Health Organization.

Section 7

Current Issues and Debates in Promoting Physical Activity Among Older People

Christina Victor

At both the individual and population levels, physical activity promotes quality of life and well-being across the life course. Older people are no exception to this observation, and there are guidelines for levels of physical activity, tailored for this population, present in the public health policies of most countries in the developed world. These generally include guidance on the amount and intensity of physical activity alongside the promotion of specific forms of exercise aimed at promoting strength and balance as a fall prevention measure. In response to the development of guidelines, there are a plethora of interventions that have been developed to get older people to be more physically active. However, in promoting physical activity for older people, at both the population and individual levels, there are several key challenges that policymakers, practitioners, and older people themselves face. In this section of the book, we address four key topics: measuring physical activity, the potential of technology to promote activity, the rise of sedentarism, and the diversity of the older population in regard to physical activity. These issues act as exemplars for the broader suite of issues that developing a more physically active (older) population needs to address.

A key question for policymakers, practitioners, and older people relates to the measurement and monitoring of physical activity. A key motivational factor in promoting physical activity is to show individuals how physically

---

C. Victor (✉)
College of Health and Life Sciences, Department of Clinical Sciences,
Brunel University London, Uxbridge, UK

(in)active they are. Policymakers and practitioners want to know how interventions do (or not) promote, enhance, and maintain levels of physical activity. Thus, a key challenge is how to measure physical activity for different functions and in different contexts. Chapter 31 by Aguilar-Farias and Hopman-Rock describes the complex science underpinning this apparently simple objective and provides us with the evidence as to the strengths and weaknesses of different approaches. Clearly, technological developments in terms of physical activity monitors offer advances in the precision with which we can monitor physical activity and can work as a motivating device to increase activity in some contexts. However, Vereijken and Helbostad (Chap. 35) remind us that there are other technological approaches which can be used to enhance activity. These authors highlight the potential of exergames to enhance activity. These technologies are in their infancy but offer specific features such as personalisation and the key element of fun which can support adherence. They are also useful for populations with specific needs such as dementia or those who are frail and for whom other forms of activity may prove challenging. These types of technologies form part of our portfolio of interventions that we can use to promote activity and are likely to achieve increased importance as future generations of elders will present an enhanced familiarity with digital technology than the current generation of elders. This serves to remind us that the nature of the older population is dynamic, and we need to ensure that our approaches to enhancing physical activity adapt appropriately.

Older people are also highly diverse in terms of age, gender, class, and ethnicity but also in terms of existing health needs. The potential of physical activity to promote well-being is well established. In Chap. 34, Liu-Ambrose considers the evidence supporting the role of physical activity in terms of primary and secondary prevention, that is, stopping individuals from getting a specific disease and then slowing/reversing the disease process for those with established disease. More specifically, Liu-Ambrose critically evaluates the evidence supporting the relationship between physical activity and cognitive health. The evidence is inconclusive and ambiguous, but there is a case for exploring this relationship further. As with the technological developments, we need to identify the most effective form of exercise that promotes cognitive health, how this links to the characteristics of the individual, and in which context. Again, this emphasises the importance of a developing research agenda around physical activity for older adults that emphasises the individual and is personalised and tailored for specific contexts. We need to focus on what physical activity interventions work, for which groups, and in which settings to promote physical and mental health. We also need to remain aware of the degree to which these types of intervention may exacerbate health inequalities within the older population.

The chapter draws attention to two important but somewhat underdeveloped areas for future research. Onambele-Pearson and colleagues in Chap. 32 discuss the emergence of sedentary behaviour as an 'independent' risk factor for ill-health. This reflects a more sophisticated conceptual engagement with the relationship between activity and sedentary behaviour. As this chapter shows, sedentarism is not simply the inverse of activity. We cannot assume that by promoting adherence to physical activity guidelines we are addressing the independent risk factor presented by sedentary behaviours. We know that older people are a major group at risk of sedentarism. However, there is a clear need for further research investigating this topic area as the paucity of research is a clear conclusion of this chapter.

There is a strong focus in physical activity research with older people to focus on the barriers that prevent them from engaging in an active lifestyle. There is also an emphasis on low rates of activity and high rates of sedentarism. However, Chap. 33 by Baker and colleagues reminds us that there are a group of highly active older people who participate in a range of sporting events. Understanding the physical activity 'life course' of these groups of highly active elders and examining what motivates them to engage in sport and physical activity may offer novel and enlightening insights on positive factors that we can promote more widely. Case studies of active elders such as masters athletes offer positive role models for older people and may offer another way of approaching increasing physical activity for older people.

31

Measurement of Physical Activity Among Older People

Nicolas Aguilar-Farias and Marijke Hopman-Rock

31.1 Introduction

Different subjective and objective methods have been used for measuring PA and SB in older adults. Subjective methods are defined as those that necessitate interpretation (e.g. questionnaire, diary, etc.), while objective methods are those that are not influenced by the individual's interpretation and perception (e.g. accelerometer, direct observation, etc.) (Swank 2012). Researchers and clinicians face special challenges when translating and interpreting results in older populations as every instrument, indistinctly of type, has advantages and limitations when using them in fieldwork (Table 31.1). For example, the most common subjective methods for measuring PA are questionnaires, but their accuracy for estimating total time spent in certain activity type during a day may be affected by different cognitive processes (such as attention and memory) that individuals experience when answering a question (van Uffelen et al. 2011). On the other hand, objective methods such as accelerometers may show high technical accuracy (i.e. inter-instrument reliability), but equations that use activity counts derived from acceleration may not be able to predict the actual Energy Expanding (EE) in activities performed by older

---

N. Aguilar-Farias (✉)
Departamento de Educación Física, Deportes y Recreación,
Universidad de La Frontera, Temuco, Chile

M. Hopman-Rock
EMGO Institute Department of Public and Occupational Health, VUmc,
Amsterdam, The Netherlands

© The Author(s) 2018
S. R. Nyman et al. (eds.), *The Palgrave Handbook of Ageing and Physical Activity Promotion*, https://doi.org/10.1007/978-3-319-71291-8_31

Table 31.1 Strengths and limitations of subjective and objective methodologies measuring physical activity (compiled from Strath et al. 2013; Swank 2012; Neuman et al. 2000; Ainslie et al. 2003)

	Strengths	Limitations
Subjective methods		
Questionnaires	Low cost Low burden Convenient/easy Applicable to large numbers of individuals Single time point assessment Valid to assess structured physical activity Can successfully rank into high/low categories Can assess different dimensions and domains	Recall and social desirability bias can occur Needs to be population and culture specific Low validity for assessing incidental or lifestyle physical activity
Diaries/logs	Low cost Detailed information on dimension and domains* Not subjected to memory or recall as much as other subjective methods Provides a good subjective measure of physical activity and energy expenditure	Very high burden on patients and participants Complex and time-consuming data reduction and analysis Similar to questionnaires, they should be population and culture specific
Proxy reports	Low cost Low burden Relatively easy to implement Can classify individuals into physical activity categories Applicable to hard-to-reach individuals (i.e. cognitively impaired)	Needs to select an adequate proxy to obtain reliable measures May not assess different physical activity domains as they may not be observable by the proxy respondent May be more valid to identify physical activity frequency than physical activity intensity May be subject to social desirability
Objective methods		
Observation	No recall necessary Provides excellent contextual information Provides detailed information on dimensions and domain	High burden on the observer Training essential to successfully administer assessment technique Can alter individual behaviour of the one being assessed

(continued)

Table 31.1 (continued)

	Strengths	Limitations
Indirect calorimetry	Highly accurate and reliable measure of physical activity and energy expenditure Suitable criterion measure of physical activity and energy expenditure	Expensive High degree of technical expertise required Short-time assessment only permissible and only one individual can be monitored at one time; large expense of measurements Systems require extensive calibration to ensure data integrity Portable systems are available and can measure for a few hours, but they are burdensome and can impact activities undertaken by patients or participants
Doubly labelled water	"Gold standard" measure for total daily energy expenditure in free-living individuals Low burden to patients or participants Applicable to a range of individuals and field conditions Energy expenditure is measured over long periods Safe and does not interfere with normal physiological conditions	Expensive Technical equipment and trained personnel required Measures of resting metabolic rate and thermic effect of food required to derive physical activity energy expenditure executed on a day High costs of oxygen-18—limits large group application Requires sophisticated equipment for analysis Error introduced if frequency is not known No information can be gained about brief or specific periods of activity Unable to discern dimensions or domains Patients required to collect urine sample
Heart rate	Low burden for short periods Relatively inexpensive Relationships strong with moderate-to-vigorous intensity Provides information on the amount of time spent in high-intensity activity Cheap and reusable	Affected by nonactivity stimuli (emotion, medication, caffeine) Weak relationship at low end of intensity realm Subject to interference with signal Large potential error in estimating energy expenditure Patients/participants may have sensitive skin Calibration requires technical expertise If individual calibration is used, may need prior physician consent

(continued)

Table 31.1 (continued)

	Strengths	Limitations
Accelerometer	Concurrent measure of movement Provides detailed intensity, frequency, and duration data Can store data for weeks at a time Low burden Relatively inexpensive	Cannot account for all activities, such as cycling, stair use, or activities that require lifting a load Upper-body activities neglected with hip or lower-back wear Data reduction transformation and processing take time Recommend seven days of monitoring to obtain habitual physical activity profile Positioning of the monitor is paramount and needs to conform to the calibration study characteristics
Pedometer	Low cost Low burden Easy data processing Applicable to large numbers of individuals Can also be used to motivate people	Simple pedometers cannot measure intensity/duration Cannot measure mode/type Not accurate for energy expenditure Depending on device, false steps can be recorded Some brands require user to write steps down If pedometer readings can be seen, likely to increase reactivity
Multisensing units	Accuracy improved compared with single sensing assessments	Higher cost Increased burden of wear for some devices Depending on device, technical expertise is essential Need to wear for a number of days to obtain a physical activity profile

*Notes: There are four dimensions and four domains. Dimensions include (1) mode or activity type, (2) frequency, (3) duration, and (4) intensity of performing activity. Domains include (1) leisure time that includes discretionary or recreational activities (e.g. sports, hobbies), (2) occupational that involves work-related activities (e.g. carrying objects, manual labour), (3) domestic activities (e.g. housework, childcare, self-care), and (4) transportation (e.g. walking, cycling, standing while riding transportation)

adults as activities may show different movement patterns as well as different daily frequency when compared with younger individuals (Strath et al. 2012; Taraldsen et al. 2012).

To better understand alternatives for measuring PA with their respective strengths and limitations, it is necessary to describe some terms (see Chap. 1). PA behaviour has four dimensions: (1) mode or activity type, (2) frequency, (3) duration, and (4) intensity of performing activity (Gabriel et al. and Woolsey

2012; Strath et al. 2013). *Mode* refers to the specific activity performed (e.g. walking, gardening, cycling) or the context of physiological and biomechanical types (e.g. aerobic activity, resistance training, stability exercise). *Frequency* is the number of sessions or activities during a specified time interval (e.g. week). *Duration* is defined as the time in minutes or hours of the activity on a given time frame (e.g. day). *Intensity* is the expression of the rate of EE, an indicator of the metabolic demand of an activity that can be quantified with physiological measures (e.g. heart rate), perceptual characteristics (e.g. rating of perceived effort; RPE), or by body movement (e.g. acceleration).

PA could also be described in terms of four domains that include (1) leisure time that includes discretionary or recreational activities (e.g. sports, hobbies), (2) occupational that involves work-related activities (e.g. carrying objects, manual labour), (3) domestic activities (e.g. housework, childcare, self-care), and (4) transportation (e.g. walking, cycling, standing while riding transportation) (Gabriel et al. 2012; Strath et al. 2013). PA domains are particularly important when understanding how PA is accrued as they define context and provide a better picture about the social aspects. This may be relevant when describing, for example, effects of a behavioural strategy on a specific context such as at work or identifying whether older adults are more active in their homes or leisure time.

Measurement tools are diverse and provide different outputs that are intended to reflect PA behaviours in all or most dimensions and domains (such as domestic work and sports activities). For this reason, some sets of definitions will be described in the following sections.

31.2 Measurement Units

31.2.1 Kilocalories

This unit is often used to describe the total amount of energy required to perform all the different PA energy expenditure (EE) executed on a day (PAEE). One litre of oxygen consumption is approximately equal to 5 kcal of energy (Katch et al. 2011). An important consideration when using kcal is that EE from ambulatory activities increases proportionally with the amount of body mass being moved. Therefore, it is common to see EE estimates for activities as kilocalories per kilogram of body mass per minute ($kcal \cdot kg^{-1} \cdot min^{-1}$) for allowing comparison between different activities or contrasting performed activities with energy intake, for example. Instruments such as accelerometers and heart rate monitors may be used to estimate PAEE in kcals with predictive equations.

31.2.2 Metabolic Equivalent

A metabolic equivalent (MET) is an estimate of intensity based on the ratio of oxygen uptake on a given activity to oxygen uptake at rest (3.5 mL·kg^{-1}·min^{-1}) (Swank 2012). METs can be converted to kilocalories (1 MET = 1 kcal·kg^{-1}·h^{-1}). It is a simple approach as METs are expressions of energy expended in multiples of resting EE. For example, three METs, which are the lower limit for moderate-intensity PA, imply that an individual is consuming three times the energy required at resting level. However, it is important to take into account that actual MET values may be different across individuals as resting metabolic rate may show different values due to age, sex, and body composition as well as energy cost derived from activities may vary depending on biomechanical changes derived from ageing or chronic conditions (Hortobagyi et al. 2003; Kozey et al. 2010; Schrack et al. 2012).

METs are often used to express total volumes of PA over a given time. PA volume is calculated by multiplying the PA intensity (METs), duration (minutes or hours), and frequency on a given time (day or week). For example, the total PA volume derived from the PA recommendation for an adult population of "doing 30 minutes of moderate-intensity PA on at least 5 days per week" is calculated as follows: 30 min (duration) × 3 METs (intensity) × 5 days (frequency) per week = 450 MET·min^{-1}·week^{-1}.

31.2.3 Physical Activity Intensities

A common measure of interest is the amount of time spent in a given PA intensity as most epidemiological and clinical evidence on PA has shown dose-response relationships with different conditions that are often expressed in these units.

Most instruments for estimating time in a given PA intensity at population level use absolute intensity measures rather than intensity in relative terms. *Absolute intensity* is determined by the external work performed (i.e. METs) and is categorised as sedentary (1–1.5 METs), light (>1.5–2.9 METs), moderate (3.0–5.9 METs), vigorous (6.0–8.9 METs), and very vigorous (≥9.0 METs) intensity (American College of Sports Medicine 2013). While *relative intensities* are determined using a percentage of an individual's level of cardiorespiratory fitness (VO$_2$max) or rating of perceived effort (RPE) (Strath et al. 2013). For example, light relative intensity is equivalent to 30–49% of the individual's maximal heart rate (HR$_{max}$) or 9–10 RPE, moderate relative intensity is equal to 50–69% HR$_{max}$ or 11–12 RPE, vigorous relative intensity is reached between 70% and 89% HR_{max} or 13–16 RPE, and very vigorous activities are performed when reaching ≥90% HR_{max} or >16 RPE.

31.3 Measurement Tools

In the following sections, the most common PA measurement tools will be described, including their advantages, limitations, and practical recommendations when using them in older adults in different settings (see also Forsen et al. 2010).

31.3.1 Subjective Methods

One of the main advantages for subjective instruments when compared with objective tools is the ability to not only measure PA dimensions but also PA domains. Therefore, these instruments should be tailored and include meaningful activities as examples (e.g. watering plants) to favour cognitive processes when answering the questions (Heesch et al. 2010; van Uffelen et al. 2011), and light intensity activities as they are highly prevalent in older adults (e.g. washing dishes) (Forsen et al. 2010).

31.3.2 Global Physical Activity Questionnaires

Global PA questionnaires (PAQ) are short (two to four items to be self-completed) and provide a quick overview of a person's PA level (Strath et al. 2013). Most instruments are designed to classify an individual as active or inactive (i.e. meeting PA guidelines of 150 min/week of moderate-to-vigorous PA) or focused on specific activities (e.g. walking). Despite their simplicity, some PAQs have shown to be reliable (Intraclass correlation (ICC) = 0.32–0.91) and associated with steps per day (r = 0.33–0.54, p < 0.0001), total accelerometer counts per day (r = 0.46–0.60, p < 0.001) (Pettee Gabriel et al. 2009), and with doubly labelled water (DLW) (Bonnefoy et al. 2001). Among these questionnaires, the Women's Health Initiative PAQ (WHI PAQ, designed for postmenopausal women) is one of those that have shown the highest reliability (ICC = 0.91, p < 0.0001), while the Stanford Usual PAQ has shown the highest correlation with DLW for both moderate and vigorous intensity PA (r = 0.65 and 0.63, respectively) (Bonnefoy et al. 2001).

The main advantage of these instruments is their simplicity and ease of administration, but they are limited when providing information about some specific domains and intensities (e.g. light PA) and estimating dose-response relationships (Ainsworth et al. 2015).

31.3.3 Short-Term Recall Questionnaires

Short-term recall questionnaires assess total volume of PA derived from dimensions and specific types of PA. Short-term recall generally has 7 to 20 items that determine PA performed in the past week (e.g. International Physical Activity Questionnaire, IPAQ; Bauman et al. 2009) or last month (e.g. CHAMPS Physical Activity Questionnaire for older adults, CHAMPS; Stewart et al. 2001). The summary score units of these instruments are often expressed in MET-min/week that are derived from time spent during a specific period in activities with predetermined EE estimates (e.g. 3.3 METs for walking or 4 METs for moderate-intensity activities in IPAQ). Then, this summary score allows the user to classify the individual as active which is 600 MET-min/week for the IPAQ (Craig et al. 2003).

Although the IPAQ was initially designed to be applied among adults aged 18–65, several studies have used the short form of this instrument for measuring PA in older populations. Grimm et al. (2012) reported that the IPAQ significantly overestimated time spent in almost all PA intensities and underestimated sitting. However, analysing group associations across measures showed significant relations in walking, total PA, and sitting ($r = 0.29$–0.36, $p < 0.05$). Agreement was 40–46% between IPAQ and accelerometer measures for meeting PA guidelines. These findings suggest that the IPAQ may not perform well at individual level but well at group-level or population-based samples. An advantage of this instrument is the large amount of population-based data that allow multiple comparisons across countries. On the other hand, the IPAQ does not consider PA reports by domains, but there is another questionnaire with similar structure that covers this issue, the Global Physical Activity Questionnaire (GPAQ) (Bauman et al. 2009).

The last limitation of self-report measures, including the IPAQ, is the inability to be sensitive to change in PA behaviour (Bauman et al. 2009). However, the CHAMPS has shown ability to detect change in PA behaviour derived from an intervention ($p < 0.001$), including changes in frequency and caloric expenditure per week for all activity types and moderate-to-vigorous PA (Stewart et al. 2001). Therefore, the CHAMPS may be useful for simply assessing the effectiveness of PA interventions in older adults.

31.3.4 PA Logs and Diaries

PA logs and diaries are instruments that require the participant or patient to log activities performed during the day (e.g. diary) or in 15-minute or 1-hour periods (e.g. logs) in a recording sheet. Most logs and diaries are scored by use of the "Compendium of Physical Activities" which includes more than 800 different activities with their respective MET values (Ainsworth et al. 2011). As individuals are required to record PA in real time or the same day, these instruments are less susceptible to recall bias, measurement bias, and social desirability (van der Ploeg et al. 2010). On the other hand, both PA logs and diaries are burdensome and may be subject to memory bias when not completed in real time. Participants who use these instruments may also change their behaviour which is described as reactivity, due to awareness of being measured or observed (Sylvia et al. 2014). A commonly used PA log is the Bouchard's Physical Activity Record (BAR) (Bouchard et al. 1983) in which participants are required to report PA for each 15-minute interval over three days. Activities are categorised on a scale of 1–9 that corresponds to a range of 1.0–7.8 METs to estimate total EE. The BAR has shown high reliability (0.86–0.95) (Bouchard et al. 1983) in adult population, but feasibility or validation studies in older populations are lacking.

Some validation efforts have been made in older adult population. Vanroy et al. (2014) validated a seven-day PA diary that used 30-minute intervals with description of the activity, position, and intensity in stroke patients. The correlation between the patients' and the observers' diaries was high for MET·minutes ($r = 0.75$, $p < 0.01$), sedentary activity levels ($r = 0.74$, $p < 0.01$), and moderate activity levels ($r = 0.71$, $p < 0.01$). However, correlation for estimating EE was not significant when comparing diary with accelerometer measures. Promising results have been reported for cell phone-based PA diaries (Sternfeld et al. 2012). A pilot study in a middle-age (45–65 years) sample showed that cell phone and paper diaries are equivalent, while being acceptable to users and reliable, with poor to moderate validity for estimating EE. Another instrument that combines a diary format with a past-day recall, the Multimedia Activity Recall in Children and Adults (MARCA), has shown high reliability and moderate validity for measuring both sedentary behaviour (Aguilar-Farias et al. 2015) and moderate-to-vigorous PA (Mace et al. 2014).

Although most logs and diaries have shown poor correlation for estimating total EE per day, these instruments appear to be feasible to implement and provide relevant contextual and time-use information that may be useful when planning, for example, behaviour change strategies. However, there are some practical considerations when using diaries or logs such as providing clear instructions and implementing mechanisms to promote compliance to fill the logs. In addition, users must consider the time and effort needed to reduce, clean, and analyse data when planning or administering resources for a study or assessment (Strath et al. 2013).

31.3.5 Proxy Reports

When patients or participants are unable to answer for themselves due to cognitive decline, unwillingness to report, inability to reach, intercurrent illness, or death (but you still need these data in studies), some data may be gathered from proxies (Hardy et al. 2009; Lynn Snow et al. 2005). Therefore, it is common to observe reliance on proxy reports as the age of the respondents in a study increases (Neumann et al. 2000). Proxy reports have been commonly used in older adults for reporting physical functioning and cognitive impairment (Magaziner et al. 1996; Middleton et al. 2010). In the last study, they used a proxy report measure for estimating PA levels in a longitudinal study that included two questions addressing the frequency and intensity of exercise. Participants were classified as a "high exerciser" (carry out PA three or more times per week, more intense than walking), a "moderate exerciser" (carry out PA three or more times per week, equal intensity to walking), or a "low exerciser" (all other exercisers) or "no exerciser", using the classification validated by the Canadian Study of Health and Aging (CSHA) (Davis et al. 2001). Although the instrument's inter-rater reliability was moderate (0.55, 95% CI 0.49–0.61), the proxy report was able to detect that people who had higher proxy-reported PA survived longer than those with lower PA levels. In both those who were cognitively impaired and those who were not, those who exercised were at a lower risk of mortality in a dose-response manner (the more they exercised the lower the risk) ($p < 0.001$). However, participants with cognitive impairment were more likely to die at any exercise level than those with normal cognition. Therefore, the authors suggested that the proxy report is not only valid but may also be a cost-effective and time-efficient tool for classifying individuals with cognitive impairment in PA categories (Middleton et al. 2010).

A key element to consider when using proxy reports for PA is that reliability on proxy reports may be influenced by both respondent characteristics and the type of data requested (Hardy et al. 2009; Neumann et al. 2000). For example, proxies who live with the participant or patient provide responses with higher reliability than those who interact with the person less often. Similarly, those proxies who are depressed or pessimistic may tend to overestimate an impairment (Neumann et al. 2000). Also, higher agreement between proxies and participants has been observed for observable variables (e.g. physical functioning) and lower agreement for subjective factors such as emotional symptoms or pain (Hardy et al. 2009; Magaziner 1997; Neumann et al. 2000). Therefore, when selecting and using a proxy report tool, it is relevant to choose a proxy with adequate knowledge of the patient or participant as well as it is recommended to use proxies for measures that have been previously validated.

31.4 Objective Methods

Objective methods provide more accurate estimates of physiological or mechanical parameters when compared with subjective methods (Westerterp 2009), which may be reflected in better ability for detecting change, for example. Also, some studies have reported stronger associations between PA and some metabolic markers or health outcomes when using objective methods compared with subjective instruments (Celis-Morales et al. 2012; Harris et al. 2009; Sabia et al. 2015). Yates et al. (2015) have reported that self-reported measures of PA may be limited when comparing ethnic groups. They found that despite PA levels were not different between ethnic groups when using objective measures (pedometer and accelerometer), differences were found with a self-report measurement tool (IPAQ; white populations reported less vigorous PA and less walking). Despite these advantages, Haskell (2012) mentioned that "being objective does not mean it is correct", as self-report methods provide valuable evidence such as contextual information that most objective methods are unable to specify as well as there are important limitations to consider when implementing data collection and interpretation (Table 31.1).

There are several objective instruments for measuring PA that have been designed to be used indistinctly of age (e.g. accelerometer). However, some researchers have suggested that tailored output interpretation of objective instruments may be required for older adults, because cognitive processes, behaviours, and physical characteristics change with ageing, thus affecting PA patterns and physiological outputs (Strath et al. 2012; Taraldsen et al. 2012; Van Domelen et al. 2014).

31.4.1 Measures of Energy Expenditure

Indirect Calorimetry Indirect calorimetry implies measuring the ventilator volume and the amounts of oxygen consumed and carbon dioxide produced (Strath et al. 2013). This method is considered the reference for measuring EE in laboratory conditions. Therefore, most subjective or objective instruments are validated against systems such as whole-body room calorimeters or computerized metabolic cart systems. In addition, portable calorimeters have allowed measuring EE in older adults in free-living environments to better understand activities performed in non-controlled conditions. However, more studies are needed to represent a wide range of meaningful activities for older adults (Hall et al. 2014).

Doubly Labelled Water Doubly labelled water (DLW) is a method that relies on the difference in elimination rates between two stable isotopes (oxygen-18, ^{18}O, and deuterium, ^{2}H) which are ingested in water (Ainslie et al. 2003). The difference in elimination through urine between these isotopes represents the carbon dioxide production during a given time in free-living conditions (4–20 days). This method is usually combined with measurements of resting metabolic rate and thermic effect of food (the energy required for digestion, absorption, and disposal of ingested nutrients) to estimate PAEE. For this reason, DLW has been commonly used as a reference for estimating total daily EE in free-living conditions (Ainslie et al. 2003; Colbert et al. 2011).

DLW has been safely applied to a range of individuals and field conditions while not interfering with normal physiological conditions (Ainslie et al. 2003). However, some considerations must be taken when selecting this method as it is expensive while requiring the participant to collect urine during the measurement process. In addition, DLW requires technical experts and sophisticated equipment for analysis, and no information can be obtained about brief periods of activity.

Direct Observation Direct observation involves watching an individual while performing physical activities at a given time. Most direct observation methods use small time intervals and coded scores for describing PA intensities to estimate EE, but they also may describe activity types, domains, location, and environmental or social context (Evenson et al. 2016; McKenzie et al. 2006; Strath et al. 2013). Tools such as the System for Observing Play and Recreation in Communities (SOPARC) have been used to produce relevant and highly reliable measures of context and activities performed in older populations from different communities (Evenson et al. 2016; Parra et al. 2010; Pleson et al. 2014).

31.4.2 Physiological Measures

Heart Rate Monitor Heart rate monitors (HRM) are the most common physiological measures in free-living environments due to their light weight and small size (Ainsworth et al. 2015; Strath et al. 2013). HRM are very useful for estimating relative intensity, but users must consider that heart rate may be influenced by external factors such as stress, emotions, or the action of medication (e.g. beta-blockers). EE from heart rate is based on the strong linear relationship observed between these parameters regardless of age or sex, including older adults (Schrack et al. 2014). HRM are excellent options for measuring activities in which accelerometers, for example, may be limited for estimating EE such as cycling or weightlifting (Chen et al. 2012, see Table 31.1).

31.4.3 Wearable Monitors

Pedometer A pedometer is a motion sensor that records movement as steps which is commonly worn on the waist; however, there are some devices designed to be used on the wrist or the ankle. There are many commercially available pedometers with different features (Floegel et al. 2016). Most pedometers are able to quantify steps and estimate distance based on a standard or customizable stride length (Martien et al. 2015). Further, new pedometers have included important features such as memory function that facilitates data extraction and minimizes bias, because some simple pedometers require the participant to log the steps and reset the device at the end of each day.

Several brands have been used in research (e.g. Omron, New Lifestyles, Yamax, SC-StepRx, StepWatch) ranging in prices from US$25 to US$2000. In general, pedometers have shown excellent reliability and higher validity for counting steps than for predicting EE (Crouter et al. 2003; Evenson et al. 2015). However, pedometers have shown low validity when counting steps at slow walking speeds (e.g. <2.5 km/h) (Crouter et al. 2003; Martien et al. 2015). Therefore, a user may be cautious when using pedometers in frail older people, but confident in their use in healthy older adults for both assessment and interventions (Cyarto et al. 2004). New technologies have emerged in the last years to minimize those sources of error such as pedometers that integrate accelerations and postures in the algorithms to estimate step count or predict EE (Ainsworth et al. 2015).

Consumer-based PA pedometers have become popular, as new models are accessible, affordable, and compatible with diverse operative systems (e.g. computers or mobile phone) showing promising results. Floegel et al. (2016) reported high reliability and low percent error for a hip-worn (Fitbit One) and wrist-worn (Jawbone UP) activity monitors for measuring steps in older adults with non-impaired and impaired ambulation during self-paced walking. However, some consumer-based devices have shown limited validity when estimating total EE (Lee et al. 2014; Nelson et al. 2016).

Accelerometer Accelerometers are small devices that record accelerations of the body in gravitational swing on one or more planes in a time-stamped format. These sensors are able to capture PA with components of frequency, intensity, and duration. Therefore, accelerometers are commonly used to predict EE or typically estimate time spent on a given PA intensity. These devices are usually attached to the body using a strap (e.g. ActiGraph, Dynaport) or sticker (e.g. ActivPAL). Accelerometers allow collecting high-resolution data from individuals for several days or weeks as they have included many improvements in terms of memory and battery in the last years (Ainsworth et al. 2015). There are many brands in the market with prices ranging from US$150 to US$600 and most provide EE estimates and steps (e.g. Actical, ActiGraph), but others provide postural information (e.g. ActivPAL, Dynaport, GENEActiv) which is important for measuring sedentary behaviour, for example.

Acceleration units are often transformed into accelerometer counts which are not comparable between accelerometer brands (Strath et al. 2013). These outcomes have been often expressed as counts on a given unit of time (e.g. counts per minute) to summarize measured activity into PA levels (i.e. sedentary, light, moderate, or vigorous) that are derived from previously validated accelerometer thresholds specific for each accelerometer brand, model, and monitor location (e.g. wrist, hip, thigh, ankle) (Schrack et al. 2016). This has been under controversy as there are too many PA cut-points affecting comparability between studies and populations when different brands are used (Schrack et al. 2016; Strath et al. 2013; Taraldsen et al. 2012). This method has shown important limitations when estimating EE as accelerometer counts on a given time (e.g. one minute) may not reflect an activity pattern, especially in free-living environments, as activities are often performed intermittently in short bouts (e.g. vacuuming) (Kamada et al. 2016). Some efforts have been made to face this limitation with the use of raw acceleration data for extracting and using the accelerometer signals with machine learning algorithms

(Schrack et al. 2016). This method of analysis has shown better performance for correctly classifying activities into intensities or types, and predict EE (Lyden et al. 2014), but requiring more complex analysis than using the cut-point method.

Multisensor Systems Multisensing assessment methods combine multiple physiological and mechanical parameters to provide more accurate estimates of PA and EE. There are different measures that may be combined in these instruments such as accelerometry, heart rate, global positioning, respiration, temperature, skin contact, and so on. The Actiheart system (CamNtech Ltd., Cambridge, UK) has shown higher accuracy for predicting EE for walking and running when combining its accelerometer and heart rate sensor than using only accelerometer (Brage et al. 2005). Other devices such as the Zephyr Bioharness (Zephyr Technology Corp., MD, USA) that include accelerometry, heart rate, global positioning, and respiration in a chest-worn strap have shown comparable results with indirect calorimetry for predicting EE in young adult population (Brooks et al. 2013). These devices can be also used to produce real-time postural and heart rate feedback in group sessions.

31.5 Considerations when Selecting a Tool

Different factors should be taken into account and balanced when selecting a PA measurement tool before implementing a protocol or starting data collection: (1) consideration of outcomes, (2) feasibility or practicality, (3) resources, (4) administration, and (5) validity of the instrument (for details see Masse and de Niet 2012; Strath et al. 2013; American Educational Research Association, American Psychological Association, National Council on Measurement in Education, & Testing 1999). We will now focus on validity only.

Validity is a unitary concept that implies the degree to which all of the accumulated evidence supports the intended interpretation of test scores for the intended purposes of an instrument (American Educational Research Association, American Psychological Association, National Council on Measurement in Education, & Testing 1999). Masse and de Niet (2012) have provided different examples for sources of validity evidence needed that should be considered when selecting a measurement tool for different situations in the field of PA. There are five sources of validity evidence: (1) *evidence based on test content* consists of determining whether the measure comprehensively represents the domains or dimensions associated with the construct;

(2) *evidence based on response processes* examines the extent to which the responses provided by the respondents demonstrate that they understood what they were asked to recall; (3) *evidence based on the behavioural stability of responses or measures* is most often referred to as assessing the consistency of responses over time; (4) *evidence based on relations with other variables* that consists of examining the relationship between measures of PA and an instrument that assesses the same construct or a construct associated to PA (e.g. minutes of activities, steps, accelerometer counts, EE); and (5) *evidence based on sensitivity to change* that aims to test whether the measure is able to detect change in PA behaviour (Masse and de Niet 2012). Each of these sources of validity evidence is required in different extent when selecting a tool. For example, in the case of surveillance aimed at monitoring levels of PA in older adults over time, we should consider all sources of validity evidence, except for evidence based on sensitivity to change as we need to produce stable estimates of PA at population level, although the estimate may be biased (e.g. a self-report method that consistently overestimates/underestimates minutes of PA or SB). On the other hand, when planning the assessment of an intervention aimed at quantifying the magnitude of change in PA, all sources of evidence should be considered, especially the evidence on sensitivity to change as some instruments may show differences with previous or basal measures, but they may not be reflecting an actual change in behaviour but reflecting measurement error or lack of stability of the instrument. In this case, some objective instruments may have the advantage versus subjective instruments as they may be able to detect smaller changes in PA (e.g. minutes vs hours), resulting in better tools for assessing the effect of an intervention at individual level, for example.

31.6 Conclusion

A lot of instruments and methods are available to measure physical activity in older adults, and careful consideration is needed to make the appropriate choice of measuring to be used depending upon the underlying reason for measuring physical activity.

Suggested Further Reading
- Strath, S. J., Kaminsky, L. A., Ainsworth, B. E., Ekelund, U., Freedson, P. S., Gary, R. A., et al. (2013). Guide to the assessment of physical activity: Clinical and research applications: A scientific statement from the American Heart

Association. *Circulation, 128*(20), 2259–2279. https://doi.org/10.1161/01.cir.0000435708.67487.da.
- University of Pittsburgh. (2016). Physical Activity Resource Center for Public Health. Retrieved from http://www.parcph.org/

References

Aguilar-Farias, N., Brown, W. J., Olds, T. S., & Peeters, G. M. (2015). Validity of self-report methods for measuring sedentary behaviour in older adults. *Journal of Science & Medicine in Sports & Exercise, 18*(6), 662–666. https://doi.org/10.1016/j.jsams.2014.08.004.

Ainslie, P., Reilly, T., & Westerterp, K. (2003). Estimating human energy expenditure: A review of techniques with particular reference to doubly labelled water. *Sports Medicine, 33*(9), 683–698.

Ainsworth, B. E., Haskell, W. L., Herrmann, S. D., Meckes, N., Bassett, D. R., Jr., Tudor-Locke, C., et al. (2011). 2011 compendium of physical activities: A second update of codes and MET values. *Medicine & Science in Sports & Exercise, 43*(8), 1575–1581. https://doi.org/10.1249/MSS.0b013e31821ece12.

Ainsworth, B., Cahalin, L., Buman, M., & Ross, R. (2015). The current state of physical activity assessment tools. *Progress in Cardiovascular Diseases, 57*(4), 387–395. https://doi.org/10.1016/j.pcad.2014.10.005.

American College of Sports Medicine. (2013). *ACSM's guidelines for exercise testing and prescription* (9th ed.). Philadelphia: Lippincott Williams & Wilkins.

American Educational Research Association, American Psychological Association, & National Council on Measurement in Education. (1999). *Standards for educational and psychological testing*. Washington, DC: American Educational Research Association.

Bauman, A., Ainsworth, B. E., Bull, F., Craig, C. L., Hagstromer, M., Sallis, J. F., et al. (2009). Progress and pitfalls in the use of the international physical activity questionnaire (IPAQ) for adult physical activity surveillance. *Journal of Physical Activity and Health, 6*(Suppl 1), S5–S8.

Bonnefoy, M., Normand, S., Pachiaudi, C., Lacour, J. R., Laville, M., & Kostka, T. (2001). Simultaneous validation of ten physical activity questionnaires in older men: A doubly labeled water study. *Journal of the American Geriatrics Society, 49*(1), 28–35.

Bouchard, C., Tremblay, A., Leblanc, C., Lortie, G., Savard, R., & Theriault, G. (1983). A method to assess energy expenditure in children and adults. *American Journal of Clinical Nutrition, 37*(3), 461–467.

Brage, S., Brage, N., Franks, P. W., Ekelund, U., & Wareham, N. J. (2005). Reliability and validity of the combined heart rate and movement sensor Actiheart. *European Journal of Clinical Nutrition, 59*(4), 561–570. https://doi.org/10.1038/sj.ejcn.1602118.

Brooks, K. A., Carter, J. G., & Dawes, J. J. (2013). A comparison of VO2 measurement obtained by a physiological monitoring device and the Cosmed quark CPET. *Journal of Novel Physiotherapies, 3.* https://doi.org/10.4172/2165-7025.1000126.

Celis-Morales, C. A., Perez-Bravo, F., Ibanez, L., Salas, C., Bailey, M. E., & Gill, J. M. (2012). Objective vs. self-reported physical activity and sedentary time: Effects of measurement method on relationships with risk biomarkers. *PLoS One, 7*(5), e36345. https://doi.org/10.1371/journal.pone.0036345.

Chen, K. Y., Janz, K. F., Zhu, W., & Brychta, R. J. (2012). Redefining the roles of sensors in objective physical activity monitoring. *Medicine & Science in Sports & Exercise, 44*(1 Suppl 1), S13–S23. https://doi.org/10.1249/MSS.0b013e3182399bc8.

Colbert, L. H., Matthews, C. E., Havighurst, T. C., Kim, K., & Schoeller, D. A. (2011). Comparative validity of physical activity measures in older adults. *Medicine & Science in Sports & Exercise, 43*(5), 867–876. https://doi.org/10.1249/MSS.0b013e3181fc7162.

Craig, C. L., Marshall, A. L., Sjostrom, M., Bauman, A. E., Booth, M. L., Ainsworth, B. E., et al. (2003). International physical activity questionnaire: 12-country reliability and validity. *Medicine & Science in Sports & Exercise, 35*(8), 1381–1395. https://doi.org/10.1249/01.MSS.0000078924.61453.FB.

Crouter, S. E., Schneider, P. L., Karabulut, M., & Bassett, D. R., Jr. (2003). Validity of 10 electronic pedometers for measuring steps, distance, and energy cost. *Medicine & Science in Sports & Exercise, 35*(8), 1455–1460. https://doi.org/10.1249/01.MSS.0000078932.61440.A2.

Cyarto, E. V., Myers, A., & Tudor-Locke, C. (2004). Pedometer accuracy in nursing home and community-dwelling older adults. *Medicine & Science in Sports & Exercise, 36*(2), 205–209. https://doi.org/10.1249/01.MSS.0000113476.62469.98.

Davis, H. S., MacPherson, K., Merry, H. R., Wentzel, C., & Rockwood, K. (2001). Reliability and validity of questions about exercise in the Canadian Study of Health and Aging. *International Psychogeriatrics, 13*(S1), 177–182.

Evenson, K. R., Goto, M. M., & Furberg, R. D. (2015). Systematic review of the validity and reliability of consumer-wearable activity trackers. *International Journal of Behavioral Nutrition and Physical Activity, 12*, 159. https://doi.org/10.1186/s12966-015-0314-1.

Evenson, K. R., Jones, S. A., Holliday, K. M., Cohen, D. A., & McKenzie, T. L. (2016). Park characteristics, use, and physical activity: A review of studies using SOPARC (system for observing play and recreation in communities). *Preventive Medicine, 86*, 153–166. https://doi.org/10.1016/j.ypmed.2016.02.029.

Floegel, T. A., Florez-Pregonero, A., Hekler, E. B., & Buman, M. P. (2016). Validation of consumer-based hip and wrist activity monitors in older adults with varied ambulatory abilities. *The Journals of Gerontology. Series A Biological Sciences and Medical Sciences.* https://doi.org/10.1093/gerona/glw098.

Forsen, L., Loland, N. W., Vuillemin, A., Chinapaw, M. J., van Poppel, M. N., Mokkink, L. B., et al. (2010). Self-administered physical activity questionnaires for the elderly: A systematic review of measurement properties. *Sports Medicine, 40*(7), 601–623. https://doi.org/10.2165/11531350-000000000-00000.

Gabriel, K. K. P., Jr., Morrow, J. R., & Woolsey, A.-L. T. (2012). Framework for physical activity as a complex and multidimensional behavior. *Journal of Physical Activity and Health, 9*(s1), S11–S18. https://doi.org/10.1123/jpah.9.s1.s11.

Grimm, E. K., Swartz, A. M., Hart, T., Miller, N. E., & Strath, S. J. (2012). Comparison of the IPAQ-short form and accelerometry predictions of physical activity in older adults. *Journal of Aging and Physical Activity, 20*(1), 64–79.

Hall, K. S., Morey, M. C., Dutta, C., Manini, T. M., Weltman, A. L., Nelson, M. E., et al. (2014). Activity-related energy expenditure in older adults: A call for more research. *Medicine & Science in Sports & Exercise.* https://doi.org/10.1249/MSS.0000000000000356.

Hardy, S. E., Allore, H., & Studenski, S. A. (2009). Missing data: A special challenge in aging research. *Journal of the American Geriatric Society, 57*(4), 722–729. https://doi.org/10.1111/j.1532-5415.2008.02168.x.

Harris, T. J., Owen, C. G., Victor, C. R., Adams, R., Ekelund, U., & Cook, D. G. (2009). A comparison of questionnaire, accelerometer, and pedometer: Measures in older people. *Medicine & Science in Sports & Exercise, 41*(7), 1392–1402. https://doi.org/10.1249/MSS.0b013e31819b3533.

Haskell, W. L. (2012). Physical activity by self-report: A brief history and future issues. *Journal of Physical Activity and Health, 9*(Suppl 1), S5–10.

Heesch, K. C., van Uffelen, J. G., Hill, R. L., & Brown, W. J. (2010). What do IPAQ questions mean to older adults? Lessons from cognitive interviews. *International Journal of Behavioral Nutrition and Physical Activity, 7*, 35. https://doi.org/10.1186/1479-5868-7-35.

Hortobagyi, T., Mizelle, C., Beam, S., & DeVita, P. (2003). Old adults perform activities of daily living near their maximal capabilities. *The Journals of Gerontology. Series A, Biological Sciences and Medical Sciences, 58*(5), M453–M460.

Kamada, M., Shiroma, E. J., Harris, T. B., & Lee, I. M. (2016). Comparison of physical activity assessed using hip- and wrist-worn accelerometers. *Gait & Posture, 44*, 23–28. https://doi.org/10.1016/j.gaitpost.2015.11.005.

Katch, V. L., McArdle, W. D., & Katch, F. I. (2011). Energy expenditure during rest and physical activity. In W. D. McArdle, F. I. Katch, & V. L. Katch (Eds.), *Essentials of exercise physiology* (4th ed.). Baltimore: Lippincott Williams & Wilkins.

Kozey, S., Lyden, K., Staudenmayer, J., & Freedson, P. (2010). Errors in MET estimates of physical activities using 3.5 ml × kg(−1) × min(−1) as the baseline oxygen consumption. *Journal of Physical Activity and Health, 7*(4), 508–516.

Lee, J. M., Kim, Y., & Welk, G. J. (2014). Validity of consumer-based physical activity monitors. *Medicine & Science in Sports & Exercise, 46*(9), 1840–1848. https://doi.org/10.1249/MSS.0000000000000287.

Lyden, K., Keadle, S. K., Staudenmayer, J., & Freedson, P. S. (2014). A method to estimate free-living active and sedentary behavior from an accelerometer. *Medicine & Science in Sports & Exercise, 46*(2), 386–397. https://doi.org/10.1249/MSS.0b013e3182a42a2d.

Lynn Snow, A., Cook, K. F., Lin, P. S., Morgan, R. O., & Magaziner, J. (2005). Proxies and other external raters: Methodological considerations. *Health Services Research, 40*(5 Pt 2), 1676–1693. https://doi.org/10.1111/j.1475-6773.2005.00447.x.

Mace, C. J., Maddison, R., Olds, T., & Kerse, N. (2014). Validation of a computerized use of time recall for activity measurement in advanced-aged adults. *Journal of Aging and Physical Activity, 22*(2), 245–254. https://doi.org/10.1123/japa.2012-0280.

Magaziner, J. (1997). Use of proxies to measure health and functional outcomes in effectiveness research in persons with Alzheimer disease and related disorders. *Alzheimer Disease & Associated Disorders, 11*(Suppl 6), 168–174.

Magaziner, J., Bassett, S. S., Hebel, J. R., & Gruber-Baldini, A. (1996). Use of proxies to measure health and functional status in epidemiologic studies of community-dwelling women aged 65 years and older. *American Journal of Epidemiology, 143*(3), 283–292.

Martien, S., Delecluse, C., Seghers, J., & Boen, F. (2015). Counting steps in institutionalized older adults during daily life activities: The validation of two motion sensors. *Journal of Aging and Physical Activity, 23*(3), 383–390. https://doi.org/10.1123/japa.2013-0223.

Masse, L. C., & de Niet, J. E. (2012). Sources of validity evidence needed with self-report measures of physical activity. *Journal of Physical Activity and Health, 9*(Suppl 1), S44–S55.

McKenzie, T. L., Cohen, D. A., Sehgal, A., Williamson, S., & Golinelli, D. (2006). System for observing play and recreation in communities (SOPARC): Reliability and feasibility measures. *Journal of Physical Activity and Health, 3*(Suppl 1), S208–S222.

Middleton, L. E., Kirkland, S. A., Mitnitski, A., & Rockwood, K. (2010). Proxy reports of physical activity were valid in older people with and without cognitive impairment. *Journal of Clinical Epidemiology, 63*(4), 435–440. https://doi.org/10.1016/j.jclinepi.2009.06.009.

Nelson, M. B., Kaminsky, L. A., Dickin, D. C., & Montoye, A. H. (2016). Validity of consumer-based physical activity monitors for specific activity types. *Medicine & Science in Sports & Exercise, 48*(8), 1619–1628. https://doi.org/10.1249/MSS.0000000000000933.

Neumann, P. J., Araki, S. S., & Gutterman, E. M. (2000). The use of proxy respondents in studies of older adults: Lessons, challenges, and opportunities. *Journal of the American Geriatrics Society, 48*(12), 1646–1654. https://doi.org/10.1111/j.1532-5415.2000.tb03877.x.

Parra, D. C., McKenzie, T. L., Ribeiro, I. C., Ferreira Hino, A. A., Dreisinger, M., Coniglio, K., et al. (2010). Assessing physical activity in public parks in Brazil using systematic observation. *American Journal of Public Health, 100*(8), 1420–1426. https://doi.org/10.2105/AJPH.2009.181230.

Pettee Gabriel, K., McClain, J. J., Lee, C. D., Swan, P. D., Alvar, B. A., Mitros, M. R., & Ainsworth, B. E. (2009). Evaluation of physical activity measures used in middle-aged women. *Medicine & Science in Sports & Exercise, 41*(7), 1403–1412. https://doi.org/10.1249/MSS.0b013e31819b2482.

Pleson, E., Nieuwendyk, L. M., Lee, K. K., Chaddah, A., Nykiforuk, C. I., & Schopflocher, D. (2014). Understanding older adults' usage of community green spaces in Taipei, Taiwan. *International Journal of Environmental Research and Public Health, 11*(2), 1444–1464. https://doi.org/10.3390/ijerph110201444.

Sabia, S., Cogranne, P., van Hees, V. T., Bell, J. A., Elbaz, A., Kivimaki, M., & Singh-Manoux, A. (2015). Physical activity and adiposity markers at older ages: Accelerometer vs questionnaire data. *Journal of the American Medical Directors Association, 16*(5), 438 e437–438 e413. https://doi.org/10.1016/j.jamda.2015.01.086.

Schrack, J. A., Simonsick, E. M., Chaves, P. H., & Ferrucci, L. (2012). The role of energetic cost in the age-related slowing of gait speed. *Journal of the American Geriatrics Society, 60*(10), 1811–1816. https://doi.org/10.1111/j.1532-5415.2012.04153.x.

Schrack, J. A., Zipunnikov, V., Goldsmith, J., Bandeen-Roche, K., Crainiceanu, C. M., & Ferrucci, L. (2014). Estimating energy expenditure from heart rate in older adults: A case for calibration. *PLoS One, 9*(4), e93520. https://doi.org/10.1371/journal.pone.0093520.

Schrack, J. A., Cooper, R., Koster, A., Shiroma, E. J., Murabito, J. M., Rejeski, W. J., et al. (2016). Assessing daily physical activity in older adults: Unraveling the complexity of monitors, measures, and methods. *Journals of Gerontology. Series A Biological Sciences and Medical Sciences, 71*(8), 1039–1048. https://doi.org/10.1093/gerona/glw026.

Sternfeld, B., Jiang, S. F., Picchi, T., Chasan-Taber, L., Ainsworth, B., & Quesenberry, C. P., Jr. (2012). Evaluation of a cell phone-based physical activity diary. *Medicine & Science in Sports & Exercise, 44*(3), 487–495. https://doi.org/10.1249/MSS.0b013e3182325f45.

Stewart, A. L., Mills, K. M., King, A. C., Haskell, W. L., Gillis, D., & Ritter, P. L. (2001). CHAMPS physical activity questionnaire for older adults: Outcomes for interventions. *Medicine & Science in Sports & Exercise, 33*(7), 1126–1141.

Strath, S. J., Pfeiffer, K. A., & Whitt-Glover, M. C. (2012). Accelerometer use with children, older adults, and adults with functional limitations. *Medicine & Science in Sports & Exercise, 44*(1 Suppl 1), S77–S85. https://doi.org/10.1249/MSS.0b013e3182399eb1.

Strath, S. J., Kaminsky, L. A., Ainsworth, B. E., Ekelund, U., Freedson, P. S., Gary, R. A., et al. (2013). Guide to the assessment of physical activity: Clinical and research applications: A scientific statement from the American Heart Association. *Circulation, 128*(20), 2259–2279. https://doi.org/10.1161/01.cir.0000435708.67487.da.

Swank, A. M. (2012). Chapter 13. Assessment of physical activity. In D. P. Swain, C. A. Brawner, & American College of Sports Medicine (Eds.), *ACSM's resource manual for guidelines for exercise testing and prescription*. Philadelphia: Lippincott Williams & Wilkins.

Sylvia, L. G., Bernstein, E. E., Hubbard, J. L., Keating, L., & Anderson, E. J. (2014). Practical guide to measuring physical activity. *Journal of the Academy of Nutrition and Dietetics, 114*(2), 199–208. https://doi.org/10.1016/j.jand.2013.09.018.

Taraldsen, K., Chastin, S. F., Riphagen, I. I., Vereijken, B., & Helbostad, J. L. (2012). Physical activity monitoring by use of accelerometer-based body-worn sensors in older adults: A systematic literature review of current knowledge and applications. *Maturitas, 71*(1), 13–19. https://doi.org/10.1016/j.maturitas.2011.11.003.

van der Ploeg, H. P., Merom, D., Chau, J. Y., Bittman, M., Trost, S. G., & Bauman, A. E. (2010). Advances in population surveillance for physical activity and sedentary behavior: Reliability and validity of time use surveys. *American Journal of Epidemiology, 172*(10), 1199–1206. https://doi.org/10.1093/aje/kwq265.

Van Domelen, D. R., Caserotti, P., Brychta, R. J., Harris, T. B., Patel, K. V., Chen, K. Y., et al. (2014). Is there a sex difference in accelerometer counts during walking in older adults? *Journal of Physical Activity and Health, 11*(3), 626–637. https://doi.org/10.1123/jpah.2012-0050.

van Uffelen, J. G., Heesch, K. C., Hill, R. L., & Brown, W. J. (2011). A qualitative study of older adults' responses to sitting-time questions: Do we get the information we want? *BMC Public Health, 11*, 458.

Vanroy, C., Vanlandewijck, Y., Cras, P., Feys, H., Truijen, S., Michielsen, M., & Vissers, D. (2014). Is a coded physical activity diary valid for assessing physical activity level and energy expenditure in stroke patients? *PLoS One, 9*(6), e98735. https://doi.org/10.1371/journal.pone.0098735.

Westerterp, K. R. (2009). Assessment of physical activity: A critical appraisal. *European Journal of Applied Physiology, 105*(6), 823–828. https://doi.org/10.1007/s00421-009-1000-2.

Yates, T., Henson, J., Edwardson, C., Bodicoat, D. H., Davies, M. J., & Khunti, K. (2015). Differences in levels of physical activity between White and South Asian populations within a healthcare setting: Impact of measurement type in a cross-sectional study. *BMJ Open, 5*(7), e006181. https://doi.org/10.1136/bmjopen-2014-006181.

32

Reducing Sedentary Behaviour Among Older People

Gladys Onambele-Pearson, Jodi Ventre, and Jon Adam Brown

32.1 Introduction

The recommended levels of physical activity (PA) are seldom reached in Western societies. In the UK, for instance, the cost of care, as a consequence of lower than recommended physical activity, is an estimated £10 billion a year to the National Health Service (NHS). 'Game plan' (Strategy-Unit & DCMS 2002) estimated that a 10% increase in physical activity in adults would benefit England at least £500 million per year and save approximately 6,000 lives a year. Interestingly, however, new research suggests that sedentary behaviour (SB) (e.g. prolonged sitting to watch TV or use a computer, regardless of whether periods of physical activity are also part of habitual lifestyle) is a distinct health risk, independent of leisure time physical activity. Indeed, sedentary behaviour has negative effects on metabolic profile (a broad-spectrum blood test assessing the risk of developing ailments such as diabetes, liver disease, kidney disease, and even hypertension), cardiovascular health, and psycho-social well-being and stimulates obesity (Tremblay et al. 2010). This has led to the phenomenon coined 'the active couch potato'(see Fig. 32.1), whereby a person may exhibit participation in bouts of medium to high physical activity, yet be highly sedentary in the intervening periods (Tremblay et al. 2010).

G. Onambele-Pearson (✉) • J. Ventre • J. A. Brown
Department of Exercise & Sport Science, Manchester Metropolitan University, Crewe, Cheshire, UK

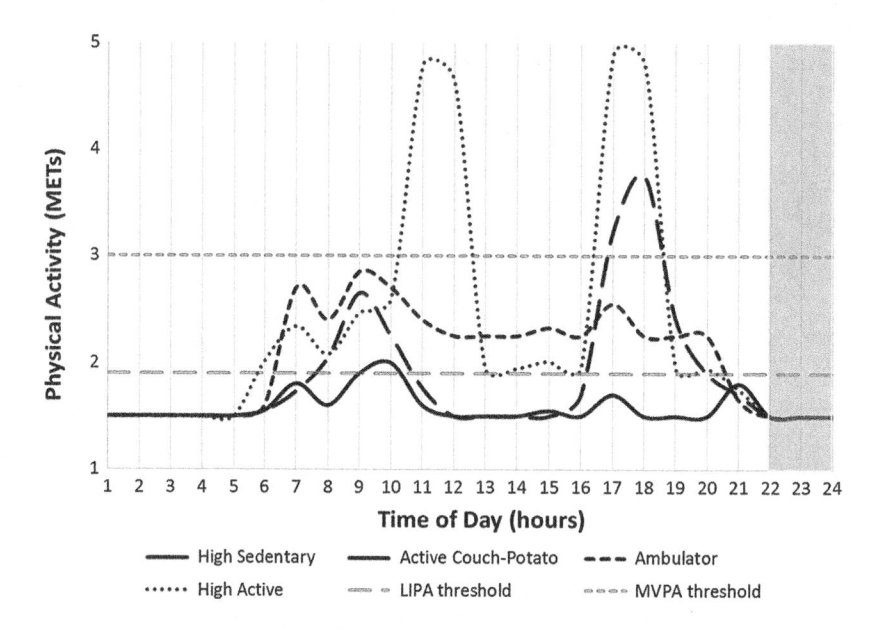

Fig. 32.1 Illustration of the four different types of physical activity patterns in adult humans. 1.0 MET is 1 kcal/kg/hour or 3.5 ml/kg/min of energy cost and is equivalent to sitting quietly

In older people in particular, sedentarism is a pressing problem as they spend a great deal of time sitting. 'Sedentary physiology' is an emerging and legitimate field of study that is complementary to, but distinct from, exercise physiology, as it aims to quantify the effects of sedentary behaviour. One definition of sedentarism is, thus, the extended engagement in behaviours characterised by minimal movement, low energy expenditure (meaning any activity requiring ≤1.5 metabolic equivalent tasks (METs) corresponding to resting metabolic rate), and rest (Owen et al. 2000; Pate et al. 2008). The following review of the literature gathers evidence that is current. Where available, the chapter emphasises data collected specifically using older persons, though the numbers of such studies are still limited.

32.2 The Effect of Sedentarism on Human Physiology

Up until recently, it was assumed that the National Health Service's (NHS 2013) recommendation that adults aged 19–64+ must carry out five bouts of 30 minutes of moderate-to-vigorous physical activity (MVPA) each week would be sufficient to ensure overall health. Disappointingly, a survey as recent as 2014 found that 47% of adults are still unable to describe the recommended guidelines for weekly physical activity (Hunter et al. 2014). This may explain the 60% of Northern Irish and 80% of English adults who are not meeting the current recommended PA guidelines (Farrell et al. 2013). In parallel, it is becoming evident that even where adults meet the NHS recommendation for habitual physical activity, this does not impact on the risk factors known to increase the incidence of cardiovascular disease (CVD). The above statistics are of great concern as they would suggest that for the segment of the population that does not meet the NHS recommendations of 150 minutes of weekly MVPA, the health prognosis must be even more worrying. In fact, exercise physiology is clear with regard to the fact that the greatest physiological benefits are from habitual physical activity rather than structured/time-limited exercise. Indeed previous authors (Turner et al. 2010) elegantly demonstrate this through a study in which at week 18 of a typical exercise intervention (which involved training for 50 minutes four times per week at 65% of maximum oxygen uptake (VO_{2max})), only 15% of the daily energy expenditure was spent during the prescribed exercises. In other words, even if a person should manage the 30 minutes daily requirements of MVPA in 16 waking hours, it is in fact what they do in the remaining 15.5 hours of daily waking time that matters most (Hamilton et al. 2008). To put this more succinctly, the greatest impact on overall health is likely to come from the habitual mobility a person adopts, rather than the generally recommended 30 minutes of structured/purposeful daily physical activity. This subtle point may be controversial to some, given the popularity of the old '30 minutes per day' recommendations.

32.2.1 Sedentary Behaviour Thresholds

In the first scale for describing sedentarism threshold, taking <5,000 steps/day is seen as a 'sedentary lifestyle index' (Tudor-Locke and Myers 2001) since persons within this mobility category exhibit a number of health concerns including obesity. Along similar lines, 'basal activity' is defined as <2,500 steps/day and 'limited activity' as 2,500–4,999 steps/day (Tudor-Locke et al. 2009).

Using a different scale, sedentary behaviour is also defined in terms of levels of energy expenditure through METs. Typically 1.0 MET (see Fig. 32.1) relates to 1 kcal/kg/hour of energy cost or 3.5 ml/kg/min and is equivalent to sitting quietly (Owen et al. 2010). Occupations such as office workers, receptionists, or supermarket cash register operators would typically spend long periods of their workday seated, thereby presenting high sedentary behaviour or sedentarism. Similarly, any person who sits for extended amounts of time to watch television, read, or even socialise with friends would equally present sedentarism. However, whilst the sedentarism threshold tends to be recognised as activities of up to 3 METs (Pate et al. 2008), this blurs the distinction between sedentary behaviour and light-intensity physical activities (LIPAs) of 1.9–2.9 METs. This is an issue since activities such as a slow-paced walk at 1.7mph which would elicit a 2.3 METs, would often not be picked up as part of the record of a person's habitual physical activity and hence lead to a person being incorrectly classified as sedentary. In fact, the overall daily energy expenditure of a person who walks at this pace to and from work, and spends their whole day standing, that is, an ambulatory (a shop worker for instance), may be even higher than that of a person who drives to work, sits at a desk all day, then attends a gymnasium for 30 minutes of MVPA, that is, an active couch potato (Owen et al. 2010). A body of work now only defines participants as sedentary if they engage in activities eliciting ≤1.5 METs) (Ainsworth et al. 2000; Rowlands et al. 2014; Tremblay et al. 2010).

This confusion of physical activity and sedentary behaviours along with current physical activity recommendations in fact means that in a recent study, approximately 90% of middle-aged men could be simultaneously described as both 'active' and 'not sufficiently active' (Thompson et al. 2009).

A third alternative scale to quantify thresholds for sedentarism utilises the accumulation of three-dimensional accelerometry-determined activity (Matthews et al. 2008). Through 3D accelerometry, it is found that sitting at a desk accumulates up to 50 counts/min, whereas driving a car accumulates up to 100 counts/min. The consensus therefore is that sedentary behaviour would be any activity resulting in ≤100 counts/min. A fourth scale is that jointly put forward by the Food and Agriculture Organization (FAO), the World Health Organization (WHO), and the United Nations University (UNU) (FAO/WHO/UNU 2001). It uses a ratio of energy expenditure and basal metabolic rate to give an estimation of physical activity levels (PAL). Thus, a PAL score of 1.40 or lower indicates a sedentary lifestyle.

It should therefore be clear from the above that, ultimately, studies should collect the entire continuum of physical activities through to sedentary behaviours in order to obtain a true picture of how health outcomes are likely to progress for a homogenous subpopulation. In other words, a person can only be described as sedentary based not only on a lack of MVPA in their lifestyle but also on levels of sedentary behaviours such as time spent lying or sitting down (Hamer and Stamatakis 2013). The importance of distinguishing between high sedentary behaviour and insufficient MVPA levels cannot be emphasised enough. Indeed it is very likely that previous studies have made erroneous statements regarding the health risks of engaging in different ambulatory lifestyles when they did not in fact systematically quantify sedentary behaviours per se (Owen et al. 2010; Pate et al. 2008). In fact, such omissions may be a significant contributor to the variability of responses to exercise training interventions both within studies and between studies, such as the HERITAGE (HEalth, RIsk factors, exercise Training And GEnetics) study (Bouchard et al. 1999). This was a large cohort study in which 130 families (both parents and at least three biological offspring) were entered in a 20-week exercise training regime, and their physiological and performance responses were used to identify genetic predisposition to the magnitude of exercise response. In the HERITAGE study, the magnitude of the training intervention-induced change in VO_{2max} showed a large variability (from no change to 1000 ml/min increase). An analysis of the typical population recruited in studies such as the HERITAGE project modelled how such variable responsiveness would come about through a range of habitual degrees of daily energy expenditure in the study population, from a few kilocalories to over 2000 Kcal daily (Thompson and Batterham 2013).

32.2.2 Health-Related Variables Shown to Be Influenced by SB

There is substantive evidence that a sedentary lifestyle, typified by a significant proportion of the day spent in a seated or reclined position, can put individuals at risk of various health limitations (Kim et al. 2013; Matthews et al. 2012). Spending long periods seated is, for example, associated with an increased chance of CVD in adults. Thus, prolonged periods of sitting to watch television has been associated with high blood pressure, heart disease, a decrease in vascular function and circulation, higher lactate and glucose levels, and in some cases, pulmonary embolism and deep vein thrombosis (de Rezende et al. 2014; Ford and Caspersen 2012; Kabrhel et al. 2011). It is also notable that a study described that participants who were monitored for four days using accelerometers and found to be sedentary for approximately 75% of the time had significant increases in the risk of poor health (van der Berg et al. 2014). Equivalent data has also been found in similar studies (Evenson et al. 2012; Matthews et al. 2008), thereby reinforcing the idea that SB has negative health effects. Up until recently, the majority of the research only pointed towards increasing MVPA in order to decrease the health risk factors of SB. However, sedentarism as an independent health risk is increasingly understood, with the suggestion that regular breaks from SB may be as effective as traditional exercise interventions (discussed below).

It should be pointed out here that there are several health factors affected by sedentary behaviours, notably an increased risk of arthritis, depression, sleep deprivation, and anxiety. It is however beyond the scope of this chapter to describe experiments for each of these conditions; as such, only a few examples are expanded on here.

32.2.2.1 Cardiovascular Disease

According to the Office for National Statistics, current mortality rates in England and Wales show that cardiovascular disease accounts for 26% of all deaths, second only to cancers (28%). Accounted in this statistic are coronary heart disease, strokes, and ischemic heart disease. Arguably, these can all, to one degree or another, be linked to a sedentary lifestyle. A 21-year longitudinal study on ~7,000 males, who self-reported lifestyle patterns and health including time spent in a car, time spent watching television, and current health conditions (Warren et al. 2010), reports that participants who spent 10 hours or more in SB compared to those spending 4 hours or less in SB had a 50% greater risk of dying from CVD. Similarly, participants who reported 23 hours or more of SB per week had a 37% greater chance of dying from CVD when compared to individuals who reported 11 hours or less per week. In parallel, a study found that individuals who reported sitting for long periods had a higher prevalence for CVD and hence mortality (Matthews et al. 2012). Counter-intuitively, the study also found that individuals who reported 7 hours or more weekly MVPA combined with 7 hours or more daily television watching had a 50% increased risk of CVD and all-cause mortality (Matthews et al. 2012). Aligned with a poor cardiovascular profile, metabolic dysfunction, which is a condition categorised by an unhealthy blood profile (high levels of triglyceride and high-density lipoprotein (HDL) cholesterol and low insulin sensitivity), is also found to be affected by SB independent of PA. Thus, a study describes that 5 days of 23.5 hours daily bed rest blunts both the insulin response and the ability of blood vessels to expand in response to increased demand (Hamburg et al. 2007).

32.2.2.2 Blood Glucose

Type 2 diabetes, a condition where the pancreas does not produce sufficient insulin or the body does not appropriately use the insulin made, is linked to a circulating glucose build up (or hyperglycaemia) instead of it being used for energy. This hyperglycaemia can increase the incidence of CVD due to the damaging cascade effect to numerous organs (Duvivier et al. 2016). Sedentary behaviours have now been associated with diabetes risk (Biswas et al. 2015; van der Berg et al. 2016). Thus, an extra hour spent sedentary relates to a 22% increased diabetes risk (van der Berg et al. 2016), whereas breaking sedentary sitting behaviour with standing or walking is associated with an improved glycaemic control in individuals with type 2 diabetes (Duvivier et al. 2016). It is notable that a threshold of uninterrupted SB is now evident (up to 30 minutes), beyond which the effects on blood glucose levels become significantly detrimental, whereas minimising prolonged bouts of SB and/or decreasing the number of long bouts of inactivity through breaks using LIPA (such as standing or walking) appears to aid glycaemic control.

32.2.2.3 Musculo-skeletal Health Profile

Whilst time spent sedentary among adults increases by half an hour every five years after the age of 65 (Townsend et al. 2015), the ability to form new bone decreases from the age of 30. The combination of the two effects would thus be a key contributor to the increased brittleness of the bone tissue in older persons (Chastin et al. 2014). Indeed, being sedentary means there is less load on the skeletal system and decreased contractions from the associated skeletal muscles through a process described in mechanostat theory. This relatively low loading affects individuals who show sedentary behaviours throughout their lives and increases their chance of having bone diseases such as osteoporosis. The femoral neck and lumbar spine in older post-menopausal women positively responds to regular breaks in sedentary behaviours by exhibiting improved bone health (Braun et al. 2016). On the other hand, higher levels of sedentary behaviours in older adults have been associated with a 33% greater risk of loss of muscle mass for each one-hour increment in overall SB, even after correcting for PA (Gianoudis et al. 2015).

32.2.2.4 Obesity and Cancer

In a sample of 7,216 children aged 7–11 years, TV watching/computer game play explained up to 44% of the variance in overweight status and up to 61% of obese status (Tremblay and Willms 2003). In 50,277 adult women, each 2 hours per day increase in TV viewing was associated with a 23% increased risk of obesity, and each 2 hours per day increase in sitting at work was associated with a 5% increased risk of obesity (Hu et al. 2003). In addition, the comparison of 3 hours vs 7 hours per day watching TV in a cohort of 488,720 adults aged 50–71 years was associated with an increased risk of colon cancer in longitudinal studies in males (Howard et al. 2008) and endometrial cancer in females (Gierach et al. 2009). It is noteworthy that the regression model used in the colon cancer risk study accounted for confounding variables including habitual physical activity, age, smoking, alcohol consumption, education, race, family history of colon cancer (yes, no, unknown), total energy, and energy-adjusted intakes (quintiles) of red meat, calcium, whole grains, fruits, and vegetables, and body mass index. Similarly, the regression model in the endometrial cancer study accounted for confounding variables including age, race/ethnicity, smoking status, parity, ever use of oral contraceptives, menopausal status, use of hormone replacement therapy, and BMI. As such, the fact that sedentarism still played a role strengthens the importance of minimising this lifestyle choice.

32.2.2.5 Psychosocial Health

Even after controlling for parental cognitive stimulation, IQ, and maternal education, data shows that TV watching before the age of three is associated with poor attention levels, language, and cognitive development including reading recognition, comprehension, and memory (Christakis et al. 2004). Similarly, 16 studies have reported a link between TV watching and decreased academic performance. For instance, high TV watching between 5 and 15 years decreases the likelihood of earning a university degree by the age of 26 years (Nunez-Smith et al. 2008). This highlights the potential continued risk of poor health in future generations of elders. Similarly in adults, the risk of mental disorder increases by 31% for an increase in TV watching from 10.5 to 42.5 hours per week (Sanchez-Villegas et al. 2008).

32.2.3 Is Sitting Always the Culprit?

Not all studies demonstrate a link between sedentarism and markers of health. It is however notable that the studies that find no sedentarism-health link tend to have measured sedentary behaviour qualitatively (Pulsford et al. 2015). Arguably, qualitative studies may not be sensitive enough to discriminate meaningful breaks in sedentary behaviour, disguising any link between sitting and mortality. Nevertheless, this low sensitivity may not explain the tendency for the disagreement between qualitative and quantitative data. Indeed a number of qualitative studies utilising retrospective, self-reporting of sedentarism have also shown a link between sedentarism and markers of health. Nonetheless, given that 20% of currently available studies data (i.e. 5533/28301 samples) report no association between objectively measured sedentary time and markers of adiposity and cardiometabolic disease risk among children and youth aged 3–19 years, it may be better to err on the side of caution and consider that SB does indeed have serious health consequences for all.

It would also appear that which element of the endo-metabolic profile is monitored has bearings on the conclusions regarding the importance of tracking sedentary behaviour. In other words, whilst some health markers have been strongly and consistently associated with sedentarism, other health markers show no change in the presence of varying degrees of SB. Indeed a study in 1,937 adults aged 21–64 years assessed body mass index, waist circumference, and plasma biochemistry including triglycerides, glucose, and insulin and found these to be strongly affected by the sleep-wake profile, whilst high-density lipoprotein (HDL) and low-density lipoprotein (LDL) were not noticeably affected (Chastin et al. 2015).

32.2.4 Evidence That Breaking Sedentarism Works

Given the health issues linked to SB, it is clear that a more mobile and hence expectantly healthier lifestyle is advisable. Sedentarism interruption, which may be an easier alternative to structured exercises, may be the way forward for widespread implementation of healthy lifestyle interventions, given that sustained adherence to structured exercise interventions is difficult to achieve in persistently sedentary populations. An increasing number of studies promote the idea that taking regular breaks from sitting can benefit an individual's health. In middle-aged persons, through finding an association between metabolic syndrome risk factors (including fasting plasma glucose, 2-h plasma glucose, serum triglycerides, HDL cholesterol, weight, height, waist circumference, and resting blood pressure) and prolonged unbroken periods of sedentary (independent of total sedentary time and/or moderate-to-vigorous intensity activity that is time-independent), a study provided early evidence of the importance of avoiding uninterrupted sitting (Healy et al. 2008). Another such study in support of the importance of breaking sedentarism proposes that diabetes, CVD, and obesity levels can decrease through addressing prolonged sitting within the workplace (Owen et al. 2010). These findings are supported by other work including one in which the authors report that reducing sedentary levels during the day is more beneficial in reducing insulin levels than an hour of physical exercise (Duvivier et al. 2013). Similarly, a recent study in 19 patients with type 2 diabetes investigated any benefits of using LIPA to break sitting time in this population and termed it the 'Sit Less' regimen (Duvivier et al. 2016). The authors reported that glucose levels improved over a 24-hour period when substituting the participants' sitting time with ambulatory activity (Duvivier et al. 2016). Even more interesting was the fact that this response was significantly better compared to both a condition where they sat throughout and another in which participants were introduced to structured exercise.

With only little research available on the most palatable and effective lifestyle intervention, it is tricky to identify the single best lifestyle protocol to recommend, if in fact one such intervention does exist. Nonetheless, there are some indications of potential avenues to pursue. Thus, even in the absence of extensive/rigorous research to support their recommendations, in 2015 an expert statement on the impact of prolonged sitting highlighted some changes needed within the workplace. These recommendations may have loosely been based on work that suggested introducing non-seated working and advocated that a review of transportation infrastructures is needed (Owen et al. 2011). A key recommendation therefore may be to utilise interventions targeting SB specifically as they appear so much better than those targeting PA (on SB-related health outcomes) (Gardner et al. 2016). Another fundamental advice would be to incrementally augment time spent standing and doing LIPA during the working day, in order to break up long periods of sitting. In other words, it may be advisable to get people to not sit longer than 28 minutes before they have to stand for 2 minutes and then they can sit again. Indeed as mentioned above, it would seem more important (and thus more practical in terms of feasibility) that we break up long periods of sitting, more so than attempting to reduce the total volume of time spent sitting (Healy et al. 2008). Another justification for the 2015 expert statement may have also been through the observation that breaking sitting with LIPA is potentially linked to a reduction in deleterious health outcomes (Owen et al. 2010). Whilst the above seem to be true for middle-aged populations, the importance of breaks in sedentarism over total sedentary time is yet to be determined where older adults are concerned.

32.2.5 Exercise Does Not Reverse the Effect of Sedentarism

Primary research data suggests that increased sedentarism is associated with 55% decreased lipoprotein lipase (LPL) activity in oxidative muscle fibres. In parallel, however, running causes no change in relative LPL activity above resting levels (Bey and Hamilton 2003), suggesting that the physiological pathway for the effects of sedentarism is distinct from those of exercise. Another case for sedentarism and exercise acting on separate physiologic targets is that presented in a study conducted over nine continuous hours (Peddie et al. 2013). The authors describe a stepwise increased blood glucose profile, expressed as the integrated area under the curve, when sedentarism is interrupted rather than continuous. Thus, the glucose profile improves from sitting continuously vs standing for 30 continuous minutes vs sitting for bouts of 30 minutes and standing for 1-minute 40-second breaks (Peddie et al. 2013). Another take-home message here would therefore be that we need to address both ends of the mobility behaviour spectrum.

32.3 Implications for Practice

32.3.1 Public Policy

With the concept of sedentarism physiology being new, it has not yet permeated general public health policy in many countries or for older adults as a group. One as yet rare example of recognition and application of the current knowledge on the issue is the 'Canadian Physical Activity Guidelines', potentially owing to the incidence of obesity increasing in Canada over the last decades (Tremblay et al. 2011). These guidelines stipulate that exercise recommendations need to be age specific to maximise specificity and effectiveness of approaches, with the age groups segregated into: children (aged 5–11 years), youths (aged 12–17 years), adults (aged 18–64 years), and older adults (aged ≥65 years). Particularly relevant to the current discussions, the guidelines in

Canada include a reference to SB guidelines, though only specific to paediatric populations (aged 0–17 years) (Tremblay et al. 2011). With research previously demonstrating that parents tend to have a significant influence on their children's habitual daily activities (Tremblay et al. 2011), the Canadian guidelines are close to being comprehensive as they also incorporate guidance directed at parents when advising actions that reduce SB time such as a reduction in recreational TV viewing time and a decrease in motorised transport time.

32.3.2 Behaviour Change

It is important to note that replacing SB with PA may necessitate the inclusion of behaviour change interventions (Gardner et al. 2014; Matei et al. 2015). For instance, a study demonstrated the importance of repetition in order to form healthy habits (Gardner et al. 2014). The repetition would ideally be incorporated in small interventions promoting PA as a way of reducing sitting. This study was conducted on the basis that inactive populations tend to have negative perception of exercise and resultantly engage in large amounts of SB in contrast to aiming to reach 150 minutes of MVPA per week. Through promoting behaviour maintenance via habit formation, behaviour change, and as such a successful adoption of a low SB lifestyle, would become more likely. In this vein, a number of previous intervention studies have been successful in reducing older adults' sedentary behaviour by up to 76 min/day less than baseline (Chang et al. 2013; Fitzsimons et al. 2013; Gardiner et al. 2011; King et al. 2013; Rosenberg et al. 2015). However, these studies tend to have features that make the scalability poor in that they are reliant on specialised training, activity monitors that are not commercially available, expensive individual behaviour coaching, or extensive group counselling. A recent study has however also demonstrated that even with limited behaviour coaching and less specialised training, sedentarism interruption interventions in older individuals can still be effective, and in this particular case, more so on weekdays than on weekends (Maher et al. 2017).

32.3.3 Scope for Integrating SB Reduction and PA Promotion Programmes

A recent workshop aimed at identifying sedentary behaviour research priorities concluded that sedentarism interventions would need to be informed by research on any potential synergy with the physiological and behavioural physical activity recommendations. The workshop also proposed that such interventions would need to: (a) be multi-level and aimed at reducing SB across all life phases and contexts, (b) harness relevant and effective strategies to increase the palatability for numerous socio-economic-cultural strata (Manini et al. 2015). Based on our current understanding, it would be reasonable to assume that a programme of healthy ageing would need to include both recommendations for sufficient engagement in MVPA (30 minutes five times per week as per normal PA recommendations) as well as strategies to incorporate breaks in sedentarism for the remainder of the waking hours (when engaging in habitual daily activities). In practical terms, this would mean taking part in one's preference of 'fast heart rate, sweat-inducing' physical activity daily (such as dancing, walking the dog, swimming, cycling, jogging, exercising at home with the help of a DVD), as well as trying to carry out normally seated activities whilst standing or standing up at regular (less than 30 minutes) intervals. To confirm the interplay between physical activity and sedentarism interruption, a large body of research is currently underway. Of note is the SITLESS project, a multi-million-pound, multi-country clinical trial aimed at reducing SB and increasing PA by enhancing existing exercise referral schemes with self-management strategies in older persons (Tully and Kee 2015).

32.4 Conclusion

The current chapter utilised the available literature, which unfortunately is still low on data gathered specifically using older populations. Nevertheless, the conclusions are useful to inform future avenues for research in aged persons. We have described that whilst sedentary activity relates to ≤ 1.5 METs, light activity is between <3 and >1.5 METs, moderate physical activity is between ≥ 3 and <6 METs, intense exercise relates to ≥ 6 METs (Owen et al. 2000), where 1 MET is representative of a resting metabolic rate, whilst 8 METs is the value of activities such as running (Owen et al. 2000; Pate et al. 2008). In view of the current literature, it could be argued that more time needs to be spent on educating the general public about the benefits of decreasing the amount of time spent sitting, instead of solely encouraging people to exercise. In any case, it is often the observation that there is a segment of the population that remains recalcitrant to the idea of taking on structured exercise. One study suggests that taking regular breaks from sitting can lower CVD risk significantly (Owen et al. 2010). In comparison, where most studies will suggest to increase MVPA, this latter body of work is unhelpful for those individuals who find partaking in regular MVPA to be an unachievable goal. What is more, not only do people under-report, and as such potentially underestimate, their habitual SB (Tucker et al. 2011) but also the general public is simply not doing enough physical activity, despite numerous public awareness campaigns. Future research is needed to design palatable methods of reducing sedentary behaviours, and these would likely involve breaking sitting with light-intensity physical activity (Owen et al. 2010), a level of activity which has proved particularly beneficial in the older person (Onambele-Pearson et al. 2010).

Suggested Further Reading

- Chastin, S. F. M., Fitzpatrick, N., Andrews, M., & DiCroce, N. (2014). Determinants of sedentary behavior, motivation, barriers and strategies to reduce sitting time in older women: A qualitative investigation. *International Journal of Environmental Research and Public Health, 11*(1), 773–791. https://doi.org/10.3390/ijerph110100773.
- Gibbs, B. B., Brach, J. S., Byard, T., Creasy, S., Davis, K. K., McCoy, S., Peluso, A., Rogers, R. J., Rupp, K., Jakicic, J. M. (2016). Reducing sedentary behavior versus increasing moderate-to-vigorous intensity physical activity in older adults: A 12-week randomized, clinical trial. *Journal of Aging Health*. pii: 0898264316635564. [Epub ahead of print].
- Prince, S. A., Saunders, T. J., Gresty, K., & Reid, R. D. (2014). A comparison of the effectiveness of physical activity and sedentary behaviour interventions in reducing sedentary time in adults: A systematic review and meta-analysis of controlled trials. *Obesity Reviews, 15*(11), 905–919. https://doi.org/10.1111/obr.12215.

References

Ainsworth, B. E., Haskell, W. L., Whitt, M. C., Irwin, M. L., Swartz, A. M., Strath, S. J., et al. (2000). Compendium of physical activities: An update of activity codes and MET intensities. *Medicine and Science in Sports and Exercise, 32*(9 Suppl), S498–S504.

Bey, L., & Hamilton, M. T. (2003). Suppression of skeletal muscle lipoprotein lipase activity during physical inactivity: A molecular reason to maintain daily low-intensity activity. *The Journal of Physiology, 551*(Pt 2), 673–682. https://doi.org/10.1113/jphysiol.2003.045591.

Biswas, A., Oh, P. I., Faulkner, G. E., Bajaj, R. R., Silver, M. A., Mitchell, M. S., & Alter, D. A. (2015). Sedentary time and its association with risk for disease incidence, mortality, and hospitalization in adults: A systematic review and meta-analysis. *Annals of Internal Medicine, 162*(2), 123–132. https://doi.org/10.7326/M14-1651.

Bouchard, C., An, P., Rice, T., Skinner, J. S., Wilmore, J. H., Gagnon, J., et al. (1999). Familial aggregation of VO(2max) response to exercise training: Results from the HERITAGE Family Study. *Journal of Applied Physiology, 87*(3), 1003–1008.

Braun, S. I., Kimb, Y., Jetton, A. E., Kang, M., & Morgan, D. W. (2016). Sedentary behavior, physical activity, and bone health in post-menopausal women. *Journal of Aging and Physical Activity*, 1–30. https://doi.org/10.1123/japa.2016-0046.

Chang, A. K., Fritschi, C., & Kim, M. J. (2013). Sedentary behavior, physical activity, and psychological health of Korean older adults with hypertension: Effect of an empowerment intervention. *Research in Gerontological Nursing, 6*(2), 81–88. https://doi.org/10.3928/19404921-20121219-01.

Chastin, S. F., Mandrichenko, O., & Skelton, D. A. (2014). The frequency of osteogenic activities and the pattern of intermittence between periods of physical activity and sedentary behaviour affects bone mineral content: The cross-sectional NHANES study. *BMC Public Health, 14*, 4. https://doi.org/10.1186/1471-2458-14-4.

Chastin, S. F., Palarea-Albaladejo, J., Dontje, M. L., & Skelton, D. A. (2015). Combined effects of time spent in physical activity, sedentary behaviors and sleep on obesity and cardio-metabolic health markers: A novel compositional data analysis approach. *PLoS One, 10*(10), e0139984. https://doi.org/10.1371/journal.pone.0139984.

Christakis, D. A., Zimmerman, F. J., DiGiuseppe, D. L., & McCarty, C. A. (2004). Early television exposure and subsequent attentional problems in children. *Pediatrics, 113*(4), 708–713.

de Rezende, L. F., Rey-Lopez, J. P., Matsudo, V. K., & do Carmo Luiz, O. (2014). Sedentary behavior and health outcomes among older adults: A systematic review. *BMC Public Health, 14*, 333. https://doi.org/10.1186/1471-2458-14-333.

Duvivier, B. M., Schaper, N. C., Bremers, M. A., van Crombrugge, G., Menheere, P. P., Kars, M., & Savelberg, H. H. (2013). Minimal intensity physical activity (standing and walking) of longer duration improves insulin action and plasma lipids more than shorter periods of moderate to vigorous exercise (cycling) in sedentary subjects when energy expenditure is comparable. *PLoS One, 8*(2), e55542. https://doi.org/10.1371/journal.pone.0055542.

Duvivier, B. M., Schaper, N. C., Hesselink, M. K., van Kan, L., Stienen, N., Winkens, B., et al. (2016). Breaking sitting with light activities vs structured exercise: A randomised crossover study demonstrating benefits for glycaemic control and insulin sensitivity in type 2 diabetes. *Diabetologia*. https://doi.org/10.1007/s00125-016-4161-7.

Evenson, K. R., Buchner, D. M., & Morland, K. B. (2012). Objective measurement of physical activity and sedentary behavior among US adults aged 60 years or older. *Preventing Chronic Disease, 9*, E26.

FAO/WHO/UNU. (2001). *Human energy requirements. Report of a joint FAO/WHO/UNU expert consultation.* Rome: FAO.

Farrell, L., Hollingsworth, B., Propper, C., & Shields, M. A. (2013). *The socioeconomic gradient in physical. Inactivity in England.* Bristol: Centre for Market and Public Organisation.

Fitzsimons, C. F., Kirk, A., Baker, G., Michie, F., Kane, C., & Mutrie, N. (2013). Using an individualised consultation and activPAL feedback to reduce sedentary time in older Scottish adults: Results of a feasibility and pilot study. *Preventive Medicine, 57*(5), 718–720. https://doi.org/10.1016/j.ypmed.2013.07.017.

Ford, E. S., & Caspersen, C. J. (2012). Sedentary behaviour and cardiovascular disease: A review of prospective studies. *International Journal of Epidemiology, 41*(5), 1338–1353. https://doi.org/10.1093/ije/dys078.

Gardiner, P. A., Eakin, E. G., Healy, G. N., & Owen, N. (2011). Feasibility of reducing older adults' sedentary time. *American Journal of Preventive Medicine, 41*(2), 174–177. https://doi.org/10.1016/j.amepre.2011.03.020.

Gardner, B., Thune-Boyle, I., Iliffe, S., Fox, K. R., Jefferis, B. J., Hamer, M., et al. (2014). 'On your feet to earn your seat', a habit-based intervention to reduce sedentary behaviour in older adults: Study protocol for a randomized controlled trial. *Trials, 15*, 368. https://doi.org/10.1186/1745-6215-15-368.

Gardner, B., Smith, L., Lorencatto, F., Hamer, M., & Biddle, S. J. (2016). How to reduce sitting time? A review of behaviour change strategies used in sedentary behaviour reduction interventions among adults. *Health Psychology Review, 10*(1), 89–112. https://doi.org/10.1080/17437199.2015.1082146.

Gianoudis, J., Bailey, C. A., & Daly, R. M. (2015). Associations between sedentary behaviour and body composition, muscle function and sarcopenia in community-dwelling older adults. *Osteoporosis International, 26*(2), 571–579. https://doi.org/10.1007/s00198-014-2895-y.

Gierach, G. L., Chang, S. C., Brinton, L. A., Lacey, J. V., Jr., Hollenbeck, A. R., Schatzkin, A., & Leitzmann, M. F. (2009). Physical activity, sedentary behavior, and endometrial cancer risk in the NIH-AARP diet and health study. *International Journal of Cancer, 124*(9), 2139–2147. https://doi.org/10.1002/ijc.24059.

Hamburg, N. M., McMackin, C. J., Huang, A. L., Shenouda, S. M., Widlansky, M. E., Schulz, E., et al. (2007). Physical inactivity rapidly induces insulin resistance and microvascular dysfunction in healthy volunteers. *Arteriosclerosis, Thrombosis, and Vascular Biology, 27*(12), 2650–2656. https://doi.org/10.1161/ATVBAHA.107.153288.

Hamer, M., & Stamatakis, E. (2013). Screen-based sedentary behavior, physical activity, and muscle strength in the English longitudinal study of ageing. *PLoS One, 8*(6), ARTN e66222. https://doi.org/10.1371/journal.pone.0066222.

Hamilton, M. T., Healy, G. N., Dunstan, D. W., Zderic, T. W., & Owen, N. (2008). Too little exercise and too much sitting: Inactivity physiology and the need for new recommendations on sedentary behavior. *Current Cardiovascular Risk Reports, 2*(4), 292–298. https://doi.org/10.1007/s12170-008-0054-8.

Healy, G. N., Dunstan, D. W., Salmon, J., Cerin, E., Shaw, J. E., Zimmet, P. Z., & Owen, N. (2008). Breaks in sedentary time: Beneficial associations with metabolic risk. *Diabetes Care, 31*(4), 661–666. https://doi.org/10.2337/dc07-2046.

Howard, R. A., Freedman, D. M., Park, Y., Hollenbeck, A., Schatzkin, A., & Leitzmann, M. F. (2008). Physical activity, sedentary behavior, and the risk of colon and rectal cancer in the NIH-AARP Diet and Health Study. *Cancer Causes & Control, 19*(9), 939–953. https://doi.org/10.1007/s10552-008-9159-0.

Hu, F. B., Li, T. Y., Colditz, G. A., Willett, W. C., & Manson, J. E. (2003). Television watching and other sedentary behaviors in relation to risk of obesity and type 2 diabetes mellitus in women. *JAMA: The Journal of the American Medical Association, 289*(14), 1785–1791. https://doi.org/10.1001/jama.289.14.1785.

Hunter, R. F., Tully, M. A., Donnelly, P., Stevenson, M., & Kee, F. (2014). Knowledge of UK physical activity guidelines: Implications for better targeted health promotion. *Preventive Medicine, 65*, 33–39. https://doi.org/10.1016/j.ypmed.2014.04.016.

Kabrhel, C., Varraso, R., Goldhaber, S. Z., Rimm, E., & Camargo, C. A., Jr. (2011). Physical inactivity and idiopathic pulmonary embolism in women: Prospective study. *BMJ, 343*, d3867. https://doi.org/10.1136/bmj.d3867.

Kim, Y., Wilkens, L. R., Park, S. Y., Goodman, M. T., Monroe, K. R., & Kolonel, L. N. (2013). Association between various sedentary behaviours and all-cause, cardiovascular disease and cancer mortality: The multiethnic cohort study. *International Journal of Epidemiology, 42*(4), 1040–1056. https://doi.org/10.1093/ije/dyt108.

King, A. C., Hekler, E. B., Grieco, L. A., Winter, S. J., Sheats, J. L., Buman, M. P., et al. (2013). Harnessing different motivational frames via mobile phones to promote daily physical activity and reduce sedentary behavior in aging adults. *PLoS One, 8*(4), e62613. https://doi.org/10.1371/journal.pone.0062613.

Maher, J. P., Sliwinski, M. J., & Conroy, D. E. (2017). Feasibility and preliminary efficacy of an intervention to reduce older adults' sedentary behavior. *Translational Behaviour Medicine, 7*(1), 52–61. https://doi.org/10.1007/s13142-016-0394-8.

Manini, T. M., Carr, L. J., King, A. C., Marshall, S., Robinson, T. N., & Rejeski, W. J. (2015). Interventions to reduce sedentary behavior. *Medicine and Science in Sports and Exercise, 47*(6), 1306–1310. https://doi.org/10.1249/MSS.0000000000000519.

Matei, R., Thune-Boyle, I., Hamer, M., Iliffe, S., Fox, K. R., Jefferis, B. J., & Gardner, B. (2015). Acceptability of a theory-based sedentary behaviour reduction intervention for older adults ('On Your Feet to Earn Your Seat'). *BMC Public Health, 15*, 606. https://doi.org/10.1186/s12889-015-1921-0.

Matthews, C. E., Chen, K. Y., Freedson, P. S., Buchowski, M. S., Beech, B. M., Pate, R. R., & Troiano, R. P. (2008). Amount of time spent in sedentary behaviors in the United States, 2003-2004. *American Journal of Epidemiology, 167*(7), 875–881. https://doi.org/10.1093/aje/kwm390.

Matthews, C. E., George, S. M., Moore, S. C., Bowles, H. R., Blair, A., Park, Y., et al. (2012). Amount of time spent in sedentary behaviors and cause-specific mortality in US adults. *The American Journal of Clinical Nutrition, 95*(2), 437–445. https://doi.org/10.3945/ajcn.111.019620.

NHS. (2013). Physical activity guidelines for adults. Retrieved from http://www.nhs.uk/Livewell/fitness/Pages/physical-activity-guidelines-for-adults.aspx

Nunez-Smith, M., Curry, L. A., Berg, D., Krumholz, H. M., & Bradley, E. H. (2008). Healthcare workplace conversations on race and the perspectives of physicians of African descent. *Journal of General Internal Medicine, 23*(9), 1471–1476. https://doi.org/10.1007/s11606-008-0709-7.

Onambele-Pearson, G. L., Breen, L., & Stewart, C. E. (2010). Influence of exercise intensity in older persons with unchanged habitual nutritional intake: Skeletal muscle and endocrine adaptations. *Age, 32*(2), 139–153. https://doi.org/10.1007/s11357-010-9141-0.

Owen, N., Leslie, E., Salmon, J., & Fotheringham, M. J. (2000). Environmental determinants of physical activity and sedentary behavior. *Exercise and Sport Sciences Reviews, 28*(4), 153–158.

Owen, N., Healy, G. N., Matthews, C. E., & Dunstan, D. W. (2010). Too much sitting: The population health science of sedentary behavior. *Exercise and Sport Sciences Reviews, 38*(3), 105–113. https://doi.org/10.1097/JES.0b013e3181e373a2.

Owen, N., Sugiyama, T., Eakin, E. E., Gardiner, P. A., Tremblay, M. S., & Sallis, J. F. (2011). Adults' sedentary behavior determinants and interventions. *American Journal of Preventive Medicine, 41*(2), 189–196. https://doi.org/10.1016/j.amepre.2011.05.013.

Pate, R. R., O'Neill, J. R., & Lobelo, F. (2008). The evolving definition of "sedentary". *Exercise and Sport Sciences Reviews, 36*(4), 173–178. https://doi.org/10.1097/JES.0b013e3181877d1a.

Peddie, M. C., Bone, J. L., Rehrer, N. J., Skeaff, C. M., Gray, A. R., & Perry, T. L. (2013). Breaking prolonged sitting reduces postprandial glycemia in healthy, normal-weight adults: A randomized crossover trial. *The American Journal of Clinical Nutrition, 98*(2), 358–366. https://doi.org/10.3945/ajcn.112.051763.

Pulsford, R. M., Stamatakis, E., Britton, A. R., Brunner, E. J., & Hillsdon, M. (2015). Associations of sitting behaviours with all-cause mortality over a 16-year follow-up: The Whitehall II study. *International Journal of Epidemiology, 44*(6), 1909–1916. https://doi.org/10.1093/ije/dyv191.

Rosenberg, D. E., Gell, N. M., Jones, S. M., Renz, A., Kerr, J., Gardiner, P. A., & Arterburn, D. (2015). The feasibility of reducing sitting time in overweight and obese older adults. *Health Education & Behavior, 42*(5), 669–676. https://doi.org/10.1177/1090198115577378.

Rowlands, A. V., Olds, T. S., Hillsdon, M., Pulsford, R., Hurst, T. L., Eston, R. G., et al. (2014). Assessing sedentary behavior with the GENEActiv: Introducing the sedentary sphere. *Medicine and Science in Sports and Exercise, 46*(6), 1235–1247. https://doi.org/10.1249/MSS.0000000000000224.

Sanchez-Villegas, A., Ara, I., Guillen-Grima, F., Bes-Rastrollo, M., Varo-Cenarruzabeitia, J. J., & Martinez-Gonzalez, M. A. (2008). Physical activity, sedentary index, and mental disorders in the SUN cohort study. *Medicine and Science in Sports and Exercise, 40*(5), 827–834. https://doi.org/10.1249/MSS.0b013e31816348b9.

Strategy-Unit, & DCMS. (2002). *Game plan*. Parliamentary copyright 2005. https://publications.parliament.uk/pa/cm200405/cmselect/cmcumeds/507/507we21.htm

Thompson, D., & Batterham, A. M. (2013). Towards integrated physical activity profiling. *PLoS One, 8*(2), e56427. https://doi.org/10.1371/journal.pone.0056427.

Thompson, D., Batterham, A. M., Markovitch, D., Dixon, N. C., Lund, A. J., & Walhin, J. P. (2009). Confusion and conflict in assessing the physical activity status of middle-aged men. *PLoS One, 4*(2), e4337. https://doi.org/10.1371/journal.pone.0004337.

Townsend, N., Wickramasinghe, K., Williams, J., Bhatnagar, P., & Rayner, M. (2015). *Physical activity statistics 2015*. Nuffield Department of Population Health, University of Oxford: Centre on Population Approaches for Non-Communicable Disease Prevention.

Tremblay, M. S., & Willms, J. D. (2003). Is the Canadian childhood obesity epidemic related to physical inactivity? *International Journal of Obesity and Related Metabolic Disorders, 27*(9), 1100–1105. https://doi.org/10.1038/sj.ijo.0802376.

Tremblay, M. S., Colley, R. C., Saunders, T. J., Healy, G. N., & Owen, N. (2010). Physiological and health implications of a sedentary lifestyle. *Applied Physiology, Nutrition, and Metabolism, 35*(6), 725–740. https://doi.org/10.1139/H10-079.

Tremblay, M. S., Leblanc, A. G., Janssen, I., Kho, M. E., Hicks, A., Murumets, K., et al. (2011). Canadian sedentary behaviour guidelines for children and youth. *Applied Physiology, Nutrition, and Metabolism, 36*(1), 59–64.; 65–71. https://doi.org/10.1139/H11-012.

Tucker, J. M., Welk, G. J., & Beyler, N. K. (2011). Physical activity in U.S.: Adults compliance with the physical activity guidelines for Americans. *American Journal of Preventive Medicine, 40*(4), 454–461. https://doi.org/10.1016/j.amepre.2010.12.016.

Tudor-Locke, C. E., & Myers, A. M. (2001). Challenges and opportunities for measuring physical activity in sedentary adults. *Sports Medicine, 31*(2), 91–100.

Tudor-Locke, C., Johnson, W. D., & Katzmarzyk, P. T. (2009). Accelerometer-determined steps per day in US adults. *Medicine and Science in Sports and Exercise, 41*(7), 1384–1391. https://doi.org/10.1249/MSS.0b013e318199885c.

Tully, M. A., & Kee, F. (2015). The SitLess study. From https://www.qub.ac.uk/research-centres/CentreofExcellenceforPublicHealthNorthernIreland/Research/PhysicalActivityResearch/TheSITlessstudy/

Turner, J. E., Markovitch, D., Betts, J. A., & Thompson, D. (2010). Nonprescribed physical activity energy expenditure is maintained with structured exercise and implicates a compensatory increase in energy intake. *The American Journal of Clinical Nutrition, 92*(5), 1009–1016. https://doi.org/10.3945/ajcn.2010.29471.

van der Berg, J. D., Bosma, H., Caserotti, P., Eiriksdottir, G., Arnardottir, N. Y., Martin, K. R., et al. (2014). Midlife determinants associated with sedentary behavior in old age. *Medicine and Science in Sports and Exercise, 46*(7), 1359–1365. https://doi.org/10.1249/MSS.0000000000000246.

van der Berg, J. D., Stehouwer, C. D., Bosma, H., van der Velde, J. H., Willems, P. J., Savelberg, H. H., et al. (2016). Associations of total amount and patterns of sedentary behaviour with type 2 diabetes and the metabolic syndrome: The Maastricht Study. *Diabetologia, 59*(4), 709–718. https://doi.org/10.1007/s00125-015-3861-8.

Warren, T. Y., Barry, V., Hooker, S. P., Sui, X., Church, T. S., & Blair, S. N. (2010). Sedentary behaviors increase risk of cardiovascular disease mortality in men. *Medicine and Science in Sports and Exercise, 42*(5), 879–885. https://doi.org/10.1249/MSS.0b013e3181c3aa7e.

33

The Role of Sport in Promoting Physical Activity Among Older People

Rachael C. Stone, Rylee A. Dionigi, and Joseph Baker

33.1 Introduction

Older adults represent the largest and fastest growing segment of the population worldwide. Given the diversity of health and fitness levels, along with abilities and personal interests, there is increased opportunity for physical activity and sport participation in later life. The general physiological benefits of physical activity (i.e., any bodily movement, including housework and walking) for older adults include, but are not limited to, enhanced cardiovascular and cognitive functioning, increased muscle mass and strength, greater self-efficacy and positive affect, as well as mitigating the risk and progression of common chronic conditions such as osteoarthritis, diabetes, cancer, and depression (Lee et al. 2012; Steinmo et al. 2014; Taylor 2014). These benefits may be even more pronounced with regular sport participation, which has been found to foster benefits that extend beyond those of traditional forms of

---

R. C. Stone (✉)
School of Kinesiology and Health Studies, Queen's University,
Kingston, ON, Canada

R. A. Dionigi
School of Exercise Science, Charles Sturt University,
Port Macquarie, NSW, Australia

J. Baker
School of Kinesiology and Health Science, York University,
Toronto, ON, Canada

exercise, such as experiencing more social connectedness with other older people, intergenerational interaction, travel, fun, sense of mastery, and positive perceptions of the ageing process (Baker et al. 2010; Dionigi et al. 2011; Gayman et al. 2017a; Jenkin et al. 2016).

Sport is a distinct form of physical activity that combines planned participation within a structure of rules and goals similar to formal exercise but also involves aspects of competition, social networking, and fun commonly associated with leisure activities (Caspersen et al. 1985). While findings regarding the extended benefits of sport have been promising, sport participation is known to greatly decrease with age. Participation rates in later life are lower than other forms of physical activity (e.g., aerobic exercise, strength training), ranging from less than 10% and up to 20% across Westernized countries (Canadian Heritage 2013; van Tuyckom et al. 2010). Reasons for not participating in sport during older adulthood include disinterest, lack of time and resources (both personal and social, e.g., monetary, equipment, and venue accessibility/policies), inability (due to illness or disability), the inconvenience of potentially relying on others for participation, and fear of injury and social judgements (Breuer et al. 2011; Canadian Heritage 2013; Grant 2002; Jenkin et al. 2016). Also, while older people play a variety of team, paired, and individual sports, the majority of sport participation in later life tends to be individual sport (i.e., track and field, golf, or swimming) as opposed to team sport (e.g., basketball or hockey; Breuer et al. 2011; Stone et al. 2012). Nevertheless, sport participation during older adulthood, especially of an individual and competitive nature, appears to have gained popularity over time as evidenced by participation rates at the World Masters Games, which take place every four years (International Masters Games Association 2016).

33.2 Masters Sport

The World Masters Games provides a forum for international sports competition during later life. Participants in these games, as well as all older adults who generally engage in competitive sport that requires continuous training, are commonly referred to as masters athletes (Ransdell et al. 2009). Involvement in masters sport typically begins between 35 and 40 years of age; however, this is largely dependent on the type of sport and diverse age estimates of when peak performance is achieved (e.g., masters athletics for swimming begins at age 25, while curling begins at age 55; Ransdell et al. 2009). Since the first World Masters Games in 1985, participation has grown from 8000 athletes to an average of 25,000 athletes at the most recent games held in 2009 and 2013 (International Masters Games Association 2016).

Given the rise in masters sport participation, a growing body of research has qualitatively examined this unique older population in terms of what predicts their participation and what can be learned from their sporting pursuits during later life (Cardenas et al. 2009; Dionigi 2002, 2005, 2006, 2007, 2008, 2016; Dionigi and O'Flynn 2007; Dionigi et al. 2010, 2011, 2013a; Gayman et al. 2017a; Heo et al. 2013; Jenkin et al. 2016; Kolt et al. 2004; Stenner et al. 2016; Tulle 2007). These studies have spanned the continuum of competitive sport participation in older adults aged 55–90 years across the United States, United Kingdom, Canada, Sweden, Australia, and New Zealand, ranging from the recreationally competitive to the elite level. The variety of sports that have been represented in this work include track and field, swimming, cycling, skiing, golf, tennis, table tennis, squash, badminton, volleyball, basketball, tae kwon do, weightlifting, shuffleboard, and orienteering. Despite the diversity of sports that has been studied, similar trends have emerged regardless of type and level of competition, suggesting inherent benefits to sport participation with more generalized implications for older adults. Some key benefits that will be discussed are resistance to stereotypes and feelings of empowerment, improving and maintaining one's health, and social connectedness and fun.

33.2.1 Resistance and Empowerment

Stereotypical Westernized depictions of older adults tend to highlight ageing as a process of inevitable physical, cognitive, psychological, and social decline. Of these depictions, physical frailty and weakness are perhaps noted most frequently within popular media formats as well as empirically from general ageing expectations of older adults (Dionigi and Horton 2012; Montepare and Zebrowitz 2002; Sarkisian et al. 2001). Consequentially, sport participation remains a largely youth-oriented sub-culture, wherein stereotypical characteristics of athletes coincide with 'youthful' characteristics, such as vigour, strength, agility, riskiness, resiliency, and a propensity for violent behaviour through competition (Bodner 2009). These characteristics are in direct contradiction to what societal norms often relay regarding expectations of older adults, such as enjoying a 'well-deserved' time of rest and relaxation while avoiding activities with inherent injury risk (i.e., sport), especially since older adults supposedly lack the physical prowess to successfully participate (Grant and O'Brien Cousins 2001; Dionigi 2008). Therefore, older adult sport participants are believed to embody the antithesis of pervasive negative age-stereotypes by actively resisting these expectations and feeling empowered by their practices (Dionigi 2006). The aforementioned body of qualitative work has consistently shown that not only can older adults participate in sport, but many are thriving and accomplishing athletic feats that continue to defy societal expectations (Baker et al. 2010; Dionigi 2015). Perhaps the most recognized example of this was Ed Whitlock, a Canadian marathon runner who in 2003 became the oldest individual to complete a marathon in under three hours at age 69 (a record he still holds). He continued to set new world records for marathon running until he passed away at the age of 86 in March 2017 (Longman 2016). Older sport participants like Ed continue to modify societal expectations of ageing by portraying characteristics of fitness, strength, self-confidence, competence, success, and productivity as well as being motivated by competing with others and themselves in terms of setting records, winning medals, and striving for personal bests. At the same time, from a broader societal perspective, Gard et al. (2017) suggest the era of the 'exceptional' older athlete (i.e., one who resists traditional norms) may have come to an end because sport is now promoted to all, regardless of age, and therefore the societal norms may be changing (i.e., older people are encouraged and made to feel obligated to remain physically active). Gard et al. also ask if sport participation among older people is becoming normalized, at least in the masters sport context, where it appears many older athletes believe there is no excuse for able older adults not remaining active. This evolving idea regarding sport and ageing has the potential to reshape social relationships between older adults given these intragenerational judgements may become more prevalent over time in conjunction with age-demographic shifts and expected participation trends (see Gard et al.). Therefore, the potential offered by older adult sport participation in re-imagining what 'normal' ageing entails has personal benefits (and challenges) for older athletes, as well as society at large.

33.2.2 Improving and Maintaining Health

Perhaps the most commonly cited motive and benefit for beginning and maintaining sport participation in older adults, as well as lifelong sport, is the desire to enhance the quality of their lives through improving and preserving physical and cognitive health. In addition to feelings of resistance and empowerment through sport, much of the aforementioned body of qualitative research has reported that older adult sport participants perceive benefits regarding their strength, endurance, flexibility, problem-solving skills, and ability to accomplish activities of daily living outside of sport (Cardenas et al.

2009; Dionigi et al. 2011; Heo et al. 2013; Kolt et al. 2004; Stenner et al. 2016).

These perceived benefits of sport have been supported quantitatively as research on older masters athletes and recreationally competitive sport participants has found that while health and performance measures decline over time, such as cardiovascular functioning (Bohm et al. 2016; Concannon et al. 2012; Tanaka and Seals 2008), lung capacity (Degens et al. 2013a, b), muscle strength (Slade et al. 2002; Wroblewski et al. 2011), and bone mass (Velez et al. 2008; Wilks et al. 2009), all decreases occurred to a lesser degree than their same-aged and gendered, non-active peers, regardless of sport and number of training hours per week. Moreover, evidence also supports the perceived benefits of sport participation during later life in terms of cognitive functioning. Research has shown older sport participants have more brain volume and better verbal and working memory (Tseng et al. 2013; Zhao et al. 2016), faster reaction time (Leach and Ruckert 2016; Zhao et al. 2016), as well as superior coordination, accuracy, and attentional resources allocated during daily tasks (Leach and Ruckert 2016) compared to their age- and gender-matched less active contemporaries. These benefits may extend beyond simply participating in sport, to the inherent connection between activity choice and time displacement whereby competitive sport participants report spending less time engaging in sedentary behaviours (e.g., long bouts of sitting idle watching television) that have been associated with all-cause mortality, compared to older adults who are inactive or who only perform leisure physical activity (Dogra and Mccracken 2016; Gayman et al. 2017b). It is important to note that not all older adults have the time, means, ability, and desire to remain active in later life. Thus, sport participation is best seen as one of many leisure opportunities that can be used to maximize quality of life, health, and functioning in later life (see Dionigi 2017), including social engagement which is explored in the next section.

33.2.3 Social Connectedness and Fun

While motivations regarding sport pursuits are often fuelled by the physical and cognitive health benefits during earlier stages of participation, over time, older athletes tend to become more driven by benefits related to social connectedness, enjoyment, and fun rather than health outcomes (Reaburn and Dascombe 2008). Qualitative literature has found that older sport participants perceive sport as a unique form of social engagement and emotional connection with other older adults sharing similar experiences (Dionigi 2016;

Eime et al. 2013; Gayman et al. 2017a; Lyons and Dionigi 2007). Older athletes often refer to feelings of camaraderie, companionship, community, and belonging to an exclusive membership through the formation of 'athletic identities' highlighted by novel opportunities for fun, fitness, travel, and social networking (Dionigi 2007, 2010, 2015, 2016; Dionigi et al. 2010, 2011; Eime et al. 2013; Lyons and Dionigi 2007; Stenner et al. 2016; Tulle 2007). The formation of this positive ageing identity may be of utmost importance to many individuals considering older adulthood commonly involves negotiating new social, psychological, and physical identities, especially while transitioning into retirement and searching for routine, structure, and purpose during later life (Sneed and Whitbourne 2005). Discovering a new identity and purpose in life through sport may prompt a perceived sense of emotional self-worth whereby older sport participants feel as if they can give back to the sport community by volunteering and coaching others (Lyons and Dionigi 2007; Stenner et al. 2016).

While relatively less quantitative research has been dedicated towards examining psychosocial outcomes of older adult sport participation, the limited evidence has supported these perceived benefits suggesting higher social functioning and connectedness, self-esteem, life satisfaction (Eime et al. 2013; Menec 2003; Reed and Cox 2007), and enjoyment (Reed and Cox 2007), as well as lower risks of depression (Stone et al. 2012) when compared to those who are leisurely active or non-active. Furthermore, claiming an athletic identity has been independently associated with more social connectedness and better performance in masters runners (Horton and Mack 2000); however, more research is necessary to corroborate these findings related to the benefits of developing an athletic identity within older adults and across sport.

Despite the potential benefits of sport participation, the notion of promoting 'sport for all', regardless of age or any other demographic factor, remains contentious (see Gard and Dionigi 2016), especially given that the majority of older adult sport participants and stakeholders tend to be White, male, well-educated, high income, and able-bodied (van Tuyckom and Scheerder 2008). Therefore, it is important to remember that sport is currently not for all and may never be, and that it is best promoted as an option for older people, not a health imperative. Nevertheless, unique promotional efforts that cater to the needs of diverse older individuals are necessary to keep up with the growing ageing population and demand for sport (Young et al. 2015). Specifically, Young et al. (2015) have suggested that participation in masters athletics is particularly incentivized by involvement opportunities, which represent perceived rewards, benefits, and special opportunities for participants through sports engagement (Scanlan et al. 2003). Therefore, promoting involvement opportunities should be an effective tool for garnering more sport participation in older adults; however, the effectiveness may be contingent on specific demographics of potential participants. For example, female masters athletes tend to be more motivated by involvement opportunities for health, fitness, and enjoyment, whereas male masters athletes tend to be more motivated by competition and rewards (Young et al. 2015). These efforts in promoting and amassing more sport participation in older adults continue to gain attention from government organizations, researchers, and sport stakeholders alike. The worldwide shift in age-demographics, growing health-economic concerns, the biopsychosocial benefits from participation, and the notion that masters athletes may represent role models of successful ageing have provided the context for masters sport to flourish.

33.3 Masters Athletes as a Model of Successful Ageing

The evidence of physical and cognitive health improvements and maintenance related to sport participation provided above has perpetuated the notion that masters athletes and older competitive sport participants represent a 'model of successful ageing' (Hawkins et al. 2003; Geard et al. 2017). The notion of successful ageing can be traced back to the 1950s, although the first large-scale empirical examinations of the phenomenon started decades later (Dillaway and Byrnes 2009; Rubinstein and de Medeiros 2015). In 1987, physician John Rowe and psychologist Robert Kahn (Rowe and Kahn, 1987) published an extremely influential paper in the journal *Science* entitled 'Human Aging: Usual and Successful' that laid the foundation for their notion of successful ageing, a notion that dominated discussions for over a decade and continues to do so. Their conceptualization was based on findings from the MacArthur Studies of Successful Aging (e.g., Seeman et al. 1994, 1995), and proposed that successful ageing reflected (a) low probability of disease and disease-related disability, (b) high cognitive and physical functioning, and (c) active engagement with life. Since their original conceptualization, descriptions of successful ageing have become increasingly more nuanced and expansive (Geard et al. 2017). Unlike the Rowe and Kahn definition, which focused on biomedical descriptions of lack of disease and maintenance of function, more recent definitions have expanded to include self-perceptions such as satisfaction and minimal disruption to daily routines (see Geard et al. 2017; Strawbridge et al. 2002).

Given the ability of older athletes to maintain high levels of function and involvement in physical activities, there is some evidence that masters athletes are more likely to 'age successfully' according to different definitions of successful ageing. For example, Peel et al.'s (2005) review of longitudinal studies found that physical activity/regular exercise was a significant predictor of multidimensional 'healthy' ageing (see similar results from Baker et al. 2009). Regarding the role of sport specifically, Menec (2003) reported on longitudinal predictors of successful ageing, including involvement in a range of activities, such as social engagement (e.g., church groups), sports/games, solitary behaviours (e.g., music, reading), and productive activities (e.g., volunteer work, housework). Successful ageing was defined via measures of happiness, life satisfaction, function (physical and cognitive), well-being, and mortality. Of all the activities Menec examined, only sports/games significantly predicted both happiness and life satisfaction.

As an activity, sport may provide an environment for enjoyment, as well as improved health and function. In their position paper on the role of sport for older adults, Baker et al. (2010) proposed that involvement in masters sport could (a) help older adults negotiate the ageing process, (b) provide continued motivation for involvement in exercise and physical activity, and (c) challenge age-related stereotypes about function and capability. However, as previously mentioned, the contentious promotion of 'sport for all' (see Gard and Dionigi 2016) that positions sport participation across the lifespan not only as a right but also an obligation may encourage older people to deny the physiological realities of old age in their 'pursuit of fitness' within contemporary consumer societies (see Bauman 2000, p. 78; Dionigi 2015). Moreover, this notion of 'obligation' may create an environment in which active older people speak judgementally about inactive older people (e.g., calling them 'lazy'; Gard et al. 2017). In turn, this may potentially lead to changes in welfare policy for older adults in assuming one can simply choose an active lifestyle (Dillaway and Byrnes 2009; Rubinstein and de Medeiros 2015) and consequentially further restrict who is specifically able to participate and subsequently accrue the benefits associated with sport participation.

It is important to note that while the ability to identify individuals 'at risk' of ageing 'unsuccessfully' according to a prescribed definition may have some diagnostic relevance for physicians and clinicians, the concept as a whole has many limitations. First is the assumption that individuals can be classified as either successful or unsuccessful agers. This dichotomous assumption runs counter to notions of ageing as a process of continuous adaptation with unique and dynamic individual constraints (Baltes and Baltes 1990). Moreover, there is emerging evidence that the outcomes of high-level sport involvement in older ages may not always be positive, as mentioned previously (Dionigi 2015, 2016, 2017; Gard et al. 2017). Furthermore, a recent study by El-Bakri et al. (2017) compared a range of life satisfaction measures among masters athletes and leisurely active and inactive older adults. Their analysis revealed that masters athletes were not different from leisurely active older adults on many aspects of life satisfaction, but were actually *lower than both groups* on others (e.g., satisfaction with family and satisfaction with friends). This finding points to the fact that sport participation is not necessarily (nor simply) a positive activity for all and that as a society we need to remember the benefits as well as the drawbacks of sport.

33.4 Moving Forward: Limitations and Future Directions

Despite these emerging results suggesting sport participation may not be as universally beneficial as commonly assumed, sport involvement does seem to confer unique benefits for its participants. Notwithstanding, there is considerable research still necessary before making any definitive conclusions. In this section we consider the limitations of previous work in this area and highlight several areas where further work is needed.

One of the most critical limitations to our understanding is the general lack of information on rates of sport participation in older adults. While governments regularly collect data on involvement in physical activity and exercise, the same cannot be said for involvement in sport specific to older adults. Collecting this type of general sport involvement data, not to mention the potential value of data on involvement in specific sports, would provide a greater understanding of the size of the population affected by sport participation. It is also important to note that the samples used in prior work have been largely homogenous with respect to ethnicity (mostly White), socioeconomic status (usually wealthy), and education levels (usually high school and above). Although this is reflective of the current population of masters athletes as a whole, this homogeneity limits the generalizability of findings for those outside these demographic groups. It also points to the finding that masters sport tends to attract like-minded individuals from a similar socioeconomic and cultural demographic (Gard et al. 2017).

Moreover, much of the work on sport participation in later life has used a rather limited range of methods and/or variables. More specifically, qualitative methods have generally been used to explore masters athletes' motives for, and benefits from, competition (see work by Dionigi and her colleagues), although some exceptions exist (e.g., Eime et al. 2013; Eman 2012; Leach and Ruckert 2016; Menec 2003; Reed and Cox 2007; Young et al. 2015). There is also a lack of research exploring masters sport participants outside of major multi-sport competitions (e.g., participants outside of those at the World Masters Games or international competitions). Just as in younger age groups, it is critical to remember that the majority of sport participation is not at elite or international levels and it is possible the reasons for participation, and the benefits derived from this participation, differ between groups at different levels (recreational, local, national) and types (individual events versus multi-sport) of competition (see Baker et al. 2006), as well as between different types of sport (e.g., team versus individual or pairs). A related area of future work is to further investigate the value of sport involvement versus regular participation in physical activity and exercise to determine whether sport participation conveys additional benefits (or costs). This question is central to the discussion of the benefits of sport participation but has been largely absent in the literature (although see El-Bakri et al. 2017; Lobjois et al. 2006, 2008 for exceptions).

Another area in need of exploration is how sport participation relates to the maximization of performance in older adults. More specifically, there is a lack of information for scientists and interested athletes to use regarding the types of coaching and training practices that would be most effective for continued improvement or performance maintenance. Prior work (e.g., Dionigi et al. 2013b; Weir et al. 2002) suggest training behaviours and competition practices change as athletes age, but the extent to which this is due to necessity (e.g., athletes are unable to train as hard as they used to) or preference (e.g., they choose activities that are more enjoyable) is not known. Furthermore, Rathwell et al. (2015) have suggested that similar to younger athletes, masters athletes coaching may be most effective when coaching strategies are tailored after assessing athletes' individual needs, preferences, and abilities, and failure to do so can result in dissatisfaction or dropout. Given these nuanced training and coaching strategies may ultimately determine continued participation in sport for older adults, further research is necessary.

Finally, there is a need for more work on the multi-dimensional nature of 'health' and the need to consider developmental outcomes (e.g., qualities that might assist ageing adults in negotiating the ageing process) outside the traditional range of biomedical indicators of function and disease (Baker et al. 2010; Geard et al. 2017). Including a broader range of health outcomes such as measures of psychological, social, emotional, and spiritual health, as well as biomedical indicators of disease and function, would provide a more comprehensive profile of how (and when) sport affects development across the lifespan.

33.5 Implications

Developing national policies and practices dedicated towards older adult sport engagement has generally not been a priority for government and sporting organizations (Jenkin et al. 2016; King and King 2010). In recognition of this emerging opportunity, Jenkin and colleagues qualitatively examined the potential implications for Australian sport organizations or clubs in implementing older adult sporting initiatives. Perceived potential benefits included interpersonal and organizational improvements (e.g., intergenerational interactions and role modelling, more volunteers, maximized facility usage, and financial contributions); however, perceived barriers pertaining to these initiatives (e.g., social stereotypes and pushback related to appropriateness of activities and accessibility issues) seemed to hinder the motivations of sporting clubs towards implementing this type of programming (Jenkin et al. 2016). While organizations may be hesitant towards independently shifting their strategic initiatives, King and King (2010) have suggested the necessary role of government infrastructures in order to create changes on a wider scale, which would include incentivizing sporting organizations to modify their recruitment pursuits. Given the previous limitations section, policy and practice need to be developed at, and collaborated between, various government structures/levels (e.g., national, regional, local) and with older people themselves. That is, older adults across the physical activity spectrum, who are the targets of health promotion polices aimed at increasing sport, physical activity, and exercise participation, need to be consulted. Their stories of sport participation (or non-participation in sport) need to inform sport promotion policies and practices (Dionigi et al. 2016). Moreover, given the biopsychosocial benefits associated with sport participation, special considerations should be dedicated towards breaking down cultural, socio-economic, and disability barriers to inclusivity in sport.

In accordance with these initiatives, the paucity of information regarding older adult sport participation could be mitigated by monitoring and evaluating the effectiveness of the policies and practices mentioned above, allowing for the development of more efficient programming based on participation rates, participant motives and barriers, and community-based factors such as accessibility, affordability, and transportation (Cosgrove and Sun 2009). Once these facets have been further investigated and integrated, research and government endeavours can better advertise and raise public awareness of potential developmental assets (e.g., positive identity, empowerment, and constructive use of time; Benson 1997) that stem from sport participation, a conceptual approach widely acknowledged within the realm of youth sport as 'positive youth development', while not associated with masters sport and older adult sport engagement (Baker et al. 2009, 2010). These developmental assets pertain to meeting needs related to autonomy and independence and fostering personal growth from enhancing cognitive and psychosocial well-being (Catalano et al. 2004). Uncovering developmental assets specific to older adult sport participation can enable policy-makers to design programmes wherein they can be effectively fostered, which according to evidence within youth-sport contexts (Fraser-Thomas et al. 2005) is more likely to result in positive outcomes and maintenance of sport participation. Therefore, implications of developing policy and practice regarding sport participation during later life may reduce the focus on a narrow biomedical approach to sport promotion and increase opportunities and access for older people to participate in sport.

33.6 Conclusion

Sport is an important element of our culture throughout the life course, and the research summarized in this chapter highlights the potential for sport participation to improve the lives of older adults who have the means, ability, and desire to participate. Framing sport participation in policy, promotion, and practice as another leisure option with biopsychosocial benefits for older adults is one way forward. As argued by Jenkin et al. (2016, p. 663):

> It is not anticipated that any policy focus on older adults will significantly increase active participation for this age group. However, any increase in older adults' sport participation either through actively playing, supporting family and friends and/or volunteering will contribute to the positive health of individuals, sport clubs and the community.

Further examination of this topic may provide important insight for the development of sport-based interventions for older adults that are grounded in empirical evidence and are therefore more likely to be embraced by practitioners and administrators, as well as older people themselves.

Further Reading

- Baker, J., Horton, S., & Weir, P. (2010). *The masters athlete: Understanding the role of sport and exercise in optimizing aging.* London: Routledge/Taylor and Francis.

- Dionigi, R. A. (2008). *Competing for life: Older people, sport and ageing.* Saarbrücken: Verlag Dr. Müller.
- Dionigi, R. A., & Gard, M. (In press). *Sport and physical activity across the lifespan: Critical perspectives.* Basingstoke: Palgrave Macmillan. isbn:9781137485618.

References

Baker, J., Côté, J., & Deakin, J. (2006). Patterns of early involvement in expert and non-expert masters triathletes. *Research Quarterly for Exercise and Sport, 77*, 413–419.

Baker, J., Meisner, B. A., Logan, A. J., Kungl, A., & Weir, P. (2009). Physical activity and successful aging in Canadian older adults. *Journal of Aging and Physical Activity, 17*, 223–235.

Baker, J., Fraser-Thomas, J., Dionigi, R., & Horton, S. (2010). Sport participation and positive development in older persons. *European Review of Aging and Physical Activity, 7*, 3–12.

Baltes, P. B., & Baltes, M. (1990). Psychological perspectives on successful aging: The model of selective optimisation with compensation. In P. B. Baltes & M. M. Baltes (Eds.), *Successful aging: Perspectives from the behavioural sciences* (pp. 1–36). Cambridge: Cambridge University Press.

Bauman, Z. (2000). *Liquid modernity.* Cambridge, UK: Polity Press.

Benson, P. L. (1997). *All kids are our kids: What communities must do to raise caring and responsible children and adolescents.* San Francisco: Jossey-Bass Higher & Adult Education.

Bodner, E. (2009). On the origins of ageism among older and younger adults. *International Psychogeriatrics, 21*(6), 1003–1014.

Bohm, P., Schneider, G., Linneweber, L., Rentzsch, A., Krämer, N., Abdul-Khaliq, H., et al. (2016). Right and left ventricular function and mass in male elite master athletes: A controlled contrast enhanced CMR study. *Circulation, 133*(20), 1927–1935.

Breuer, C., Hallmann, K., & Wicker, P. (2011). Determinants of sport participation in different sports. *Managing Leisure, 16*(4), 269–286.

Canadian Heritage. (2013). *Sport participation 2010.* Her majesty the queen in right of Canada. Catalogue No. CH24-1/2012E-PDF. isbn:978-1-100-21561-7.

Cardenas, D., Henderson, K. A., & Wilson, B. E. (2009). Physical activity and senior games participation: Benefits, constraints, and behaviors. *Journal of Aging and Physical Activity, 17*(2), 135–153.

Caspersen, C. J., Powell, K. E., & Christenson, G. M. (1985). Physical activity, exercise, and physical fitness: Definitions and distinctions for health-related research. *Public Health Reports, 100*(2), 126–131.

Catalano, R. F., Berglund, M. L., Ryan, J. A. M., Lonczak, H. S., & Hawkins, J. D. (2004). Positive youth development in the United States: Research findings on evaluations of positive youth development programs. *The Annals of the American Academy of Political and Social Science, 591*(1), 98–124.

Concannon, L. G., Grierson, M. J., & Harrast, M. A. (2012). Exercise in the older adult: From the sedentary elderly to the masters athlete. *PM & R, 4*(11), 833–839.

Cosgrove, C., & Sun, B. (2009, January). Age-friendly initiatives: Breaking down barriers offers benefits for all. *Active Living: Newsletters*, N6–N7.

Degens, H., Maden-Wilkinson, T. M., Ireland, A., Korhonen, M. T., Suominen, H., Heinonen, A., et al. (2013a). Relationship between ventilatory function and age in master athletes and a sedentary reference population. *Age, 35*(3), 1007–1015.

Degens, H., Rittweger, J., Parviainen, T., Timonen, K. L., Suominen, H., Heinonen, A., & Korhonen, M. T. (2013b). Diffusion capacity of the lung in young and old endurance athletes. *International Journal of Sports Medicine, 34*(12), 1051–1057.

Dillaway, H. E., & Byrnes, M. (2009). Reconsidering successful aging: A call for renewed and expanded academic critiques and conceptualizations. *Journal of Applied Gerontology, 28*, 702–722. https://doi.org/10.1177/0733464809333882.

Dionigi, R. A. (2002). Resistance and empowerment through leisure: The meaning of competitive sport participation to older adults. *Society & Leisure, 25*(2), 303–328.

Dionigi, R. A. (2005). A leisure pursuit that 'goes against the grain': Older people and competitive sport. *Annals of Leisure Research, 8*(1), 1–22.

Dionigi, R. A. (2006). Competitive sport as leisure in later life: Negotiations, discourse, and aging. *Leisure Sciences, 28*(2), 181–196. https://doi.org/10.1080/01490400500484081.

Dionigi, R. A. (2007). Resistance training and older adults' beliefs about psychological benefits: The importance of self-efficacy and social interaction. *Journal of Sport and Exercise Psychology, 29*(6), 723–746.

Dionigi, R. A. (2008). *Competing for life: Older people, sport and ageing*. Saarbrücken: Verlag Dr. Müller.

Dionigi, R. A. (2010). Masters sport as a strategy for managing the aging process. In J. Baker, S. Horton, & P. Weir (Eds.), *The Masters athlete: Understanding the role of sport and exercise in optimizing aging* (pp. 137–155). London: Routledge.

Dionigi, R. A. (2015). Pathways to masters sport: Sharing stories from sport 'continuers', 'rekindlers' and 'late bloomers'. In E. Tulle & C. Phoenix (Eds.), *Physical activity and sport in later life: Critical approaches* (pp. 54–68). London: Palgrave.

Dionigi, R. A. (2016). The competitive older athlete: A review of psychosocial and sociological issues. *Topics in Geriatric Rehabilitation, 32*(1), 55–62.

Dionigi, R. A. (2017). Leisure and recreation in the lives of older people. In M. Bernoth & D. Winkler (Eds.), *Healthy ageing and aged care* (pp. 204–220). Melbourne: Oxford University Press.

Dionigi, R. A., & Horton, S. (2012). The influence of leisure on discourses of aging. In H. J. Gison & J. F. Singleton (Eds.), *Leisure and aging: Theory and practice* (pp. 27–39). Champaign: Human Kinetics.

Dionigi, R. A., & O'Flynn, G. (2007). Performance discourses and old age: What does it mean to be an older athlete? *Sociology of Sport Journal, 24*, 359–377.

Dionigi, R. A., Horton, S., & Baker, J. (2010). Seniors in sport: The experiences and practices of older World Masters Games competitors. *International Journal of Sport and Society, 1*, 55–68.

Dionigi, R. A., Baker, J., & Horton, S. (2011). Older athletes' perceived benefits of competition. *The International Journal of Sport and Society, 2*(2), 17–28.

Dionigi, R. A., Horton, S., & Baker, J. (2013a). Negotiations of the ageing process: Older adults' stories of sports participation. *Sport, Education and Society, 18*(3), 370–387.

Dionigi, R. A., Horton, S., & Baker, J. (2013b). How do older masters athletes account for their performance preservation? A qualitative analysis. *Ageing & Society, 33*(2), 297–319.

Dionigi, R. A., Gard, M., Horton, S., Baker, J., & Weir, P. (2016). Sport, ageing, and the physical activity spectrum: Implications for policy. *Journal of Aging and Physical Activity, 24*, S49.

Dogra, S., & Mccracken, H. (2016). Self-reported sedentary time among masters and recreational athletes aged 55 years and older. *Journal of Exercise, Movement, and Sport, 48*(1), 161.

Eime, R. M., Young, J. A., Harvey, J. T., Charity, M. J., & Payne, W. R. (2013). A systematic review of the psychological and social benefits of participation in sport for adults: Informing development of a conceptual model of health through sport. *International Journal of Behavioral Nutrition and Physical Activity, 10*, 135.

El-Bakri, R., Stone, R. C., Patelia, S., & Baker, J. (2017). *Is participation in competitive sport during older adulthood associated with greater life satisfaction?* Manuscript under review.

Eman, J. (2012). The role of sports in making sense of the process of growing old. *Journal of Aging Studies, 26*(4), 467–475. https://doi.org/10.1016/j.jaging.2012.06.006.

Fraser-Thomas, J. L., Côté, J., & Deakin, J. (2005). Youth sport programs: An avenue to foster positive youth development. *Physical Education & Sport Pedagogy, 10*(1), 19–40.

Gard, M., & Dionigi, R. A. (2016). The world turned upside down: Sport, policy and ageing. *International Journal of Sport Policy and Politics, 8*, 737–743.

Gard, M., Dionigi, R. A., Horton, S., Baker, J., Weir, P., & Dionigi, C. (2017). The normalisation of sport for older people? *Annals of Leisure Research, 20*, 253–272.

Gayman, A. M., Fraser-Thomas, J., Dionigi, R. A., Horton, S., & Baker, J. (2017a). Is sport good for older adults? A systematic review of psychosocial outcomes of older adults' sport participation. *International Review of Sport and Exercise Psychology, 10*(1), 164–185.

Gayman, A. M., Fraser-Thomas, J., Spinney, J. E. L., Stone, R. C., & Baker, J. (2017b). Leisure-time physical activity and sedentary behaviour in older people: The influence of sport involvement on behaviour patterns in later life. *AIMS Public Health, 4*(2), 171–188.

Geard, D., Reaburn, P., Rebar, A., & Dionigi, R. A. (2017). Masters athletes: Exemplars of successful aging? *Journal of Aging and Physical Activity, 25*, 490–500.

Grant, B. C. (2002). Physical activity: Not a popular leisure choice in later life. *Society and Leisure, 25*(2), 285–302.

Grant, B. C., & O'Brien Cousins, S. (2001). Ageing and physical activity: The promise of qualitative research. *Journal of Aging and Physical Activity, 9*(3), 237–244.

Hawkins, S. A., Wiswell, R. A., & Marcell, T. J. (2003). Exercise and the master athlete—A model of successful aging? *Journal of Gerontology A: Biological Science and Medical Science, 58*(11), M1009–M1011. https://doi.org/10.1093/gerona/58.11.M1009.

Heo, J., Culp, B., Yamada, N., & Won, Y. (2013). Promoting successful aging through competitive sports participation: Insights from older adults. *Qualitative Health Research, 23*(1), 105–113.

Horton, R., & Mack, D. (2000). Athletic identity in marathon runners: Functional focus or dysfunctional commitment? *Journal of Sport Behavior, 23*(2), 101.

International Masters Games Association. (2016). Retrieved January 22, 2017, from https://imga.ch/en/data/24

Jenkin, C., Eime, R. M., Westerbeek, H., O'Sullivan, G., & van Uffelen, J. G. Z. (2016). Are they 'worth their weight in gold'? Sport for older adults: Benefits and barriers of their participation for sporting organisations. *International Journal of Sport Policy and Politics, 8*(4), 663–680. https://doi.org/10.1080/19406940.2016.1220410.

King, A. C., & King, D. K. (2010). Physical activity for an aging population. *Public Health Reviews (2107–6952), 32*(2), 401–426.

Kolt, G. S., Driver, R. P., & Giles, L. C. (2004). Why older Australians participate in exercise and sport. *Journal of Aging and Physical Activity, 12*(2), 185–198.

Leach, S. J., & Ruckert, E. A. (2016). Neurologic changes with aging, physical activity, and sport participation. *Topics in Geriatric Rehabilitation, 32*(1), 24–33.

Lee, I. M., Shiroma, E. J., Lobelo, F., Puska, P., Blair, S. N., & Katzmarzyk, P. T. (2012). Effect of physical inactivity on major non-communicable diseases worldwide: An analysis of burden of disease and life expectancy. *Lancet, 13*(9838), 219–229. https://doi.org/10.1016/S0140-6736(12)61031-9.

Lobjois, R., Benguigui, N., & Bertsch, J. (2006). The effect of aging and tennis playing on coincidence-timing accuracy. *Journal of Aging and Physical Activity, 14*, 74–97.

Lobjois, R., Benguigui, N., Bertsch, J., & Broderick, M. P. (2008). Collision avoidance behavior as a function of aging and tennis playing. *Experimental Brain Research, 184*, 457–468.

Longman, J. (2016). *85-year-old marathoner is so fast that even scientists marvel.* Retrieved January 23, 2017, from https://www.nytimes.com/2016/12/28/sports/ed-whitlock-marathon-running.html?_r=0

Lyons, K., & Dionigi, R. A. (2007). Transcending emotional community: A qualitative examination of older adults and masters' sports participation. *Leisure Sciences, 29*(4), 375–389.

Menec, V. H. (2003). The relation between everyday activities and successful aging: A 6-year longitudinal study. *The Journal of Gerontology B: Psychological Sciences & Social Sciences, 58*(2), S74–S82.

Montepare, J. M., & Zebrowitz, L. A. (2002). A social-developmental view of ageism. In T. D. Nelson (Ed.), *Ageism: Stereotyping and prejudice against older persons* (pp. 77–125). Cambridge, MA: MIT Press.

Peel, N. M., McClure, R. J., & Bartlett, H. P. (2005). Behavioral determinants of healthy aging. *American Journal of Preventive Medicine, 28*, 298–304.

Ransdell, L. B., Vener, J., & Huberty, J. (2009). Masters athletes: An analysis of running, swimming and cycling performance by age and gender. *Journal of Exercise Science & Fitness, 7*(2), S61–S73.

Rathwell, S., Callary, B., & Young, B. W. (2015). Exploring the context of coached masters swim programs: A narrative approach. *International Journal of Aquatic Research and Education, 9*(1), 70–88.

Reaburn, P., & Dascombe, B. (2008). Endurance performance in masters athletes. *European Review of Aging and Physical Activity, 5*(1), 31.

Reed, C. E., & Cox, R. H. (2007). Motives and regulatory style underlying senior athletes' participation in sport. *Journal of Sport Behavior, 30*, 307–329.

Rowe, J. W., & Kahn, R. L. (1987). Human aging: Usual and successful. *Science, 237*, 143–150.

Rubinstein, R. L., & de Medeiros, K. (2015). Successful aging. Gerontological theory and neoliberalism: A qualitative critique. *The Gerontologist, 55*, 34–42. https://doi.org/10.1093/geront/gnu080.

Sarkisian, C. A., Hays, R. D., Berry, S. H., & Mangione, C. M. (2001). Expectations regarding aging among older adults and physicians who care for older adults. *Medical Care, 39*, 1025–1036.

Scanlan, T. K., Russell, D. G., Beals, K. P., & Scanlan, L. A. (2003). Project on elite athlete commitment (PEAK): II. A direct test and expansion of the sport commitment model with elite amateur sportsmen. *Journal of Sport and Exercise Psychology, 25*, 377–401.

Seeman, T. E., Charpentier, P. A., Berkman, L. F., Tinetti, M. E., Guralnik, J. M., Albert, M., Blazer, D., & Rowe, J. W. (1994). Predicting changes in physical performance in a high-functioning elderly cohort: MacArthur studies of successful aging. *Journal of Gerontology, 49*, M97–M108.

Seeman, T. E., Berkman, L. F., Charpentier, P. A., Blazer, D. G., Albert, M. S., & Tinetti, M. E. (1995). Behavioral and psychosocial predictors of physical performance: MacArthur studies of successful aging. *The Journals of Gerontology Series A: Biological Sciences and Medical Sciences, 50*, M177–M183.

Slade, J. M., Miszko, T. A., Laity, J. H., Agrawal, S. K., & Cress, M. E. (2002). Anaerobic power and physical function in strength-trained and non-strength-trained older adults. *Journal of Gerontology & Medical Science, 57A*, M168–M172.

Sneed, J. R., & Krauss Whitbourne, S. (2005). Models of the aging self. *Journal of Social Issues, 61*, 375–388.

Steinmo, S., Hagger-Johnson, G., & Shahab, L. (2014). Bidirectional association between mental health and physical activity in older adults: Whitehall II prospective cohort study. *Preventive Medicine, 66*, 74–79.

Stenner, B. J., Mosewich, A. D., & Buckley, J. D. (2016). An exploratory investigation into the reasons why older people play golf. *Qualitative Research in Sport, Exercise and Health, 8*(3), 257–272.

Stone, R. C., Meisner, B. A., & Baker, J. (2012). Mood disorders among older adults participating in individual and group active environments: "Me" versus "Us," or both? *Journal of Aging Research*. https://doi.org/10.1155/2012/727983.

Strawbridge, W. J., Wallhagen, M. I., & Cohen, R. D. (2002). Successful aging and well-being: Self-rated compared with Rowe and Kahn. *The Gerontologist, 42*, 727–733.

Tanaka, H., & Seals, D. R. (2008). Endurance exercise performance in masters athletes: Age-associated changes and underlying physiological mechanisms. *The Journal of Physiology, 586*(1), 55–63.

Taylor, D. (2014). Physical activity is medicine for older adults. *Postgraduate Medical Journal, 90*(1059), 26–32.

Tseng, B. Y., Uh, J., Rossetti, H. C., Cullum, C. M., Diaz-Arrastia, R. F., Levine, B. D., et al. (2013). Masters athletes exhibit larger regional brain volume and better cognitive performance than sedentary older adults. *Journal of Magnetic Resonance Imaging, 38*(5), 1169–1176.

Tulle, E. (2007). Running to run: Embodiment, structure and agency amongst veteran elite runners. *Sociology, 41*(2), 329–346.

Ungerleider, S., Golding, J. M., & Porter, K. (1989). Mood profiles of masters track and field athletes. *Perceptual and Motor Skills, 68*(2), 607–617.

United Nations. (2013). *World population ageing 2013*. Department of Economic & social affairs – Population division. Retrieved January 23, 2017, from http://www.un.org/en/development/desa/population/publications/pdf/ageing/WorldPopulationAgeing2013.pdf

van Tuyckom, C., & Scheerder, J. (2008). "Sport for all?" Social stratification of recreational sport activities in the EU-27. *Kinesiologia Slovenica, 14*(2), 54–63.

van Tuyckom, C., Scheerder, J., & Bracke, P. (2010). Gender and age inequalities in regular sports participation: A cross-national study of 25 European countries. *Journal of Sports Sciences, 28*(10), 1077–1084.

Velez, N. F., Zhang, A., Stone, B., Perera, S., Miller, M., & Greenspan, S. L. (2008). The effect of moderate impact exercise on skeletal integrity in master athletes. *Osteoporosis International, 19*(10), 1457–1464.

Weir, P. L., Kerr, T., Hodges, N. J., McKay, S. M., & Starkes, J. L. (2002). Master swimmers: How are they different from younger elite swimmers? An examination of practice and performance patterns. *Journal of Aging and Physical Activity, 10,* 41–63.

Wilks, D. C., Winwood, K., Gilliver, S. F., Kwiet, A., Chatfield, M., Michaelis, I., et al. (2009). Bone mass and geometry of the tibia and the radius of master sprinters, middle and long distance runners, race-walkers and sedentary control participants: A pQCT study. *Bone, 45*(1), 91–97.

Wroblewski, A. P., Amati, F., Smiley, M. A., Goodpaster, B., & Wright, V. (2011). Chronic exercise preserves lean muscle mass in masters athletes. *The Physician and Sports Medicine, 39*(3), 172–178.

Young, B. W., Bennett, A., & Séguin, B. (2015). Masters sport perspectives. In M. M. Parent & J. L. Chappelet (Eds.), *Routledge handbook of sports event management: A stakeholder approach* (pp. 136–162). London: Routledge.

Zhao, E., Tranovich, M. J., DeAngelo, R., Kontos, A. P., & Wright, V. J. (2016). Chronic exercise preserves brain function in masters athletes when compared to sedentary counterparts. *The Physician and Sports Medicine, 44*(1), 8–13.

34

Physical Activity as a Strategy to Promote Cognitive Health Among Older People

Teresa Liu-Ambrose

34.1 Introduction

With the world's ageing population increasing, it is imperative we identify efficient (i.e., effective and economical) strategies that can promote healthy ageing at a population level. Maintaining cognitive capacity is vital to healthy ageing, functional independence, and quality of life. According to the World Health Organization and the Alzheimer's Disease International (2012), one new case of dementia is detected every four seconds worldwide. Individuals with cognitive impairment and dementia have reduced quality of life as they lose their functional independence (Barrios et al. 2013). As the proportion of the population over 65 years continues to increase, dementia will place increasing demands and costs on the health and social care system, as well as caregivers. Thus, the societal value of identifying and developing effective intervention and prevention strategies cannot be overstated (Brookmeyer et al. 2007). If the onset or progression of dementia were delayed by one year, there would be nine million fewer cases worldwide by 2050 (Brookmeyer et al. 2007).

Effective drug treatment of dementia remains a major challenge (Raschetti et al. 2007). As a result, there is much interest in lifestyle approaches for preventing or treating dementia. Notably, a 10–25% reduction in modifiable risk

T. Liu-Ambrose (✉)
Againg, Mobility, and Cognitive Neuroscience Laboratory, Department of Physical Therapy, University of British Columbia, Vancouver Coastal Health Research Institute, Vancouver, BC, Canada

factors such as smoking, mid-life obesity, hypertension, type 2 diabetes, depression, and physical inactivity would prevent as many as three million cases of dementia worldwide (Barnes and Yaffe 2011).

As such, there is strong interest in physical activity as a primary behavioural prevention strategy against cognitive decline. Notably, physical activity significantly reduces the risk of developing chronic conditions that are associated with cognitive impairment and dementia (Barnes and Yaffe 2011), such as hypertension and type 2 diabetes, for both Alzheimer's disease (AD) and vascular cognitive impairment—the two most common types of dementia.

In this chapter, we will provide an overview of the current evidence, with a particular focus on randomized controlled trials, for the role of physical activity in promoting cognitive health (i.e., maintaining mental capacity and performance) in older adults, discuss the possible underlying mechanisms, and conclude with limitations and future directions for this rapidly expanding line of research. As we delve into the specific randomized controlled trials, one should consider the following factors along with the study findings: (1) type of exercise training, (2) training durations, (3) training intensity, (4) training frequency, (5) sample size, and (6) target population.

34.2 Critical Review

Epidemiological studies have largely focused on assessing the association between the amount of physical activity and cognitive health. Historically, physical activity in epidemiological studies has been recorded by self-report questionnaires that typically ask participants to recall their level of physical activity over the last seven days. A key strength of self-report questionnaires is its high feasibility of administration to a large number of research participants. However, they are prone to social desirability biases (people providing answers they think the researcher will want to hear rather than providing honest answers) and thus, may provide inaccurate estimates of physical activity. More recent studies have begun to successfully employ objective measures of physical activity using monitoring devices, such as accelerometers and pedometers (Gow et al. 2012). These studies tend to demonstrate a greater magnitude of benefit of physical activity on cognitive and brain outcomes than studies using self-report questionnaires (Middleton et al. 2011).

34.2.1 What Is Currently Known?

34.2.1.1 Epidemiology Studies

Accumulating data from epidemiological research indicates substantial benefits of regular physical activity for cognitive function (Buchman et al. 2012; Erickson et al. 2011a; Lee et al. 2015; Sattler et al. 2011; Weuve et al. 2004; Yaffe et al. 2001). Epidemiological studies are observational in nature and examine whether engagement in physical activity is associated with longitudinal changes in cognitive function or risk for dementia. Overall, epidemiological studies demonstrate a consistent relationship between higher physical activity levels and reduced risk of developing dementia or of cognitive decline. A meta-analysis of 16 prospective epidemiological studies on the incidence of neurodegenerative disease found more physical activity at baseline reduced the risk of developing dementia (resulting from all causes) by 28% and of developing AD by 45%, even after controlling for confounding variables (Hamer and Chida 2009). Another more recent meta-analysis of 15 prospective studies among individuals without dementia found that high levels of physical activity reduced the risk of cognitive decline by 38%, while low to moderate levels reduced the risk by 35% (Sofi et al. 2011).

Moreover, using structural magnetic resonance imaging (MRI), Erickson and colleagues (2011a) provide insight as to how much regular physical activity is required as well as how it promotes cognitive health. In 299 adults (mean age 78 years) from the Cardiovascular Health Cognition Study, Erickson and colleagues (2011a) assessed the association between grey-matter volume, physical activity, and cognitive impairment in community-dwelling older adults with normal cognitive function. Grey matter is composed of neuronal cell bodies, dendrites, and synapses, whereas white matter is composed of axons and myelin. AD has long been thought of as a grey-matter disease with severe grey-matter atrophy seen first in the entorhinal cortex and hippocampus (Janke et al. 2001). Baseline physical activity was quantified as the number of blocks walked, the equivalent of a distant of 100 metres (approximately) in one week, and structural MRIs were acquired nine years later. Clinical adjudication for cognitive impairment occurred 13 years after baseline. Erickson and colleagues (2011a) demonstrated that greater physical activity, walking 72 blocks, at baseline is associated with greater volumes of frontal, occipital, entorhinal, and hippocampal brain regions nine years later. Moreover, greater grey-matter volume was associated with a twofold reduction in the risk for cognitive impairment.

Results from studies with objective measures of physical activity provide additional support for the positive association between physical activity and cognitive function. For example, Buchman and colleagues (2012) reported that greater total daily physical activity as assessed by ten days of continuously monitored actigraphy (physical activity detected from sensors worn on the body) was associated with a twofold reduced risk of AD over a four-year period in 716 older adults, even after controlling for self-reported physical activity.

In regard to providing specific physical activity recommendations to promote cognitive health in older adults, a major limitation of epidemiology studies is that they do not distinguish between different types of physical activity. Broadly, there are two main types of physical activity: (1) aerobic exercise training (e.g., running), aimed at improving cardiovascular health, and (2) resistance training (e.g., lifting weights), aimed at improving muscle mass and strength. Yet, each type of exercise training has its own distinct physiology and benefits (Wanderley et al. 2013).

To some extent, Lee and colleagues (2015) recently addressed this gap in epidemiology evidence by examining the amount and type of physical exercise that might reduce the future risk of dementia in community-living older people. This six-year observational study included a total of 15,589 community-living Chinese adults aged 65 years and older with no history of stroke, clinical dementia, or Parkinson disease when they completed the baseline health assessment. Self-reported habitual physical exercise patterns in the past one month, including the frequency, duration, and type of exercise, at baseline and three years later were analysed. The type of exercise training was then classified as: (1) aerobic (i.e., jogging, running, swimming, hiking, ball games, and cycling), (2) mind-body (e.g., Tai Chi and yoga), (3) stretching and toning (i.e., strolling and shaking limbs), and (4) others. The study outcome was incident dementia six years from baseline. Lee and colleagues (2015) found that compared with those who developed dementia, those who remained dementia-free performed more aerobic and mind-body exercises regardless of type or duration of activity. However, stretching-and-toning exercises did not reduce the risk of dementia. A key limitation of this study is the lack of quantification of resistance training.

34.2.1.2 Randomized Controlled Trials

Randomized controlled trials are studies in which participants are randomly allocated to one of several experimental groups. One of the experimental groups is the standard of comparison or control. To reduce both known (e.g., socialization) and unknown confounding effects, it is recommended that randomized controlled trials of targeted exercise training and cognitive health use an active control arm that provides light stretching or low-intensity exercise training (Nagamatsu et al. 2011). Results from randomized controlled studies further corroborate the association between targeted exercise training (i.e., aerobic exercise and resistance training) and cognitive health. Accordingly, four meta-analyses of randomized controlled trials (where the results of several trials are combined) concluded that targeted exercise training has cognitive benefits for older adults (Barha et al. 2017a; Colcombe and Kramer 2003; Etnier et al. 2006; Heyn et al. 2004). Notably, in the systematic review and meta-analyses by Barha and colleagues (2017a), it was shown that aerobic training, resistance training, and multimodal training (i.e., both aerobic and resistance training) were beneficial for executive functions—particularly in randomized controlled trials with a higher percentage of women. This suggests that women may benefit more from targeted exercise training than men. Hence, more research is needed to better understand factors, such as biological sex, that may moderate the benefit of targeted exercise training on cognitive health (Barha et al. 2017b).

A key challenge of epidemiological data is the interpretation of causality. For example, it is possible that those individuals who engage in more physical activity have a more robust genetic profile against cognitive impairment and dementia. Thus, evidence from randomized controlled trials is critical in providing insight to the causal direction between physical activity and cognitive health.

Kramer and colleagues (Colcombe et al. 2003, 2004, 2006; Kramer et al. 1999) conducted seminal work in demonstrating the benefit of aerobic exercise training on cognitive and brain health in older adults. In a sample of 124 cognitively healthy, but low-fit older adults that were randomized to six months of either an aerobic exercise intervention (i.e., brisk walking) or to a stretching-and-toning control condition, Kramer and colleagues (Kramer et al. 1999) demonstrated that the aerobic exercise group, compared with control group, significantly improved executive functions. Executive functions are cognitive abilities that allow individuals to interact with their environment in an efficient, effective manner, particularly under novel circumstances. They include cognitive abilities such as decision making and problem solving. Executive functioning decline substantially with ageing as does the volume of brain regions that support them (West 1996). Thus, the results of this randomized controlled trial suggest that even cognitive processes that are highly susceptible to age-related changes appear to be amendable to aerobic exercise interventions.

Colcombe and Kramer (2003) then conducted a meta-analysis of 18 randomized controlled trials that included aerobic exercise as an intervention. They concluded that targeted aerobic exercise training has robust but selective benefits for cognition, with the largest aerobic exercise-induced benefits occurring for executive functions. Notably, Colcombe and Kramer (2003) also found that aerobic-based training programs combined with resistance training had a greater positive effect on cognition than aerobic training alone.

More recently, in a randomized controlled trial with 120 older adults, Erickson and colleagues (2011b) demonstrated that three times per week of one-hour aerobic exercise training increased hippocampal volume by 2%, which led to improvements in spatial memory. These are notable findings given that after the age of 55, the hippocampus atrophies by 1–2% per year (Raz et al. 2005) and this loss of volume increase the risk for developing cognitive impairment. Moreover, Erickson and colleagues (2011b) found that increased hippocampal volume is associated with greater serum levels of brain-derived neurotrophic factor (BDNF). BDNF is a protein and key neurotrophic growth factor in brain plasticity. Brain plasticity refers to the capacity of the brain to change, even with age, if given the appropriate environmental stimuli, thoughts, and emotions.

It is well recognized that the majority of randomized controlled trials to date has focused on aerobic exercise training, defined as cardiovascular exercise where the heart rate is raised (Colcombe and Kramer 2003). Yet, not all older adults have the necessary mobility to participate in targeted aerobic exercise training at the recommended intensities and duration. Thus, other types of targeted exercise training, such as resistance training, must be considered and evaluated. Auspiciously, there is a growing interest in the role of resistance training (Liu-Ambrose and Donaldson 2009), and recent research findings indicate that it is beneficial for both cognitive and functional brain plasticities (Best et al. 2015; Liu-Ambrose et al. 2010, 2012; Nagamatsu et al. 2012). These findings are not be surprising given that resistance training, similar to aerobic exercise, reduces the risk of developing chronic conditions (Cornelissen and Fagard 2005; Hovanec et al. 2012; Strasser et al. 2010; Taaffe et al. 2007; Williams et al. 2007) that are associated with cognitive impairment and dementia, and promotes neurotrophic factors that are beneficial for the brain (Cassilhas et al. 2007, 2012). Specifically, in humans, resistance training is associated with increased blood levels of insulin growth factor-1 (IGF-1), while aerobic exercise training is associated with increased levels of BDNF (Cassilhas et al. 2007, 2016; Erickson et al. 2011b).

Aside from its neurocognitive benefits, resistance training may be a particularly important mode of exercise for seniors as it specifically moderates sarcopenia (age-related loss in both muscle mass and strength), whereas aerobic exercise training does not. The multifactorial deleterious sequelae of sarcopenia include increased falls and fracture risk as well as physical disability. For more than a decade in the United States, resistance training has been recommended for adults, particularly seniors, as a primary prevention intervention, and increasing the prevalence of resistance training is an objective of Healthy People 2010 (United States Department of Health and Human Services 2010).

At initial review of randomized controlled trials of resistance training, the results may appear equivocal, or less consistent than those of aerobic exercise training. However, it should be noted that most studies with negative results have small sample sizes (i.e., 13–23 participants per experimental group), short intervention periods (i.e., 8–16 weeks), and training protocols that did not require progressive loading or were of moderate intensity (Dustman et al. 1984; Kimura et al. 2010; Perrig-Chiello et al. 1998; Tsutsumi et al. 1997).

A key randomized controlled trial supporting the notion that resistance training is beneficial for cognitive function was conducted by Cassilhas and colleagues (2007). They demonstrated that resistance training three times per week for 24 weeks significantly improved several measures of cognitive function among 62 community-dwelling senior men aged 65–75 years. Notably, comparable benefits were observed for both high- and moderate-intensity groups, defined as 80% and 50% of single-repetition maximum lift (i.e., 1 RM), respectively. Results from this study suggest that even moderate-intensity resistance training for a relatively short time period, such as six months, can have a significant impact on cognitive function. Using a protocol similar to that of Cassilhas and colleagues (2007), Busse and colleagues (2008) showed that resistance training may also be beneficial for sedentary older adults at greater risk for Alzheimer's disease—those with objectively mild memory impairment.

Extending the work of Cassilhas and colleagues (2007), Liu-Ambrose and colleagues (2010) found that both once- and twice-weekly moderate-intensity resistance training significantly improved the executive processes of selective attention and conflict resolution in senior women. Specifically, community-dwelling senior women participated in a 12-month randomized controlled trial that required them to engage in resistance training either one or two days per week. The intensity of the training stimulus was at a work range of six to eight repetitions to fatigue with a 60-second rest between each set, two sets in total. Compared with a balance and tone control group, those in the resistance training groups performed significantly better on the Stroop Colour-Word Test at trial completion. For the Stroop Colour-Word Test, there were three conditions. First, participants were instructed to read out words printed in black ink (e.g., BLUE). Second, they were instructed to read out the colour of coloured-X's. Finally, they were shown a page with colour words printed in incongruent coloured inks (e.g., the word 'BLUE' printed in red ink). Participants were asked to name the ink colour in which the words are printed (while ignoring the word itself). There were 80 trials for each condition and we recorded the time participants took to read each condition. The ability to selectively attend and control response output was calculated as the time difference between the third condition and the second condition. Smaller time differences indicate better selective attention and conflict resolution.

Changes in functional activation in the cortex were also examined in each of the three groups (Liu-Ambrose et al. 2012). Interestingly, only the twice-weekly resistance training group showed increased neural activation in two key regions of cortex integral for response inhibition—the anterior portion of the left middle temporal gyrus and the left anterior insula extending into the lateral occipital frontal cortex. Thus, while resistance training once per week may improve executive functions at a behavioural level, twice-weekly training may be required for functional plasticity at the neural level.

There is also emerging evidence that resistance training may impact pre-existing pathology in the brain. In a secondary analysis of the 12-month randomized controlled trial of progressive resistance training mentioned above (Liu-Ambrose et al. 2010), Bolandzadeh, Liu-Ambrose, and colleagues (Bolandzadeh et al. 2015) provided preliminary evidence that compared with balance and tone training (i.e., control), twice-weekly moderate-intensity resistance training (for 40 minutes) significantly reduced the progression of white matter lesions in the brain. White matter lesions appear as hyperintensities on T2-weighted magnetic resonance imaging (MRI) and are markers of (but not specific to) cerebral small-vessel disease (Huijts et al. 2013). These covert lesions are highly prevalent in older adults (Kuo and Lipsitz 2004), with epidemiological studies reporting a prevalence of 85% or greater (de Leeuw et al. 2001; Liao et al. 1996; Longstreth et al. 1996), and are significantly associated with impaired cognitive function and mobility. Bolandzadeh and colleagues (2015) also showed that reduced white matter lesion progression over 12 months was significantly associated with maintenance of gait speed. However, the magnitude of correlation between white matter lesion progression and gait speed was similar to that of white matter lesion progression and executive functions ($r = -0.31$, $P = 0.049$ for gait speed versus $r = 0.30$, $P = 0.06$ for executive functions). These results provide novel insights as to how resistance training may promote both mobility and cognitive outcomes in older adults at risk for functional decline.

The results from Bolandzadeh and colleagues (2015) as well as Busse and colleagues (2008) suggest that beneficial effects of targeted exercise training on cognitive and functional brain plasticity are not restricted to cognitively healthy older adults. In particular, there is now much interest in assessing the effect of exercise in individuals at risk for dementia, such as those with mild cognitive impairment (MCI). Mild cognitive impairment is a well-recognized risk factor for dementia. Longitudinal studies report that older adults with MCI develop AD at a rate of 10–30% annually (Busse et al. 2003; Petersen et al. 1999), compared to 1–2% of older adults without MCI (Petersen et al. 1999). Mild cognitive impairment is characterized by cognitive decline that is greater than expected for an individual's age and education level, but does not significantly interfere with everyday function (Petersen et al. 2001). Thus, MCI represents a critical window of opportunity for intervening and altering the trajectory of both cognitive decline and loss of functional independence in older adults.

Lautenschlager and colleagues (2008) conducted one of the first high-quality randomized controlled trials of physical activity in those with MCI. In 170 adults aged 50 years or older who reported memory problems but did not meet criteria for dementia, they demonstrated that a 24-week home-based programme of physical activity significantly improved cognitive function as measured by the Alzheimer's Disease Assessment Scale-Cognitive Subscale (ADAS-Cog). The physical activity intervention focused on encouraging participants to partake at least 150 minutes of moderate-intensity physical activity per week. Participants in the intervention group improved 0.26 points (95% confidence interval, 0.89–0.54) and those in the usual care group deteriorated 1.04 points (95% confidence interval, 0.32–1.82) on the ADAS-Cog at the end of the intervention.

Baker and colleagues (2010) examined the efficacy of high-intensity aerobic exercise training on cognitive function in older adults with MCI. They randomized 33 older adults with MCI to either an aerobic exercise training group or to a stretching control group for four days per week for six months. The aerobic exercise group trained under the supervision of a fitness trainer at 75–85% of heart rate reserve for 45–60 minutes per day, four days per week for six months. The stretching control group carried out supervised stretching activities according to the same schedule but maintained their heart rate at or below 50% of their heart rate reserve. Interestingly, compared with the stretching control group, they found that the aerobic exercise significantly improved cognitive function in women, but not in men. It is noteworthy that this sex-specific effect was also reported in two meta-analyses (Barha et al. 2017a; Colcombe and Kramer 2003).

The potential benefit of targeted aerobic training for older adults with MCI is further demonstrated by Liu-Ambrose and colleagues (2016) who demonstrated that thrice-weekly training significantly improved global cognitive function, as measured by the ADAS-Cog (Rosen et al. 1984), among older adults with MCI primarily due to vascular pathology. Moreover, reduction of cardiovascular risk factors may be an important pathway by which aerobic exercise improves cognitive function as reduced diastolic blood pressure was significantly associated with improved ADAS-Cog performance. Moreover, in a subset of individuals who underwent functional MRI, there was evidence of neural efficiency (Hsu et al. 2017), which can be defined as the level of activity a neural network requires in order to complete the task at hand (Barulli and Stern 2013). Specifically, among this subset, thrice-weekly aerobic training resulted in improved executive functions and reduced neural activation of associated brain regions; reduced activity was significantly associated with improved executive performance (Hsu et al. 2017).

Zheng and colleagues (2016) published a systematic review and meta-analysis of 11 randomized controlled trials of aerobic exercise training on cognitive function in older adults with MCI. Meta-analysis showed that aerobic exercise training significantly improved global cognitive ability as measured by Mini-Mental State Examination or Montreal Cognitive Assessment. In regard to specific cognitive domains, aerobic exercise training only had a small but positive effect on short-term recall (memory).

The results of Zheng and colleagues (2016) extend the results of an earlier systematic review by Ohman and colleagues (2014). Ohman and colleagues (2014) assessed the evidence from 22 randomized controlled trials of all types of targeted exercise training. Overall, targeted exercise training had positive effects on global cognition, executive functions, attention, and delayed recall among older adults with MCI. However, among those with dementia, there was generally no effect of targeted exercise training on cognitive function.

Current evidence also suggests that resistance training is a promising strategy for promoting cognitive health among older adults with MCI. In 86 older women with MCI, Nagamatsu and colleagues (2012) demonstrated that six months of twice-weekly moderate-intensity resistance training significantly improved the executive cognitive processes of selective attention and conflict resolution compared with balance and tone training (i.e., control). They also found improvements in associative memory—the ability to remember items that were previously presented simultaneously. In conjunction, regional patterns of functional plasticity were found in the resistance training group.

Notably, the improvements observed in executive performance were after only six months of resistance training in those with MCI, compared with 12 months in otherwise cognitively healthy seniors (Liu-Ambrose et al. 2010). Thus, it appears that the benefits of moderate-intensity resistance training can be observed earlier in those with a larger opportunity for change or improvement (i.e., older adults with MCI). In a full factorial randomized controlled trial, Suo and colleagues (2016) also found that resistance training benefited cognitive function in adults aged 55 years or older with MCI. Specifically, they found that six months of moderate-intensity resistance training (i.e., three sets of eight repetitions) significantly improved ADAS-Cog scores as well as expanded grey matter in the posterior cingulate. Moreover, resistance training also reduced progression of white matter lesions.

Overall, the current evidence suggests that moderate amounts and intensity of exercise—both aerobic and resistance training—may improve cognitive outcomes in older adults with and without MCI. Nevertheless, more research is required to better understand the magnitude, generalization, persistence, and mechanisms of benefit (Gates et al. 2013; Ohman et al. 2014) as well as the type of exercise training to prescribe (Nagamatsu et al. 2014). Notably, higher-quality randomized controlled trials are needed. As such, future randomized controlled trials should be designed with sufficient training duration (i.e., = or > 6 months), intensity, frequency, and sample size and include possible mechanistic outcomes (e.g., growth factors, cortisol, etc.). Moreover, future trials need to ensure bias is minimized (i.e., blinding, allocation concealment, control groups with equal engagement with researchers and peers as the training groups, and reduce contamination). Finally, in order to compare and summarize results across trials, it would be helpful to establish a set of standardized set of cognitive measures and standardized exercise protocols among researchers.

34.2.2 Knowledge Gaps to Be Addressed by Future Research

A large degree of variation still exists in exercise efficacy for improving cognitive function in humans, as several meta-analyses of RCTs have found modest to minimal or no effects of engaging in targeted exercise training (Kelly et al. 2014; Young et al. 2015). To maximize its effectiveness and promote adherence, it is imperative to use evidence-based recommendations to personalize targeted exercise recommendations. However, we currently lack the prerequisite knowledge regarding potential factors that moderate exercise efficacy. A better understanding of *what type* of exercise regime is most beneficial for cognitive performance and for *whom*, and *how* each type of exercise exerts its influence on the brain will lead to tailored strategies that go beyond the one-size-fits-all approach, allowing exercise to be prescribed precisely as medication for healthy cognitive ageing.

34.3 Implications for Practice

Findings to date reinforce current American College of Sports Medicine (ACSM) overall recommendation for most adults to engage in at least 150 minutes of moderate-intensity exercise each week. Specifically, clinicians should consider encouraging patients to undertake both aerobic exercise training (e.g., running, aimed at improving cardiovascular health) and resistance training (e.g., lifting weights, aimed at improving muscle mass and strength) not only for 'physical health' but also because of the almost certain benefits for 'brain health'. Individuals interested in taking up resistance training should consult with their family physician and may wish to review the *ACSM Position Stand: Progression Models in Resistance Training in Healthy Adults* (Kraemer et al. 2002).

34.4 Conclusions

In summary, research in the area of exercise neuroscience over the last decade provide an optimistic outlook to our future in dementia prevention. It really may be as simple as keeping the ageing population as physically active for as long as possible. Some may still argue the evidence is still not quite there yet—that we need larger and longer trials with hard outcomes. However, can we afford to keep waiting given the impending crisis that both our health-care system and society will face? Furthermore, is there any other intervention strategy that could be feasibly implemented at the population level with equal benefits as exercise?

Suggested Further Reading

- Forbes, D., Forbes, S. C., Blake, C. M., Thiessen, E. J., & Forbes, S. (2015). *Exercise programs for people with dementia*. Cochrane Database of Systematic Reviews, CD006489. https://doi.org/10.1002/14651858.CD006489.pub4.

- Global Council on Brain Health (GCBH). (2016). The brain-body connection: GCBH recommendations on physical activity and brain health. http://www.aarp.org/health/brain-health/global-council-on-brain-health/
- Northey, J. M., Cherbuin, N., Pumpa, K. L., et al. Exercise interventions for cognitive function in adults older than 50: A systematic review with meta-analysis. *British Journal of Sports Medicine*. Published Online First: 24 April 2017. https://doi.org/10.1136/bjsports-2016-096587.

References

Baker, L. D., Frank, L. L., Foster-Schubert, K., Green, P. S., Wilkinson, C. W., McTiernan, A., et al. (2010). Effects of aerobic exercise on mild cognitive impairment: A controlled trial. *Archives of Neurology, 67*(1), 71–79.

Barha, C. K., Davis, J. C., Falck, R. S., Nagamatsu, L. S., & Liu-Ambrose, T. (2017a). Sex differences in exercise efficacy to improve cognition: A systematic review and meta-analysis of randomized controlled trials in older humans. *Frontiers in Neuroendocrinology, 46*, 71. https://doi.org/10.1016/j.yfrne.2017.04.002.

Barha, C. K., Galea, L. A., Nagamatsu, L. S., Erickson, K. I., & Liu-Ambrose, T. (2017b). Personalising exercise recommendations for brain health: Considerations and future directions. *British Journal of Sports Medicine, 51*(8), 636–639. https://doi.org/10.1136/bjsports-2016-096710.

Barnes, D. E., & Yaffe, K. (2011). The projected effect of risk factor reduction on Alzheimer's disease prevalence. *Lancet Neurology, 10*(9), 819–828.

Barrios, H., Narciso, S., Guerreiro, M., Maroco, J., Logsdon, R., & de Mendonca, A. (2013). Quality of life in patients with mild cognitive impairment. *Aging and Mental Health, 17*(3), 287–292. https://doi.org/10.1080/13607863.2012.747083.

Barulli, D., & Stern, Y. (2013). Efficiency, capacity, compensation, maintenance, plasticity: Emerging concepts in cognitive reserve. *Trends in Cognitive Science, 17*(10), 502–509. https://doi.org/10.1016/j.tics.2013.08.012.

Best, J. R., Chiu, B. K., Liang Hsu, C., Nagamatsu, L. S., & Liu-Ambrose, T. (2015). Long-term effects of resistance exercise training on cognition and brain volume in older women: Results from a randomized controlled trial. *Journal of the International Neuropsychological Society, 21*(10), 745–756. https://doi.org/10.1017/S1355617715000673.

Bolandzadeh, N., Tam, R., Handy, T. C., Nagamatsu, L. S., Hsu, C. L., Davis, J. C., et al. (2015). Resistance training and white matter lesion progression in older women: Exploratory analysis of a 12-month randomized controlled trial. *Journal of the American Geriatrics Society, 63*(10), 2052–2060. https://doi.org/10.1111/jgs.13644.

Brookmeyer, R., Johnson, E., Ziegler-Graham, K., & Arrighi, H. (2007). Forecasting the global burden of Alzheimer's disease. *Alzheimer's and Dementia, 3*, 186–191.

Buchman, A. S., Boyle, P. A., Yu, L., Shah, R. C., Wilson, R. S., & Bennett, D. A. (2012). Total daily physical activity and the risk of AD and cognitive decline in older adults. *Neurology, 78*(17), 1323–1329.

Busse, A., Bischkopf, J., Riedel-Heller, S. G., & Angermeyer, M. C. (2003). Mild cognitive impairment: Prevalence and incidence according to different diagnostic criteria. Results of the Leipzig longitudinal study of the aged (LEILA75+). *British Journal of Psychiatry, 182*, 449–454.

Busse, A. L., Filho, W. J., Magaldi, R. M., Coelho, V. A., Melo, A. C., Betoni, R. A., & Santarém, J. M. (2008). Effects of resistance training exercise on cognitive performance in elderly individuals with memory impairment: Results of a controlled trial. *Einstein, 6*(4), 402–407.

Cassilhas, R. C., Lee, K. S., Fernandes, J., Oliveira, M. G., Tufik, S., Meeusen, R., & de Mello, M. T. (2012). Spatial memory is improved by aerobic and resistance exercise through divergent molecular mechanisms. *Neuroscience, 202*, 309–317.

Cassilhas, R. C., Tufik, S., & de Mello, M. T. (2016). Physical exercise, neuroplasticity, spatial learning and memory. *Cellular and Molecular Life Sciences, 73*(5), 975–983. https://doi.org/10.1007/s00018-015-2102-0.

Cassilhas, R. C., Viana, V. A., Grassmann, V., Santos, R. T., Santos, R. F., Tufik, S., & Mello, M. T. (2007). The impact of resistance exercise on the cognitive function of the elderly. *Medicine & Science in Sports & Exercise, 39*(8), 1401–1407.

Colcombe, S. J., & Kramer, A. F. (2003). Fitness effects on the cognitive function of older adults: A meta-analytic study. *Psychological Science, 14*(2), 125–130.

Colcombe, S. J., Erickson, K. I., Raz, N., Webb, A. G., Cohen, N. J., McAuley, E., & Kramer, A. F. (2003). Aerobic fitness reduces brain tissue loss in aging humans. *Journal of Gerontology A, Biological Sciences and Medical Sciences, 58*(2), 176–180.

Colcombe, S. J., Erickson, K. I., Scalf, P. E., Kim, J. S., Prakash, R., McAuley, E., et al. (2006). Aerobic exercise training increases brain volume in aging humans. *Journal of Gerontology A, Biological Sciences and Medical Sciences, 61*(11), 1166–1170.

Colcombe, S. J., Kramer, A. F., Erickson, K. I., Scalf, P., McAuley, E., Cohen, N. J., et al. (2004). Cardiovascular fitness, cortical plasticity, and aging. *Proceedings of the National Academy of Sciences U S A, 101*(9), 3316–3321.

Cornelissen, V. A., & Fagard, R. H. (2005). Effect of resistance training on resting blood pressure: A meta-analysis of randomized controlled trials. *Journal of Hypertension, 23*(2), 251–259.

de Leeuw, F. E., de Groot, J. C., Achten, E., Oudkerk, M., Ramos, L. M., Heijboer, R., et al. (2001). Prevalence of cerebral white matter lesions in elderly people: A population based magnetic resonance imaging study. The Rotterdam scan study. *Journal of Neurology, Neurosurgery, & Psychiatry, 70*(1), 9–14.

Dustman, R. E., Ruhling, R. O., Russell, E. M., Shearer, D. E., Bonekat, H. W., Shigeoka, J. W., et al. (1984). Aerobic exercise training and improved neuropsychological function of older individuals. *Neurobiology of Aging, 5*(1), 35–42.

Erickson, K. I., Raji, C. A., Lopez, O. L., Becker, J. T., Rosano, C., Newman, A. B., et al. (2011a). Physical activity predicts gray matter volume in late adulthood: The cardiovascular health study. *Neurology, 75*(16), 1415–1422.

Erickson, K. I., Voss, M. W., Prakash, R. S., Basak, C., Szabo, A., Chaddock, L., et al. (2011b). Exercise training increases size of hippocampus and improves memory. *Proceedings of the National Academy of Sciences U S A, 108*(7), 3017–3022.

Etnier, J. L., Nowell, P. M., Landers, D. M., & Sibley, B. A. (2006). A meta-regression to examine the relationship between aerobic fitness and cognitive performance. *Brain Research Reviews, 52*(1), 119–130.

Gates, N., Fiatarone Singh, M. A., Sachdev, P. S., & Valenzuela, M. (2013). The effect of exercise training on cognitive function in older adults with mild cognitive impairment: A meta-analysis of randomized controlled trials. *The American Journal of Geriatric Psychiatry, 21*(11), 1086–1097.

Gow, A. J., Bastin, M. E., Munoz Maniega, S., Valdes Hernandez, M. C., Morris, Z., Murray, C., et al. (2012). Neuroprotective lifestyles and the aging brain: Activity, atrophy, and white matter integrity. *Neurology, 79*(17), 1802–1808. https://doi.org/10.1212/WNL.0b013e3182703fd2.

Hamer, M., & Chida, Y. (2009). Physical activity and risk of neurodegenerative disease: A systematic review of prospective evidence. *Psychological Medicine, 39*(1), 3–11.

Heyn, P., Abreu, B. C., & Ottenbacher, K. J. (2004). The effects of exercise training on elderly persons with cognitive impairment and dementia: A meta-analysis. *Archives of Physical Medicine and Rehabilitation, 85*(10), 1694–1704.

Hovanec, N., Sawant, A., Overend, T. J., Petrella, R. J., & Vandervoort, A. A. (2012). Resistance training and older adults with type 2 diabetes mellitus: Strength of the evidence. *Journal of Aging Research, 2012,* 284635. https://doi.org/10.1155/2012/284635.

Hsu, C. L., Best, J. R., Davis, J. C., Nagamatsu, L. S., Wang, S., Boyd, L. A., et al. (2017). Aerobic exercise promotes executive functions and impacts functional neural activity among older adults with vascular cognitive impairment. *British Journal of Sports Medicine.* https://doi.org/10.1136/bjsports-2016-096846.

Huijts, M., Duits, A., van Oostenbrugge, R. J., Kroon, A. A., de Leeuw, P. W., & Staals, J. (2013). Accumulation of MRI markers of cerebral small vessel disease is associated with decreased cognitive function. A study in first-ever lacunar stroke and hypertensive patients. *Frontiers in Aging Neuroscience, 5,* 72. https://doi.org/10.3389/fnagi.2013.00072.

Janke, A. L., de Zubicaray, G., Rose, S. E., Griffin, M., Chalk, J. B., & Galloway, G. J. (2001). 4D deformation modeling of cortical disease progression in Alzheimer's dementia. *Magnetic Resonance Medicine, 46*(4), 661–666.

Kelly, M. E., Loughrey, D., Lawlor, B. A., Robertson, I. H., Walsh, C., & Brennan, S. (2014). The impact of exercise on the cognitive functioning of healthy older adults: A systematic review and meta-analysis. *Ageing Research Reviews, 16*, 12–31. https://doi.org/10.1016/j.arr.2014.05.002.

Kimura, K., Obuchi, S., Arai, T., Nagasawa, H., Shiba, Y., Watanabe, S., & Kojima, M. (2010). The influence of short-term strength training on health-related quality of life and executive cognitive function. *Journal of Physiological Anthropology, 29*(3), 95–101.

Kraemer, W. J., Adams, K., Cafarelli, E., Dudley, G. A., Dooly, C., Feigenbaum, M. S., et al. (2002). American College of Sports Medicine position stand. Progression models in resistance training for healthy adults. *Medicine & Science in Sports & Exercise, 34*(2), 364–380.

Kramer, A. F., Hahn, S., Cohen, N. J., Banich, M. T., McAuley, E., Harrison, C. R., et al. (1999). Ageing, fitness and neurocognitive function. *Nature, 400*(6743), 418–419.

Kuo, H. K., & Lipsitz, L. A. (2004). Cerebral white matter changes and geriatric syndromes: Is there a link? *Journal of Gerontology A, Biological Sciences and Medical Sciences, 59*(8), 818–826.

Lautenschlager, N. T., Cox, K. L., Flicker, L., Foster, J. K., van Bockxmeer, F. M., Xiao, J., et al. (2008). Effect of physical activity on cognitive function in older adults at risk for Alzheimer disease: A randomized trial. *Journal of the American Medical Association, 300*(9), 1027–1037. https://doi.org/10.1001/jama.300.9.1027.

Lee, A. T. C., Richards, M., Chan, W. C., Chiu, H. F. K., Lee, R. S. Y., & Lam, L. C. W. (2015). Intensity and types of physical exercise in relation to dementia risk reduction in community-living older adults. *Journal of the American Medical Directors Association, 16*(10), 899.e891–899.e897. https://doi.org/10.1016/j.jamda.2015.07.012.

Liao, D., Cooper, L., Cai, J., Toole, J. F., Bryan, N. R., Hutchinson, R. G., & Tyroler, H. A. (1996). Presence and severity of cerebral white matter lesions and hypertension, its treatment, and its control. The ARIC study. Atherosclerosis risk in communities study. *Stroke, 27*(12), 2262–2270.

Liu-Ambrose, T., Best, J. R., Davis, J. C., Eng, J. J., Lee, P. E., Jacova, C., et al. (2016). Aerobic exercise and vascular cognitive impairment: A randomized controlled trial. *Neurology, 87*(20), 2082–2090. https://doi.org/10.1212/WNL.0000000000003332.

Liu-Ambrose, T., & Donaldson, M. G. (2009). Exercise and cognition in older adults: Is there a role for resistance training programmes? *British Journal of Sports Medicine, 43*(1), 25–27.

Liu-Ambrose, T., Nagamatsu, L. S., Graf, P., Beattie, B. L., Ashe, M. C., & Handy, T. C. (2010). Resistance training and executive functions: A 12-month randomized controlled trial. *Archives of Internal Medicine, 170*(2), 170–178.

Liu-Ambrose, T., Nagamatsu, L. S., Voss, M. W., Khan, K. M., & Handy, T. C. (2012). Resistance training and functional plasticity of the aging brain: A 12-month randomized controlled trial. *Neurobiology of Aging, 33*(8), 1690–1698.

Longstreth, W. T., Jr., Manolio, T. A., Arnold, A., Burke, G. L., Bryan, N., Jungreis, C. A., et al. (1996). Clinical correlates of white matter findings on cranial magnetic resonance imaging of 3301 elderly people. The Cardiovascular Health Study. *Stroke, 27*(8), 1274–1282.

Middleton, L. E., Manini, T. M., Simonsick, E. M., Harris, T. B., Barnes, D. E., Tylavsky, F., et al. (2011). Activity energy expenditure and incident cognitive impairment in older adults. *Archives of Internal Medicine, 171*(14), 1251–1257. https://doi.org/10.1001/archinternmed.2011.277.

Nagamatsu, L. S., Davis, J. C., & Liu-Ambrose, T. (2011). Commentaries on viewpoint: Control arms in exercise training studies: Transitioning from an era of intervention efficacy to one of comparative clinical effectiveness research. A PROPOSED ALTERNATIVE TO AN INACTIVE CONTROL ARM: LOW-IMPACT EXERCISE GROUPS. *Journal of Applied Physiology, 111*(3), 949–950.

Nagamatsu, L. S., Flicker, L., Kramer, A. F., Voss, M. W., Erickson, K. I., Hsu, C. L., & Liu-Ambrose, T. (2014). Exercise is medicine, for the body and the brain. *British Journal of Sports Medicine, 48*(12), 943–944. https://doi.org/10.1136/bjsports-2013-093224.

Nagamatsu, L. S., Handy, T. C., Hsu, C. L., Voss, M., & Liu-Ambrose, T. (2012). Resistance training promotes cognitive and functional brain plasticity in seniors with probable mild cognitive impairment. *Archives of Internal Medicine, 172*(8), 666–668.

Ohman, H., Savikko, N., Strandberg, T. E., & Pitkala, K. H. (2014). Effect of physical exercise on cognitive performance in older adults with mild cognitive impairment or dementia: A systematic review. *Dementia and Geriatric Cognitive Disorders, 38*(5–6), 347–365. https://doi.org/10.1159/000365388.

Perrig-Chiello, P., Perrig, W. J., Ehrsam, R., Staehelin, H. B., & Krings, F. (1998). The effects of resistance training on well-being and memory in elderly volunteers. *Age and Ageing, 27*(4), 469–475.

Petersen, R. C., Doody, R., Kurz, A., Mohs, R. C., Morris, J. C., Rabins, P. V., et al. (2001). Current concepts in mild cognitive impairment. *Archives of Neurology, 58*(12), 1985–1992.

Petersen, R. C., Smith, G. E., Waring, S. C., Ivnik, R. J., Tangalos, E. G., & Kokmen, E. (1999). Mild cognitive impairment: Clinical characterization and outcome. *Archives of Neurology, 56*(3), 303–308.

Raschetti, R., Albanese, E., Vanacore, N., & Maggini, M. (2007). Cholinesterase inhibitors in mild cognitive impairment: A systematic review of randomised trials. *PLoS Medicine, 4*(11), e338.

Raz, N., Lindenberger, U., Rodrigue, K. M., Kennedy, K. M., Head, D., Williamson, A., et al. (2005). Regional brain changes in aging healthy adults: General trends, individual differences and modifiers. *Cerebral Cortex, 15*(11), 1676–1689.

Rosen, W. G., Mohs, R. C., & Davis, K. L. (1984). A new rating scale for Alzheimer's disease. *American Journal of Psychiatry, 141*, 1356–1364.

Sattler, C., Erickson, K. I., Toro, P., & Schroder, J. (2011). Physical fitness as a protective factor for cognitive impairment in a prospective population-based study in Germany. *Journal of Alzheimers Disease, 26*(4), 709–718.

Sofi, F., Valecchi, D., Bacci, D., Abbate, R., Gensini, G. F., Casini, A., & Macchi, C. (2011). Physical activity and risk of cognitive decline: A meta-analysis of prospective studies. *Journal of Internal Medicine, 269*(1), 107–117. https://doi.org/10.1111/j.1365-2796.2010.02281.x.

Strasser, B., Siebert, U., & Schobersberger, W. (2010). Resistance training in the treatment of the metabolic syndrome: A systematic review and meta-analysis of the effect of resistance training on metabolic clustering in patients with abnormal glucose metabolism. *Sports Medicine, 40*(5), 397–415. https://doi.org/10.2165/11531380-000000000-00000.

Suo, C., Singh, M. F., Gates, N., Wen, W., Sachdev, P., Brodaty, H., et al. (2016). Therapeutically relevant structural and functional mechanisms triggered by physical and cognitive exercise. *Molecular Psychiatry, 21*, 1633. https://doi.org/10.1038/mp.2016.19.

Taaffe, D. R., Galvao, D. A., Sharman, J. E., & Coombes, J. S. (2007). Reduced central blood pressure in older adults following progressive resistance training. *Journal of Human Hypertension, 21*(1), 96–98. https://doi.org/10.1038/sj.jhh.1002115.

Tsutsumi, T., Don, B. M., Zaichkowsky, L. D., & Delizonna, L. L. (1997). Physical fitness and psychological benefits of strength training in community dwelling older adults. *Applied Human Science, 16*(6), 257–266.

U.S. Department of Health and Human Services. (2000). *Healthy people 2010: Understanding and improving health* (2nd ed.). Washington, DC: U.S. Government Printing Office. http://www.who.int/mental_health/publications/dementia_report_2012/en/

Wanderley, F. A. C., Moreira, A., Sokhatska, O., Palmares, C., Moreira, P., Sandercock, G., et al. (2013). Differential responses of adiposity, inflammation and autonomic function to aerobic versus resistance training in older adults. *Experimental Gerontology, 48*(3), 326–333.

West, R. L. (1996). An application of prefrontal cortex function theory to cognitive aging. *Psychology Bulletin, 120*(2), 272–292.

Weuve, J., Kang, J. H., Manson, J. E., Breteler, M. M. B., Ware, J. H., & Grodstein, F. (2004). Physical activity, including walking, and cognitive function in older women. *Journal of the American Medical Association, 292*(12), 1454–1461.

Williams, M. A., Haskell, W. L., Ades, P. A., Amsterdam, E. A., Bittner, V., Franklin, B. A., et al. (2007). Resistance exercise in individuals with and without cardiovascular disease: 2007 update: A scientific statement from the American Heart

Association Council on Clinical Cardiology and Council on Nutrition, Physical Activity, and Metabolism. *Circulation, 116*(5), 572–584. https://doi.org/10.1161/circulationaha.107.185214.

World Health Organization, & Alzheimer's Disease International. (2012). *Dementia: A public health authority.* http://www.who.int/mental_health/publications/dementia_report_2012/en/.

Yaffe, K., Barnes, D., Nevitt, M., Lui, L. Y., & Covinsky, K. (2001). A prospective study of physical activity and cognitive decline in elderly women: Women who walk. *Archives of Internal Medicine, 161*(14), 1703–1708.

Young, J., Angevaren, M., Rusted, J., & Tabet, N. (2015). Aerobic exercise to improve cognitive function in older people without known cognitive impairment. *Cochrane Database Systematic Reviews, 4*, CD005381. https://doi.org/10.1002/14651858.CD005381.pub4.

Zheng, G., Xia, R., Zhou, W., Tao, J., & Chen, L. (2016). Aerobic exercise ameliorates cognitive function in older adults with mild cognitive impairment: A systematic review and meta-analysis of randomised controlled trials. *British Journal of Sports Medicine, 50*, 1443. https://doi.org/10.1136/bjsports-2015-095699.

35

The Potential for Technology to Enhance Physical Activity Among Older People

Beatrix Vereijken and Jorunn L. Helbostad

35.1 Introduction

The development and use of tools and technology is one of the most distinguishing hallmarks of the human race. Early tools were first and foremost an extension of our physical abilities, allowing us to expand our reach, work our fields and crops more easily, and kill our prey from increasing distances. As tools and subsequently technology became gradually more and more advanced, they allowed us to do things not originally part of our skill set, such as fly, move at speeds faster than running, and lift loads multiple times our body mass. Extensive industrialisation in the last century has allowed us to increasingly replace human labour with machine work, thereby reducing demands on physical activity at the work place. In addition, the rapidly evolving information and communication technologies (ICT) in the last decades have turned working hours increasingly to sedentary office hours for a large part of the work force. Developments in transportation technology have allowed us to shift from physically active transport modes such as walking and cycling to sedentary modes of transport such as trains, cars, and planes (see Chap. 25 in this volume) with implications for levels of physical activity in the older population.

B. Vereijken (✉) • J. L. Helbostad
Department of Neuromedicine and Movement Science, Norwegian University of Science and Technology, Trondheim, Norway

Technological developments have enabled us to spend less time and effort on our survival, take up jobs that are less physically demanding, and thereby have more spare time for leisure activities, such as arts, sports, and entertainment. However, what we do in our spare time has gradually become less energetic and more sedentary as well. Many adults in the Western society spend on average 2–4 hours watching television daily, and the amount of accumulated sitting time throughout a typical day is even higher. These combined developments have led to today's situation where worldwide, approximately 30% of adults (Hallal et al. 2012; WHO 2017) do not comply with WHO's recommendations regarding physical activity of at least 150 minutes of moderate-intensity aerobic physical activity throughout the week (WHO 2010). Moreover, estimates of inactivity in adults vary between regions and countries and could be as high as 50–60% in high-income countries and further increase with age in all WHO regions (Hallal et al. 2012). According to a recent review on sedentary behaviour in older adults, about 60% report sitting for more than four hours per day (Harvey et al. 2013). When measured objectively with body-worn accelerometers, sedentary behaviour accumulated throughout the day reached a shocking 8.5 hours in over 65% of older adults (Stamatakis et al. 2012).

In sum, technological developments have facilitated a gradual reduction in physical activity and concomitant increase in inactivity, with associated detrimental effects on health (Murtagh et al. 2015). Can we reverse this development and use technology to enhance rather than reduce physical activity? What types of technology are available that may serve this purpose? To what extent is this technology suited for older people and what challenges remain? The current chapter will examine the evidence for these and additional questions regarding the potential of technology to enhance physical activity in older people.

35.2 Types of Technology to Enhance Physical Activity

In this first part of the chapter, we will look at what types of technology have been used to enhance physical activity. Although many different types of technology can be used to enhance and promote physical activity, we will describe the two arguably most common types, namely, exercise games or exergames that can instruct and motivate physical activity and wearable self-monitoring devices that can track and give feedback about several aspects of physical activity. For an in-depth discussion regarding the opportunities and barriers that transportation technology provides for promoting physical activity in later life, see Chap. 25 in this volume.

35.2.1 Exercise-Based Games or Exergames

Although exergames can come in different guises and appearances, so far, the majority has been in the form of screen-based video games. Such video games are played using bodily movements to control the game, hence the label exergames. The first commercial exergame to hit the market was Dance Dance Revolution or DDR (GetUpMove.com) in 2004, promoted mainly as a weight loss tool for children and adolescents. Players stood in the centre of an electronic mat and, to the beat of music, tapped their feet on specified areas to all four sides according to arrows on the screen (up/down and left/right, corresponding to steps to be made forward, backward, left, and right, respectively). DDR signalled the start of a new trend where video games were sold for the purpose of playful exercising. Before long, DDR was followed by the introduction of Nintendo Wii in 2006 and PlayStation Move from Sony in 2009. Whereas DDR relied on an electronic mat to detect the players' movements, Nintendo Wii and PlayStation Move made use of hand-held controllers (Lee 2008), enabling players to move more freely while gaming and allowing for a wide range of sports activities to be enacted in the comfort of one's living room. The introduction of the Kinect for Xbox 360 from Microsoft in 2010 heralded yet a new generation of exergames, where the combination of depth and RGB cameras (i.e., cameras that capture the three basic colour components red, green, and blue) with concomitant technology allowed detection of full-body motion in 3D without the need for additional controllers to play the game (Zhang 2012).

These early generations of exergames were explicitly aimed at the entertainment and exercise of young people in particular, and their distinctive characteristics of demanding interfaces, frenzied visual displays, and excited auditory accompaniment were found to be largely incompatible with the needs and preferences of older adults (Nawaz et al. 2014, 2016). Nevertheless, at least for a while several of these early games were quite popular during family gatherings, with older people playing together or in competition with their grandchildren. An occasional game console also found its way into nursing homes, leading to anecdotal tales of older people starting to play games and purportedly improving several aspects of their physical functioning.

It did not take long before exergames were more formally recognised as a potential tool to explicitly enhance physical activity in general and to administer and monitor specific exercises in the context of rehabilitation in particular, in both young and older adults. This led to an increase in the use of exergame technology for these purposes, as well as the development of new exergame concepts and systems specifically designed to meet the needs and preferences of older people. However, many of these games were developed for research purposes, and so far, few are available in the market for the general older user. Further below, we will take a closer look at the appeal of technology as a tool to enhance physical activity, and what the challenges are when this technology is to be used by older people. But first, we will take a look at a second general type of technology used to enhance physical activity, namely, self-monitoring devices.

35.2.2 Self-Monitoring Devices

Recent technological developments have made it possible to continuously monitor our own movements and heart rate by the use of small wearable sensors. Activity monitoring using a belt around the chest has existed for many years and is commonly used to track heart rate during endurance training sessions. After a training session, signals can be transferred wirelessly to a web-based computer or smartphone application for processing and presentation of results. Other wearable sensors, including accelerometers and lately also gyroscopes and magnetometers, are commonly used in research aimed at monitoring activity over multiple days. Outcomes from such methods are typically related to energy expenditure or activity classification. This kind of monitoring requires sensors to be worn or fixed to the body over longer time periods, for example, a week, and has not been adopted by the general public for tracking their physical activity.

With the introduction of smartphones, a new generation of tracking devices became available for the consumer market. The first mobile applications date back to the end of the twentieth century and came in the guise of calculators, calendars, arcade games, and so on. But the release of the Apple iPhone in 2007 opened up new possibilities because of proprietary mobile platforms, increased storing and battery capacity, and since then the number of smartphone applications (so-called apps) has exploded. Smartphones are in fact small computers that include multiple sensors such as accelerometers, gyroscopes, and magnetometers that inform about the orientation of the device, barometers that detect changes in altitude, light sensors for the estimation of heart rate, cameras, as well as geo-sensors (GPS) for the tracking of geographical position. These sensor systems can monitor many aspects of behaviour, physical activities, and location of the activities, and subsequently provide feedback about these aspects to the user. Interested readers are referred to Chap. 31 in this volume for more information about the use of such sensor systems in the measurement of physical activity. Improved internal memory and battery capacity and near-global access to the Internet also helped make smartphone-based physical activity apps increasingly popular, in that the collected information can be stored, sent, and received and the information shared and compared with other users of the same system. The latter allows for both competition and collaboration with others, both of which can function as important motivators to continue the activity (e.g., Aarhus et al. 2011; Peng and Hsieh 2012). However, there are some challenges to using smartphones to track physical activity in that they are not always worn on the body and when worn, they can be worn at different places on the body, such as in a pocket, in a shoulder bag, or held in the hand. This makes it challenging to develop generic algorithms that can estimate aspects of physical activity accurately, such as energy expenditure, sitting time, walking time, and number of steps. This problem can be addressed by creating reference datasets that can be used to validate different sensors, sensor locations, and algorithms (cf. Bourke et al. 2017).

The latest generation of activity trackers are in the form of wristbands and smartwatches. Wristbands typically include acceleration sensors and derive information about energy expenditure, positions, activities such as sleeping time and sitting time, and number of steps. Wrist sensors do not have an interface; therefore the monitored activity needs to be transferred to smartphone applications for reading and processing of results. Smartwatches are a different story. In addition to being digital yet ordinary watches, they are also small computers that include several of the sensors and sending and receiving systems that are included in smartphones. Because watches and wristbands are worn most of the day, they are better suited for collecting information about heart rate and activity levels during the day. However, heart rate monitoring by such systems is still less reliable than measurements from chest sensors; therefore most applications also allow monitoring from additional devices. Another important limitation with wristbands or smartwatches as activity trackers is the reliable estimation of both energy expenditure and activity recognition. As arm movements are involved in most activities during the day, as well as upper body movements and communication, it is challenging for generic algorithms to interpret movement signals correctly. Finally, most applications for smartphones, wristbands, and smartwatches were not developed specifically for older adults. Although their needs are different from younger generations (Holzinger et al. 2007), the usability of the user interfaces for older adults has been assessed insufficiently, and the information and feedback derived from such systems has had minimal validation with older age groups.

35.3 The Potential of Technology to Increase Physical Activity

Technology has great potential to support healthy, active ageing, but wherein lies the appeal of technology as a tool to increase physical activity? Within the context of treatment and rehabilitation, it is easy to argue why we need to turn towards the increased use of technology. Ongoing demographic changes in our society increasingly shift the population away from the working force and increasingly towards the silver generation (EU 2011). In addition, we become older on average than ever before, but not all extra years come in the guise of healthy years (Murray et al. 2012), so we need to count on additional years lived with disease and disability (WHO 2011). This creates a challenging situation in which more people will need more healthcare that has to be provided by fewer people. Increased use of technology in general and welfare technology in particular has been heralded as a necessary part of future healthcare to be able to provide everyone with the care they need. But what about outside the healthcare system, what could be the broader appeal of technology there?

35.3.1 Apps and Games Are Fun

One of the first factors often mentioned when talking about the use of technology to enhance physical activity is the fun factor. Enjoyment improves adherence and has been identified as one of the predictors of the effectiveness of an exercise programme (Bird et al. 2015). Being affordable and easily available, both exergames and self-monitoring devices capitalise on making exercise and physical activity fun to do, either indoors or outdoors, alone or with others. Points can be scored, performance and progress can be tracked, and records can be broken and shared. Furthermore, one has the choice to play and exercise alone, together with other people, or against others in a competition. There is some evidence that the fun factor holds true for older people as well. For example, Nap et al. (2009) found that older people played computer-based physical and/or cognitive games for fun, for enjoyment, and to have some private time away from everyday life. Furthermore, a recent Australian study reported that older adults found exergaming appealing and providing them with improved motivation to be physically active (Bird et al. 2015). The potential for social interaction seems to be closely related to the appeal of exergames as well and is often mentioned by older people as a desirable characteristic of, for example, exergames (Lewis and Rosie 2012; Nawaz et al. 2014). As social isolation and loneliness tend to increase with age, technology can be used to promote social interaction with peers as well as with other age groups, also for those not eager or able to leave their homes because of disease or disability, or something as mundane as the weather. However, few if any studies have investigated whether these reported perceptions of fun using exergames or self-monitoring devices last over longer periods of time, and it remains to be established whether the use of technology leads to long-term adherence to a physically active life style. But anecdotal evidence on the use of gaming and training apps suggests that interest can fade quickly, even in the case of temporarily hugely popular games such as Pokémon GO.

35.3.2 Technology Allows for Personalisation

A second more serious factor for using technology to increase physical activity is the potential to personalise games and devices to the users' own needs and preferences. For example, many training apps allow the users to set their own goals. Subsequent feedback messages about performance serve a dual role as information on how the users are closing in on personal goals and as motivation to continue by maintaining users' interest and involvement and by building confidence (Baranowski et al. 2013). According to behaviour change theory, these are important elements to strengthen adherence, thereby promoting the formation of new habits (Gardner et al. 2012). Personalisation can also be done with respect to the functions the user wishes to target during physical activity, such as strength, balance, flexibility, or endurance. In addition, many games, apps, and other training devices include an option to challenge cognitive functions. As advanced age may be accompanied by cognitive decline, this possibility is relevant in the case of older users, and evidence suggests that the combination of physical and cognitive exercise has indeed a beneficial effect on cognitive functioning (Anderson-Hanley et al. 2012). A recent meta-analysis that included both physical and cognitive computer games provides further evidence that playing such games has a positive effect on older adults' functional mobility, balance, balance confidence, executive function, and information processing speed (Zhang and Kaufman 2015).

Finally, modern technological solutions allow for a high degree of flexibility, such that physical and cognitive challenges can be increased or decreased by the user, depending on, for example, their form on the day and prior level of achievement. In sum, the potential of technology to personalise both the content and intensity of the physical activity offered to the user can provide a strong incentive, perhaps paralleled only by a personal trainer or therapist.

35.3.3 Has Technology Succeeded in Enhancing Physical Activity?

As described above, technology has great potential to increase physical activity. To what extent has technology made good on this potential so far? What is the evidence for its effectiveness to enhance physical activity and improve functioning? Despite the relative newness of the field, a large and steadily growing number of studies has been published in the form of case reports and descriptive studies, clinical studies that compared technology-based interventions with treatment as usual, and narrative and systematic reviews that provided comprehensive overviews over the use of technology and combined evidence for its effectiveness to enhance physical activity and improve physical, cognitive, and social functioning. The picture that emerges from this large body of original studies and reviews is surprisingly consistent.

Regarding exergames, most studies report equal or better effects of exergaming interventions in terms of effectiveness and adherence compared to other training forms (e.g., Bleakley et al. 2015; Skjæret et al. 2016). However, reported effects were generally small and possibilities for comparison and meta-analysis across studies limited because of large variation in study designs and outcome measures collected (e.g., Larsen et al. 2013). Furthermore, the majority of studies were conducted in clinical and laboratory settings, focusing on the rehabilitation of specific physical functions (most prominently balance) in specific patient groups (such as stroke survivors) (cf. Skjæret et al. 2016). So far, only one systematic review focused specifically on the effectiveness of exergame use at home by older adults, finding similar positive but weak evidence (Miller et al. 2014).

There is less accumulated evidence regarding the effectiveness of smartphone applications to improve physical activity. Although there are many apps available on all major smartphone platforms, relatively few have been rigorously tested in research. Here as well, findings suggest that apps can be efficacious in promoting physical activity but that the effect is rather modest (e.g., Coughlin et al. 2016). Furthermore, there is some evidence for a dose-response effect, with higher app usage being associated with improved outcome, and multi-component interventions tended to be more effective than stand-alone app interventions (Schoeppe et al. 2016).

A common set of themes was highlighted across studies and reviews on exergames and apps, emphasising in particular the need for higher-quality intervention studies that are conducted on larger samples sizes over longer periods of time. Preferably, more consistent outcome measures should be used to enable meta-analyses and thereby provide stronger evidence for the effectiveness of technology to enhance physical activity and improve functioning.

35.4 The Challenges for Technology

This section of the chapter discusses several challenges for technology to function as an effective tool to enhance physical activity in older adults. We address whether older adults are ready for technology, the acceptability and usability of technology by older adults, automatic adaptation to the user, and safety of using the technology by older adults.

35.4.1 The Readiness of Older Adults for Technology

Before we discuss the challenges related to using technology to promote physical activity in older people, we want to address the reverse question first: Are older people ready for—and willing to use—technology? Are older people as technophobic as sometimes claimed or is this an unfounded stereotype? When it comes to using digital technology, there are certainly several legitimate barriers for older people. Today's seniors did not grow up with this technology as subsequent generations have done, so there may be lack of knowledge and experience, feelings of embarrassment, and issues with ease and comfort of use (Hawley-Hague et al. 2014; Heinz et al. 2013). Such concerns in turn may prompt well-meaning carers, relatives, and friends to discourage and shield older adults from participating in technology-based activities in a potentially misguided effort to protect them from disappointment or harm. In addition, older age is often accompanied by increasing limitations in physical and cognitive capacity and higher prevalence of disabilities and chronic diseases, in turn causing difficulties with reading, learning, and manipulating small objects. This makes use of digital technology more challenging for older people than for their younger counterparts—but not impossible. Although early adopters of new systems and technologies continue to be mostly younger people, newer evidence suggests that older people are quickly catching up in using technology. Recent surveys in the USA report that over 75% of those aged 65 and older have a mobile phone, over 50% use smartphones or tablets, and approximately 25% play computerised physical activity and/or cognitive games (Duggan 2015; Smith 2014). Surveys on digital inclusion from the UK report similar numbers, with roughly 50% using the Internet as of 2012, and their numbers projected to rise to as much as 90% by 2020 (Green and Rossall 2013). This is in line with recent evidence that older people are eager to learn how technology can help them maintain independence and high quality of life (Heinz et al. 2013). Furthermore, there is accumulating evidence that not only well-functioning older adults but also those with cognitive disabilities such as dementia can learn to play computerised games independently (e.g., Astell et al. 2014) and benefit from using such technology (e.g., Cutler et al. 2016). Finally, today's older generation is not the same as tomorrow's older generation, so even technology that will reach the market in the near future will face a more digital-ready older population. All in all, older people seem to be ready enough for technology, but is the technology ready enough for them?

35.4.2 Acceptability and Usability of Technology

One of the biggest challenges for any technology concerns the acceptability and usability of the technology by the intended users, in this case older people. As mentioned before, most of the technological solutions on the market today were not purpose-designed for older people. Off-the-shelf exergames, fitness apps, and performance trackers are largely aimed at the population in general or at younger people in particular. Those technologies that were purpose-designed for older people were mainly developed to provide training of specific physical functions as part of a rehabilitation programme such as balance training (van Diest et al. 2013, 2016; Wüest et al. 2014), not to promote physical activity in general. If older people are to accept technology as a tool to help them increase their physical activity, it must represent a clear benefit to them (Devos et al. 2015) and fit with their goals, expectations, and lifestyles (Hawley-Hague et al. 2014).

Usability is a separate issue and refers to the ease of use of products and systems, matching the latter to the needs and requirements of the user. The international standard ISO 9241–11 defines usability as the extent to which a system or product can be used by specified users to achieve specified goals with effectiveness, efficiency, and satisfaction in a specified context of use (Travis 2013). One way to achieve usability is by actively involving users and other stakeholders in the development of the technology, so-called co-design (Sanders and Stappers 2008). Although the question of usability is an important one, it has received relatively little attention in research and design, particularly with respect to older people. In the context of exergames, focus has mainly been on the relation between the games and the player in different contexts, as well as on the design aspects of the game (IJsselsteijn et al. 2007), not its actual usability for older adults. The same applies to most mobile physical activity trackers that were developed for younger people to monitor their training sessions and track everyday life activities, such as step counts and total energy expenditure during the day. Whether these functionalities and the user interfaces of present applications fit the preferences and needs of older adults has yet to be shown but seems questionable.

35.4.3 Automatic Personalised Adjustment

Both exergames and self-monitoring devices contain a variety of sensors that allow the monitoring of a wealth of behavioural, biological, and environmental data. Subsequently, this data can be used to calculate several characteristics of the physical activity, such as the frequency and intensity of activity, steps taken, and heart rate, as well as deduce specific patterns of movements, activity, and sleeping. This information can be fed back to the user in the form of performance feedback, information about progression, and motivational messages. However, despite this wealth of information and possibilities, most existing applications to date are one-dimensional and address a single function only, such as cardiovascular fitness or number of steps taken. Especially in the case of older adults, individual needs are likely to be complex and to consist of several dimensions, requiring multi-functionality of the technology. Furthermore, good cardiovascular health for an older adult likely means something else than for their younger counterparts, with different requirements and cut-off levels. This necessitates the further development of algorithms that can be applied to the sensor data to not only extract more advanced information from the user but also individualise the feedback and messages that are fed back to the user. As noted above, current technology has the potential to be used to personalise an exergame or a device to the specific goals, needs, and preferences of an individual user. However, at the moment, the users themselves still need to decide what activity to do, when, how much, and often on what difficulty level as well. The real challenge for personalised adjustment lies in making this process automatic and implemented within the technology. This would include making the level of challenge, instructions, feedback, and motivational messages all contingent on actual performance of the user on a moment-to-moment basis (Skjæret et al. 2015).

35.4.4 Engendering Behavioural Change

Our bodies were made to move, and muscles, bone, and tissue alike grow stronger and retain their functionality better when we use and challenge our bodies on a regular basis. But as mentioned above, today's society increasingly allows and facilitates a sedentary existence. Although most people, young and older, are aware of the importance of physical activity, most do not meet weekly physical activity recommendations, and inactivity further increases with age (Murtagh et al. 2015). An occasional burst of training is not enough to alleviate the effects of sedentariness; to that end, return to an active lifestyle is necessary. For most people that are not active enough, there is a need for behavioural change where daily routines are made more active and challenging. We should take the stairs rather than the elevator, walk or cycle to work rather than drive, and stand rather than sit at the office. Technology can support us making a lasting change in our daily routines by giving us information, instructions, reminders, feedback, motivational and encouraging messages, praise and rewards, and so on (Michie et al. 2013). However, few if any of the extant technology have capitalised on these opportunities, and most of these potential functionalities remain to be implemented in products available on the consumer market.

35.4.5 The Safety of Using Technology

The last challenge we want to address is the safety aspect when older people use technology independently to be—or to become—physically more active. Although safety is a crucial aspect particularly in the case of older users, this has received comparatively little attention in the consumer market. Most off-the-shelf exergames, fitness trackers, and health apps were not developed specifically with older people in mind as the intended user, and both national and international safety regulations lag behind the fast developments in this area. In contrast, safety is an explicit issue when it comes to conducting research because of strict ethical standards and requirements to have research protocols evaluated and approved before a study can start. To the extent that research has investigated the use of technology in older adults, there is some evidence about its potential safety or lack thereof. A recent integrative review of the use of exergames in exercise and rehabilitation of older adults revealed that 70% of the reviewed studies used a safety measure during interventions, such as personal supervision, availability of support surfaces, or use of a safety harness (Skjæret et al. 2016). However, only half of these studies reported on whether adverse events had actually occurred. On a more positive note, none of these studies reported any serious adverse events during the intervention, and the few adverse events that were reported ranged from mild discomfort to musculoskeletal pain (Skjæret et al. 2016). These findings are in line with an earlier Cochrane review on VR and interactive video gaming in stroke rehabilitation where only a few mild adverse events were reported that consisted of transient dizziness, headache, and pain (Laver et al. 2015). Although these studies support the contention that exergames can be safely used, only three of the intervention studies in Skjæret et al. (2016) were conducted in an unsupervised home environment, so we lack sufficient evidence to draw firm conclusions on whether or not independent technology use by older adults is safe. In addition to safety as such, even mild adverse events such as pain or discomfort could have a negative effect on a person's interest and motivation to continue being physically active. However, this potential effect of adverse events has received little attention so far.

35.5 Implications for Practice

The previous section highlighted several important challenges for technology to function as a tool to enhance physical activity in older adults. Most of the identified challenges hold true for current technology to be used by today's older adults. But developments go fast and innovations follow each other closely. In addition, today's typical 70-year-old is a far cry from a typical 70-year-old a bare century ago and is likely as different from tomorrow's typical 70-year-old as well. As technology continues to develop and to become yet more accessible and affordable, devices and products such as exergames, physical activity monitors, and health apps will become more widely used as well, by young and older people alike. Some of the developments we can predict, some innovations might take us by surprise. However, it will remain relevant to ask whether a specific piece of technology offers what a potential user is looking for, whether its use is feasible, acceptable, and safe for that specific user, and what is required for it to be effective given the goals of the user. Another relevant question is related to how 'smart' the product really is. Can it adjust its features automatically to the needs and preferences of the user even if these can change on a moment-to-moment basis? Will it know when to send motivational messages and reminders and when to back off? Today's products are not this smart yet but the technology exists to implement these functionalities.

35.6 The Way Forward for Activating Technology

Technology continues to develop fast and innovations and improvements in functionality follow each other ever more closely. Although these fast developments might be challenging in their own right for older technology users, they also carry with them the promise that several of the challenges with current technology discussed above might meet solutions in the near future. Both capabilities in general and battery life in particular of self-monitoring devices are continually updated and improved. As technological solutions continue to decrease in size and increase in functionality and flexibility, future possibilities of smartwatches and other smart devices are only just appearing on the horizon.

As for exergames, their future might be found partly in increased personalisation and automated challenge adjustment, guiding players through exercises and activities that correspond best with their needs and preferences, and providing them with the appropriate feedback and encouragement. The other part of the future likely entails moving away from screen-based playing, and instead turning objects, surroundings, and situations increasingly into possibilities for games, so-called gamification of the environment. If successful, large-scale gamification could make it fun again to capitalise on opportunities for playful activities, thereby truly helping to stimulate people of all ages to become more active both inside and outside their own homes.

A final example of the way forward that we want to address is related to virtual reality (VR) and augmented reality (AR). VR has been around for a while and has found its way to rehabilitation settings in particular to help patients recover specific functions, for example, after stroke (Laver et al. 2015) or in Parkinson's disease (Dockx et al. 2016). However, VR is dependent on large screens in front of the subject to give a feeling of submersion in a virtual world, or on glasses that block vision of the real world and instead offer a window onto a virtual world. This makes most VR solutions expensive and dependent on continual supervision or a safety harness, and thereby inappropriate for the consumer market and unsupervised use at home. In contrast, AR is a more recent technology that projects virtual objects on otherwise clear glasses, allowing them to 'appear' in the real world. As simulations become more authentic and interactions with virtual objects more convincing, AR might well have boundless possibilities for enhancing physical activity in all ages.

35.7 Conclusion

The use of technology has enormous potential to help enhance physical activity in older people. However, to date this potential has been realised only partly at best. There is insufficient evidence whether the use of exergaming and health apps leads to better long-term adherence and more solid behavioural change towards a more active, healthy lifestyle than traditional forms of exercise or formal guidelines on how one should be living a healthy life. Similarly, most commercially available apps and exergames lack a solid foundation in research, despite popular claims that they are evidence-based. And perhaps most important of all, existing devices and solutions have rarely been developed with the participation of the older user in the design process, or even with an older user in mind. These factors make current technological products and systems largely inappropriate for—and unsought by—older adults. Fortunately, the identified shortcomings can be addressed, and research into technology as well as the design and continued development of technology increasingly focus on the needs and preferences of the end user. Formulating what the latter are is an important step towards realising the potential of technology to enhance physical activity in older adults.

Suggested Further Reading
- Hall, A. K., & Marston, H. R. (2014). Games for health in the home: Gaming and older adults in the digital age of healthcare. In J. van Hoof, G. Demiris, & E. J. M. Wouters (Eds.), *Handbook of smart homes, health care and well-being* (pp. 579–588). Cham: Springer International Publishing.
- Helbostad, J. L., Vereijken, B., Becker, C., Todd, C., Taraldsen, K., Pijnappels, M., Aminian, K., & Mellone, S. (2017). Mobile health applications to promote active and healthy ageing. *Sensors, 17*, 622.
- King, A. C., Hekler, E. B., Grieco, L. A., Winter, S. J., Sheats, J. L., Buman, M. P., Banerjee, B., Robinson, T. N., & Cirimele. J. (2013). Harnessing different motivational frames via mobile phones to promote daily physical activity and reduce sedentary behavior in aging adults. *PLoS One, 8*(4), e62613.

References

Aarhus, R., Grönvall, E., Larsen, S. B., et al. (2011). Turning training into play: Embodied gaming, seniors, physical training and motivation. *Gerontechnology, 10*(2), 110–120.

Anderson-Hanley, C., Arciero, P. J., Brickman, A. M., Nimon, J. P., Okuma, N., Westen, S. C., Merz, M. E., Pence, B. D., Woods, J. A., Kramer, A. F., & Zimmerman, E. A. (2012). Exergaming and older adult cognition: A cluster randomized clinical trial. *American Journal of Preventive Medicine, 42*(2), 109–119.

Astell, A., Alm, N., Dye, R., Gowans, G., Vaughan, P., & Ellis, M. (2014). Digital video games for older adults with cognitive impairment. *International Conference on Computers for Handicapped Persons* (pp. 264–271). Cham: Springer.

Baranowski, M. T., Bower, P. K., Krebs, P., Lamoth, C. J., & Lyons, E. J. (2013). Effective feedback procedures in games for health. *Games For Health: Research, Development, and Clinical Applications, 2*(6), 320–326.

Bird, M. L., Clark, B., Millar, J., Whetton, S., & Smith, S. (2015). Exposure to "exergames" increases older adults' perception of the usefulness of technology for improving health and physical activity: A pilot study. *JMIR Serious Games, 3*(2), e8.

Bleakley, C. M., Charles, D., Porter-Armstrong, A., McNeill, M. D., McDonough, S. M., & McCormack, B. (2015). Gaming for health: A systematic review of the physical and cognitive effects of interactive computer games in older adults. *Journal of Applied Gerontology, 34*(3), 166–189.

Bourke, A. K., Ihlen, E. A. F., Bergquist, R., Wik, P. B., Vereijken, B., & Helbostad, J. L. (2017). A physical activity reference data-set recorded from older adults using body-worn inertial sensors and video technology—The ADAPT study data-set. *Sensors, 17*(3), 559.

Coughlin, S. S., Whitehead, M., Sheats, J. Q., Mastromonico, J., & Smith, S. A. (2016). Review of smartphone applications for promoting physical activity. *Jacobs Journal of Community Medicine, 2*, 021.

Cutler, C., Hicks, B., & Innes, A. (2016). Does digital gaming enable healthy aging for community-dwelling people with dementia? *Games and Culture, 11*(1–2), 104–129.

Devos, P., Min Jou, A., De Waele, G., & Petrovic, M. (2015). Design for personalized mobile health applications for enhanced older people participation. *European Geriatric Medicine, 6*(6), 593–597.

Dockx, K., Bekkers, E. M. J., van den Bergh, V., Ginis, P., Rochester, L., Hausdorff, J. M., Mirelman, A., & Nieuwboer, A. (2016). Virtual reality for rehabilitation in Parkinson's disease. *Cochrane Database of Systematic Reviews, 12*, CD010760.

Duggan, M. (2015). *Gaming and gamers*. Washington, DC: Pew Research Center.

EU. (2011). *Demography report 2010 – Older, more numerous and diverse Europeans*. Luxembourg: Publications Office of the European Union.

Gardner, B., Lally, P., & Wardle, J. (2012). Making health habitual: The psychology of 'habit-formation' and general practice. *The British Journal of General Practice, 62*(605), 664–666.

Green, M., & Rossall, P. (2013). *Digital inclusion evidence report*. London: Age UK.

Hallal, P. C., Andersen, L. B., Bull, F. C., Guthold, R., Haskell, W., & Ekelund, U. (2012). Global physical activity levels: Surveillance progress, pitfalls, and prospects. *The Lancet, 380*(9838), 247–257.

Harvey, J. A., Chastin, S. F. M., & Skelton, D. A. (2013). Prevalence of sedentary behavior in older adults: A systematic review. *International Journal of Environmental Research and Public Health, 10*(12), 6645–6661.

Hawley-Hague, H., Boulton, E., Hall, A., Pfeiffer, K., & Todd, C. (2014). Older adults' perceptions of technologies aimed at falls prevention, detection or monitoring: A systematic review. *International Journal of Medical Informatics, 83*(6), 416–426.

Heinz, M., Martin, P., Margrett, J. A., Yearns, M., Franke, W., Yang, H. I., Wong, J., & Chang, C. K. (2013). Perceptions of technology among older adults. *Journal of Gerontological Nursing, 39*(1), 42–51.

Holzinger, A., Searle, G., & Nischelwitzer, A. (2007). On some aspects of improving mobile applications for the elderly. In C. Stephanidis (Ed.), *Universal access in HCI: Coping with diversity* (pp. 923–932). Beijing: Springer.

IJsselsteijn, W. A., Nap, H. H., de Kort, Y. A. W., & Poels, K. (2007). Digital game design for elderly users. *Proceedings of Futureplay 2007* (Toronto, 14–18 November 2007, pp. 17–22).

Larsen, L. H., Schou, L., Lund, H. H., & Langberg, H. (2013). The physical effect of exergames in healthy elderly—A systematic review. *Games for Health Journal, 2*(4), 205–212.

Laver, K. E., George, S., Thomas, S., Deutsch, J. E., & Crotty, M. (2015). Virtual reality for stroke rehabilitation. *Cochrane Database for Systematic Reviews, 12*, CD008349.

Lee, J. C. (2008). Hacking the Nintendo Wii remote. *IEEE Pervasive Computing, 7*(3), 39–45.

Lewis, G. N., & Rosie, J. A. (2012). Virtual reality games for movement rehabilitation in neurological conditions: How do we meet the needs and expectations of the users? *Disability and Rehabilitation, 34*(22), 1880–1886.

Michie, S., Richardson, M., Johnston, M., Abraham, C., Francis, J., Hardeman, W., Eccles, M. P., Cane, J., & Wood, C. E. (2013). The behavior change technique taxonomy (v1) of 93 hierarchically clustered techniques: Building an international consensus for the reporting of behavior change interventions. *Annals of Behavioral Medicine, 46*(1), 81–95.

Miller, K. J., Adair, B. S., Pearce, A. J., Said, C. M., Ozanne, E., & Morris, M. M. (2014). Effectiveness and feasibility of virtual reality and gaming system use at home by older adults for enabling physical activity to improve health-related domains: A systematic review. *Age and Ageing, 43*(2), 188–195.

Murray, C. J., Vos, T., Lozano, R., Naghavi, M., Flaxman, A. D., Michaud, C., et al. (2012). Disability-adjusted life years (DALYs) for 291 diseases and injuries in 21 regions, 1990–2010: A systematic analysis for the Global Burden of Disease Study 2010. *Lancet, 380*(9859), 2197–2223.

Murtagh, E. M., Murphy, M. H., Murphy, N. M., Woods, C., Nevill, A. M., & Lane, A. (2015). Prevalence and correlates of physical inactivity in community-dwelling older adults in Ireland. *PLoS One, 10*(2), e0118293.

Nap, H. H., de Kort, Y. A. W., & IJsselsteijn, W. A. (2009). Senior gamers: Preferences, motivations and needs. *Gerontechnology, 8*(4), 247–262.

Nawaz, A., Skjæret, N., Ystmark, K., Helbostad, J. L., Vereijken, B., & Svanæs, D. (2014). Assessing seniors' user experience (UX) of exergames for balance training. *NordiCHI '14: Fun, Fast, Foundational* (pp. 578–587). New York: ACM.

Nawaz, A., Skjæret, N., Helbostad, J. L., Vereijken, B., Boulton, E., & Svanæs, D. (2016). Usability and acceptability of balance exergames in older adults: A scoping review. *Health Informatics Journal, 22*, 911–931.

Peng, W., & Hsieh, G. (2012). The influence of competition, cooperation, and player relationship in a motor performance centered computer game. *Computers in Human Behavior, 28*, 2100–2106.

Sanders, E. B.-N., & Stappers, P. J. (2008). Co-creation and the new landscapes of design. *CoDesign, 4*(1), 5–18.

Schoeppe, S., Alley, S., Van Lippevelde, W., Bray, N. A., Williams, S. L., Duncan, M. J., & Vandelanotte, C. (2016). Efficacy of interventions that use apps to improve diet, physical activity and sedentary behaviour: A systematic review. *International Journal of Behavioral Nutrition and Physical Activity, 13*, 127.

Skjæret, N., Nawaz, A., Ystmark, K., Dahl, Y., Helbostad, J. L., Svanæs, D., & Vereijken, B. (2015). Designing for movement quality in exergames: Lessons learned from observing senior citizens playing stepping games. *Gerontology, 61*(2), 186–194.

Skjæret, N., Nawaz, A., Morat, T., Schoene, D., Helbostad, J. L., & Vereijken, B. (2016). Exercise and rehabilitation delivered through exergames in older adults: An integrative review of technologies, safety and efficacy. *International Journal of Medical Informatics, 85*(1), 1–16.

Smith, A. (2014). *Older adults and technology use*. Washington, DC: Pew Research Center.

Stamatakis, E., Davis, M., Stathi, A., & Hamer, M. (2012). Associations between multiple indicators of objectively-measured and self-reported sedentary behaviour and cardiometabolic risk in older adults. *Preventive Medicine, 54*, 82–87.

Travis, D. (2013). *ISO 9241 for beginners* (9th ed.). London: Userfocus.

van Diest, M., Lamoth, C. J., Stegenga, J., Verkerke, G. J., & Postema, K. (2013). Exergaming for balance training of elderly: State of the art and future developments. *Journal of Neuroengineering and Rehabilitation, 10*, 101.

van Diest, M., Stegenga, J., Wörtche, H., Verkerke, G., Postema, K., & Lamoth, C. (2016). Exergames for unsupervised balance training at home: A pilot study in healthy older adults. *Gait & Posture, 44*, 161–167.

WHO. (2010). *Global recommendations on physical activity for health*. Geneva: WHO.

WHO. (2011). *Global health and aging*. Bethesda: NIH.

WHO. (2017). *Physical activity*. Factsheet 385. http://www.who.int/mediacentre/factsheets/fs385/en/

Wüest, S., Borghese, N. A., Pirovano, M., Mainetti, R., van de Langenberg, R., & de Bruin, E. D. (2014). Usability and effects of an exergame-based balance training program. *Games for Health Journal, 3*(2), 106–114.

Zhang, Z. (2012). Microsoft Kinect sensor and its effect. *IEEE Multimedia, 19*(2), 4–10.

Zhang, F., & Kaufman, D. (2015). Physical and cognitive impacts of digital games on older adults: A meta-analytic review. *Journal of Applied Gerontology, 35*(11), 1189–1210.

Erratum to: Physical Environments That Promote Physical Activity Among Older People

Jelle Van Cauwenberg, Andrea Nathan, Benedicte Deforche, Anthony Barnett, David Barnett, and Ester Cerin

The book was inadvertently published with incorrect affiliations of the authors in chapter 22. The chapter has been updated with the correct affiliation of the authors as given below.

Affiliations were changed from
Jelle Van Cauwenberg, Department of Public Health, Ghent University, Ghent, Belgium
Anthony Barnett, Research Foundation Flanders, Brussels, Belgium
David Barnett, Research Foundation Flanders, Brussels, Belgium
Ester Cerin, Research Foundation Flanders, Brussels, Belgium

to

Jelle Van Cauwenberg, Department of Public Health, Ghent University, Ghent, Belgium
Research Foundation Flanders, Brussels, Belgium
Anthony Barnett, Institute for Health and Ageing, Australian Catholic University, Melbourne, VIC, Australia
David Barnett, Institute for Health and Ageing, Australian Catholic University, Melbourne, VIC, Australia
Ester Cerin, Institute for Health and Ageing, Australian Catholic University, Melbourne, VIC, Australia

---

The updated online version of this chapter can be found at https://doi.org/10.1007/978-3-319-71291-8_22

Glossary

Acceptability The combined effect of *antecedents* of performing a behaviour, such as attitudes towards the behaviour or perceived norms regarding the behaviour: the more positive these are, the more likely a behaviour is to be performed. These include positive factors such as enjoyment, as well as negative factors, such as low perceived value.

Action planning Action planning describes the process of planning in advance when, where, and how a specific behaviour will be performed (e.g., 'Every day after I finish my breakfast, I will go out to the park and walk for 20 minutes.').

Active ageing Active ageing is a reconstruction of ageing which focuses on enabling the participation and presence of people as they move through the life course in all aspects of social and economic life. As such it acts as a critique of previous understandings of old age which naturalised disengagement in old age and promoted ageism. It has been argued recently that, in line with the erosion of State welfare and the greater reliance on individual responsibility, active ageing as a policy framework, and within it physical activity, has become a normative target which older people should attain to reduce the burden of population ageing.

Active transport Walking, bicycle riding, or other muscle-powered methods of getting from place to place. Often used to distinguish task-oriented travel from bicycle riding or walking for pleasure or sport.

Activities of daily living Activities of daily living refer to the performance of daily tasks such as eating, bathing, dressing, toileting, transferring/walking, and continence.

Adherence The degree to which an individual's health-related behaviour corresponds with medical advice. Note that there are often good reasons why older people do not do as much physical activity as recommended to them.

Affordance Opportunities (or threats) afforded to users by specific environmental features. Depending on the user, a feature such as tree may afford shelter, a hiding place, something to lean on, or a climbing frame, or it may pose a threat to a cyclist.

Aged embodiment Aged embodiment refers to the ways in which the ageing body is experienced by older men and women. This includes both the individual sensate experiences of the body and the socio-cultural expectations, representations, and uses of the ageing body.

Ageing in place As defined by the US Centers for Disease Control is: 'The ability to live in one's own home and community safely, independently, and comfortably, regardless of age, income, or ability level' (https://www.cdc.gov/healthyplaces/terminology.htm).

Ageism A reliance on stereotypical notions of what older adults are like. These perceptions are usually negative, or consider older adults to be less capable, weak, frail, and not as cognitively capable as younger people.

Agency Agency refers to the ability of individuals to make independent actions and choices. Contrastingly, structure refers to the societal factors which provide the context in which individuals make decisions and engage in particular actions. These factors include class, race, gender, age, and so on. Bourdieu links both of these concepts through his concept of habitus.

Aspirational design Design or planning aimed at flourishing rather than merely at the mitigation or removal of harms.

Athletic identity A self-conceptualisation that is formed by experience, relations with others and involvement in sport activities.

Autonomous motivation The ultimate version of self-determination theory contrasts autonomous versus controlled motivation based on the extent of identification with a goal. It is assumed that autonomous motivation leads to longer-term engagement in behaviour.

Barriers Factors that are known to prevent or reduce the likelihood of individuals undertaking physical activity. Barriers can be personal (including psychological, financial), social (including no family or other support), or environmental (no access to a programme or suitable, safe location to undertake activity).

Behaviour change taxonomy A classification system for behaviour change techniques.

Behaviour change technique (BCT) A component of an intervention designed to change behaviour and which cannot be further reduced and is specified such that it can be clearly identified, implemented, and replicated.

Built environment The man-made space open to people to walk in and the buildings fronting public spaces.

Capital Capital is a concept used by the sociologist Pierre Bourdieu to denote the range of resources we have at our disposal as social actors commensurate with our habitus (social location). In his early work Bourdieu describes three main forms of capital: economic capital, social capital, and cultural capital. These operate like a currency which can be accumulated, transformed, and transmitted within social groups to gain recognition.

Cardiac rehabilitation A coordinated approach to facilitate recovery after a cardiac event and promote ongoing self-management and prevention, comprising physical activity, health education, and behaviour modification strategies.

Cardiovascular disease Diseases that affect the heart or blood vessels. Cardiovascular diseases include coronary artery disease, cerebrovascular disease, and peripheral arterial disease.

Care models to increase activity Designing care structures and environments to encourage physical activity as part of everyday functions and tasks. This might involve promotion of more frequent usual activity, longer durations of usual activity, switching to a more active method to achieve a goal or adding intensity to existing activity periods.

Cognitive impairment Signs of compromised cognitive functioning demonstrated by scoring below a pre-defined threshold in a validated test of cognition (e.g., Mini Mental State Examination score of <24).

Community-dwelling older people Older people who are living at their own or other's home, either independently or dependent on care support, who are not resident in a formal care facility.

Comorbidities Comorbidities include any known pathological condition or disease.

Continuity theory A conceptual framework used to describe the continuation of a regular behaviour, activity, or action over a period of time. 'Continuity' entails consistent behaviours and maintenance of relationships and activities over a length of time, and in gerontology has been applied as a concept to identify adaptations in midlife and among older people.

Coping planning Coping planning is a barrier-focussed prospective self-regulation strategy where an individual imagines possible threats and/or obstacles towards successful implementation of action plans and creates concrete plans to cope with the respective barriers.

Cost-effectiveness A ratio of the difference in costs and the difference in effects (or outcomes) of a given intervention compared with another intervention or control condition.

Disability Disability is an umbrella term, covering impairments, activity limitations, and participation restrictions. An impairment is a problem in body function or structure; an activity limitation is a difficulty encountered by an individual in executing a task or action, while a participation restriction is a problem experienced by an individual involved in a life situation (http://www.who.int/topics/disabilities/en/).

Discourse Discourse is a term used by Michel Foucault to show that how we ask questions about society, imagine solutions to problems, and articulate explanations—in other words what is deemed as the truth of a phenomenon—are formed in very specific historical contexts. We always think and act within discourses. The concept of discourse can therefore be used to examine how individuals came to possess ideas and opinions of certain topics.

Ecological model of physical activity promotion Theoretical approaches that incorporate determinants from more than one level of influence on physical activity. The levels differ by model but usually include an individual level (biological and psychological factors), social and community network level (implementation of programmes), and general socioeconomic, cultural, and environmental conditions level (landscape and built environment architecture and culture).

Effectiveness The effectiveness of an intervention considers the performance of the intervention under 'real world' conditions. Factors considered when determining effectiveness include provider acceptance and target audience adherence. In the context of physical activity guidelines, the effectiveness of the guidelines refer to the external validity of recommending specific levels of physical activity outside of research in everyday life (Weed 2016).

Efficacy The efficaciousness of an intervention refers to the performance of an intervention under controlled conditions. Evidence for the efficacy of physical activity in conferring a range of health benefits and reducing all-cause morbidity and mortality has been well-established (Weed 2016).

Embodiment Embodiment is concerned with the bodily aspects of human experience. That is, the body is not only a physiological entity; the way we use or treat our bodies is shaped by the social and cultural context in which we live. The body is always social and this is in evidence in how it is regulated, represented, and experienced.

Ethnicity or ethnic group Is a population group whose members identify with each other on the basis of common nationality, shared cultural traditions, dress, and group history. In some cases ethnicity includes shared language or religion. Ethnicity is in essence self-defined by the individual.

Exercise A subcategory of physical activity. This refers to physical activity to improve or maintain physical fitness that is planned, structured, and repetitive.

Exergames Videogames that are played using bodily movements to interact with the game console and control the game. Exergames involve physical exertion and are therefore seen as a form of exercise. Exergaming relies on technology to track bodily movements or reactions.

Experientially similar others In older adults, these are individuals who share common experiences (e.g., through life events, living environments, age, gender, race, or health status). According to adult development theories, experientially similar others are a good choice to provide effective social support for physical activity.

Fascination Effortless engagement with the experience of being in a particular setting and a key construct in restorative environment theory.

Fast-track surgery Components in fast-track surgery comprise patient information, 'stress-reduced' surgery, efficient postoperative pain treatment, perioperative care (i.e., the care that is given before, during, and after surgery) focusing on medical treatment (including thromboprophylaxis, oxygen therapy, etc.), early mobilisation, and oral nutrition to enhance recovery, decrease morbidity, and reduce hospital length of stay.

Figuration A conceptual tool which refers to the webs of tensile, interdependent power relationships within which social agents, or I-units, are situated. These relationship networks enable or constrain social agency or actions. Figurations can be thought of as a form of social organisation, possessing a power-structure structure resulting from the aggregation of the actions of all agents within the web.

FITT principle An acronym commonly used to describe the four key variables underpinning any exercise prescription: frequency, intensity, type and time. Depending on the type of exercise, a different application of these variables determines the physiological responses to exercise that are anticipated.

Frailty Frailty is a term widely used to denote a multidimensional syndrome of loss of reserves (energy, physical ability, cognition, health) that gives rise to vulnerability after a stressor event, which increases the risk of adverse outcomes, including falls, delirium, and disability. The phenotype of physical frailty is characterised by three or more of five factors: unintentional weight loss, self-reported exhaustion, low physical activity, slow gait speed, and low muscle strength.

Functional decline Functional decline refers to a decrease in physical and/or cognitive function and occurs when a person is unable to perform simple activities of daily living, for example, during hospitalisation.

Gamification Refers to turning an ordinary task, activity, object, or environment into a game by adding game characteristics to them, such as competition and achievement.

Gender A social construction of individuals as male or female and adhering to traits of masculinity and femininity. This is often associated with biological sex, but gender is a more fluid term, and individuals may have a gender identity which does not align with their sex at birth.

Gender ideology A reflection of rigid notions of how males and females 'should' behave, based on stereotypical definitions of gender.

Habitus A concept utilised by several social theorists including Norbert Elias and Pierre Bourdieu to describe the intersection of external socio-cultural processes with agency, or the intended actions of individuals. Commonly, habitus is used to describe how external social norms are 'internalised,' that is, can begin to become part of an individual's unconscious decision making processes or 'second nature.' At the same time, individuals can 'act back' upon socio-cultural processes and contest and can change them throughout the life course.

Health psychology The study of cognitive (thought-related) processes and behaviours related to health and prevention of illness.

Hospital setting Hospitals provide medical treatment to people of all ages with a variety of health conditions. They include acute and rehabilitation hospitals. Each has a different patient, staffing, and environmental profile, which have implications for promoting physical activity.

Instructor Someone who delivers a programme of exercises to either a group of people or provides one-to-one instruction to individuals.

Interactionist (ecological) approaches As contrasted with 'deterministic' approaches, interactionist (or 'ecological') interpretation of causality avoids the assumption of linear causation of and outcome by any one factor. Rather, outcomes are assumed to derive from transactional relationships and multiple influences (environmental, mental, social, biological) from which changes emerge over time.

Internalised ageism The phenomenon whereby older adults themselves view age in stereotypical (and negative) ways. For example, that older people are not able to be productive or competent. Internalised ageism infers a shame about ageing and can keep people from seeing their potential.

Land use mix The diversity of different land uses or destinations within an area. Having a variety of land uses means that people live closer to destinations used for activities, which provides the opportunity to walk or cycle.

Leadership (within the exercise context) Leadership of an exercise programme focuses on the interaction with the participant when teaching the programme.

Legible space In order to walk and cycle, spaces need signals to users that they should be there through clearly marked walking or cycling space, benches to wait on, and attractive use of materials.

Light-intensity (or baseline) physical activity Low-energy expenditure activities (e.g., slow walking, light housework, stretching) with minimal effect on breathing (only increases the amount of oxygen utilisation up to three times than seen at rest).

Long-term care An institution that provides permanent accommodation as well as the necessary care services within the same location.

Masters athlete Athletes participating in sport beyond the age of peak performance. The age of masters competition varies by sport, generally starting at around 35 years of age.

Mastery experience Mastery experience occurs when a person successfully performs a behaviour. Mastery experience is generally recognised as being the strongest source of information for self-efficacy judgements.

Measurement units These could be kilocalories (kcal) or Metabolic equivalent (MET).

Measurement tools These could be subjective (questionnaires, logs, diaries, or proxy reports) or objective (indirect calorimetry, doubly labelled water, direct observation, heart rate monitoring, or any kind of wearable monitors).

Meta-analysis A statistical analysis that combines results of multiple individual studies in order to test the pooled data for statistical significance.

Mobility Mobility is a person's capacity to physically navigate oneself through activities of daily living and to be able to walk or travel to the destinations necessary to achieve everyday tasks.

Mode of exercise Refers to the types of exercise that can be prescribed. Modes of exercise most commonly prescribed in exercise guidelines for older people are cardiovascular, strengthening, balance, flexibility, and functional activity.

Moderate-intensity physical activity Moderate-energy expenditure activities (e.g., brisk or uphill walking, low impact aerobics, aqua aerobics, dancing) which increase breathing rate but during which the participant can still hold a conversation (3–6 times greater oxygen consumption relative to rest).

Multisectoral Multisectoral models of policy development and health promotion recognise that no single sector or agency can adequately address complex health issues. Multisectoral efforts involve organisational coordination and collaboration across key public, private, and non-governmental stakeholders.

Musculoskeletal disorders Injuries, damage, or disorder of the joins or other tissues in the upper/lower limbs or the back.

Needs Things or activities required for well-being—whether objectively or subjectively defined. One person may feel a need to walk or run every day, while another may feel no such need, but everyone needs some physical activity to maintain bodily health and mental well-being.

Objective data Data obtained from instruments that measure movement, speed, and/or expenditure of energy during physical activity.

Older people There is no consensus on when old age begins. However, old age is often interpreted in the literature to begin around the age of 65 years.

Osteoarthritis A joint disease characterised by the breakdown of joint cartilage and underlying bone that is often referred to as the 'wear and tear' arthritis. Symptoms often include joint pain and swelling as well as stiffness and reduced joint range of motion.

Osteopenia A state of a bone mineral density loss and weakened bones that has not reached the extent of osteoporosis. Often there are no physical symptoms experienced by people with osteopenia, although it can be detected with bone density testing.

Osteoporosis A state of having substantial bone mineral density loss and bone weakness with an elevated risk of fractures. People with osteoporosis may be unaware that they have the condition until a fracture occurs. Osteoporosis is a major contributor to bone fractures among older adults.

Outcome expectancy Outcome expectancies have the form of if-then assumptions that refer to expected consequences of actions or behaviours that differ in the degree of desirability and probability. Classically, outcome expectancies ascribe value to an action due to presumed positive psychological effects, body image, or health benefits. In old age, outcome expectancies for physical activity should preferably be proximal, emotional, and realistic with high chances of fulfilment.

Outdoor physical activity Any physical activity that occurs under an open sky in built or natural environments. Examples include walking, structured exercise, cycling, gardening, and so on.

Pandemic (Of a disease) prevalent throughout an entire country, continent, or the entire world; epidemic over a large area.

Participation Involvement in a life situation (World Health Organization 2002).

Person-environment compatibility The match between an individual's needs and the environmental setting.

Phenomenological Derived from Phenomenology, is a philosophical movement which emphasises that human experience is shaped in constant interaction with the world via perception. Our bodies mediate between us and the wider world and are fully involved in how we develop our subjectivity, that is, our sense of who we are and how we fit in the world. Thus, our actions are always intentional, but mostly at a pre-conscious level because our intentions become deeply internalised during our everyday engagement with the world.

Physical activity Body movement that increases energy expenditure from the contraction of skeletal muscles. This may include unplanned physical activity that does not have physical fitness as the objective.

Physical activity behaviour Consists of (1) mode or activity type, (2) frequency, (3) duration, and (4) intensity of performing activity.

Physical activity guidelines This usually refers to the World Health Organization recommendations that adults engage in at least 150 minutes per week of moderate-intensity aerobic physical activity or 75 minutes of vigorous aerobic physical activity. These activities are to be in bouts of ten minutes or more. National guidelines are usually similar.

Physical activity policy Physical activity policies may include legislative actions, guidelines, regulations, or standards at any level (governmental, community, school, etc.) that have the potential to affect the physical activity behaviour of people and/or the physical activity environment (Physical Activity Policy Research Network 2010).

Physical capital Physical capital is a form of capital coined by the sociologist Pierre Bourdieu and works in conjunction with the other types of capital identified in his early work. It is the recognition that our bodies are affected by social structures, that is, we possess physical resources which reflect our habitus (social location). These physical resources are not equally distributed and range from our body phenotype to our competence to engage in specific activities such as sport and exercise.

Physical deconditioning Physical deconditioning is defined as an integrated physiological response of the body to a reduction in metabolic rate, that is, to a reduction in energy use or exercise level.

Physical environmental factors Any identifiable aspect of the natural and built world that might be relevant to understanding causality. This may include tangible, physical items (such as pavements, trees, or grass), as well as atmospheric and other processes (such as wind, rain, or noise). They can be classified into four different features: destination (e.g., shops, services, parks, and public transit), functional (e.g., street connectivity, pedestrian infrastructure), safety (e.g., traffic safety, safety from crime), and aesthetic (e.g., cleanliness, greenery, pollution) (Pikora et al. 2003).

Population attributable risk The number (or proportion) of cases with a certain condition that would not occur in a population if the risk factor (e.g., physical inactivity) was eliminated.

Postural stability Postural stability is defined as the capacity of being able to stand in an upright position while efficiently completing a task.

Postural strategies Postural strategies includes the motor actions used to maintain balance during the upright standing position.

Pre-frailty Pre-frailty is an intermediate stage between non-frail and frail status, though there is no consensus on how it should be measured (Sternberg et al. 2011). Using the frailty phenotype approach, pre-frailty is indicated by meeting one or two of five criteria (Fried et al. 2001).

Pre-reflective Pre-reflective describes actions which occur without extensive cognitive consideration. Closely linked to habitus, these actions are understood as natural, normal, and ordinary so require little consideration before action proceeds.

Prevalence estimates In physical activity research, estimates of the proportion of a population meeting physical activity guidelines for maintaining or enhancing health.

Progressive resistance exercise A method of increasing the strength of a weak or injured muscle by gradually increasing the resistance against which the muscle works, such as by using graduated weights. The minimum load must be such that the person can perform the exercise no more than 20 times until fatigue, and higher loads are more efficient.

Prospective cohort study A research study that follows over time groups of individuals who are alike in many ways but differ by a certain characteristic (e.g., physically active versus physically inactive) and compares them for a particular outcome.

Psychological restoration The renewal of a psychological, physiological, or social resource that has become depleted.

Psychosocial The combination of psychological and social factors.

Public realm The open space that people use to walk or cycle in between buildings. This may include street furniture, pavements, and cyclepaths, for example, as well as natural formations including topography.

Pulmonary rehabilitation A comprehensive intervention based on a thorough patient assessment that includes, but is not limited to, exercise training, education, and behaviour change, designed to improve the physical and psychological condition of people with chronic respiratory disease and to promote the long-term adherence to health-enhancing behaviours.

Quality-adjusted life year A generic measure of disease burden, including both the quality and the quantity of life lived. The ratio ranges from 0 (death) to 1 (optimal quality of life).

Quality of life The individual's perception of their position in life in the context of the culture and value systems in which they live and in relation to their goals, expectations, standards, and concerns. It is a broad-ranging concept affected in a complex way by the persons' physical health, psychological state, level of independence, social relationships, and their relationship to salient features of their environment.

Race Refers to the concept of dividing people into populations or groups on the basis of various sets of physical characteristics (which usually result from genetic ancestry) such as skin, hair, or eye colour. Race presumes shared biological or genetic traits, whether actual or asserted. However, the scientific basis of racial distinctions is very weak.

Randomised controlled trial A study in which participants are assigned by chance to separate groups that compare different treatments/ interventions; neither the researchers nor the participants can choose which group. Using chance to assign people to groups means that the groups will be similar and that the treatments they receive can be compared objectively.

Restorative environment Any environment that permits or promotes psychological restoration.

Risk perception Risk perceptions typically deal with an anticipated health problem, which set the stage for the motivational contemplation process. To make people take protective actions, general risk perceptions must be converted to personal risk perceptions. Risk communication must take care of persistent biases in risk perceptions, such as unrealistic optimism.

Rotator cuff A group of four muscles and their tendons including the supraspinatus, infraspinatus, subscapularis, and teres minor. The rotator cuff plays an important role in stabilising the shoulder. Painful rotator cuff conditions may or may not be associated with a prior traumatic injury.

Sarcopenia Sarcopenia is a syndrome characterised by progressive and generalised loss of skeletal muscle mass and muscle function (low muscle strength or performance) with a risk of adverse outcomes such as physical disability, poor quality of life, and death (a practical clinical definition by European Working Group on Sarcopenia in Older People) (EWGSOP) (Cruz-Jentoft 2010).

Sedentary A person who, for the greater proportion of their waking hours, engages in physical activities eliciting up to 1.5 times the oxygen consumption compared to their resting state. It can also include people who are only sporadically active but are highly inactive the remainder of the time.

Sedentary behaviour Sedentary behaviours (from the Latin *sedere*, 'to sit') include sitting during commuting, in the workplace and the domestic environment, and during leisure time. Sedentary behaviours such as TV viewing, computer use, or sitting in an automobile typically are in the energy-expenditure range of 1.0 to 1.5 METs (multiples of the basal metabolic rate).

Self-efficacy Self-efficacy is the belief that one is able to accomplish a behaviour despite the presence of setbacks and barriers.

Self-identity Having an identity means being situated in a specific role. According to identity theory, people's goals are based on their identities, and in pursuing these goals, people strive to maintain consistency between identity and behaviour. The more people agree that physical activity is part of their identity, the more active they are, and the more they intend to maintain their activities.

Self-monitoring According to control theory, self-monitoring refers to the comparison of an individual's current behaviour against a set goal standard. If discrepancies are encountered, then effort is initiated to adjust the behaviour to bring it in line with the goal standard.

Self-monitoring devices Devices such as smartphones, smartwatches, fitness trackers, and apps that contain a variety of sensors that allow the monitoring of behavioural, biological, and environmental data, such as steps taken, heart rate, and energy expenditure, that are fed back to the user as information about performance.

Self-perceptions of ageing Self-perceptions of ageing entail the way we view and evaluate our own ageing and are associated with health and well-being and even longevity. It appears that self-perceptions of ageing are an important determinant of productive, cognitive, and motivational dynamics that leads to adoption and maintenance of health behaviours. As a result, people with favourable views on ageing show higher levels of physical activity.

Self-regulation Self-regulation refers to control processes that actively modulate behaviour to bring it in line with set goals and standards. Important self-regulatory strategies are self-monitoring, action planning, and coping planning.

Sensors Objects or devices that detect or measure physical properties such as heat, light, sound, motion, force, tension, and so on. Sensors embedded in wearable devices include accelerometers, gyroscopes, magnetometers, and barometers.

Social class Generally conceptualised as being related to income and education. Socioeconomic status (SES) and social class are typically used interchangeably.

Social cognitive theory This theory tries to explain human behaviour with its core concepts: self-efficacy, outcome expectancies (e.g., losing weight, gaining fitness, or being socially approved via physical activity) and goals. It further assumes that behaviour and social cognitions can either be hindered or facilitated by factors in a person's environment (e.g., sports facilities close by).

Social constructionism An umbrella term applied to theoretical perspectives that analyse the socially created basis of social life through the actions of individuals and social groups. Often ascribed to the Chicago School of sociology and the phenomenologically inspired sociology of Alfred Schütz, social constructionism posits that society is actively created by humans in everyday life and interaction. The everyday world is thus conceptualised as 'produced' rather than existing as a 'thing' independent of human interaction.

Social contacts (ties) Those individuals with whom older people spend time with and give and lend support to; adult development theory suggests older adults' choice and number of social contacts is a voluntary and adaptive process, focusing on emotional satisfaction.

Subjective norm A person's subjective norm is his or her impression of what important social partners believe the person ought to do. Subjective norms are useful for predicting older adults' intentions to be physically active, and thus, only have an indirect effect on behaviour.

Sources of self-efficacy Social cognitive theory suggests that self-efficacy can best be increased by addressing the following four hypothesised sources: mastery experience, vicarious experiences, verbal persuasion, and somatic and affective states.

Sportification of society 'Refers to a growing number of people that have become involved in sport activities over the past decades and to the related diversification of activities and settings' (Tischer et al. 2011, p. 83).

Standards (levels) of evidence Frameworks that have been developed to help structure how evidence is gathered, interpreted, and assessed. Several different frameworks exist, with some specific to the evaluation and interpretation of scientific literature and others specific to the development of policy or clinical practice guidelines. All attempt to reduce bias in these endeavours through the application of tightly defined criteria to the evaluative process.

Street connectivity Represented by the intersection density, that is, the ratio between the number of true intersections (three or more legs) to a given land area (Frank et al. 2010). Higher intersection density is associated with more direct travel paths between destinations that are closer to the Euclidean ('as the crow flies') distance between destinations and offers a greater number of alternative routes from one destination to another (Transportation Research Board 2005).

Streets Small residential or commercial roads shared by people walking and cycling as much as they are for vehicles.

Strength training/resistance training A type of exercise that requires the body muscles to exert a force against some form of resistance, such as weights (including the older person's own body weight), stretch bands, water, or immovable objects. Regular strength training will increase lean muscle tissue and improve muscle strength, resulting in both physical and psychological benefits for the individual.

Structured exercise programmes A series of activities performed with the sole purpose of engaging participants in exercise. This activity could be performed in a class environment or by an individual alone or with supervision.

Subjective data Data obtained from surveys. Often called self-report data. Termed 'subjective' because those completing surveys must make judgements about the meaning of questions asked and instructions given in the survey as well as about the intensity of their physical activities and the lengths of time devoted to those activities.

Successful ageing A state of ageing that reflects a health and disease profile, and/or level of life satisfaction that is above typical levels for older adults.

Symbolic interactionism A major strand of sociological theory with roots in pragmatism and also the work of the sociologist, Max Weber, who argued that people act on the basis of their interpretations of the world and the meaning that things hold for them. The American, George Herbert Mead, is a key figure within symbolic interactionism and highlighted the centrality of meaning and people's 'definition of the situation' in social action. People interpret and give meaning to each other's actions and responses, including their imagined responses to an individual's behaviour.

Telerehabilitation The delivery of rehabilitation services at a distance using telecommunications technology as a delivery medium.

Translational research Translational research aims to 'translate' findings from laboratory research into practice, including the development and adoption of best practices in community-based interventions. A common example of translational research would be studies of the cost-effectiveness of public health interventions.

Type 2 diabetes A condition characterised by high blood glucose levels caused by either a lack of insulin or the body's inability to use insulin efficiently. Type 2 diabetes develops most often in middle-aged and older adults but can appear in young people.

Usability Defined by the international standard ISO 9241-11 as the extent to which a system or product can be used by specified users to achieve specified goals with effectiveness, efficiency, and satisfaction in a specified context of use. Thus, usability refers to the ease of use of products and systems, to what extent the latter are matched to the needs and requirements of the user.

Vigorous intensity physical activity High-energy expenditure activities (e.g., running, swimming front crawl, fast cycling) greatly increasing the breathing rate, where the participant would not be able to say more than a few words without pausing for breath (above six times greater oxygen consumption relative to rest).

Walkability Describes the ease of walking in a neighbourhood. This is often related to the proximity of shopping, access to necessary services, safety, in terms of crime and the ability to navigate through traffic safely, attractiveness of area, and walkways that are wide, safe, and well-maintained.

Willingness-to-pay threshold The hypothetical limit to resources that the society is willing to allocate to medical interventions. It reflects how much a society is willing to pay to achieve a certain health gain for one person, for example, to prevent one person from developing a certain condition or to increase a person's quality of life.

World Masters Games The largest sporting event in the world, held every four years for participants at the masters level of competition.

References

Chodzko-Zajko, W. J., Proctor, D. N., Fiatarone Sing, M. A., Minson, C. T., Nigg, C. R., Salem, G. J., et al. (2009). Exercise and physical activity for older adults. *Medicine & Science in Sports & Exercise, 41*, 1510–1530.

Cruz-Jentoft, A. J., Baeyens, J. P., Bauer, J. M., Boirie, Y., Cederholm, T., Landi, F., Martin, F. C., Michel, J. P., Rolland, Y., Schneider, S. M., Topinková, E., Vandewoude, M., & Zamboni, M. (2010). European working group on sarcopenia in older people. Sarcopenia: European consensus on definition and diagnosis:

Report of the European working group on sarcopenia in older people. *Age and Ageing, 39*(4), 412–423.

Frank, L. D., Sallis, J. F., Saelens, B. E., Leary, L., Cain, K. L., Conway, T. L., & Hess, P. M. (2010). The development of a walkability index: Application to the neighborhood quality of life study. *British Journal of Sports Medicine, 44*(13), 924–933. https://doi.org/10.1136/bjsm.2009.058701.

Fried, L. P., Tangen, C. M., Walston, J., Newman, A., Hirsch, C., Gottdiener, J., et al. (2001). Frailty in older adults: Evidence for a phenotype. *The Journals of Gerontology. Series A, Biological Sciences and Medical Sciences, 56*, M146–M156.

Physical Activity Policy Research Network. (2010). https://paprn.wustl.edu/about-us/Pages/WhatisPhysicalActivityPolicy.aspx

Pikora, T., Giles-Corti, B., Bull, F., Jamrozik, K., & Donovan, R. (2003). Developing a framework for assessment of the environmental determinants of walking and cycling. *Social Science & Medicine, 56*(8), 1693–1703. https://doi.org/10.1016/s0277-9536(02)00163-6.

Sternberg, S. A., Schwartz, A. W., Karunananthan, S., Bergman, H., & Mark Clarfield, A. (2011). The identification of frailty: A systematic literature review. *Journal of the American Geriatrics Society, 59*(11), 2129–2138.

Tischer, U., Hartmann-Tews, I., & Combrink, C. (2011). Sport participation of the elderly-the role of gender, age, and social class. *European Reviews of Aging and Physical Activity, 8*(2), 83–91.

Transportation Research Board. (2005). *Does the built environment influence physical activity? Examining the evidence*. Retrieved from Washington, DC. http://onlinepubs.trb.org/onlinepubs/sr/sr282.pdf

Weed, M. (2016). Evidence for physical activity guidelines as a public health intervention: Efficacy, effectiveness, and harm – A critical policy sciences approach. *Health Psychology and Behavioral Medicine, 4*, 56–69. https://doi.org/10.1080/21642850.2016.1159517.

World Health Organization. (2002). *Towards a common language for functioning, disability and health: ICF, the international classification of functioning, disability and health*. Geneva: World Health Organization.

Index[1]

NUMBERS AND SYMBOLS

1-repetition maximum (1-RM), 90, 148
6-minute walk test, 129

A

Accelerometer, 33–35, 44, 135, 188, 275, 280, 383, 590, 631, 635, 637–639, 641, 643–646, 657, 694, 714, 716
Acceptability, 106, 208, 222, 240, 291–298, 300, 301, 303, 304, 306, 307, 403, 721–723
Action planning, 220, 275–278, 281–283, 285
Active ageing, 2, 9, 53, 146, 343, 469, 479, 527, 535, 545, 601, 718
Active travel, 4, 31, 32, 65, 300, 452, 507–510, 519–521
Activity classification, 716
Activity counselling, 127, 131–133
Activity monitor/tracker, 135, 361, 478, 628, 644, 664, 717, 723, 725
Activity patterns, 14, 26, 467, 473, 478, 554, 644, 654
Adherence, 5, 6, 27, 28, 31, 35, 87, 104, 106, 110, 112, 114, 130, 133, 134, 155, 156, 191, 218, 262, 279, 281, 282, 304, 305, 329, 341, 363–365, 369, 391, 415, 469, 628, 629, 661, 718–720, 727
Adoption of physical activity programmes, 315, 393
Adverse events, 84, 90, 173, 175, 366, 373, 387, 390, 395, 725
Aerobic exercise, 4, 5, 46, 50, 87, 92, 147, 149, 153, 155, 192, 194, 674, 696–699, 701, 702, 704
Aesthetics, 425, 437, 439, 448, 457, 458, 491, 493, 494, 510, 516, 520
Affective depletion, 486
Affordance, 423, 428, 433, 434, 437, 438, 485, 488

---

[1] Notes: Page numbers followed by 'n' refer to notes.

Ageing, 1, 2, 7, 9, 14, 45, 47, 52, 53, 84, 103, 136, 146, 185, 208, 231, 241–243, 251, 253, 256, 257, 260–262, 277, 278, 280, 281, 296, 298, 302, 303, 305, 319, 321, 322, 328–330, 338, 342, 343, 352, 401, 410, 413, 423, 424, 439, 468–471, 478, 479, 527, 531–546, 552, 554–565, 571, 572, 574–576, 580, 583, 584, 594, 595, 598–601, 636, 641, 665, 674–676, 678–682, 704, 718

Ageing in place, 470–472, 475, 478

Ageism/ageing stereotypes, 241, 321, 322, 328, 331

Allotments, 492

American College of Sports Medicine (ACSM), 34, 85, 86, 91, 108, 589, 636, 704

Applications, apps, mobile apps, 716

Assessment of function during hospitalisation, 197

Assisted living, 252, 359, 360, 468, 475–477

Atrophy, 83, 94, 194, 197, 695

Attention Restoration Theory (ART), 486, 487

Attribution, 233

Augmented reality (AR), 726

Automatic adjustment, automatic adaptation, 721, 723

Autonomous motivation, 253, 254, 261

Autonomy, 5, 67, 155, 219, 221, 254, 278, 294, 302, 307, 339, 385, 584, 601, 684

B

Balance, 5, 12, 27, 46, 47, 50, 53, 66, 69, 85–88, 91–93, 95, 106–113, 148, 150, 152–155, 168, 169, 171, 178, 190, 196, 212, 213, 215, 219, 272, 298, 304, 342, 351, 362, 369, 404, 406, 408, 410, 434, 469, 474–476, 491, 558, 560, 590, 610, 627, 699, 700, 702, 719, 720, 722

Balance confidence, 719

Barriers and enablers, 108, 114, 313, 359, 363, 365–367, 392, 521

Barriers for physical activity during hospital admission, 198, 328

BCT, *see* Behaviour Change Technique

Behaviour change, 10, 13, 63, 103, 114, 131, 132, 134, 177, 211–224, 234, 235, 237, 241, 242, 255, 259, 260, 262, 273, 276, 291, 298, 313, 342, 412, 413, 424, 469, 470, 478, 479, 519, 535, 594, 614, 639, 664, 719

Behaviour change taxonomy, 211, 221, 235, 277, 297

Behaviour Change Technique (BCT), 12, 177, 207–209, 211, 221–223, 232, 235–237, 242, 274, 275, 277, 278, 284, 297–299, 306, 345

Behaviour change theory, 211–224, 234, 235, 273, 342, 719

Bias of unrealistic optimism, 259

Biophilia hypothesis/biophilic design, 435

Blue space, 494, 495, 497, 498

Body/Embodiment, 1, 3, 4, 6, 12, 21, 48, 49, 84, 87–89, 108, 110, 147, 153, 166, 167, 169, 170, 173–175, 196, 197, 258, 259, 261, 281, 282, 303, 347, 367, 408, 414, 428, 432, 441, 488, 512, 527, 531–546, 555, 560, 562–564, 574, 590, 593, 635, 636, 644, 656, 659–661, 665, 675, 676, 696, 713, 714, 716, 717, 720

Bone health, 659
Botanical gardens, 492, 493, 498, 499
Built environment, 3, 13, 14, 223, 325, 327, 374, 424, 425, 431, 432, 467, 471, 476–478, 485, 493, 514–516, 578, 618
Burden of disease, 62, 63, 72
Bus use, 518

C

Cachexia, 83
Cancer, 1, 21, 47, 48, 54, 62, 65, 72, 107, 258, 292, 338, 352, 402, 508, 658, 660, 673
Capability, Opportunity, Motivation - Behaviour (COM-B), 10, 222, 223
Cardiac rehabilitation (CR), 128, 130, 133, 134, 137, 192, 278, 342, 558
Cardiovascular disease (CVD), 21, 22, 44, 49, 53, 54, 65, 105, 106, 123, 126, 130, 133, 216, 219, 258, 338, 352, 508, 655, 657–659, 662, 665
Cardiovascular fitness, 111, 112, 723
Care staff, 347, 362, 365, 366, 369, 370, 372
Centers for Disease Control and Prevention (CDC), 28, 29, 34, 615
Chronic diseases, 25, 26, 34, 52–54, 104, 127, 132, 134, 137, 166, 258, 303, 341, 382, 405, 534, 721
Chronic obstructive pulmonary disease (COPD), 45, 124, 125, 129, 132–135, 338, 392
Chronic respiratory disease, 125, 130
Co-design, co-production, 436
Cognitive decline, 51, 283, 299, 490, 491, 515, 640, 694, 695, 701, 719
Cognitive fatigue, 486, 487
Cognitive function, 43, 51, 54, 256, 413, 695, 696, 699–703, 719
Cognitive health, 489, 628, 676, 677, 679, 693–704
Cognitive status, 388
COM-B, see Capability, Opportunity, Motivation-Behaviour
Community-based physical activity, 11, 304, 328, 411, 615–620
Community-dwelling older people, 11, 401–416
Compatibility, 486, 487, 499
Consequences of bed rest, 314
Continence, 363, 364, 373
Continuity, 306, 350, 454, 515, 528, 552–555, 557–565
Control belief, 235
Control Theory, 272, 273, 284, 285
COPD, see Chronic obstructive pulmonary disease
Coping appraisal, 404
Coping planning, 220, 275–279, 283, 285
Cost-effectiveness of interventions, 425
CR, see Cardiac rehabilitation
CVD, see Cardiovascular disease
Cycling, 50, 85, 87, 89, 106, 107, 113, 208, 252, 448, 452, 455–457, 507–510, 516–521, 574, 635, 643, 675, 696, 713

D

Dance, 87, 93, 109, 110, 302, 362, 369, 372, 411
Delivery (of interventions, physical activity), 127, 295, 299, 307, 340, 349, 381, 411, 599

Dementia, 1, 51, 61, 65, 70–73, 107, 151, 193, 348, 352, 359, 361, 366, 382, 402, 485, 491, 497, 498, 515, 590, 607, 628, 693–698, 701, 702, 704, 722
Demography, 189, 429
Diabetes, 6, 21, 29, 45, 46, 49, 53, 54, 62, 65, 86, 126, 216, 218, 258, 508, 595, 653, 659, 662, 673, 694
Digital games/exercise games, exergames, 14, 151, 628, 714–716, 718–727
Digital technology, 628, 721
Disability, 1, 2, 46, 50, 52–54, 62, 108, 110, 124, 125, 145, 150, 154, 174, 185, 186, 188, 189, 193–195, 198, 402, 415, 468, 498, 554, 593, 674, 679, 683, 699, 718, 719, 721, 722
Discontinuity, 406, 553, 554
Disease, 6, 12, 21–23, 25, 26, 34, 43–47, 52–54, 62, 63, 65, 72, 80, 83, 84, 104, 107, 110, 123–134, 137, 149–151, 153–156, 166, 167, 172, 174–176, 179, 185, 186, 188, 194, 197, 257, 258, 282, 303, 338, 341, 382, 392, 405, 508, 534, 541, 593, 599, 607, 608, 628, 653, 657–659, 661, 679, 682, 694–696, 699, 700, 718, 719, 721, 726

E

Ecological model, 10, 11, 23, 207, 322, 325, 434
Effectiveness, 22, 23, 64, 65, 68, 70–72, 109, 110, 129, 147, 151, 167, 169, 207, 208, 238, 274, 277, 278, 281, 283–285, 297–299, 314, 322, 338, 388, 394, 411, 477, 599, 608–611, 613–615, 619, 620, 638, 663, 679, 683, 703, 718, 720–722

Efficiency, 609, 702, 722
Emotional satisfaction, 67, 319
Empowerment, 339, 528, 562, 563, 601, 675, 676, 683
Encouraging messages, 724
Endurance, 47, 66, 85, 91, 110, 124, 127, 150, 152, 154, 178, 196, 362, 363, 402, 574, 676, 716, 719
Energy expenditure, 3, 89, 125, 635, 641, 642, 654–657, 716, 717, 723
Enjoyment, 110, 112, 114, 253, 262, 282, 295, 300, 304, 307, 345, 407, 410, 413, 414, 428, 439, 494, 495, 581, 677–680, 718
Environmental determinism, 430
Environmental features, 9, 427, 428, 438, 449, 450, 473, 476
Environmental gerontology, 423, 450
Established-Outsider Relationships, 559–561
Ethnic group/Ethnicity, 218, 323, 330, 499, 528, 534, 552, 556, 577, 578, 584, 590, 594, 596, 599–601, 628, 641, 660, 681
Evidence-based, 26, 103, 137, 147, 155, 156, 171, 191, 338, 342, 349, 352, 412, 427, 432, 529, 578, 584, 611, 613, 614, 617, 618, 620, 703, 727
Executive function, 281, 299, 697, 698, 700, 702, 719
Exercise, 27, 45, 66, 79, 84–94, 104, 105, 109–111, 148, 190–193, 218, 231, 272, 296, 313, 321, 328, 337–352, 361–363, 382, 402, 414, 415, 428, 469, 519, 534, 552, 589, 615, 627, 635, 655, 663, 674, 714
Exercise in hospitalised persons, 190–193
Exercise prescription, 79, 80, 84–92, 95, 104, 105, 170–172, 174, 175
Exercise science, 2, 12, 534, 560

Exercise training, 5, 49, 50, 88, 124–127, 129–131, 135–137, 146, 147, 150, 194, 342, 657, 694, 696–699, 701–704
Experience, 34, 72, 106, 132, 136, 145–147, 167, 170, 176, 189, 190, 215–217, 219, 231, 236–243, 257, 260, 261, 278, 283, 293–296, 301, 303, 306, 315, 320, 322, 323, 325, 327, 331, 341–350, 365, 367, 384, 388, 394, 395, 404, 433–435, 439, 440, 449, 455, 486, 488–490, 495–497, 499, 527, 528, 531–533, 535, 536, 538, 540, 541, 544, 545, 551, 552, 554, 555, 557–560, 563–566, 572–576, 581, 583, 589–601, 608, 611, 612, 620, 631, 677, 721
Extrinsic motivation, 220, 253

F

Falls, 12, 46, 47, 50, 68, 69, 85, 86, 88, 91, 93, 94, 107–112, 150–154, 169, 190, 215, 219, 261, 272, 338, 342, 352, 363–366, 369, 370, 372, 373, 384, 387, 388, 390, 402, 406, 410, 473, 474, 476, 477, 491, 499, 508, 515, 590, 699
Fascination, 487, 490, 498, 499
Feedback, 112, 131, 133, 135, 217, 237–239, 258, 262, 272–274, 297, 299, 339, 340, 344–346, 351, 365, 392, 394, 410, 411, 415, 434, 552, 645, 714, 717–719, 723, 724, 726
Fitness, 4, 14, 29, 49, 85, 87, 92, 105–107, 110–112, 149, 153, 173, 178, 186, 234, 252, 261, 280, 284, 298, 344, 409, 489, 494, 517, 538, 564, 578, 620, 636, 673, 676, 678–680, 701, 723

Fitness apps, 722
Fitness trackers, 724
FITT principle, 80, 84–92
Flexibility for aerobic training/strength training, 149
Fractures, 46, 71, 80, 108, 151, 167–172, 188, 191–193, 197, 373, 388, 470, 476, 699
Frailty, 1, 12, 152, 155, 165, 185, 283, 314, 315, 360, 363, 366, 370, 371, 401–416, 533, 560, 675
Frequency of exercise, 88
Function, 6, 14, 33, 35, 43, 45, 46, 48, 49, 51–54, 67, 79, 83, 93, 94, 104, 124, 126, 127, 129, 135, 145, 147, 153–155, 166, 170–174, 176, 185, 187–190, 192, 193, 196–198, 217, 219, 256–258, 272, 273, 281, 299, 305, 319, 343, 344, 362–365, 404, 407–409, 411, 413, 415, 436, 437, 477, 591, 610, 627, 643, 657, 679, 680, 682, 695–702, 717, 719–723, 725, 726
Functional capacity, 67, 83, 106, 107, 123, 124, 137, 190, 296, 361, 447, 577
Functional mobility, 84, 86, 88, 148, 150, 719
Functional task training, 169, 362

G

Games/Gamification, 726
Gardens, 30, 31, 89, 433, 436, 438, 439, 457, 474–476, 490–493, 497–499, 514
Gender, 9, 21, 22, 30, 32, 33, 218, 238, 323, 325, 344, 429, 433, 450, 499, 518, 528, 534, 535, 537–540, 545, 552, 556, 571–584, 590–592, 594, 596, 597, 599–601, 628

Goal setting and staff training, 364–365
Green exercise, 431
Green space, 326, 424, 433, 489, 490, 492–495, 499
Gyroscopes, 716

H

Habit Formation, 306, 664
Habitus, 534, 538, 563
Health, 21, 25, 43–47, 49, 50, 61, 63–65, 79, 83, 103, 124–126, 145, 165, 186, 207, 211, 234, 235, 251, 277, 292, 314, 337, 346, 360, 381, 406, 412–414, 424, 429, 453, 488, 489, 507, 527, 534, 552, 589, 607, 627, 641, 653, 657–660, 673, 676, 677, 693, 714
Health action process approach (HAPA), 212, 220–222, 235, 273
Health apps, 724, 725, 727
Health Belief Model (HBM), 212, 218, 219, 235, 259
Health care costs/utilisation/professionals, 13, 61–65, 70–73, 147, 303
Healthy ageing, 1, 413, 555, 572, 665, 680
Heart failure, 45, 126, 130, 194
Heart rate monitor (HRM), 635, 643
Home-based physical activity, 300, 305
Hospital, 13, 63, 68, 71, 125, 132, 152, 171, 185, 188–193, 195–198, 238, 314, 315, 338, 349, 359, 381, 382, 384–394, 401, 507
Hospitalisation-associated disability, 188, 195, 198
Human Physiology, 654–663

I

Implementation, 3, 13, 113, 147, 151, 176, 216, 252, 275–277, 313–315, 331, 364, 388, 393–395, 402, 414–416, 584, 612, 615–617, 661
Inactivity, 12, 21, 25–36, 43, 44, 47, 48, 50, 61–63, 72, 73, 83, 125, 126, 146, 152, 166, 185–189, 193, 195, 198, 214, 313, 367, 383–385, 387, 393, 394, 428, 534, 561, 607, 615, 616, 618, 621, 659, 694, 714, 724
Independence, 1, 7, 66, 83, 85, 150, 171, 189, 197, 296, 302, 304, 305, 362, 365, 366, 383, 384, 390, 395, 408, 415, 471, 475, 488, 515, 534, 684, 693, 701, 722
Information and communication technology (ICT), 713
Information-Motivation-Behavioural-Skills Model (IMB), 212, 218
Instructor, 14, 110, 111, 253, 293, 302, 313, 314, 324, 337–352, 405, 408, 539, 575, 576, 615
Intensity of strength training/exercise, 88–91, 153, 640, 703
Intention, 4, 11, 13, 113, 213, 215, 216, 219–221, 255, 256, 258–260, 273, 275–277, 281–283, 367, 404
Interactionist approaches, 430
Interdependency chains, 558
Intergenerational, 257, 327, 329, 490, 492, 494, 499, 674
Intrinsic motivation, 219, 253

J

Just Walk It, 619

L

Life History, 536
Life-Span Theory of Control, 278–280
Lifestyle, 4, 8, 9, 12, 21, 22, 29, 44, 45, 50, 51, 53, 65–67, 72, 123, 127, 146, 153, 155, 166, 167, 169, 178, 214, 218, 231, 296, 304–307, 323, 404, 410, 427, 474, 477, 489, 541, 553, 558, 561, 565, 572, 629, 643, 653, 655–658, 660–662, 664, 680, 693, 722, 724
Lifestyle drift, 558, 565
Light physical activity, 301
Locus of control, 232, 233
Loneliness, 327, 436–438, 490, 492, 507, 595, 596, 719
Long term care, 70, 72, 73, 84, 154, 314, 315, 338, 343, 347–349, 352, 359–374, 468, 590

M

Magnetometers, 716
Maintenance of physical activity programmes, 132, 207–209, 255, 260, 292, 293, 298, 300–306, 317, 410, 411, 472
Managing expectations, 302
Masters athletes, 538, 629, 674, 677, 679–682
Mastery experience, 236, 237, 239, 240, 242, 243, 257
Measurement of activity levels, 26, 361, 590, 656
Media, 9, 177, 219, 257, 352, 439, 440, 528, 581–584, 598, 610, 613, 615, 619, 675
Memory, 7, 51, 147, 280, 281, 299, 486, 488, 489, 491, 495, 497, 499, 552, 562, 631, 639, 643, 644, 660, 677, 698, 699, 701, 702, 717

Mental health, 1, 21, 49, 50, 54, 110, 256, 298, 408, 424, 428, 492, 508, 580, 628
Mental imagery, 237
Mild cognitive impairment (MCI), 701–703
Mindfulness, 498
Mini mental state examination (MMSE), 360, 362, 364, 702
Mobile phone, 35, 137, 155, 283, 284, 499, 644, 722
Mobility, 12, 46, 50, 68, 84–86, 88, 126, 145, 150, 152, 153, 190, 192, 193, 196–198, 272, 298, 303–305, 366, 387, 390, 394, 395, 408, 410, 415, 424, 427–441, 450, 468–470, 474–476, 478, 479, 485, 488–491, 493–499, 507, 508, 511, 518, 521, 579, 655, 663, 698, 700, 701, 719
Moderate physical activity, 126, 239, 294, 507, 665
Mood, 67, 104, 107, 111, 273, 303, 305, 361, 363, 365, 433, 486–488, 491, 498
Morbidity, 62, 65, 66, 107, 123, 125, 151, 192, 196, 534, 596
Mortality, 1, 43, 44, 47, 49, 52, 54, 62, 65, 66, 68, 84, 107, 123, 125, 126, 130, 151, 193, 198, 297, 410, 490, 508, 534, 640, 658, 661, 677, 680
Motivation, 5, 10, 112, 113, 131, 153, 166, 177, 195, 207–209, 213, 217–221, 223, 235, 253–255, 258, 261, 262, 273, 278, 285, 293, 299, 304, 305, 313, 318, 324, 337, 344, 347, 348, 350, 351, 364, 370, 392, 408, 409, 433, 434, 437, 472, 486, 489, 490, 493, 498, 535, 581, 599, 677, 680, 683, 719, 725

Motivational interviewing, 131, 132, 236, 392, 578
Motivational messages, 326, 723, 725
Motivators for physical activity during hospital admission, 581
Movement patterns, 634
Multigenerational playgrounds, 494
Multiple-comorbidities, 366
Multiple component interventions, 152
Multisectoral, 616, 617, 620

N

Nature relatedness/nature deficit disorder, 435
Needs, vi, 2, 3, 7, 12, 13, 22, 30, 33, 34, 52, 63–66, 70, 72, 73, 79, 85, 88, 91–94, 103, 124, 125, 132, 133, 152, 155, 156, 165, 166, 177, 178, 190, 192, 195–198, 208, 212–214, 216, 217, 219–221, 223, 232, 237, 239, 254, 257, 262, 263, 276, 277, 279, 282, 284, 291–293, 296, 298, 300–302, 304, 306, 313–315, 319, 321, 323–325, 331, 338, 339, 341, 342, 344–347, 349, 350, 352, 359, 371–373, 387–395, 405, 411, 414–416, 424, 425, 427–429, 432, 433, 436, 437, 441, 451, 454, 458, 459, 467–473, 477, 478, 485–487, 489–491, 493, 495, 497–499, 511, 512, 514–517, 519–521, 528, 529, 531, 534–536, 541, 546, 552, 560, 562, 564–566, 576, 578, 579, 581, 583, 584, 589, 590, 600, 601, 612, 613, 616, 619, 620, 627–629, 640, 646, 663–665, 678, 681–684, 703, 704, 715–719, 721–727
Neuromuscular diseases, 148, 153, 154

Non-communicable diseases, 43, 53, 65, 607
Number of steps, 187, 383, 389, 717, 723

O

Obesity, 21, 29, 43, 47–49, 54, 107, 146, 173, 489, 508, 519, 529, 593, 615, 653, 655, 660, 662, 663, 694
Occupational therapy, 191, 423
Osteoarthritis, 46, 80, 94, 109, 110, 112, 172–174, 178, 283, 360, 383, 614, 673
Osteoporosis and osteopenia, 46, 80, 167–170, 174, 659
Outcome expectancy, 215, 217, 220, 221, 234, 240, 255, 259–262
Outdoor gyms/senior playgrounds, 494
Outdoor physical activity, 427, 436
Overload, 80, 93, 95, 108, 172, 178

P

Pacing, 134, 301, 302, 371
Parkinson's disease, 110, 150, 151, 726
Pedestrian and bicycle infrastructure, 454–455
Pedestrian crossings, 450, 511
Pedestrian safety, 578
Pedometer, 28, 33, 106, 132, 133, 135, 137, 274, 275, 298, 345, 383, 411, 590, 641, 643, 644, 694
Perceived behavioural control (PBC), 215, 233, 255
Perceived social environment, 214, 327, 328
Perceived Value (of physical activity), 295, 299, 301, 304, 305
Perception of ageing, 7, 302–303, 575
Performance trackers, 722
Personalisation, 215, 628, 719, 720, 726

Person environment fit, 433, 434, 472, 473, 477, 486
Physical activity behavior, 489
Physical Activity Careers, 540, 543
Physical activity measurement tools/units/monitors/trackers, 53, 63, 81, 89, 135, 628, 644, 694, 717, 722–724
Physical fitness, 4, 92, 149
Physical frailty, 314, 401–416, 675
Physical inactivity, 12, 21, 25–36, 43, 44, 47, 48, 50, 61–63, 72, 73, 83, 125, 126, 146, 166, 185–189, 193, 195, 198, 313, 384, 607, 615, 616, 618, 621, 694
Physical inactivity during hospitalisation, 188, 195
Physical limitations, 8, 253, 254, 262, 280, 283, 284, 293, 296, 297, 407
Physiotherapists, 12, 68, 155, 238, 362, 366, 383, 387, 389, 390, 406
Play, 4, 13, 14, 45, 50, 52, 67, 71, 73, 110, 167, 185, 273, 313, 320, 322, 330, 337, 341, 343, 345, 346, 349, 352, 367, 392, 431, 433, 469, 477, 488, 489, 494, 517, 533, 538, 542, 545, 583, 642, 660, 674, 684, 715, 718, 719, 722, 726
Positivity effect, 241
Praise, 724
Pre-frailty, 401
Progression, 3, 150, 151, 155, 156, 171, 179, 341, 344, 402, 479, 673, 693, 700, 703, 723
Psychological restoration, 485, 486, 492
Psychological wellbeing, 70, 495, 499
Public parks, 14, 497
Pulmonary rehabilitation (PR), 89, 128–130, 133–137

Q
Quality of life (QOL), vi, 2, 7, 21, 48, 49, 61, 62, 65–73, 103, 107, 110, 123, 126, 127, 129, 130, 133–135, 137, 154, 174, 222, 363, 401, 477, 479, 488, 491, 508, 519, 529, 534, 595, 627, 677, 693, 722

R
Race, 149, 323, 552, 594, 660, 713
Randomized Clinical Controlled (RCT) Trials, 129, 135, 186, 190, 195, 212, 216, 218, 363, 364, 608, 609, 613, 614, 703
Rating of perceived exertion, 89, 90
Recovery, 46, 80, 93–95, 108, 170–172, 189, 191–193, 220, 233, 371, 385, 392, 486, 487, 489
Rehabilitation, 4, 46, 79, 89, 127–130, 133, 134, 152, 155, 156, 170–172, 176, 191–193, 195, 237, 238, 278, 338, 342, 349, 350, 364, 381–384, 387, 390, 558, 559, 581, 716, 718, 720, 722, 724–726
Relational self, 556
Reminders, 113, 136, 391, 394, 406, 439, 495, 724, 725
Residential care home, 359, 488, 491, 497
Resistance training, 45, 46, 67, 84, 87, 107, 127, 148, 150, 155, 169, 362, 367–369, 635, 696–704
Restorative environment, 485–500
Reward, 220, 253, 260, 284, 292, 678, 679, 724
Rheumatic diseases, 80, 174–176
Risk perception, 220, 221, 257–259, 262

Roads, 186, 450, 458, 509–511, 513, 515, 516, 521, 574
Role model, 214, 238, 251, 257, 261, 262, 307, 320, 329, 330, 346, 599, 629, 679
Rotator cuff, 176

S

Safety, 69, 81, 90, 155, 171, 179, 259, 326, 330, 342, 348, 371, 388–390, 395, 416, 429, 437, 438, 448, 451, 455–457, 475, 476, 495, 509, 510, 512, 578–581, 584, 721, 724–726
Salutogenic environments, 435
Sarcopenia, 48, 83, 155, 185, 360, 534, 699
Satisfaction, 67, 191, 254, 257, 305, 319, 326, 342, 344, 477, 491, 553, 575, 678–681, 722
Sedentary behaviour/sedentary time/sedentariness/sitting time, 53, 145, 146, 148–150, 152, 208, 214, 261, 294, 296, 297, 301, 307, 314, 360, 361, 474, 477, 478, 528, 580, 607, 618, 621, 628, 629, 639, 644, 653–666, 677, 714, 717, 724
Selection, optimisation, and compensation, 278, 279
Self Determination Theory (SDT), 212, 219, 220, 222, 253, 254, 580
Self-efficacy
  initiation, 207, 209, 220, 233, 243
  maintenance, 207, 209, 220, 233, 243
  recovery self-efficacy, 233
Self-identity, 252, 253, 256, 300, 302
Self-monitoring, 127, 131–133, 135, 137, 213, 237, 273–275, 283–285, 298, 345, 351, 411, 415, 714, 716–719, 723, 726
Self-perceptions of ageing, 241, 253, 256, 257, 260, 302

Self-regulation, 208, 223, 254, 271–285, 298, 299, 489, 540
Sensors, 155, 477, 643–645, 696, 716, 717, 723
Smartphones/Smartwatches, 177, 345, 351, 716, 717, 720, 722, 726
Social class, 323, 528, 571–584
Social Cognitive Theory (SCT), 212, 217, 218, 222, 234, 242, 252, 254, 259, 273, 292, 324, 325, 330
Social constructionism, 532, 555–557
Social contacts (or social ties), 241, 295, 297, 300, 305, 318–320, 328, 329, 489, 490, 492
Social ecological model, 325
Social functioning and participation, 69, 127, 449, 678, 720
Social interaction, 146, 241, 300, 307, 318, 319, 324, 339, 348, 366, 407, 409, 413, 437, 439, 467, 471, 488, 489, 493, 497, 498, 556, 719
Social isolation, 303, 318, 437, 490, 719
Socially inclusive design, 436
Social support, 104, 171, 188, 213, 214, 216, 218, 223, 234, 283, 284, 293, 298, 313, 314, 317, 320–328, 341, 345, 348, 382, 406, 407, 416, 468, 493, 572, 581, 584, 593, 595
Socio-ecological model, 432, 434, 448, 450, 451, 457, 546n1
Socio-economic status (SES), 11, 292, 293, 303, 306, 528, 572, 573, 576–578, 580, 581, 600, 614, 681
Socioemotional Selectivity Theory (SST), 260, 282, 283, 298, 299, 318–320, 326
Somatic and affective states, 239
Sources of self-efficacy, 235–243
Specificity, 80, 92, 93, 108, 151, 663
Sport, 2, 4, 22, 32, 91, 105, 109, 111, 256, 293, 303, 404, 431, 438,

Index

448, 454, 507, 534, 536, 538, 539, 542, 545, 564, 572–576, 581, 596, 616, 618, 629, 635, 673–684, 714, 715
Stages of Change, 212, 273
Step counts, step counters, 130, 132, 134, 135, 219, 273, 282, 361, 473, 643, 723
Streets, 326, 330, 384, 423, 425, 433, 435, 437, 438, 447–452, 454, 456–459, 473, 485, 488, 489, 493, 494, 499, 511–516, 520, 618
Strength, 4, 44, 66, 83, 107, 108, 124, 149, 168, 185, 257, 276, 300, 342, 362, 384, 402, 430, 458, 469, 491, 529, 534, 574, 590, 612, 627, 632, 660, 673, 694, 719
Stress Reduction Theory (SRT), 487
Stroke, 45, 105, 108, 148, 149, 151, 152, 238, 258, 338, 352, 360, 382, 384, 392, 470, 508, 639, 658, 696, 720, 725, 726
Subjective norm, 208, 215, 218, 253, 255, 256, 261
Surveillance, 26, 29–31, 36, 451, 457, 612, 616, 646
Symbolic interactionism, 555–557

T

Tablets, 722
Tai Chi, 47, 49, 66, 68, 87, 93, 109–112, 150, 152, 168, 173, 362, 369, 372, 408, 696
Technology, 14, 106, 133, 135, 137, 155, 177, 283, 284, 430, 431, 439, 440, 471, 477–479, 627, 628, 643, 713–727
Telerehabilitation, 133
Theory of Planned Behaviour (TPB), 212, 215, 216, 254, 255, 259, 273
Therapeutic gardens, 497

Threat appraisal, 257, 259, 404
Toileting, 171, 188, 363, 364, 370
Training/Training apps, 4, 5, 36, 45–47, 49–51, 53, 67, 84–88, 90–94, 105–109, 114, 124–127, 129–132, 135–137, 146–150, 152–155, 168, 169, 173, 191–196, 222, 272, 301, 304, 314, 322, 338, 341–347, 350–352, 362, 364, 365, 367–370, 372, 387, 389, 390, 394, 405, 407, 415, 469, 474, 517, 543, 571, 590, 615, 618, 619, 635, 655, 657, 664, 674, 677, 682, 694, 696–704, 716, 719, 720, 722–724
Transport, 10, 14, 81, 223, 301, 302, 314, 350, 373, 391, 405, 406, 410, 411, 416, 429, 430, 434, 450, 452–454, 456, 457, 507, 508, 511, 512, 516, 518, 519, 538, 579, 664, 713
Transtheoretical Model of Change (TTM), 212–215, 219
TTM, *see* Transtheoretical Model of Change
Types of exercise, 85–88, 111, 150, 168, 169, 172, 175, 408, 409

U

Under-stimulation, 372, 487
Uptake, 52, 89, 112, 114, 123, 129, 132, 186, 187, 192, 235, 255, 293, 315, 337–339, 341, 343–347, 349, 363, 366, 367, 372, 392, 393, 405–407, 409, 416, 593, 636, 655
Urban environments/streets, 14, 487–489, 493, 494, 513
Usability, 394, 520, 718, 721–723
User interface, 718, 723

V

Vicarious experience, 237–240
Videogames, 715
Virtual reality (VR), 151, 155, 440, 725, 726
Vital signs, 197, 198
Volition, 213, 220, 260, 271

W

Walking/Walkability, 4, 12, 148, 214, 322, 326, 330, 429, 441, 451, 452, 493, 579–581, 583, 584
Welfare technology, 718
Wellbeing, 1, 2, 12, 21, 22, 66, 67, 70, 72, 125, 197, 224, 284, 365, 384, 424, 427–430, 434, 436, 439, 440, 487–490, 493–497, 499, 507, 519, 590, 598, 627, 628
WHO, *see* World Health Organization
Woodlands, 492
World Health Organization (WHO), 1, 5, 7, 9, 27, 28, 31, 32, 43, 44, 69, 86, 91, 124, 130, 151, 154, 155, 255, 294, 296, 298, 447, 468, 470, 507, 590, 607, 610, 621, 656, 693, 714, 718

Printed in Great Britain
by Amazon